LEGACY

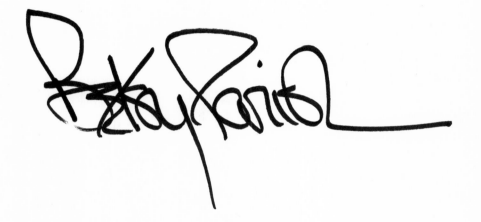

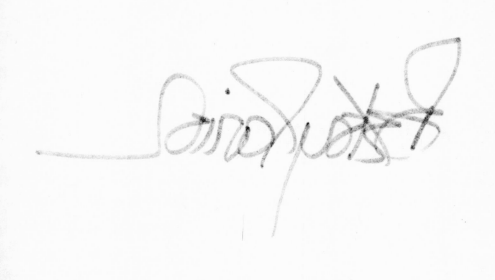

LEGACY

50 Years of Loving Care

Texas Children's Hospital
1954 – 2004

Betsy Parish

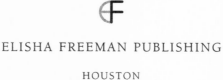

ELISHA FREEMAN PUBLISHING

HOUSTON

Elisha Freeman books may be purchased for educational, business, or sales promotional use. For information, please write:
Marketing Department, Elisha Freeman Publishing, 661 Bering Drive, #503, Houston, Texas 77057.

FIRST EDITION: October 2006
Designed by Peter Layne
Printed on acid-free paper

Library of Congress Control Number: 2006927326

Hardcover:
ISBN: 0-9786200-5-4
ISBN 13: 978-0-9786200-5-9

Softcover:
ISBN: 0-9786200-4-6
ISBN 13: 978-0-9786200-4-2

9 8 7 6 5 4 3 2 1

Unless otherwise noted, photographs are courtesy of Texas Children's Hospital.

The graphics on pages 1, 95, 121 and 641 are from a 1993 photograph of the wall "hand painted" by patients
and staff members in the Gulf Coast Regional Blood Center in the Abercrombie Building at Texas Children's Hospital.

This book is dedicated to children all over the world.

CONTENTS

Preface ix

PART I - INSPIRATION

1. The Founders 3
2. The Administration 25
3. The Leadership 43
4. The First Physician-in-Chief 57
5. The Second Physician-in-Chief 74

PART II - IMAGES

PART III - REALIZATION

6. Allergy and Immunology 123
7. Auxiliary 142
8. Cardiology 163
9. Child Life 191
10. Congenital Heart Surgery 207
11. Critical Care 241
12. Diabetes Care Center 257

13. Diagnostic Imaging 276

14. Emergency Center 294

15. Gastroenterology, Hepatology and Nutrition 314

16. Genetics. 334

17. Hematology-Oncology. 354

18. Infectious Diseases. 384

19. Junior League of Houston 418

20. Learning Support Center. 439

21. Meyer Center for Developmental Pediatrics. 459

22. Neonatology 478

23. Neurology 505

24. Nursing. 529

25. Pulmonary Medicine 547

26. Renal. 569

27. Rheumatology 596

28. Surgery 620

Notes 643

Index 673

Appendix 686

Acknowledgments 695

PREFACE

LEGACY IS A NARRATIVE HISTORY of the first 50 years at Texas Children's Hospital in Houston, Texas.

Among the first few hospitals to open in the Texas Medical Center, the originally small Texas Children's Hospital has evolved into one of the largest, full-care pediatric hospitals in the United States.

Legacy is a testament to this accomplishment, told from the participants' points of view. Gleaned from hundreds of personal interviews, oral histories, and archival documents, the stories in *Legacy* personify dedication, commitment, and contribution. These personal accounts also serve to illustrate how this ambitious endeavor to treat children in the community continually expanded its boundaries, eventually encompassing the treatment of children all over the world.

It is an awe-inspiring saga, rich in detail and worthy of more than just one book. Therefore, rather than attempting to summarize all of the noteworthy chronological events, *Legacy* presents a general overview, giving an in-depth look only at selected areas. The book is divided into three parts: the first presents the circumstances surrounding and the personalities involved with the inspiration, the founding, the administration, and the leadership of Texas Children's Hospital, including the strategic inclusion of the first two physicians-in-chief; the second features photographs taken at memorable moments during the hospital's first five decades; and the third documents how the founders' dreams and the legacy of loving care came to be realized. That realization is illustrated in a series of historical profiles of selected areas and services, each enveloped by the personal recollection of an experience within that particular area or service.

A recurring theme in *Legacy* is the unbridled expansion of Texas Children's Hospital, both in its facilities and in its patient population. Since its fiftieth anniversary in 2004, the hospital has continued its phenomenal growth in size and reputation. In 2006, Texas Children's Hospital is internationally recognized as one of the best full-care pediatric hospitals in the nation and is ranked as one of the top five pediatric hospitals in the United States by both *Child* magazine and *U.S. News & World Report*. This is the seventh consecutive year *U.S. News & World Report* has ranked Texas Children's Hospital among its top ten pediatric hospitals.

It is highly unlikely that the founders of Texas Children's Hospital ever imagined how fully their hopes and dreams would be realized. Since its opening in 1954 as a 106-bed facility for specialized pediatric care, Texas Children's Hospital has evolved into a 639 licensed-bed, full-care pediatric center accredited with commendation by the Joint Commission on Accreditation of Healthcare Organizations.

The symbiotic relationship with Baylor College of Medicine first established by the founders continues to flourish today. As a result, Texas Children's Hospital is the primary training site for one of the largest pediatric residencies in the nation. Consistently ranked among the nation's best, the department of pediatrics at Baylor College of Medicine is committed to providing superior programs of instruction for medical students and residents; advancing specialty knowledge in the medical sciences, particularly with regard to the health problems of children; and maintaining its role as a major contributor to research training and scientific activities that enhance the health of children—not only at Texas Children's Hospital, but also at pediatric facilities throughout the world.

Texas Children's Hospital is no longer conjoined with St. Luke's Episcopal Hospital, as initially planned by the founders. Instead, it is the singular guiding force of the Texas Children's Hospital Integrated Delivery System, a defined network of healthcare services that includes Texas Children's Pediatric Associates, Texas Children's Health Centers, Texas Children's Health Plan, and Texas Children's International.

As envisioned by the founders, the Texas Children's Hospital board of trustees in 2006 comprises men and women who are recognized leaders in their professions and in the community.* The board works closely with the executive leadership team at Texas Children's Hospital to set the overall course and direction of the hospital, instituting and funding new programs and services, and assuring high-quality healthcare.

A steady growth in patient population throughout the existence of Texas

---

* See appendix.

Children's Hospital is a pattern that shows no signs of diminishing in 2006. Each year at Texas Children's Hospital, there are approximately 20,000 children admitted as patients and more than 300,000 outpatient visits. Surgeons at Texas Children's Hospital perform approximately 20,000 procedures with general anesthesia each year, and more than one million tests are administered annually in the clinical chemistry laboratory. Approximately 60,000 clinical examinations take place in the radiology department and there are more than 80,000 visits to the emergency center each year. In total, patient encounters number more than 2 million annually at Texas Children's Hospital.

In tandem with its steadily increasing physical size and patient population, Texas Children's Hospital has developed an equally impressive and internationally recognized level of excellence and sophistication. The hospital's leading-edge technology features the most modern and complex diagnostic and therapeutic equipment, including its own operating rooms, MRI unit, CT scanners, interventional radiology unit, EEG laboratory, nuclear medicine unit, and cardiac catheterization laboratory. Together with Baylor College of Medicine, Texas Children's Hospital participates in approximately 400 research projects and benefits from more than $90 million in annual extramural grant support awarded to pediatric physician-scientists. Baylor College of Medicine faculty members at Texas Children's Hospital earned the top spot among all medical schools in the country in receiving competitive grant funding for pediatric research through the National Institutes of Health in 2003 and 2004.

Financial support for Texas Children's Hospital also comes from the community that helped build it in 1954. Following the 2001 completion of its $345 million expansion project, the most ambitious in the history of the Texas Medical Center, the main campus of Texas Children's Hospital became a four-building complex connected by walkways and tunnels. The original hospital building, named the Abercrombie Building in 1990, now functions primarily as an administrative, learning, and resource center.

The new 20-story West Tower at Texas Children's Hospital opened in June 2001 and houses inpatient services, the emergency center, and the operating rooms. Inpatient services include general level of care units, some of which are dedicated to individual specialties such as hematology-oncology, cardiology, and pulmonary disease, as well as special units such as pediatric intensive care, neonatal intensive care, and level 2 nurseries. The general care patient rooms are single-bed units with facilities for parents to stay, and there are a number of appropriately furnished play areas, including separate recreational facilities for adolescent patients.

The adjacent 16-story Clinical Care Center opened in October 2001 and is the outpatient building designed to accommodate a variety of general medical, surgical, and subspecialty clinics.§ The 12-story Feigin Center, originally opened in 1991 to house the outpatient clinics, was renovated in 2001 to house more than 200,000 square feet of bench laboratory space. Construction of an additional six floors on the Feigin Center for Pediatric Research began in 2006.

Future expansion projects are on the drawing board. Announced in 2006 are plans to establish the Texas Children's Neurological Research Institute, a research-based center of excellence in pediatric neurosciences that will be focused on children with mental or neurological disorders. Another new program introduced in 2006 is the high-risk obstetrics and perinatology service. Implemented to improve neonatal outcomes through diagnosis, treatment, and research in the newborn center, heart center, children's nutrition and research center, and fetal surgery center, the program will help bridge the gap between the obstetrician's concerns for the expectant mother and the care of her newborn by a pediatrician.

Current plans also include the development of a Texas Children's Hospital facility in the rapidly expanding suburb of West Houston. In response to the growing needs of children and families in that community, this new facility will offer pediatric subspecialty outpatient services, as well as both primary and secondary inpatient care. Offering convenient neighborhood access to an array of treatments previously only available in the Texas Medical Center, the West Houston Texas Children's Hospital campus eventually will encompass 54 acres.

With new facilities planned for the future and extensive inpatient and outpatient facilities already in place, in 2006 Texas Children's Hospital is both a primary community hospital and a tertiary referral center designed and equipped to meet the unique needs of infants and children. Texas Children's Hospital's staff consists of more than 1,600 board-certified primary-care physicians, pediatric subspecialists, pediatric surgical subspecialists, and dentists. The staff also includes more than 6,000 members of the highly skilled nursing and support staff.

Serving as service chiefs and staff physicians in Texas Children's Hospital's more than 40 patient care centers are professors from among the 535 full-time faculty members of the department of pediatrics at Baylor College of Medicine. In addition, Baylor College of Medicine has 160 pediatric house staff

§ See appendix.

members, 160 fellows in pediatric subspecialty training, and 35 residents and fellows in pediatric surgical subspecialty training at Texas Children's Hospital.

Since its inception in 1954, Texas Children's Hospital has been committed to research. The hospital has become internationally known for its expertise and breakthrough developments in the treatment of childhood cancer, cardiac disorders, diabetes, asthma, HIV/AIDS, and newborn diseases. Convinced that future advances will dwarf those of the past, more than 200 physicians and scientists at Baylor College of Medicine and Texas Children's Hospital are involved in current research projects devoted to seeking cures for childhood diseases and conditions.

One of Texas Children's Hospital's major strengths is its ability to attract and care for pediatric patients with various backgrounds and diverse medical problems. For 50 years, patients have come to Texas Children's Hospital with disorders as common as pneumonia and gastroenteritis and as complex as congenital heart disease and inborn errors of metabolism. Many of these children are referred to the special services of Texas Children's Hospital from across the United States, from Central and South America, and from all over the world.

Although there have been countless embellishments and alterations to the Texas Children's Hospital first envisioned by the founders, one specific detail remains unchanged. Just as the founders planned, all of the children and their families who come to Texas Children's Hospital are treated with loving care—just as they always have been and just as they always will be.

Legacy is a celebration of this enduring aspect of Texas Children's Hospital. It is a tribute to the founders who inspired that legacy of loving care, to the individuals who instigated the legacy, to those who are contributing to the legacy, and to those who are charged with perpetuating the legacy into the future.

Betsy Parish
October 1, 2006

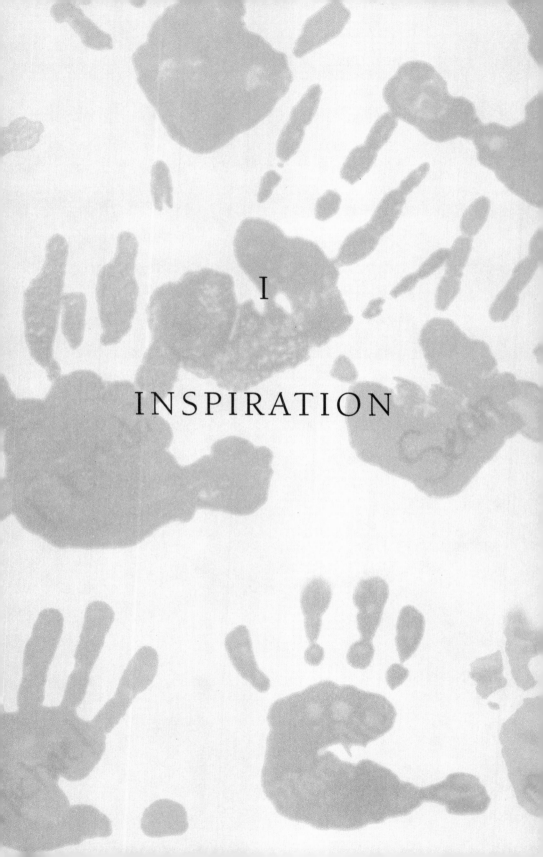

I

INSPIRATION

1

🖐 THE FOUNDERS 🖐

Texas Children's Hospital had an unusual beginning.

Rather than evolving from another institution or a smaller structure, like most other children's hospitals, the 106-bed Texas Children's Hospital originated from an idea held by only one man in 1944.

The initial concept of building a new hospital to provide loving care to children in Houston belonged to pediatrician Dr. David Greer. That such a singular vision eventually became Texas Children's Hospital was attributable to the enthusiastic support of his fellow pediatricians, the generosity of community leaders, and the dedicated efforts of an extraordinary set of individuals.

One of Houston's first pediatricians in 1919, Greer had been among the nine who founded the Houston Pediatric Society in 1933 with the stated purpose of disseminating knowledge of pediatrics among its members and to the community as a whole. Because Houston pediatricians traditionally spent the mornings making house calls and the afternoons seeing patients in the office, the new organization held informal dinner meetings, the first medical group to do so in Houston.

A frequent subject of discussion at those evening gatherings was the limited scope of pediatric services available in Houston hospitals. Although membership in the newly formed Houston Pediatric Society quickly grew to 35 during the early 1940s, the pediatric services in Houston hospitals remained unchanged, consisting of a few beds in The Methodist Hospital, Baptist Hospital, St. Joseph's infirmary, and Hermann Hospital. As for pediatric outpatient services, the only one available was at Hermann Hospital, where Greer and Dr. James Park alternated as chief of staff.

The supply of beds and pediatric services in these Houston hospitals did not reflect the existing demand. These shortcomings were reflected in statistical records concerning the care and treatment of sick children throughout Texas. Records from the 1930s indicate that Texas had an infant mortality rate one-third higher than that of any other state in the nation. As children in Texas continued to die of complications from whooping cough and pneumonia, doctors had limited resources to treat them. "Aspirin, diuretics, transfusions, prayer, and very little else," Dallas pediatrician Dr. Gladys Fashena recalled.[1]

This dilemma in Houston was intensified in the 1930s by the city's continuing growth. By 1941, Houston had become the clear leader of finance and industry on the Gulf Coast.[2] With its new industrial economy, the city experienced an unprecedented increase in population, quickly becoming one of the state's largest urban centers. The inadequacy of the healthcare services available in the community was a growing concern to Houston's civic and industrial leaders.

One such industrial leader planted the seeds for improved medical care in 1936. Funded with $300,000 from the estate of banker, cotton magnate, and philanthropist Monroe Dunaway Anderson, a charitable foundation bearing Anderson's name was created for "the support of hospitals and similar institutions for the care of people and the diffusion of knowledge and understanding among people." After Anderson's death in 1939, an additional $19 million bequest from his estate enabled the trustees of the M. D. Anderson Foundation to begin laying the groundwork for a medical center in Houston.[3]

Within two years, the trustees of the M. D. Anderson Foundation secured the cornerstone for Houston's new medical center. In 1941, the Texas legislature authorized the University of Texas to establish a hospital for cancer research and treatment, appropriating $500,000 for that purpose. The M. D. Anderson Foundation trustees seized the opportunity to be of service. They approached members of the University of Texas Board of Regents and offered them a deal: the M. D. Anderson Foundation would not only match the state's $500,000 funds, but also provide free land for the facility. There was one stipulation: the hospital had to be located in Houston and named for Anderson.

This benevolent offer was accepted. In 1942, university officials announced that the Texas State Cancer Hospital was to be named the M. D. Anderson Hospital for Cancer Research of the University of Texas. Planned to open in 1944, the new hospital was to be located in existing temporary facilities purchased and provided by the M. D. Anderson Foundation in Houston and moved to a newly constructed, permanent structure in the medical center at a future date.

Next, the M. D. Anderson Foundation trustees focused their attention on attracting a medical school to their proposed medical center. Unable to convince the University of Texas to relocate its medical branch from Galveston, the trustees began to look elsewhere. In Dallas, they heard rumors of a possible relocation plan for that city's Baylor University College of Medicine and immediately drafted an enticing invitation.

The trustees' financial offer to Baylor University officials in Waco was generous: $1 million for a permanent building for the medical school in the center, and another $1 million, payable over ten years, in research funding. The offer was accepted and Baylor University College of Medicine, later known as Baylor College of Medicine, signed an agreement on May 8, 1943.[4] The medical school immediately moved to Houston, set up temporary headquarters in an abandoned Sears & Roebuck warehouse on Buffalo Drive, and began classes shortly thereafter. One student, who later became a successful Houston doctor, often replied to compliments about his medical expertise with: "Not bad for a guy who got his medical degree at Sears, is it?"[5]

With Baylor College of Medicine as one of the two guaranteed occupants for the proposed medical center, the M. D. Anderson Foundation trustees set out to purchase the necessary property. What they wanted to buy—134.359 acres of land located south and east of Hermann Hospital—was owned by the city of Houston and had been designated as parkland. Undaunted by this restriction, the trustees approached City Hall with their proposal for the property's future use. Stressing the economic benefits of a medical center and pointing out the civic pride that such a center would generate, the trustees successfully convinced the city officials to put the foundation's proposal for purchase of the land to a citywide vote.

In a special election in 1943, Houston voters approved the sale. The trustees purchased the property and Houston's medical center finally had a permanent home. What to name the center was the next question. The decision made by the trustees was based on sound reasoning, according to Dr. Richard E. Wainerdi, president and chief executive officer of the Texas Medical Center since 1984. "It would be a medical center like no other," Wainerdi stated. "It would consist of many different hospitals, academic institutions of all kinds, and various support organizations—a city of medicine such as envisioned by Æsclepius in ancient Greece. It would be on land purchased by the M. D. Anderson Foundation and made available without cost to institutions so that they would come and build here. Seed money would also be provided, and people from all over Texas would be asked to help fund it. Hence, the name was to be the Texas Medical Center, not the Houston Medical Center."[6]

The Texas Medical Center was chartered under the laws of the State of Texas in 1945, the same year that the groundbreaking ceremony for the Baylor College of Medicine in the Texas Medical Center took place. The previous year, when the M. D. Anderson Foundation trustees began to deed parcels of Texas Medical Center land to the various medical facilities approved for inclusion in 1944, Greer made a timely presentation to the Houston Pediatric Society. He told his fellow members that the three glaring deficiencies in the medical treatment of children in Texas had an obvious solution. The first problem was that there were too few beds for children in Houston's existing hospitals; the second was that there was nowhere in Texas where doctors could receive pediatric training; and the third was that there was no place for research in children's diseases in Texas.[7] The one solution to all three problems was a children's hospital, one that would offer a balanced combination of care, teaching, and research. And, Greer proposed, that hospital should be built in the newly named Texas Medical Center.

All members of the Houston Pediatric Society enthusiastically embraced Greer's innovative idea, voting to establish a small committee to research the possibilities and promote the idea in the community. Asked to chair this hospital committee was Greer, who enthusiastically accepted the challenge. He knew that this was an ambitious task, even though the need for a children's hospital in Houston was abundantly clear to him and to everyone on the committee. All agreed that because Houston was rapidly becoming a major American city, it should have a children's hospital like those that most major American cities already had.

Convincing others in the community of this obvious need was not an easy task for Greer and his committee of pediatricians. Because the medical specialty of pediatrics was in its infancy and pediatric departments had been slow to develop in medical schools, trained specialists were few in number. Often the subject of ridicule from other physicians who labeled them "baby feeders" and "baby doctors," pediatricians dedicated to caring for children were not taken seriously in the medical community at that time. Undaunted by these misperceptions, members of the Houston Pediatric Society proceeded with the challenge of creating a community groundswell to build a children's hospital.

The timing of their efforts exacerbated the difficulty, particularly because the city of Houston was feeling the impact of World War II. The outbreak of the war had disrupted the healthcare system available to Houstonians, and many physicians had enlisted in, or were drafted into, the military, forcing those who remained to do "double duty." Nurses, too, joined the war effort and were in short supply between 1941 and 1945.

The war years also saw a severe shortage of building materials, preventing civilian hospitals and clinics from expanding. Future expansion, however, was inevitable—especially since Houston's population continued to grow rapidly, from 384,510 people in 1941 to 476,000 in 1946. This was the result of increased war-related activity at the Port of Houston and nearby petroleum refineries, as well as general migration into the city.[8]

The postwar boom also affected the Houston Pediatric Society. With more than half of its members in the service during the war, the society was forced to regroup in 1946. At its first postwar meeting, members pledged to double their efforts to establish a children's hospital. "The membership of the Houston Pediatric Society was keenly aware of, and disturbed by, Houston's lack of a modern specialized children's hospital affording them advanced facilities and therapies," Greer recalled. "In fact, there was not to our knowledge any other comparable city in the United States without such an institution. We became increasingly aware that we, as the trained and organized physicians for care of children in our city, were primarily responsible for the innovations of a movement to remedy the situation."[9]

As a result of that Houston Pediatric Society meeting, president Dr. Raymond Cohen appointed additional members, including himself, to the hospital committee and asked Greer to continue serving as its chairman. Other members selected to join Greer and Cohen in these efforts to establish a children's hospital were Dr. A. Lane Mitchell, Dr. John K. Glenn, and Dr. George W. Salmon. "We didn't know much about what we were after, except we wanted a children's hospital," Cohen remembered. "Nobody had any money, but we all had ideas."[10]

Big ideas were the norm for Houstonians in 1946. The postwar boom was immediate and entrepreneurs raced to be the first to develop something new. Downtown Houston was quickly turning into a citywide construction site, with excavations and building cranes on practically every corner. Skyscrapers were seemingly built overnight, causing some wags to quip: "If you leave your car on a parking lot overnight, you might return to find it 16 stories up on a new building."[11]

The postwar period in Houston was an exciting time, one that seemed to be endless. "I think I'll like Houston if they ever get it finished," observed Oveta Culp Hobby, the legendary Houstonian who was the first director of the Women's Army Auxiliary Corps.[12]

Along with the excitement of the new, the end of the war also brought back a familiar sense of normalcy, especially in the medical community. Returning physicians resumed their practices and returning nurses resumed their careers. And, as anticipated, Houston's medical facilities began planning for expansion.

Impetus for improving the quality of healthcare was provided by the sulfa drugs and antibiotics, the new surgical techniques, an emphasis on specialized medical training, and other medical advances that had improved healthcare for soldiers and support personnel during the war. Across the United States, many communities resolved to upgrade their healthcare facilities and expand hospital access to more of their citizens.

Houston was ahead of other communities in this respect, thanks to the previous and ongoing efforts of the M. D. Anderson Foundation at the Texas Medical Center. However, the foundation wasn't the only major benefactor of the Houston health community, just the first of many. During one week in 1945, in less than 48 hours, oilman and philanthropist Hugh Roy Cullen and his wife, Lillie, gave four gifts of $1 million each to four Houston hospitals. Although it was an all-time record in philanthropy at that time, Cullen appeared nonchalant about his generosity.[13]

After giving $1 million to Hermann Hospital and Baptist Memorial Hospital, Cullen explained: "Giving away money is no particular credit to me. Most of it came out of the ground—and while I found the oil in the ground, I didn't put it there. I've got a lot more than Lillie and I and our children and grandchildren can use. I don't think I deserve any great credit for using it to help people. It's easier for me to give a million dollars now than it was to give five dollars to the Salvation Army 25 years ago."[14]

And, after presenting these unexpected gifts to The Methodist Hospital and the yet-to-be-built St. Luke's Episcopal Hospital in the Texas Medical Center, Cullen told members of the Texas Hospital Association at a March 1947 meeting in Houston's Music Hall: "Both Lillie and I are pretty selfish about our giving. We want to see our money spent, so we can enjoy the spending. A lot of our friends are much less selfish than we are. They are willing to let their heirs or trustees distribute their money after they are dead and gone, when they won't even get the kick out of giving it away."[15]

True to Cullen's word, the Cullen family became known for contributing large sums of money to hospitals in Houston. When asked why he and his wife had given so much to the medical community, Cullen replied: "In our opinion, there is no more worthy cause than caring for people who are suffering—the sick and disabled, who often cannot help themselves," he replied, adding one of his typical political barbs. "Graft and pork barrels, and other kinds of leakage that occur when the government spends our money do not exist when we give directly to hospitals."[16]

To emphasize that point, Cullen announced in 1947 that he and his wife had formed The Cullen Foundation, in which they had placed oil properties with an estimated worth of $160 million. The largest charitable foundation in the South, and one of the largest in America, The Cullen Foundation was established for the sole purpose of making "the Texas Medical Center and University of Houston the kind of institutions Texans will be proud of," Cullen said.[17]

The newly established Cullen Foundation issued one of its first checks to Baylor College of Medicine in 1947. In response to a request from college trustees, the foundation donated $800,000 for use in the completion of the Baylor College of Medicine building in the Texas Medical Center. Named the Roy and Lillie Cullen Building and opened in the fall of 1947, it stood at the head of M. D. Anderson Boulevard and became the first completed structure in the Texas Medical Center. "To Mr. and Mrs. Cullen, Baylor will ever owe a debt of sincere gratitude," said college dean Dr. Walter H. Moursund. "In very large measure the progress of the medical college since coming to Houston has been and is being made possible by their generous philanthropies."[18]

Such generosity was not unusual in Houston—in fact, it was one of the city's defining characteristics. Philanthropy had been a trademark responsibility of wealthy Houstonians since the city's inception in 1836. "Houston was lucky," said renowned Houston philanthropist and patron of the arts Miss Ima Hogg. "The first people who got rich here, in the days long before oil, were nice people. They gave their money to schools, hospitals, charities, parks, the library, and the arts. They set the pattern. This is what Houstonians do once they get a little money."[19]

Exactly how to approach such altruistic Houstonians was unknown to Greer and the pediatricians on the Houston Pediatric Society children's hospital committee. One reason for the dilemma was that they did not know who they were or where to find them. This was because Houston was a town in which Southern gentility was the rule in the 1940s. With the exception of oil wildcatters, who were nouveau rich one day and nouveau poor the next, one's personal wealth was understated and never publicized.

The elusiveness of individual benefactors had become a major concern to Greer and Cohen, who sought the advice of community leaders.

Among those contacted were Rabbi Hyman Judah Schachtel of Congregation Beth Israel and Dr. Jack Ehlers, a physician and surgeon who counted Cullen and Houston businessman James S. Abercrombie among his patients.

In what later proved to be a turning point, Ehlers agreed not only to serve on Greer's committee, but also to tell Abercrombie about the Houston Pediatric Society and its efforts to promote a children's hospital for Houston.[20] Both Schachtel and Ehlers suggested the inclusion of laymen on the committee and urged the pediatricians to contact Leopold L. Meyer, a tireless community leader and humanitarian whose organizational and fund-raising skills were well known and highly respected.

The decision to act on that advice was pivotal. When Greer asked Meyer to serve on the Houston Pediatric Society children's hospital committee in 1947, Meyer accepted. His immediate participation marked a turning point and the committee gained the momentum and direction needed to achieve its goal.

It was not Meyer's first time to serve as a catalyst for success. Born in Galveston to a prosperous merchant, he had graduated from Tulane University before returning to Galveston to run his family's store after the illness and subsequent death of his father. Meyer moved to Houston in 1918 to accept a position with Foley Brothers Dry Goods Company, where he quickly became executive vice-president and a national authority on retail credit. When Federated bought Foley's in 1946, Meyer departed. He and his siblings then opened Meyer Brothers, Inc., a chain of clothing stores. As chairman of the board of that successful retail operation, Meyer devoted himself to the community and to charitable fund-raising projects.

In the early 1920s, Meyer was one of the founders of Houston's Community Chest, the forerunner of the United Fund. He was also chairman of the board of the Houston Civic Music Association, an officer of the Houston Symphony Society, and a director of the Houston Fat Stock Show, which later became the Houston Livestock Show and Rodeo. Meyer helped organize the Friends of the Library at the University of Houston in the early 1940s and re-organized the Houston Retail Merchants Association, serving as its president from 1942 until 1944. "I've spent my whole life begging. I believe I am recognized as the most professional beggar in the city of Houston," Meyer said in retrospect.[21]

With Meyer's tireless community involvement and history of "professional" begging, it was successfully argued in the postwar years that there wasn't a leading citizen in Houston whom Meyer didn't know, or who didn't know him. That included members of the legendary group of powerful Houstonians who met regularly and helped shape the city's future in George and Herman Brown's Suite 8F at the Lamar Hotel. As a resident of the Lamar Hotel, Meyer was practically a charter member. And within that influential group consisting of the Browns, Jesse H. Jones, Gus Wortham, Judge Jim Elkins, Lamar Fleming, Oveta Culp Hobby, James S. Abercrombie, and others, Abercrombie was Meyer's closest friend.

Known to his friends as "Mr. Jim," Abercrombie was many things during his lifetime: oil field worker, wildcatter, industrialist, inventor, and philanthropist. At the start of the 1920s, he went into business for himself, borrowing money to buy his own drilling rig. He was the first person to drill a well off the Louisiana coast. In 1922, a well in the Hull oil field blew out, destroying his derrick. Despite the fact that Abercrombie had used the best blowout preventor then available, he resolved to design a better one—and did so.

Abercrombie and Harry S. Cameron had purchased a small machine shop in 1920 for $17,000, primarily to repair Abercrombie's growing inventory of oil drilling equipment. Named Cameron Iron Works, Inc., the company was soon manufacturing a blowout preventor designed by Abercrombie himself. It was more advanced than anything then available—indeed, its basic design is still in use today throughout the world.

Following Cameron's death in 1928, Abercrombie assumed control of the company and guided it through decades of spectacular growth. Cameron Iron Works recorded sales of less than $28,000 and profits of less than $5,000 in its first year of operations; for the period 1961 to 1970, it recorded sales of $822 million and profits of more than $46 million. Abercrombie's ownership of Cameron Iron Works, together with his vast oil holdings and other interests, made him one of Houston's wealthiest citizens; his experiences earlier in life made him one of its most selfless.[22]

During a conversation in Suite 8F during 1945, after Abercrombie had hosted and underwritten the successful "Houston Holidays" benefit horse show at his Pin Oak Stables, Meyer made a proposal. Because the show was to raise funds to bring veterans from McCloskey General Hospital in Temple to Houston for a brief vacation, why not upgrade and expand that fund-raising event to make it "the best in the country"? To this, Abercrombie laughed and said: "Everything has to be the best for you, Lep. Would you run some sort of a horse show organization if we set it up—would you be president?" Meyer accepted and the Houston Horse Show Association was granted a state charter, with Meyer serving as president and Abercrombie as chairman of the board.[23]

The location for the Pin Oak Charity Horse Show was Pin Oak Stables, built in 1938 by Abercrombie for his daughter, Josephine E. Abercrombie, an accomplished equestrian since the age of six. Located on a 100-acre track on Post Oak Road near the city of Bellaire in the undeveloped western fringes of Houston, the property had a stable for the more than two dozen top-caliber horses owned by Josephine, along with a small but adequate riding ring.[24]

By the time that the second Houston Holidays fund-raising horse show was held on May 23, 1946, there had been some dramatic changes made by the newly chartered Houston Horse Show Association. Gone were the original stables, replaced by a handsome new plant consisting of a 10,000-seat stadium, fireproof stalls, a fine arena, and additional barns. The capacity crowd on hand for what was now called the Pin Oak Charity Horse Show consisted of a virtual "Who's Who" of Houston. With its hundreds of volunteer workers, sold-out box seats, and impressive showcasing of exhibitors and competitors, it was the beginning of an annual spring tradition that, with a few alterations, would last for more than 30 years.[25]

Another very important development at the Pin Oak Charity Horse Show took place in 1947. With the war over and veterans no longer being treated at McCloskey Hospital, the "Houston Holidays" group disbanded, leaving the Pin Oak Charity Horse Show without a charity. Greer and Meyer recognized this chance to promote the Houston Pediatric Society committee's idea for a children's hospital. The two began to institute a plan. They approached the Junior League of Houston, the women's organization that had sponsored a prenatal and children's health clinic in the city since 1927, and asked the organization to market the show and raise start-up funds for the children's hospital. Members of the league enthusiastically agreed to the request, appointing Mrs. George H. Black as the show's chairwoman. Priced at $1.20 for admission seats and $3 for box seats, tickets went on sale on May 15, 1947.[26]

As first stipulated with the Houston Holidays group in 1945 and 1946, Abercrombie insisted that he pay all expenses of the 1947 horse show and that gross receipts go to Greer's children's hospital fund, the one that Ehlers had told him about. This was agreed. After the four-day show concluded on June 1, 1947, the Junior League of Houston presented Greer's committee with a $30,000 check, the gross proceeds from the first Pin Oak Charity Horse Show benefiting the children's hospital.[27]

This 1947 event marked the beginning of a long relationship between Pin Oak Charity Horse Show and Texas Children's Hospital, one that continued uninterrupted until 1985 and resumed in 2005. Although the Junior League of Houston was no longer involved, the annual benefit horse show continued under the auspices of Meyer and Abercrombie's Houston Horse

Show Association. It was the hospital's major fund-raising event and Houston's most eagerly anticipated social event of the spring, with annual contributions reaching a peak in 1974. When the show moved from its original quarters at Pin Oak to the newly built air-conditioned arena next to the Astrodome in 1975, enthusiasm for the indoor event stagnated and the association was severed in 1985. Twenty years later, the Pin Oak Charity Horse Show resumed its association with Texas Children's Hospital.

It was the proceeds from the 1947 Pin Oak Charity Horse Show that enabled the Houston Pediatric Society children's hospital committee to establish the Texas Children's Foundation. With cash in the coffers, the Texas Children's Foundation was formally chartered on August 20 to develop plans for a new pediatric hospital and to secure community support for the project. Elected as first president was Greer, with Meyer serving as treasurer. Other members of the board of trustees were businessman George Butler, socialites Nina Cullinan and Martha Lovett, physician Ehlers, and pediatricians Cohen, Glenn, Mitchell, and Salmon, the original members of the children's hospital committee formed in 1946.

The trustees of the newly formed Texas Children's Foundation shared unbridled enthusiasm about their goal. "At this point, it was nothing more than a dream and a remote hope that at some future date Houston would be blessed with a sorely needed children's hospital," Meyer recalled. "The board members were laymen and women as well as specialists and scientists and their discussions, which often lasted late into the night, reflected almost religious zeal and devotion for the wellbeing of living and unborn children."[28]

In order to fulfill the mission of the Texas Children's Foundation, one of Greer's first actions as president of the Texas Children's Foundation was to send telegrams requesting pertinent information from 14 children's hospitals across the country. To each institution he pledged to hold in strict confidence all information received about cost figures, patient census, outpatient visits, and all other sensitive matters. Simultaneously, other trustees of the foundation contacted United States Representative Albert Thomas of Houston, asking for his help in obtaining architectural plans for large children's hospitals from the government. In response, the U.S. Public Health Service provided the Texas Children's Foundation with a number of hospital diagrams, along with a note stating that nothing was available relating exclusively to pediatric hospitals.

The trustees' disappointment with the lack of information from the government was superseded by the excitement of welcoming Baylor College of Medicine's new chief of pediatrics, Dr. Russell J. Blattner, who arrived in July 1947 from St. Louis. Blattner, who had a reputation for exceptional teaching and research abilities, enthusiastically shared the view of local pediatricians that a children's hospital was needed in Houston. Convinced that a new children's hospital should focus on teaching and research, as well as treating sick children, Blattner set out to build a strong relationship between Baylor College of Medicine and the Texas Children's Foundation, one that ultimately proved to be mutually advantageous. From the moment he arrived in Houston, Blattner began taking small steps towards that goal.

One giant leap in making the hospital a reality was the solicitation of the Texas Medical Center for land on which it might be built. The long awaited answer to this request came on June 3, 1948, from Dr. E. W. Bertner, acting president of the Texas Medical Center.[29] Bertner's letter formally notified the Texas Children's Foundation that the Texas Medical Center board of trustees had allocated a 5.75-acre tract of land in the medical center for the site of a children's hospital.

"The conveyance of this land to your institution will be for the purpose of your erecting thereon and maintaining a hospital of the first class," Bertner's letter read. "While the quantity of land in mind for conveyance to your institution is considerably more than ordinarily would be needed for a single hospital, it is the thought of our trustees that such land will be useful for use in conjunction with your hospital for parking space and similar necessary uses, as well as for possible future expansion."[30]

For members of the Texas Children's Foundation board, Bertner's letter served as an impetus to accelerate its planned program. "Designation of the site is the first step in our program," Greer said in 1948. "We are now going ahead with our plans to study children's hospitals in other cities and utilize the latest advances in such institutions in developing our own proposed hospital."[31]

To determine how to make Houston's new pediatric hospital truly state-of-the-art, the Texas Children's Foundation offered to pay Blattner and Houston architect Milton Foy Martin to tour existing children's hospitals throughout the country. Many years later, Blattner recalled telling the foundation's trustees that "there wasn't enough money in the world to pay me to spend three months of my first year away from my new job, but that I would do it for nothing if I was on the team." Soon after, Blattner was elected to the Texas Children's Foundation's board of trustees, which was later proven to be another fortuitous decision.[32]

Using funds raised at the 1947 Pin Oak Charity Horse Show, Blattner and Martin began their travels. The purposes of the trip, as outlined in August 1948, were "to see at first-hand the available facilities in Mexico, Canada, and the rest of the United States, note the unusual and desirable features and attempt to incorporate these in the new children's hospital; to gain ideas from people who had experience in working in children's hospitals; and to study the integration of children's hospitals with other hospitals such as will be necessary between the Texas Children's Hospital and the other institutions in the Texas Medical Center."[33]

Blattner and Martin's tour to myriad pediatric hospitals lasted from August until early October. In cities including Baltimore, Boston, Cincinnati, Denver, Los Angeles, Mexico City, New York, Philadelphia, Portland, Seattle, and Toronto, they photographed lecture halls, child-friendly wall hangings, recreational facilities, sun therapy rooms, laboratories, and other features they considered essential to the type of modern pediatric hospital they envisioned for Houston.

After returning to Houston, Martin and Blattner presented their findings to the Texas Children's Foundation trustees. Included in this precisely detailed report were Blattner's keen observations and cogent input, which proved to be invaluable to the planning of the future hospital, according to fellow foundation trustee Salmon. Although Greer had been the first to propose building a children's hospital, Blattner ultimately was "the one that put it together," Salmon said.[34]

In a tribute to Blattner and Martin's efforts, several three-ringed notebooks containing photographs taken during their travels in the fall of 1948 were preserved. These records remain housed in the Blattner Conference Room at Texas Children's Hospital.

Blattner also influenced the thinking of the Texas Children's Foundation trustees regarding how the new hospital should be organized and, in particular, how to avoid any duplication of functions and facilities with others in the expanding Texas Medical Center. Many concurred that Houstonians might be hesitant to support multiple efforts, prompting the Texas Children's Foundation trustees to explore a variety of options, including cooperative arrangements with other medical institutions.[35]

One possible arrangement, first discussed in early 1948, would have allied Texas Children's Hospital with the Hedgecroft Clinic, the Houston facility that cared for polio victims. Treating Houston's many polio victims had stretched the Hedgecroft Clinic's resources to the limit, and fears of a looming polio epidemic made an alliance with another medical facility all the more urgent. Through May and June of 1948, the clinic and the Texas

Children's Foundation discussed a possible cooperative arrangement. As the number of polio cases continued to rise, the trustees eventually distanced the Texas Children's Foundation from the Hedgecroft Clinic and its sole focus on polio.[36]

At about the same time, Texas Children's Foundation trustees began discussions with the Arabia Temple Shrine to determine if the two institutions, the proposed Texas Children's Hospital and the Arabia Temple Crippled Children's Clinic, might benefit by operating a joint medical facility. Meetings between the Shriners and foundation trustees dragged on for months in the fall of 1948 and into the spring and summer of 1949. At one point, it was hoped that a single building could meet the needs of crippled children, house the Junior League's outpatient clinic, and handle large numbers of pediatric polio patients for short periods of time.

By August 1950 it became apparent that differences in the type of work to be undertaken by the two institutions would make separate facilities necessary. The Arabia Temple Crippled Children's Clinic announced that it would remain singularly focused on caring for its orthopedic patients, and would construct a small facility connected to Hermann Hospital for that purpose. "We are for the Texas Children's Foundation 100 percent. It's just that their work with children is entirely different from ours," Phillip Johnson, potentate of the Houston Arabia Temple Shrine, told the news media when the 50-bed Arabia Temple Crippled Children's Clinic was eventually dedicated in February 1952.[37]

In the fall of 1950, Meyer announced that the Texas Children's Foundation "has ceased to exist now that its job has been completed. All of its surplus funds on hand, approximately $130,000, being largely proceeds from the annual events of the Houston Horse Show Association and gifts from well-wishers, have been surrendered to Texas Children's Hospital." Meyer, treasurer of the foundation, became president of the Texas Children's Hospital board; Abercrombie became its chairman.[38]

The transition marked the precise moment when the seemingly impossible effort begun by the Houston Pediatric Society was transformed into the attainable mission of aggressive businessmen and industrial leaders. Texas Children's Hospital, Inc., was incorporated with the following Houstonians as its charter members: J. S. Abercrombie, Herman Brown, James A. Elkins, Jr., Lamar Fleming, Jr., W. J. Goldston, J. W. Link, Jr., Douglas B. Marshall, Leopold L. Meyer, Herman Pressler, and William B. Smith. Although no members of the Houston Pediatric Society served as trustees, their active participation in the detailed planning of the new hospital was a certainty.

As he had done in the past, Meyer continued to spearhead the fund-raising efforts for the next several years with his usual gusto, but without much luck. "We spun our wheels for an awfully long time. And then lightning struck," Meyer recalled. "Abercrombie came to visit me."[39]

Meyer and his wife, Adelena, were vacationing at the Biltmore Hotel in Phoenix, Arizona in the spring of 1952. They had invited Abercrombie, Ralph McCullough, and Morrow Cummings and their wives to join them for a weekend of golf, gin rummy, and "big talk." Meyer recalled thinking it was "fish or cut bait time." He managed to get Abercrombie away from the crowd to tell him that architect Martin had given him an estimated cost of $2.5 million for Texas Children's Hospital.[40]

Abercrombie did not tell Meyer that he had already discussed the details and cost estimates with Martin during a previous meeting at the Houston home of Texas Children's Foundation trustee Ehlers. He did, however, ask one question: "This hospital, would it be open to every sick or hurt child? No restrictions on religion, color, whether or not you could pay?"[41]

"Absolutely," Meyer replied. "We'll have it written in the by-laws."[42]

"Well, let's build it," Abercrombie said. "I'll put up one million dollars in seed money and you can go out and rustle up the rest. It's a good cause."[43]

Meyer was ecstatic. "He was the best man I ever knew. I loved him like a brother. He was modest to a fault and charitable beyond reason," Meyer said later. "I wanted to name the hospital Abercrombie, or dedicate a wing or a portion of the building to him. He wouldn't hear of it."[44]

What Abercrombie did hear were Meyer's questions concerning the hospital's future needs and how it would be supported financially. "Well, the horse show should continue to help," Abercrombie replied, having decided that the Pin Oak Charity Horse Show would benefit Texas Children's Hospital every year in the foreseeable future. "And I would think that there'll be contributions, once we're underway. Other than that, you bring me the amount of the deficit every year-end. I'll handle it for five years, anyhow."[45]

This promise of support was fulfilled ten times over. Abercrombie continued to be generous to the hospital long after his self-imposed five-year commitment had expired. The always-grateful Meyer recalled: "He did pay the deficit until he died, practically."[46]

Indeed "Mr. Jim's" generosity, and that of his beloved wife, "Miss Lillie," extended well past their own lifetimes. In late 1967, they announced the creation of a trust to benefit Texas Children's Hospital for decades to come. The trust they established guaranteed that the hospital would have the funds necessary to expand its facilities, cover its expenses, and provide charity care.

When the trust was finally dissolved, the hospital realized a significant inheritance that continued to ensure that it would have the financial resources needed to carry out its obligations to the community in perpetuity.[47]

When Abercrombie died in January 1975, *Intercom,* the official publication of St. Luke's Episcopal Hospital and Texas Children's Hospital, began his obituary with this tribute: "Had it not been for this man, Texas Children's Hospital would not exist today."[48]

Abercrombie's willingness to help others was the result of his early years in the oil fields. In a 1953 *Houston Post* profile, he recalled that one of his early rigs cost him "about $13,000. I didn't have it all in cash but a bank made me a loan. Then shortly afterwards, when things got tough, the bank foreclosed. I would have lost my drilling rig if it had not been for the help of a friend."[49]

An alternative explanation, mentioned in his *Houston Post* obituary, was that "the cause of children was a natural for Abercrombie, who said that when he was a teenager in the oil fields, he saw so many poor and sick children that if he ever made money he would do something to help."[50]

Abercrombie's daughter had a simpler and more personal viewpoint of her father's altruistic support of Texas Children's Hospital. "He just adored children," Josephine Abercrombie said. "He was the seventh of nine children himself and his family had very little money. He just believed that children were the future of the country, and that they needed help and attention." She recalled that her father often told her how grateful he was for the good things that had happened to him, and how much he wanted to give something back. As she approached young adulthood, she remembers her father telling her: "You've been blessed in life, and you've got to give something back. You can't always take all the time."[51]

As one of the recipients of Abercrombie's legendary philanthropy in 1952, the Texas Children's Hospital trustees received $1 million for the $2.5 million building fund.

Meyer knew that raising the additional $1.5 million was not an impossible task for him—he had done it before for many other organizations. And, sure enough, with his trademark determination and persistence, Meyer did it again. A little more than a year after his 'fish or cut bait" conversation with Abercrombie, he had succeeded in raising the needed $1.5 million.

This was but one of the many successes achieved by the Texas Children's Hospital board of trustees. Imbued with an inordinate amount of business acumen, the trustees instituted a strategic plan for the future. Despite the intense, and ultimately unsuccessful, discussions with the

Hedgecroft Clinic and the Shriners, the trustees still believed that some type of joint undertaking made financial sense. Talks began with St. Luke's Episcopal Hospital, which was planning to build a new general hospital in the Texas Medical Center. The St. Luke's Episcopal Hospital project had stalled and been restarted a couple of times since it was first considered in 1941. Negotiations between the boards of Texas Children's Hospital and St. Luke's Episcopal Hospital centered on the feasibility of constructing a jointly administered complex of two separate hospitals that would be attached by a "connecting link" housing shared facilities.[52]

Shared facilities and joint administration did not otherwise exist in the Texas Medical Center. Indeed, such an arrangement was unique in the southwestern United States. Under the plan that was proposed, both hospitals would remain separate, with separate boards of trustees and medical staffs. They would share certain services and departments to reduce the duplication of equipment and to cut operating and personnel costs. Additionally, both Texas Children's Hospital and St. Luke's Episcopal Hospital would join with The Methodist Hospital in operating shared power and laundry facilities that would serve all three hospitals. Corridors on the first, second, and third floors would connect Texas Children's Hospital with St. Luke's, which, in turn, would be connected to The Methodist Hospital by an underground tunnel.[53]

On October 18, 1950, the boards of Texas Children's Hospital and St. Luke's Episcopal Hospital signed a commitment contract. After extensive discussion, and after carefully considering the pros and cons of such a joint arrangement, Abercrombie, chairman of the Texas Children's Hospital board, and George B. Journeay, president of the St. Luke's board, announced that the two hospitals would construct adjoining buildings in the Medical Center and would operate under a system of joint administration, an arrangement that would continue for almost 35 years.[54]

Given the new joint arrangement with St. Luke's Episcopal Hospital, the Texas Children's Hospital board worked with the Texas Medical Center to arrange an exchange of acreage. The original land given to the Texas Children's Foundation was sandwiched on the land between Hermann Hospital and Baylor College of Medicine. Handing back that property, the Texas Children's Hospital board asked for and received a new parcel adjacent to the land given to St. Luke's Episcopal Hospital.

Such tangible progress was welcomed by Blattner, who wrote to his sister-in-law: "After years of planning ... we have now reached the stage where Mr. Abercrombie has charged us with the responsibility of getting the plans for the Children's Hospital underway as soon as possible."[55]

The realization that a children's hospital in Houston was within reach created great excitement among local pediatricians, particularly Greer, who watched in awe as the pace of progress quickly accelerated. When Abercrombie told the news media on October 26, 1950, "We are definitely started now, and we do not expect to stop until this hospital ranks with the greatest of children's hospitals anywhere," Greer and members of the Houston Pediatric Society rejoiced in their good fortune of having Abercrombie and all the other prominent businessmen in charge of their quest.

The momentum of Abercrombie's board was unstoppable. Less than six months after its formation, the boards of trustees from Texas Children's Hospital and St. Luke's Episcopal Hospital presided over the ceremonies held on February 20, 1951, to dedicate their conjoined site in the Texas Medical Center.

Within weeks of the dedication ceremonies, Abercrombie began to have discussions with Howard T. Tellepsen, head of the company slated to build St. Luke's Episcopal Hospital. Tellepsen had previously agreed to build St. Luke's Episcopal Hospital at cost plus 1 percent, to cover his over-head, a fact already known to Abercrombie and the Texas Children's Hospital board of trustees. When Tellepsen offered to do the same for Texas Children's Hospital, Abercrombie graciously accepted. Meyer signed the contract with the Tellepsen Construction Company in Abercrombie's office on May 17, 1951.[56]

Although construction of Texas Children's Hospital was scheduled to begin in July, the groundbreaking took place months earlier. Surrounded by nurses, physicians, and Texas Medical Center dignitaries, four children with miniature shovels turned the first earth on the site for Texas Children's Hospital on May 23, 1951. Blessing the occasion was Houston Rabbi Hyman Judah Schachtel, one of the first Houstonians to support Greer's Houston Pediatric Society children's hospital committee in 1947, who said: "May all children who come here aching and in pain leave healed; and all those who come in tears leave smiling."

The smiles in the audience belonged to an eclectic gathering of Houston pediatricians, physicians, socialites, and civic leaders who were bonded by the common goal of building a children's hospital in Houston. Each knew that the ceremonial groundbreaking was more than just a photo opportunity. Instead, it signified that their collective dream, one that had been years in the making, was one step closer to fulfillment.

Construction officially began on July 16, 1951. With the cacophonous sounds of bulldozers hard at work as their reassuring background music, the board's strategic planning for the hospital shifted into high gear. Of utmost importance to the trustees was the need to intensify community involvement in Texas Children's Hospital. Although the annual Pin Oak Charity Horse Show effectively showcased its initial efforts and raised significant funds, the donor base required further expansion.[57]

To help achieve this goal, the board of trustees turned to an outside public relations firm, the Gulf State Advertising Agency. Intrigued with the idea of raising funds and promoting awareness of Texas Children's Hospital, agency executives began looking at other hospital fund-raising brochures for inspiration. After finding most efforts to be "very stilted, and prosaic," an agency executive suggested a different, lighter approach—one that included soliciting ideas from cartoonists. The board of trustees approved this unique idea and the result was beyond what anyone could have possibly expected.

Unveiled by Abercrombie and Meyer on January 21, 1952, was a spectacular fund-raising brochure illustrated by Walt Disney Productions, which donated the company's services. Adorning the four-color cover was an artist's rendering of Texas Children's Hospital and its landscaped grounds filled with young children at play with Disney cartoon characters Mickey and Minnie Mouse, Donald Duck, and the bluebirds from *Snow White and the Seven Dwarfs*.[58]

The inside pages of the brochure encouraged potential contributors to look over the floor plans and select a specific item, area, or need to support. Blood bank facilities cost $4,250. Elevators were listed at $45,000 each. Construction of the linen room was listed as a $1,750 expense, while some much bigger items, such as the auditorium/lecture room, required an expenditure of $75,000. For those able to give far less, wheelchairs for $90 and silverware sets for $25 were also listed.

Mailed to more than 10,000 people in the Houston area, the unique brochure also garnered coverage by the local media. One newspaper ran a picture of Abercrombie and Meyer's January announcement of the completed brochure. The March 16, 1952, edition of the *Houston Post* extended its exposure by featuring a full-page copy of the Disney cover and documenting its popularity in an article titled "Texas Children's Hospital Catches Popular Fancy!"[59]

With a rapidly expanding base of community support, in 1952 the Texas Children's Hospital board of trustees turned its attention to support from the Texas Medical Center. Unanswered since the formation of the Texas Children's Foundation in 1947 was the question of whether Texas

Children's Hospital would align itself with the Baylor College of Medicine, or remain independent.

Blattner's efforts to build a strong relationship between Baylor College of Medicine and Texas Children's Hospital had begun the moment he arrived in Houston in 1947. His ultimate goal was an affiliation, an idea supported by many, but not all, members of the Houston Pediatric Society. Some, Greer chief among them, wanted "their" new hospital to be independent and worried about the role that Baylor faculty members would play at the new hospital.

In the intervening years since his arrival, Blattner had made significant headway in his efforts to cement the affiliation of Baylor and Texas Children's Hospital. His inclusion on the Texas Children's Foundation board and his subsequent travels on its behalf, his detailed report from his travels, and his genuine interest and support of the children's hospital helped forge a highly favorable relationship between the Houston Pediatric Society and pediatric faculty members at Baylor College of Medicine. In later years, Greer often voiced his opinion about how Blattner's "addition to the board of the foundation was a decisive factor in our final and complete accomplishment."

Convincing the board of trustees to agree to the affiliation was another challenge, one in which Blattner eventually prevailed. Based on the common objectives of giving complete care to pediatric patients, providing pediatric education, and instigating worthwhile pediatric research, the formal affiliation agreement between Texas Children's Hospital and the Baylor College of Medicine was signed by the trustees of both institutions on June 28, 1952.[60]

The agreement included the naming of Blattner as physician-in-chief of Texas Children's Hospital. Blattner's first administrative decisions reinforced the confidence that local pediatricians had placed in him. From the moment he assumed his new role, he implemented measures to make all members of the Houston Pediatric Society members of the active staff at the new hospital when it opened. He also established a rule to ensure that the president of the Houston Pediatric Society would automatically serve as the head of the new hospital's medical staff. Additionally, the medical executive committee at Texas Children's Hospital was to be established to monitor the medical policies of the hospital and to be an arm of the medical staff. Practicing physicians outnumbered Baylor College of Medicine faculty members on that committee.[61]

All of Blattner's newly announced plans met with the approval of the Houston Pediatric Society, as well as faculty members of Baylor College of Medicine. "Blattner made the local pediatricians feel wanted," said Dr. Irvin

Kraft, a child psychiatrist at Baylor College of Medicine and Texas Children's Hospital. "He worked to involve local pediatricians not affiliated with Baylor in the affairs of the hospital, thereby minimizing the perception that Baylor might be taking total control of the project."[62]

While Blattner continued to build the medical staff and to establish policies, construction of Texas Children's Hospital progressed at a rapid pace. At the formal dedication ceremonies on May 15, 1953, Meyer unveiled the cornerstone of Texas Children's Hospital. For the eclectic group of Houston pediatricians, physicians, socialites, civic leaders, and businessmen whose names were duly inscribed on the cornerstone, it was a historic moment—so, too, for the thousands upon thousands of anonymous Houstonians who had supported and contributed to the building of Texas Children's Hospital.

In reality, the ceremony represented more than the beginnings of the brick-and-mortar building. It was the cornerstone of the very concept of Texas Children's Hospital. From its inception in 1944, Greer's idea to build a children's hospital had received immeasurable support from Houstonians —individually and collectively, recognized and anonymous, young and old, sick and well, rich and poor. In essence, they, along with the countless members of the Houston Pediatric Society, community leaders, social luminaries, volunteers, physicians, nurses, patients and their families, were the founders of Texas Children's Hospital.

All were represented in the gathered crowd that included one of the most generous supporters of Texas Children's Hospital, Abercrombie, at the dedication ceremonies. Although he was not among the many dignitaries who spoke, his unmistakable influence was voiced by master of ceremonies Meyer: "Embodied within the walls of our structure are the broader concepts of the fatherhood of God and the brotherhood of man, for this hospital shall live and abide within the resolution that any child in the State of Texas in need of medical care and attention, regardless of race, color, creed, or capacity to pay shall find in Texas Children's Hospital a refuge from the ravages of disease and illness and the hope for health and happiness."[63]

Nine months later, the community-held dream of providing loving care to children in a very special Houston hospital was fulfilled. With interior columns painted like peppermint candy, colorful furnishings, 106 specially designed beds for patients, loungers for parents staying overnight, custom medical equipment, snack bar, child-friendly décor, and a 180-seat auditorium, Texas Children's Hospital opened on February 1, 1954.

Although there was no fanfare or formal ceremony to officially commemorate this occasion, there was just cause for a citywide celebration. With the opening of this three-story state-of-the-art pediatric facility in the Texas Medical Center, an extraordinary group of Houston individuals had accomplished a remarkable feat in a relatively short period of time.

From its unusual beginning as only an idea held by one Houston pediatrician, Texas Children's Hospital had fully evolved into a community-supported, brick-and-mortar reality in less than ten years.

2

THE ADMINISTRATION

Having been in and out of hospitals with kidney problems for most of her life, three-year-old Lamaina Leigh Van Wagner entered another one on February 1, 1954.

Referred by her pediatrician and admitted at 3 a.m., she spent the night in room 411. After being examined the next morning by her doctor, she was dismissed. Although the experience lasted less than 24 hours, it was historic. Her brief visit officially marked the opening of Texas Children's Hospital.

Too young at the time to realize the significance of this event, Van Wagner deemed it memorable for a strictly personal reason. More than three decades later, she fondly recalled that it was the first time she had not been frightened at a hospital. "They gave me loving attention," she explained. "I remember an enormous playroom. I had never seen anything like it before in a hospital."[1]

Neither had the 12 other children who gained admittance during the first 48 hours of the hospital's opening, nor the thousands who soon followed. Designed to capture a child's fantasy as well as offer expert medical care, this unique facility quickly captured the media's attention as well.

Rather belatedly documented in a front-page story in the February 4, 1954, issue of the *Houston Chronicle* was the fact that Texas Children's Hospital had "opened its doors to the first patients without fanfare" on February 1 and that "the little girl who became the first patient in the history of the Texas Medical Center institution has already gone home."[2]

The newspaper also reported that the "$2,000,000 haven for children" was open only on a "limited basis." Pediatricians who attended the Harris County Medical Society meeting on February 3 heard the news of the hospital's opening, but "many of the city's doctors didn't know it opened."

An explanation for this low-keyed approach, attributed to an unidentified hospital spokesperson, was the following: "You don't just throw open the doors to a hospital, it's more like breaking in a new car. You move slowly but make certain everything is operating as it should. No patient will be accepted who can not presently be cared for at this time."[3]

What the newspaper did not report was that such policy decisions fell under the auspices of the board of trustees of Texas Children's Hospital. From its inception in 1950, the board assumed responsibility as the sole authority with jurisdiction over the hospital's operation. It was the board's duty to supervise not only the construction of the bricks and mortar, but also the management of the completed facilities.

It was an impressive task for an equally impressive board. Each of the trustees was recognized as a pillar of the community.[4] They "were pretty practical minded people who were successful businessmen ten or more years older than I," recalled Herman Pressler, the youngest member of the board. "Most of the trustees were really close associates and friends and intimates of Jim Abercrombie. The board was built around him."[5]

During the years that the hospital was in the planning stages, the trustees began laying the groundwork for its operation. No detail was considered too small to merit their attention and few, if any, pertinent subjects escaped discussion. "Mr. Abercrombie never said much," recalled Pressler. "Mr. Meyer kind of ran the board meetings, and he really kind of ran the institution. Most of us just helped him or just approved whatever he and Mr. Abercrombie suggested. Mr. Abercrombie was putting up the money, and he and Mr. Meyer had ideas of what they wanted to do."[6]

One area of concentration for the entire board during this period was the recruitment of supervisory personnel for the nursing staff. After signing a contract in 1951 with Bonnie Shoemate of Clovis, New Mexico, the board loaned her $630 to secure advanced training in pediatric work for one year at Children's Hospital Boston. Shoemate completed that training and officially joined the hospital's payroll on May 15, 1953.

By early 1954, Shoemate had equipped the nurses' stations in Texas Children's Hospital. She then began a two-week training program for her staff of 11 nurses and eight nurses' aides in preparation for the hospital's imminent opening. In a January 26 report to the board, Shoemate announced: "The nursing staff is ready to go."[7]

Also reporting directly to the board of trustees was the hospital's first chief administrator, Lee C. Gammill, who was hired in 1950. Responsible for overseeing the management of Texas Children's Hospital, the jointly administered St. Luke's Episcopal Hospital, and the two hospitals' "connecting link," Gammill planned for all facilities to open at the same time. Because construction delays necessitated a later opening date for St. Luke's, the chief administrator was able to devote his full attention to the activities taking place at Texas Children's during its opening hours.

"We had a lot of 'little detail' things happen our first day," Gammill reported to the board. "I was like a 'cat on a tin roof,' but everything went off smoothly. At breakfast the second day with mamas feeding their babies in our rocking chairs and one nurse feeding a child—it was a sight to justify our efforts."[8]

Gammill, who had answered to the boards of both Texas Children's Hospital and St. Luke's Episcopal Hospital during the planning and construction phases, continued to do so after the hospitals opened. He supervised the special arrangements made for the pediatric-sized furniture, fixtures, and equipment needed at Texas Children's Hospital, as well as the multipurpose needs of the shared facilities. Gammill also assisted in efforts to staff both hospitals.

In every area, the stated goal for employees was to provide unequaled service to patients. Exemplifying this mission was the kitchen. Tapped to serve as head chef was Donald Gladu, who had recently worked for four years at the famed Shamrock Hotel, the nearby Houston landmark. Gladu's arrival was highly touted, and the chef lived up to expectations when he began to introduce highly inventive children's meals in a hospital setting. Patients at Texas Children's Hospital were able to select their food for the next day from special menus that also had "little figures ... for them to color." Each day brought the opportunity to order such specialties as "kitty cat salad" or "pirate pudding."

One particularly memorable item was the "elephant sandwich." Fashioned in the form of a pachyderm from a peanut-butter-and-jelly sandwich, the treat featured a rolled carrot as the elephant's trunk and a banana resting on top. When delivered on a tray to a sick child's bed, there were smiles all around—not only from the patients and their families, but from the doctors and nurses as well. Everybody "got such a kick out of that sandwich," one dietitian recalled.[9]

The kitchen's creativity and presentation were an integral part of both hospitals' patient-oriented mission, as was emphasized in one of the first issues of the joint in-house newsletter, *Intercom:* "Food is a symbol of security to the patient and provides him with reassurance as well as nourishment, and sometimes it is difficult to determine which is the more important."[10]

Another reassuring service for patients and their families at Texas Children's Hospital was the remarkable policy that allowed parents to stay in the hospital room with their sick children. One of the first hospitals in the country to offer such family-centered care, Texas Children's Hospital benefited from the positive publicity generated by the policy.

One mother from El Campo who accompanied her daughter to the hospital had returned home full of praise, as was reported in the local newspaper. Enthusiastically endorsing the hospital, she spoke of the "contemporary modern building with the entire front construction of plate glass, brick, and aluminum," the "colorfully furnished children's toy areas," and the "courteous and helpful" volunteers who "even helped pack and load up my car."

From another parent interviewed about her experiences at the new hospital came this hometown newspaper report: "For us country folks, the new and comfortable Texas Children's Hospital had many startling innovations. We were waterless until an aide came to the rescue and pushed a lever under the lavatory with her knee. 'Think nothing of it,' laughed the girl in her orange jumper uniform. 'When I first came here and saw a nurse filling glasses of water with both hands, I thought she was saying a magic word to get the water to spout.'"[11]

While the modern new facilities inspired awe in patients and their families, Texas Children's Hospital also garnered praise from the Houston community at large. Promoted annually since 1950 at the fund-raising Pin Oak Charity Horse Show, which generated thousands of dollars in donations over the years, Texas Children's Hospital developed a large following of benevolent supporters. In addition, community response to the brochure designed by Walt Disney Productions in 1950 was immeasurable. Listing specific dollar donations for items ranging from silverware ($25) and wheelchairs ($90) to elevators ($45,000) and other high-ticket items, the whimsically illustrated solicitation inspired individuals and corporations to donate generously.

Unsolicited contributions from individuals and corporations became a regular occurrence after the hospital opened. The H. R. Cullen family donated a freezer full of chickens, capons, and turkeys during the hospital's first month. From the family-owned Sakowitz Brothers department store came a donation of all the pennies, nickels, dimes, and quarters thrown by children into its wishing well in the downtown store's Sky Terrace since its 1950 opening. Amounting to a significant amount of money, the donation covered the cost of furnishing an entire patient room at Texas Children's Hospital.

To the delight of many young patients, Adelena Meyer, wife of board president Leopold L. Meyer, gave a collection of doll clothes. Labeled "A Fan Harriet Original" in honor of the Meyers' late daughter, Fan Harriet, who had died at the age of 15 in 1939, each outfit was designed and created by Meyer. These creations, along with other elaborately dressed dolls, were placed on display in the Junior League Diagnostic Clinic to be admired, but not touched.[12]

Other contributions, large and small, continued to arrive at Texas Children's Hospital during its first few months of operation. Also growing in number was the patient population. Still structurally incomplete in June 1954, Texas Children's Hospital had by that time logged 511 admissions. Licensed as a 106-bed hospital, it boasted an occupancy level of 50 percent. Given the fact that the still-under-construction St. Luke's Episcopal Hospital remained unopened, the low occupancy was disappointing but not unexpected.

What did come as a surprise was the sudden resignation of Gammill. Claiming ill health, he immediately resigned as chief administrator in June. Named to replace him as acting director by the hospitals' two boards was Gammon Jarrell, who continued Gammill's previous duties at Texas Children's Hospital. The August 4 opening of St. Luke's Episcopal Hospital, the completion of the two hospitals' connecting link, and the inauguration of the surgical suite of operating rooms became Jarrell's responsibilities.

Six months later, Jarrell relinquished his duties to Dr. Maynard W. Martin. A pediatrician with extensive hospital administrative experience, Martin was recruited by both boards and was named chief administrator for joint operations in November 1954. His arrival was heralded by the medical staff at Texas Children's Hospital, who optimistically welcomed their fellow pediatrician.

"When they were searching for someone who would have the knowledge of administration and who had the understanding of medical problems, they were very fortunate to get him to come here," recalled physician-in-chief Dr. Russell J. Blattner. "Actually, a great deal of the credit for the smooth running of this rather complicated situation we must give to Dr. Martin."[13]

From the beginning of his 18-year tenure at Texas Children's Hospital, Martin enthusiastically embraced the founders' vision of creating and maintaining a hospital for the care of children afflicted with unusual diseases. He also wholeheartedly subscribed to the belief that "two autonomous hospitals can share physical facilities and voluntarily work together for the common good." Comparing his first year's efforts to "the shakedown cruise of a large ship" in which a major goal was to be the "training and stabilization of personnel," Martin launched his efforts to organize an administrative team in 1955.[14]

First to be inducted was Emma Moody Foreman, one of the two hospitals' newly hired employees. "Because of my experience with medical terminology as a surgical secretary, I was offered a position in medical records initially," she recalled. "I had worked only a few days when I was asked if I would help Dr. Martin in administration, whose secretary had left unexpectedly. When I started, he and I were the only employees in the department for a while."[15]

At that time, St. Luke's Episcopal Hospital had been open for just six months and the year-old Texas Children's Hospital, with only three stories and 106 beds, was small in size and staff. "You knew practically everyone by sight, if not personally," said Foreman. "The hospital was surrounded by lots of open land with old trees draped with Spanish moss. Access to the hospital was easy and there was even an overabundance of parking space."[16]

As both hospitals began to grow in census and in stature, Foreman's secretarial workload escalated at an equally rapid pace. Under Martin's direction were the hospitals' jointly operated facilities, including administration, operating rooms, emergency room, central supply, radiology, dietary, personnel department, building and grounds, and maintenance. Martin was also responsible for administering each hospital as an independent facility, answering to both boards equally. For Foreman, this translated into a daunting amount of paperwork. "In the beginning, I not only provided the secretarial support for Dr. Martin, but also did the work of both boards of trustees and both medical staffs," she said. "It was excellent experience, but assistant administrators and additional support staff were soon added."[17]

Wanting to offer improved "service to the patient," Martin sought the hospital boards' approval for increasing the size of his staff. With a growing patient population at St. Luke's Episcopal Hospital and the daily census at Texas Children's Hospital in 1956 nearing 80 percent, he strongly felt that the quality of care and support services also needed to grow. The boards concurred.

Martin proceeded to enlarge his administrative staff. His search for a second assistant ended in 1956 with the hiring of 30-year-old Newell E. France, who later recalled his first interview: "I was impressed that there was a children's hospital in association with an adult general hospital, and that the administrator for the two was a pediatrician who was one of about 20 medical administrators nationally at that time."[18]

France soon found Martin to be "an absolute master" in administration and a "total delegator." One responsibility that Martin delegated to France was the nationwide search for a director of nursing for both hospitals. The process lasted for more than a year and produced only limited results. "Nursing candidates couldn't quite see how a joint nursing director, differentiate pediatric and adults and all that, was going to be possible," he recalled.[19]

One potential contender was Mrs. Opal M. Benage, RN, BSN, MSN, from Little Rock, Arkansas. "She came to visit the hospital and meet with me," France recalled. "She did not apply for the position, but she said she would let me know and went back to Arkansas. For the next year, she would come back and visit, and her visits became more and more frequent. Meanwhile, I'm being the director of nursing and making a lot of mistakes, like over-staffing. By the time she accepted the position in 1959, half the hospital thought she'd already been at work. She immediately began to correct the mistakes I had made."[20]

Gathering all the nursing personnel from every shift for a mandatory meeting in the auditorium, Benage introduced herself, discussed her background, and explained what she planned and hoped to accomplish at Texas Children's Hospital and St. Luke's Episcopal Hospital. What Benage did next was particularly memorable to France, who recalled her bluntly saying the following: "About one-third of you know you don't belong here. Think about it, and we'll have a book in the nursing office for you to sign for your termination. Another third of you have potential, but you will have to accept intensive training, and those of you who can't devote that kind of time both on and off duty don't belong here. Another not quite a third of you are doing a fine job, and that's particularly true at Texas Children's Hospital."[21]

The result of Benage's speech was measurable. "We lost half the staff and started all over again," said France. "She was a strict disciplinarian, but she was known to be fair and always available, 24 hours a day. Whenever I put a page in for her, there was always a quick response, whether she was in the hospital, at home, or vacationing in Las Vegas, her favorite thing to do. She was a great lady and was with the hospitals more than 25 years."[22]

From the start of her career at Texas Children's Hospital, Benage championed the emerging concept of family-centered care. She was acutely aware of the distinct needs of hospitalized children and their families, introducing unique nursing policies to serve them more effectively. "She was far ahead of her time in many things," recalled fellow nurse Ruth Sylvester, RN, whom

Benage placed in charge of the joint operating rooms and services. "She insisted that we allow parents into the intensive care unit any time they wanted to be there. She also insisted that we let parents into the recovery room to see the patients after surgery. None of us wanted that, but, as it turned out, it was the best thing possible for the children and their families."[23]

Along with her compassion for patients and their families, Benage brought her no-nonsense style of management to the hospitals. She quickly gained the reputation of being "tough as nails" and a stickler for minute details. The professional appearance of the nursing staff was of utmost importance to her. "She was as neat as a pin and never looked like she sat down," said Florence Dickey, LVN. "When she was walking down the hallway and you saw her, in a minute, she could just sweep you from head to toe and if your shoe strings weren't clean, or your uniform wasn't all together, she'd let you know about it."[24]

To Benage, rigid conformity to the strict dress-code rules was flexible only if the needs of patients demanded relaxation. When a group of Texas Children's Hospital nurses suggested that colorful pinafores be worn over their white uniforms as a way to decrease patient anxiety, Benage wholeheartedly supported the innovation. With her authorization, the idea was implemented in 1960. As a result, hospitalized children and their families soon found themselves surrounded not by the crisp white uniforms of the past, but by a virtual rainbow of colors, stripes, and playful prints. The reaction from both patients and nurses was immediate and gratifying. Explaining why she felt that she suddenly looked "more friendly" to her patients, one nurse explained: "The children are not as afraid of colors as they were of that white."[25]

Experiencing this "unfailingly cheerful and gay atmosphere" at Texas Children's Hospital was a steadily increasing number of patients. Their personal details and financial circumstances were documented daily by administrative secretary Foreman. "Private rooms were $16 a day and semi-private rooms were $11," she recalled. "Word soon spread around that the hospital cared for children with no regard for race, color, or creed, or ability to pay. When both hospitals were fully opened, the census rapidly grew."[26]

Also growing was the two hospitals' reputation for high-quality patient care. Within the first few years of their existence, both Texas Children's Hospital and St. Luke's Episcopal Hospital received full accreditation from the newly formed Joint Commission on Accreditation, which was responsible for setting national standards for hospital operation and patient care. "Since that time, Texas Children's Hospital has continued to merit accreditation," said Foreman. "Even though there are more numerous and stringent standards, Texas Children's Hospital always is commended for the high quality of patient care."[27]

To accommodate the increasing patient population and to meet the needs created by advances in medical care and breakthroughs in medical technologies, in the late 1950s the board of trustees began considering possibilities for expanding Texas Children's Hospital—even though the facilities were less than a decade old. To board president Meyer, expansion was inescapable, both at that time and whenever deemed necessary in the future: "Children from all corners of the globe come to our Texas Children's Hospital for treatment, care, and cure; as time goes on, our problem will be to accommodate all who need what we have to offer."[28]

There was also a need to expand the 293-bed St. Luke's Episcopal Hospital. Experiencing an acute shortage of beds for its patients in the late 1950s, that hospital's board of trustees also accepted the foregone conclusion of expansion. The resulting plans for additional space and equipment necessary for the required support services involved considerable reconfiguring of the existing "connecting link" shared with Texas Children's Hospital.

Recognizing the economies of constructing both hospitals simultaneously, as in the beginning, each of the boards voted to commence the joint project in 1961. Although agreeing to begin building together, the boards remained uncertain as to exactly what the new additions were to be—not to mention what the expansion was to cost and which board was responsible for raising what amount of money.

Further complicating future construction plans was the chartering of the Texas Heart Institute by Dr. Denton A. Cooley in 1962. A medical and surgical institute devoted exclusively to treatment, education, and research in the field of cardiovascular diseases, the Texas Heart Institute was to be a joint facility of St. Luke's Episcopal Hospital and Texas Children's Hospital and was to share the hospitals' joint facilities.

Enthusiastically welcomed by the boards of trustees of both hospitals, the creation of the Texas Heart Institute necessitated a change in the expansion plan. Officially announced on July 22, 1962, by both hospital boards was a newly enlarged plan that included the proposed construction of a $6 million ten-story building to house the institute.

To expedite these construction plans and to assume corporate responsibility for the management of the Texas Heart Institute after its completion was a totally separate board of trustees, formed by the institute in August 1962. The trustees of all three institutions began to hammer out the details of the hospitals' proposed expansion. "Originally, the plan contemplated was to comprise ten floors at a cost of $18 million," recalled Meyer of that five-year process. "Periodically, however, the plans were expanded to encompass 26 floors at a cost of $50 million, including, of course, the Texas Heart Institute."[29]

The exponential rise in costs also reflected other adjustments necessitated by outside influences. One major cause for altering the plans was the changing healthcare needs of the community prompted by the implementation of the federal legislation for Medicare and Medicaid on July 1, 1966. Another major occurrence impacting the fluid design plans was the escalating availability in the 1960s of federal funds for medical research. The possibility of acquiring such future funding inspired the allocation of space for additional research facilities and support services in both hospitals.

With the inclusion of these and other mutually agreed-upon additions, the three boards agreed to proceed with construction. However, one trustee felt that in their zealous mission to prepare for the future, the combined boards had inadvertently disregarded the past—in particular, the property line established in the original joint operating contract between St. Luke's Episcopal Hospital and Texas Children's Hospital.

Originally executed in 1950 by Texas Children's Hospital trustee Herman Pressler, a Humble Oil executive and attorney, "the contract really was something like a joint operating contract of oil, a basic thing," he explained. "We did it in a very simple sort of way. The tracts that Texas Medical Center had given the two institutions adjoined, the west line of St. Luke's with the east line of Texas Children's. So, we just provided that two-thirds of the connecting link would be on St. Luke's property, and one-third would be on Texas Children's property. If we ever wanted to sever this relationship of a joint administration, we could just build a wall along that property line and they could go their way and we could go our way. When we were planning the new additions, I called our board's attention to the fact that we were not following this property line."[30]

In response to Pressler's concerns that "some of the building on our side of the line would be occupied and used by St. Luke's and vice-versa, and that we should work out an agreement between the institutions," the Texas Children's Hospital board instructed him to "work out such an agreement." After accepting that assignment in 1966, Pressler spent the next fourteen years spearheading efforts to reach a new agreement. In the meantime, he recalled, "We were still operating under the old law, as they say."[31]

Undaunted by Pressler's warning of a potential property-line dispute,

Meyer instead championed an optimistic view of further expansion needs. In a meeting with Texas Medical Center's Colonel W. B. Bates, Meyer stated "there is no doubt that by 1985 Texas Children's Hospital, St. Luke's Episcopal Hospital, and the Texas Heart Institute will be cramped within the confines of the land." He received Bates' commitment to provide additional acreage "contingent upon the need for such acreage in a reasonably early future."[32]

The immediate need of the boards of St. Luke's Episcopal Hospital, Texas Children's Hospital, and the Texas Heart Institute in 1966 was for the funds necessary to execute the expansion plans. To expedite the collection of contributions, each board appointed its own chairman to spearhead a three-pronged effort in the community.

Once again, the community responded with generous financial support. The long-awaited construction commenced after a groundbreaking ceremony on June 26, 1967, that was presided over by Texas Governor John Connally. The resulting national publicity about "the largest hospital expansion program West of the Mississippi" inspired one out-of-state physician to pen this congratulatory note to Meyer: "I suspect that it is only in Texas that one adds a 20-story addition to a three-story building, but then I have become accustomed to Texans doing things in a big way."[33]

In actuality, plans called for the addition of four stories to Texas Children's Hospital, bringing it to seven stories, and the building of a 26-story tower and underground facilities for the joint use of Texas Children's Hospital, St. Luke's Episcopal Hospital, and the Texas Heart Institute. With the resulting number of beds totaling more than 1,000, the hospital complex was to triple in size. "Construction began in 1967 and was completed five years later in 1972," said France, who was named administrator of the three entities in 1964 when Martin became executive director.

Recalling how both hospitals continued to deliver quality patient care during construction, France said: "It was the boards' requirement that construction be carried out on all six sides simultaneously; that's the four external sides, the top, and the excavation underneath. It was a 24-hour, enormous, and coordinated task for the medical staff and personnel to work among the dust and rubble and to suffer great inconveniences, and yet carry out programs that continued to grow."[34]

During this often-chaotic period, there were also new programs introduced by necessity. "We had no way of staffing the new building when it was going to be done," France explained. "At that time, the nursing shortage was terrible. Methodist Hospital was importing Philippine nurses and housing them. Opal Benage came to me and said, 'We are just going to have to train our own staff,' so we established a student vocational nursing school for both hospitals at St. Luke's in 1969. Over 400 graduates of the school during its four-year run remained to staff St. Luke's and Texas Children's."[35]

With this in-house-trained supplement, France noted that the number of beds utilized during construction of Texas Children's Hospital never decreased as it gradually increased to the projected 254. Though often inconvenienced by the altered physical surroundings, patients continued to receive quality care. France credited this astonishing administrative feat to Martin. "He was our leader," France said. "He was a magnificent teacher and, of course, recognized the only way to go through such an enormous construction program was to delegate authority and responsibility, which he did so well."[36]

One unexpected responsibility of the administrative staff in 1968 was "to feed and nurture all the media" who flocked to St. Luke's Episcopal Hospital after the initial heart transplant performed by Cooley on May 3, 1968. The first such operation in the United States, the procedure was to be followed by nine more before August of that year. As these transplants proceeded, the number of journalists multiplied into the hundreds. To meet the demands of the press, as well as those of patients and the two hospitals in the midst of construction, the administrative staff worked on a revolving shift basis, eight hours on and 12 hours off.[37]

These and other extraordinary adaptations to daily routines became ordinary occurrences during the five years of construction. Under the masterful direction of Martin, hospital services continued uninterrupted. The coexistence of patients and their families, television crews, doctors, construction workers, nurses, journalists, volunteers, and the hospitals' support staff became commonplace.

Behind the scenes, Martin proved himself to be unequaled. "He had probably one of the most difficult administrative positions that anybody could have," said Texas Children's Hospital trustee Pressler. "He had three boards to please. And these boards are composed of men that are not reticent about expressing their ideas. We've all got pretty definite ideas, and we're not easily convinced they aren't right. There were a lot of pulling, frictions between the institutions on a lot of things that he was in between them on. And he just did an outstanding job of getting along with everybody, and reconciling conflicts and frictions. In fact, there were a lot of us that thought Dr. Martin just kind of hung the moon."[38]

Therefore, when Martin began to suffer from ill health and submitted his resignation to the hospitals' boards in 1969, the trustees rejected his request. They convinced him to remain until construction was completed in May 1972. After an extensive national search for a successor, the three boards offered the position to France.

"Texas Children's Hospital has been singularly fortunate in having had a level-headed Dr. Maynard W. Martin for 18 years, ably assisted by Mr. Newell E. France, a uniquely qualified successor to Dr. Martin upon his retirement," said Meyer in 1974. "These two men, with very competent assistants, not the least important of whom are Mr. John E. Creighton and Mrs. Opal M. Benage, have cooperated to the end that Texas Children's Hospital is recognized, after only 20 years, as equal in rank with Children's Hospital Boston, which has been in existence for nearly 100 years."[39]

As the newly named executive director of the expanded Texas Children's Hospital, France was charged by the board to begin instituting the staff restructuring necessitated by the hospital's evolving role. "In accomplishing all of these things, the mission of Texas Children's Hospital changed from being a children's hospital dedicated to children with difficult diagnostic problems, to a concept of being a general hospital for children," said France. "This was a philosophy that had far-reaching consequences, in that the mix of patients, which was 80 percent medicine and 20 percent surgical before the expansion, was to become 52 percent surgical and 48 percent medicine."[40]

This shift in the patient population brought not only increased occupancy, but also an acute awareness of Texas Children's Hospital's lack of ancillary support services. "Meyer telephoned me one day and asked that I write on a piece of paper for him all those things which Texas Children's Hospital could not provide for children, and that he expected to receive a blank piece of paper," said France, recalling Meyer's determination that the hospital become a more comprehensive children's center.[41]

To transform Texas Children's Hospital into a sophisticated research and teaching center, France continued the efforts he and physician-in-chief Blattner had begun in the mid-1950s. "He pioneered the pediatric department at Baylor College of Medicine, and we had set about, Dr. Blattner and I, in really programming how to bring faculty aboard and how to introduce pediatric subspecialties to the community," France said. "In our planning, we rarely had any difficulty in coming up with a plan. All we lacked was the time to do it, how much it cost, and where the money was going to come from."[42]

One source of funds was the community. As they had since the first years of Texas Children's Hospital, Meyer, France, and Blattner promoted the hospital's work whenever they could. "People like Herman Pressler would create those opportunities for us with all kinds of groups," recalled France. "Mr. Meyer, Dr. Blattner, and I believed in our product and we did a lot of speech making."[43]

Another possible source of support was federal funds. In pursuit of research grants similar to the one received in 1964 to establish the Clinical Research Center at Texas Children's Hospital, France often accompanied Blattner to his meetings in Washington, D.C., with representatives from the National Institutes of Health. By 1977, their efforts resulted in more than $900,000 in extramural grant support at Texas Children's Hospital.

Also in the national arena, France pursued the establishment of administrative guidelines for children's hospitals. To address the major issues of concern to Texas Children's Hospital—the third-largest of 101 children's hospitals across the country—France became a founding trustee of the National Association of Children's Hospitals and Related Institutions (NACHRI) in 1969. "These issues of concern were universal and had to do with Medicaid legislation, reimbursement problems, the decline of census in children's hospitals, the enormous growth in outpatients, new techniques, and modalities of delivering care," said France. "In 1977, we were one of the few children's hospitals in the nation that had a 9 percent growth factor per year in its census, rather than decreasing or reaching a plateau."[44]

Other impressive statistics at Texas Children's Hospital in 1977 included 2,800 admissions, 9,000 emergency room visits, and full utilization of the 234 inpatient beds. This accelerated growth exacerbated an ongoing problem: achieving financial stability. "St. Luke's seemed to be the more economically viable of the two in those days," said Texas Children's Hospital trustee George A. Peterkin, Jr. "We were bleeding badly. We were not only losing money, we didn't have any money and were on C.O.D. with vendors, and we owed a lot of money to St. Luke's because we could not meet our expenses. In effect, we were an unsecured creditor of St. Luke's."[45]

This was a devastating turn of events for Texas Children's Hospital founder Meyer, whose failing health had prompted him to retire from the board in 1974. Although aware that children's hospitals traditionally experienced deficits, Meyer was nonetheless extremely apprehensive about possible repercussions of the limited cash flow. "I remember one of the last times I saw him before he died in 1982," recalled Peterkin. "He broke into tears, fearing that we wouldn't take care of every child who showed up at the door."[46]

Peterkin believed that this crisis was averted with the arrival in 1977 of Dr. Ralph D. Feigin, the second physician-in-chief at Texas Children's

Hospital. "Dr. Feigin had a vision, and he wanted nothing less than excellence in education, research, and clinical care," said Peterkin. "He would settle for nothing less than excellence, and he was willing to do it within the realm of not running the hospital broke. He was conscious of you do what's within your means. Dr. Blattner was perfect for the founding and formation of the hospital in those days. And then, in more modern times in the 1970s, the game changed and Dr. Feigin is perfect for these times."[47]

Within months of his arrival at Texas Children's Hospital, Feigin had implemented efforts to achieve his mission. When recruiting new faculty and staff members, he anticipated their needs would tax the space available in the hospital complex. With Feigin and his newly enlarged staff's accelerated development of new services and programs—along with the expansion of those already in existence—the need for more physical space became increasingly evident.

Complicating matters was the confusing overlap of space utilized by both hospitals, together with the absence of an updated ownership and operating agreement between St. Luke's Episcopal Hospital and Texas Children's Hospital. The property-line issues that trustee Pressler had warned of during pre-construction in the late 1960s became a reality. In 1980, both boards of trustees at last signed a new agreement that superseded all previous agreements and was retroactive to October 1, 1978.

Although its immediate effects were minimal, the agreement would have a profound impact. "Hospital activity and board involvement became so intense that I became executive assistant for trustee affairs, with responsibilities focused on providing support to the boards of trustees of Texas Children's Hospital, St. Luke's Episcopal Hospital, and the Texas Heart Institute and for assisting the executive director in all matters related to board involvement," recalled longtime administrative secretary Foreman.[48]

Many changes in the operation of both Texas Children's Hospital and St. Luke's Episcopal Hospital soon followed. After Newell France resigned in 1983, Mike Grafton served as interim executive director of both hospitals through 1984. During the search for a new joint executive director, St. Luke's Episcopal Hospital trustees decided to hire their own separate chief executive officer. As a result of this decision, Alex White became the first executive director of Texas Children's Hospital, a position he held from January 1985 until 1987.

The appointment of an individual executive director for each hospital in 1984 marked the beginning of the separation of the two hospitals' joint services. For the next three years, the two boards engaged in lengthy negotiations to conclude the previous joint-operating agreement and to initiate a new separation agreement. In 1987, with a signed agreement finalizing the further separation of all joint services, a new era officially began at Texas Children's Hospital.

"The decision to separate the shared services was a momentous one," said executive assistant Foremen. "To make that decision, the Texas Children's Hospital Board of Trustees had to make a commitment to build, staff, and open facilities including operating rooms and radiology, emergency room, and outpatient facilities in a short four-year time frame under the terms of the separation agreement with St. Luke's Episcopal Hospital."[49]

This commitment necessitated an immediate centralization of services for surgical patients at Texas Children's Hospital. With the exception of cardiovascular surgery, there would be a single location on the fourth floor for the preoperative, intraoperative, and postoperative care of all pediatric surgical and surgical subspecialty patients. Pediatric renal and liver transplantation surgery would also be conducted in the newly designated area.

As the enormous repercussions of the separation became increasingly apparent, the board searched for someone to fill the newly created position of executive director and chief executive officer of Texas Children's Hospital. The lengthy recruitment process failed to produce the right candidate, but it was a problem that was quickly solved.

"Dr. Feigin courageously and voluntarily assumed for more than two years the extra responsibilities as executive vice president and interim executive director in addition to his own heavy duties as physician-in-chief," Foreman reported.[50]

For Feigin—who knew firsthand the particular needs and wants of patients, physicians, and staff—the opportunity to bring his vision for Texas Children's Hospital closer to fruition was both exhilarating and exhausting.

"I literally worked day and night, seven days a week," Feigin recalled. "We were losing money, but I thought it could be turned around. We started our own pharmacy department, and the whole central supply, and our own operating rooms, and everything else—even while we still were in St. Luke's operating rooms. We had our own cost centers and we turned the hospital from a negative position to $16 million profit margin, a very serious positive position."[51]

Credited with ensuring the institution's financial viability was Sally I. Nelson, executive vice president and chief financial officer. Joining Texas Children's Hospital after the separation from St. Luke's Episcopal Hospital in 1987, Nelson found that the billing system was broken and the operating loss stood at more than $17 million. In tandem with the board's Kirby Attwell, chairman of the finance committee, Nelson crafted a plan to generate cash flow and to manage expenses more aggressively. By squeezing costs from both administrative and clinical processes to preserve margins, within two years their plan brought Texas Children's Hospital back to breakeven. When income levels eventually surpassed expenses, Nelson and Attwell championed the reinvestment of profits back into facilities, staff, new technologies, patient care, research, and education.

Financial success brought new challenges to the board. With the development of various new support and ancillary departments, high census and high occupancy levels continued. Texas Children's Hospital began to experience severe capacity constraints. With limited internal space available for future growth, the board declared the imminent need for a major capital expansion project.

Announced on July 15, 1988, the plans included the construction of two new buildings. The first, a multistory facility with underground parking, was designed to accommodate the consolidation of all ambulatory care and research programs. The second, a five-story facility constructed concomitantly to the existing hospital, was to provide a new private entrance to Texas Children's Hospital. In this building was a sizeable pediatric emergency center, a ten-room surgical suite with adjoining support service areas, and adequate space for the expansion of intensive care services for newborns and children. Built on a foundation that could support the eventual construction of a patient room tower, the building also boasted adjacent parking for both patients and physicians.

"We embarked on a $149 million facilities modernization and development program," board member Peterkin said, recalling the program's projected completion date of late 1991 or early 1992. "With the addition of 1,016,400 square feet of space and total of 450 licensed beds, Texas Children's Hospital was to become the largest pediatric hospital in the United States."[52]

Within a year of the announcement, all plans had been completed. The groundbreaking for the two new buildings took place on July 20, 1989. In addition to the new facilities, eight new departments were under development—including the only dedicated pediatric emergency center in the area.

With construction underway, the board's next priority was to find an executive director and chief executive officer to lead Texas Children's Hospital into the twenty-first century. Convinced that the hospital's future accomplishments were dependent on the effectiveness of its administration, the board searched for an outstanding leader.

The challenge for that new leader was to expand the reach of Texas Children's Hospital while remaining firmly rooted in the institution's traditions. In the 35 years since its opening day in 1954, Texas Children's Hospital had weathered dramatic and difficult changes, both in its physical surroundings and in its internal organization, but it had remained the same in one essential area.

Throughout its history of unprecedented growth, even during the often-tumultuous years during the separation from St. Luke's Episcopal Hospital and the establishment of independent facilities, Texas Children's Hospital never wavered from its commitment to quality family-centered patient care.

Because of that steadfast mission, first patient Lamaina Leigh Van Wagner's recollections of her experience at Texas Children's Hospital were echoed by all the patients who followed her: "They gave me loving attention."

3

✋ THE LEADERSHIP ✋

THE FOUNDATION FOR THE FUTURE GROWTH of Texas Children's Hospital was cemented into place in October 1989.

As the concrete pump truck began pouring the slab for the one-million-square-foot expansion project, the board of trustees of Texas Children's Hospital also secured the necessary cornerstone for the solid foundation of its infrastructure. It was Mark A. Wallace, the newly appointed executive director and chief executive officer of Texas Children's Hospital. Wallace's arrival marked the beginning of a new chapter in the history of Texas Children's Hospital, in which it would become one of the largest independent pediatric hospitals in the nation.

That these two events occurred during the same week was symbolic, but not strategically planned. The appointment of Wallace marked the successful culmination of the board's lengthy and extensive search for a leader. Surprisingly, after devoting years to scouring the country for a candidate, the trustees had found exactly what they were looking for right in their own neighborhood. However, finding Wallace was only the first hurdle. Convincing him to accept the position and come to Texas Children's Hospital was another.

Recognized nationally by his peers in 1987 as an emerging leader in healthcare, Wallace was a senior vice president of patient services at The Methodist Hospital in the Texas Medical Center. With more than 12 years of valuable experience in healthcare administration at Methodist, he maintained a strong sense of loyalty to that institution. Arriving there at the age of 24, he was the youngest assistant vice president in the history of the hospital. Named a vice president at the age of 26, Wallace became senior vice president at 30. His responsibilities included the consolidation of the two largest clinical operating divisions at the hospital into a single all-encompassing patient services division with direct responsibility for 1,527 licensed beds and 18 medical services. As senior vice president, he was responsible for a combined operating unit comprising 54 departments and employing more than 4,200 employees.

Wallace's significant accomplishments did not go unnoticed. At the age of 35, he became one of the few healthcare executives in the country who advanced to fellowship status in the American College of Healthcare Executives. He also received the 1988 Profile in Excellence Award for alumni achievement from Oklahoma Baptist University.

Such credentials impressed the search committee. Members found Wallace to be a uniquely talented individual, one with the potential to be a major leader in the healthcare field. When an executive search firm asked Wallace about his availability for a position elsewhere, he responded with polite refusals. But the committee's interest in Wallace was undaunted.

Although reluctant to consider a career change, Wallace eventually accepted an invitation to meet with two members of the board's search committee for another stated purpose—to share his thoughts on the profile that Texas Children's Hospital needed in a chief executive officer. It was during that first encounter with trustees George A. Peterkin, Jr., and William K. McGee, Jr., that Wallace learned of the hospital's mission. He became enthralled with the possibilities and potentialities.

"George and Bill started sharing with me their vision for Texas Children's Hospital, and that got me excited," Wallace recalled. "I saw that they were going to move away from being in the shadow of St. Luke's, and that they were really going to embark on a journey which would allow them to be one of the preeminent children's hospitals in the United States, if not the world. I really got enthralled in possibly being a part of that."[1]

Wallace also noted a unique aspect of the board, one that separated it from other hospitals. "They are people who are very caring and compassionate about Texas Children's Hospital," he said. "They are good business people who have the legal, ethical, and moral responsibility to be the stewards of the assets of the organization, but they do it in a unique manner of care and compassion and sensitivity for children, for families, and for this community."[2]

Subsequent meetings with the entire search committee and the Texas Children's Hospital board of trustees fueled Wallace's growing interest in the board's vision for Texas Children's Hospital. He soon came to embrace the vision as his own. After these encounters, Wallace knew "this was something that I wanted to come and be a part of, so I came over here and brought my ambition, my vision, my motivation, and my energy level and my youth and inexperience."[3]

With his arrival at Texas Children's Hospital on October 9, 1989, the 36-year-old Wallace became the youngest chief executive officer in the Texas Medical Center. Not hampered by his inexperience as a chief executive officer and anxious to lead, Wallace "was committed to the challenge of leadership and was not going to be deterred in any way."[4]

Wallace was unfazed when executives at The Methodist Hospital warned him that he would be unable to work with physician-in-chief Dr. Ralph D. Feigin. Wallace dismissed such pessimism, relying instead on his trademark optimism and determination to succeed. The result, based on mutual motivation and admiration, was the immediate establishment of an effective working relationship and a lasting friendship between Wallace and Feigin.

"Dr. Feigin and I shared a vision of excellence," he said. "We both had arrived in the Texas Medical Center in 1977, so I already knew him. What he had been able to build in his 12 years at Texas Children's Hospital before my arrival in 1989 was comprehensive excellence in the medical staff."[5]

From the onset of their professional relationship, there was shared mutual respect between these established leaders. Wallace regarded Feigin as one of the great men of medicine, while Feigin's dual role as interim chief executive officer and physician-in-chief for more than two and a half years afforded him a deeper appreciation of the challenges faced by Wallace. Individually unique, each strove towards the same goal of making Texas Children's Hospital the preeminent pediatric hospital in the world. Together, they knew that future successes were dependent on leadership.[6]

Indeed, Wallace's management philosophy was based on his belief that leadership was the secret to success in all endeavors, particularly those in hospital administration. In his first address to the full board of trustees, he shared his philosophy, management style, and vision for Texas Children's Hospital. He stated that leadership was of paramount importance in achieving the goal of becoming the preeminent pediatric hospital in the country—a center of excellence in patient care, education, and research.

"Leadership is the sum of vision, structure, and people, with people being by far the most important ingredient," he stated. "People make the difference, but if they don't have vision and structure, the good people will leave. In this business, you can't do anything by yourself."[7]

In this premier speech, and in subsequent ones, Wallace clearly defined his role of chief executive officer as one of leadership involving decision making by consensus building among the board, medical staff, and management. He announced the establishment of specific goals in important areas: providing outstanding care and service; developing a successful nurse recruitment and retention program; implementing a strategic management process; managing and completing the building project; achieving or exceeding the goal of the hospital's capital campaign; selecting the correct vendor for the management information system; and implementing that system.[8]

Wallace's major operational priority was to search for new opportunities to provide outstanding service to patients, families, and visitors. Achieving that goal required the development and implementation of an overall service program that paid meticulous attention to operating details. Wallace emphasized improved service and customer relations.

Working closely with Feigin and the more than 1,000 staff physicians, Wallace fostered cohesive relationships to ensure the provision of quality care to patients and their families. Within one year of his arrival, admissions increased more than 7.2 percent to 13,692. Texas Children's Hospital was providing medical care to children from 38 other states and 27 other countries. This escalating patient population produced increased excess revenues over expenses that were 170 percent over budget. Performance for fiscal year 1991 was projected at 214 percent over budget.

With the expansion of services and operating capacity afforded by the completion of the facilities in 1991, Wallace warned that the unparalleled growth had tremendous ramifications for staffing. The expansion and potential doubling of the patient population, together with the prevailing shortage of nurses, presented a particularly difficult problem for the nursing service. Wallace's solution was to create and implement a comprehensive management and staff-driven nurse recruitment and retention program. He aimed to create an environment where nurses wanted to build a career, not just hold a job.

Motivated by that goal, Wallace embarked on a national search for a vice president of nursing who could establish such a program. Just as the board's extensive search efforts led to finding him in the Texas Medical Center, Wallace found his search also led him back to the familiar neighborhood and Susan M. Distefano, a nurse manager at Hermann Hospital's Turner Neonatal Intensive Care Unit.

"I kept hearing the name Susie Distefano, and about how she was such a young, dynamic leader," said Wallace, who arranged for an interview. From the first 30 seconds of their meeting, Wallace knew that "this person is it. She's dynamic. She's young. She's courageous and not afraid to lead. She had the right vision and she had the right attitude. So I said, 'Do you want the job?' Fortunately, she took it, and within a matter of a year she had totally turned nursing around at Texas Children's Hospital."[9]

Other dynamic leaders were recruited to the administrative team. Wallace challenged all of his executives, new and established, to create the tone, the environment, and the culture of excellence that would allow Texas Children's Hospital to achieve its mission and fulfill its vision.

"I have many expectations for Texas Children's Hospital executives," Wallace stated, listing three distinct categories—attitude, competence, and conduct. "Attitude is a commitment to our hospital's direction and philosophy, its style and tone. Competence is the ability to carry out stated goals and objectives with innovation and initiative. I encourage each executive to take charge of his or her area and to take the lead in professional conduct."[10]

The way in which executives conducted the hospital's day-to-day business was transformed by Wallace. Planning for the future, he adopted the maxim of management theorist Peter Drucker that "the best way to predict the future is to create it." To focus energies, strategies, and resources on creating a vision, Wallace instituted strategic management practices. Honing the identity of Texas Children's Hospital, he championed a new way of thinking, a new way of communicating, and a new way of leading. By analyzing the ideals, hopes, and dreams of patients, medical staff, employees, trustees, and the medical school, he began instituting the strategic planning processes necessary to establish the future direction of Texas Children's Hospital.

Having established the "people" and "vision" part of his philosophy, Wallace shifted his focus to the "structure" elements. First, he helped stabilize the newly independent Texas Children's Hospital by assisting in the creation and development of eight new departments. These services included dietary, nuclear medicine, emergency, physical therapy, and occupational therapy—all of which had previously been shared with or purchased from St. Luke's Episcopal Hospital.

Next, Wallace aided in the selection and implementation of a new information system. The financial performance of the hospital had been adversely affected by the existing system, particularly in the area of accounts receivable, where the billing processes were delayed by up to 90 days. Wallace developed guiding principles for formalizing the system selection process to ensure that the $5.5 million system that was eventually acquired would offer efficiency, sophisticated integration, and a high level of functionality.

For the expansion project that was already in progress at the time of his arrival at Texas Children's Hospital, Wallace developed and implemented a protocol to ensure that all phases would be completed in a timely fashion and within budgetary guidelines. "I quantified what the cost of the project was going to be with the building and grounds committee and Ben Brollier, and it was more than the board expected," Wallace recalled. "Since the board already had borrowed $130 million in tax exempt revenue bonds, we had to put together some off-balance-sheet financing to pay for the rest."[11]

The resulting capital campaign, tagged "Building for Children," became Wallace's responsibility. Entrusted by the board to spearhead efforts to raise more than $67.5 million, Wallace was given five years to accomplish the task. He worked closely with Holcombe Crosswell, who successfully concluded the campaign in less than two years. Exceeding its goal by more than $2 million, the campaign raised a total of $69.2 million almost exclusively from local sources, including hospital employees and the medical staff.

When Texas Children's Hospital employees donated more than $215,000 to that campaign, Wallace declared that the precise value of their generosity was measureless. "While that's only a small percentage of the total amount donated, employees' contributions demonstrate to outsiders the commitment of the hospital's work force," he said. "And that probably helped us raise millions and millions and millions of dollars."[12]

The success of this first major capital campaign at Texas Children's Hospital "illustrates the extraordinary level of commitment and dedication to the mission of Texas Children's Hospital that Mark has been able to instill in the hospital and the community," Peterkin said. "Mark focuses on goal setting, board participation, achievement, and recognition. He offers a shared vision, creates a supportive environment, and then steps aside to allow his employees to accomplish common goals."[13]

Peterkin also had unbridled praise for Wallace's handling of the expansion project, which was completed earlier than expected in 1991. "Under his direction, the two buildings have been completed ahead of schedule and under budget," he said. "In today's climate of endless budget overruns, this is indeed an impressive accomplishment."[14]

Although keenly focused on the future, Wallace and the board of trustees of Texas Children's Hospital never lost sight of past accomplishments. In 1990, they enacted a lasting tribute to James Smither Abercrombie and Lillie Frank Abercrombie, two of the hospital's founders and strongest supporters. The original hospital structure that had opened in 1954 was renamed the Abercrombie Building in honor of the couple. Renovated to complement the newly constructed Clinical Care Center and the critical care and surgical West Tower, the Abercrombie Building was connected to both buildings and contained restyled patient rooms and family support areas.

In the administration of this newly enlarged and fully independent campus of multiple facilities that comprised Texas Children's Hospital, Wallace continually stressed the need to accelerate the quality of service provided to patients and their families. He introduced methods to increase efficiency in the delivery of services, to facilitate access to the facilities, and to nurture the development of a "professional, friendly, polite, courteous, helpful, hard-working, upbeat, concerned, caring, and open" organization.[15]

"Mark believes implicitly that delivery of the highest quality service is the cornerstone of an effective healthcare institution," Peterkin said. "He believes friendly, professional, and courteous service is the standard by which all else is judged. It sets the tone and gives patients the confidence that the clinical care they receive will be equally outstanding."[16]

To instill this philosophy, Wallace encouraged employee participation and expanded the existing Patient Relations Is Demonstrating Excellence (PRIDE) task force to assist in the identification of opportunities to improve service. Under his direction, the task force developed enhancement programs throughout the hospital.

The PRIDE task force identified and implemented improvements in the elevator service, in programs to assist physicians with medical records, and in the use of the hospital's new information system. Further recommendations helped to improve the quality of service. For example, employee orientation and training programs were revamped to emphasize the special needs of pediatric patients.

"Employee participation in hospital-wide issues is indicative of Mark's leadership style, particularly his role as a motivator," Peterkin said. "He is proud of the accomplishments of the hospital's employees and management team and personally sees to the appropriate recognition of individual achievement."[17]

Equally vital to Wallace's philosophy was the concept of teamwork. He believed that a sense of unity was essential to achieving the vision of Texas Children's Hospital, and that unity was derived from an awareness that everyone in the organization believed in and worked towards the same goal. To foster this awareness, Wallace established a strong sense of direction, encouraging employees to participate in the hospital's ongoing development.

To instill his philosophy of service within the management team, Wallace championed an inverted organizational chart, rather than a standard one. This creative tool illustrated his belief in serving those executives who reported directly to him, while they, in turn, served their direct employees. This chain of respect, rather than command, ultimately linked everyone in the organization to the shared responsibility of providing quality service to patients and their families.

"We're not here just to make Texas Children's Hospital a flagship for pediatric care," Wallace said. "We're here to impact children's lives and the lives of their families. That's a mission that is much mightier than just trying to grow the number of beds that a hospital has and increase an organization's balance sheet."[18]

Wallace's dedication had an evident impact on the employees, medical staff, and volunteers at Texas Children's Hospital. Following his arrival, there was a renewed sense of camaraderie among staff and a growing sense of pride in the institution. Visitors quickly sensed and often commented on the high morale. Spreading rapidly throughout Texas Children's Hospital, Wallace's trademark enthusiasm was both contagious and uplifting.

"Through his creative and innovative leadership, Mark is able to inspire in his employees the level of dedicated commitment that is necessary to attain the hospital's vision of preeminence and ensure its future success," Peterkin stated. "Mark, himself, is motivated by his own personal sense of accomplishment in developing and leading an outstanding medical institution which also responds to the more personal, service-related needs of young patients and families."[19]

Recognition of Wallace's efforts was not limited to his colleagues at Texas Children's Hospital. Honored for demonstrating outstanding leadership qualities and "accomplishing more than most healthcare executives hope to achieve in a lifetime," he received the Robert S. Hudgens Memorial Award and was named the Young Healthcare Executive of the Year by the American College of Healthcare Executives in 1992.[20]

Further affirmation of Wallace's leadership skills came in 1992, when Texas Children's Hospital received full accreditation, with no type 1 recommendations, from the Joint Commission on Accreditation of Healthcare Organizations (JCAHO). After receiving identical accreditation in 1995, 1998, and 2002, Texas Children's Hospital became the only children's hospital in the United States to attain this recognition in four successive surveys.

These accolades arrived at a time of astounding growth at Texas Children's Hospital. Immediately following the opening of the new facilities in 1991, Wallace discovered that activity levels had "just exploded literally." Although the addition of more than one million square feet had doubled the hospital's previous capacity, conditions were already becoming crowded. "We were full," said Wallace. "The operating rooms were full. The clinics in the Clinical Care Center were full. The emergency room was full. The reception we received from the medical community, the patients, and families was just phenomenal."[21]

When an incredible financial performance accompanied this patient population explosion in the early 1990s, memories of the financial woes of the 1980s faded, but were not forgotten. "George Peterkin once put it this way at a board meeting, 'We are experiencing an embarrassment of riches,'" Wallace recalled. "The rating agencies loved that story. They upgraded us. We have had two upgrades since the initial rating on the bonds that were issued in 1991."[22]

Also upgraded was Wallace's original business plan for Texas Children's Hospital. Once deemed ambitious, the plan had been surpassed. The scope for future achievements became unlimited. The immediate need for additional space inspired Wallace's idea for an off-site building to house support services. Opened in 1994 and dedicated to the memory of Leopold L. Meyer, the six-story building bore Meyer's name as a tribute to his countless contributions during the formative years of Texas Children's Hospital. The Leopold L. Meyer Building commemorated the inspired dreams and hopes of all the founders of Texas Children's Hospital and served to symbolize how dramatically their original concept had been expanded.

"All of a sudden, we had a whole new idea about how great this organization could become," Wallace said, recalling how the "embarrassment of riches" necessitated the inspiration and creation of the Meyer Building. "We launched another strategic planning process and facilities modernization and development program in the mid-1990s to develop new strategies for the future."[23]

The impending need for new strategies soon became evident. As Texas Children's Hospital continued its evolution under Wallace's leadership in the 1990s, the healthcare industry was going through a revolution caused by the advent of managed care. Hospitals and hospital-based clinics could no longer expect to receive traditional fees for their services, creating a mandate for effective cost management in healthcare.

To Wallace and his team of executives, this newly emerging paradigm of managed care necessitated the development of a new business plan, one that ensured the continuation of the hospital's newly embraced financial fluidity. So that the institution could compete effectively in the future, Wallace envisioned a unique concept for corporate restructuring at Texas Children's Hospital.

As the architect of the integrated delivery system (IDS), Wallace unveiled his blueprint for restructuring in 1996. Once again, he utilized an unexpected organizational chart to emphasize his philosophy of service to the community. "Dace Reinholds, the director of governance affairs, was very helpful in the creation of the IDS structure," Wallace explained. "We wanted to have Texas Children's Hospital on the top of the organizational chart, basically serving as the holding company for the IDS. Symbolically, I thought it was very important for the hospital to be on top. I didn't want anyone to think we viewed any other corporation as being more important than the hospital."

Other hospitals across the country developed integrated delivery systems, but theirs did not follow this strategy. "Later, when other hospitals began to dismantle their systems piece by piece, ours remained strategically sound," he explained. "What we said we wanted to do proved to be pretty much the right strategy."[24]

The IDS at Texas Children's Hospital was developed to provide patients from across the country and around the world with the finest pediatric care through community physicians, managed care, and hospital care. It encompassed a total of seven previously independent or non-existent corporations. Representing eight strategic areas—managed care, clinical services, operations, finances, information systems, facilities, marketing, and advocacy—this restructuring broadened the corporate scope of Texas Children's Hospital.

With Texas Children's Hospital as its umbrella, the IDS covered Texas Children's Pediatric Associates, a certified nonprofit health corporation with the purpose of acquiring, managing, and affiliating with pediatric services; TCH System, Inc., a new entity created to direct the overall integration of the business activities of the other IDS corporations; Texas Children's Health Plan, a new entity established to facilitate the IDS development and administration of the pediatric health maintenance organization (HMO), the nation's first, and for providing quality pediatric care and ensuring access to care and insurance coverage for children; Texas Children's Home Health Services, a new entity created to provide improved access to pediatric home health services in the community; Texas Children's International, developed to support pediatric healthcare efforts internationally; and TCH Insurance Co., Ltd., a single-parent, captive insurance company established to provide liability coverage to Texas Children's Hospital and all affiliated corporations.

Although comprising multiple entities with diverse functions, Texas Children's Hospital IDS maintained its singular goal and established a unified identity in its rapidly expanding community. "All of this restructuring means a lot to me and to the board of trustees, but it doesn't matter to the moms, the pops, and the kids," Wallace said. "It's not important for patients and their families to understand the intricacies of an integrated delivery system. They just need to know it means access and coverage for kids. To them, we are, and will continue to be, Texas Children's Hospital, period."

Within the healthcare industry, the complex identity of the Texas Children's IDS became known, as did Wallace's overall responsibilities for its leadership and management. Heralding the development and confirming the viability of the IDS was the receipt of accreditation with commendation from the JCAHO following its initial survey in 1998.

In addition to overseeing the IDS, Wallace continued to develop and implement policies and programs as delegated by the board; to develop and recommend strategic objectives; and to coordinate efforts with Dr. Feigin and a medical staff of more than 1,550 physicians to provide the highest possible standard of medical care and service. To ensure the continued success of Texas Children's Hospital, Wallace envisioned an expanded horizon.

"We kept pushing out our vision, because we no longer thought of ourselves as being just a local hospital," said Wallace. "We wanted to be on the national and international stage, to serve patients and families from all over the world. We developed Texas Children's International to recruit international patients, and eventually attracted and treated more patients from outside of the United States than any other children's hospital in the United States."[25]

Increased national and international media awareness of Texas Children's Hospital quickly followed. While other hospitals across the country suffered a decrease in clinical activities and in occupancy during the late 1990s, the clinics and the 456 beds at Texas Children's Hospital remained full to capacity.

When patient demand continued to increase, the board of trustees made another newsworthy announcement in 1999. It was a $345 million four-year expansion project, one of the nation's largest building projects for a healthcare facility. The most ambitious expansion project in the history of the Texas Medical Center, the proposed addition of 1.2 million square feet was to double the existing size of Texas Children's Hospital, making it one of the largest independent pediatric hospitals in the United States.

Included in the plans was a 15-story inpatient addition to the West Tower, licensed for 715 beds, and the construction of a new 16-story outpatient center. Also announced was a dedicated research hub to be located in the planned renovation of the Feigin Center, the former Clinical Care Center renamed to honor the contributions of Dr. Feigin and his wife, Dr. Judith Z. Feigin, in 1997.

The $345 million needed for the expansion was to be funded through a combination of debt and an $80 million capital campaign. Appointed by the board to spearhead the "Building for Children" campaign was Wallace.

Newly appointed as president and chief executive officer—becoming the first person to assume that position at Texas Children's Hospital—Wallace proclaimed the expansion project to be "Texas Children's most significant undertaking since our founding in 1954."[26]

Ambitious in scope, the project exemplified both the mission and the vision of Texas Children's Hospital. "We are committed to providing quality healthcare to our patients," Wallace said, reiterating the hospital's mission of excellence in patient care, education, and research. As for the hospital's vision to be the preeminent pediatric hospital in the world, Wallace stated: "This project will allow us to grow, adapt, and implement new, customized services to continue to set the highest standards for pediatric medicine."[27]

Wallace acknowledged the successful issuance in 1999 of Texas Children's Hospital bonds to finance a major portion of the expansion, crediting chief financial officer Sally Nelson with selling the ambitious capital expansion plan to credit analysts. Attributed to sound management practices that produced a strong financial position, the highest ratings possible came from three of the country's leading rating agencies. Both Standard & Poor's and Fitch IBCA issued AA ratings and Moody's Investor Service gave an Aa2 rating, the first such rating for a children's hospital in the United States and the highest for any Texas hospital.[28]

Singular status recognition came to Texas Children's Hospital for an altogether different reason in 2001 during Tropical Storm Allison, one of the worst storms in Houston's history. Flooding from that storm's 22 inches of rain paralyzed the Texas Medical Center, causing billions of dollars in damages to every institution—except Texas Children's Hospital, where damage was limited to the flooding of one basement. This apparent good fortune was in fact due to foresight.

Just months before Allison, as the result of intense planning and study of the flood plain and watershed in the Texas Medical Center, the board of Texas Children's Hospital approved an engineering plan to install five submarine-style doors in tunnels leading to and from its facilities. Constructed of aerospace aluminum—the same material as the space shuttle—and weighing more than 2,500 pounds each, the strategically placed doors blocked more than six million gallons of floodwater. In the months following the storm, the design and implementation of this unique plan was to garner engineering awards in Texas and media attention around the world.

An immediate assessment of the submarine doors, as well as the overall flood alert system, came from Wallace: "In comparison to neighboring hospitals, we sustained a minimum amount of damage, thanks to the preparation and foresight of our facilities and operations teams. The intense planning, the study and design of construction barriers, the staff preparation, and flood alert system training protected our patients and families."[29]

Although saved from the flooding, everyone at Texas Children's Hospital shared the inconveniences experienced by others in the Texas Medical Center who found themselves stranded without electricity or running water. It was an untenable position to which the community quickly responded. Truckloads of water and food to establish and staff mobile kitchens arrived from Houston merchants, as did countless citizens who donated flashlights, batteries, and sump pumps. Many of these volunteers were off-duty employees of Texas Children's Hospital and members of their families—including children.

Overwhelmed by such unsolicited generosity, Nelson, speaking on behalf of Texas Children's Hospital, told the media: "This heartwarming response from the community has reminded us of how caring our neighbors are and how highly they regard the work we do at Texas Children's. We are extremely grateful to all of them."[30]

The high esteem in which Texas Children's Hospital was held was not limited to the local community. In 2001, *Child* magazine instituted a survey to ascertain the "Top Ten Children's Hospitals," publishing the results taken from 54 participating hospitals across the nation. In fifth place was Texas Children's Hospital.

The achievement was shared with equal pride by every member of the Texas Children's Hospital team, which comprised more than 6,000 employees and 1,625 board-certified primary-care physicians, pediatric subspecialists, pediatric-surgical specialists, and dentists. Energized by the recognition and inspired by the collective sense of accomplishment, each realized the importance of his or her individual contribution to the team effort.

In all respects, this winning attitude was precisely what Wallace had envisioned a decade earlier as being the prerequisite culture for the future of Texas Children's Hospital. Rather than merely predict that future, he and Feigin and the entire team at Texas Children's Hospital had assumed the responsibility for creating it.

As one of the architects of that plan, Wallace reflected on what had taken place since his arrival in 1989. "What's happening at Texas Children's Hospital is that every opportunity that we have to perform, this organization just knocks it out of the ballpark," he said. "The successive accreditations, the bond rating, the ranking as one of the top ten children's hospitals, the quality of patient care, the improved services, the massive expansion project, and the list goes on and on. We had such momentum, such confidence. The board, Dr. Feigin, the medical staff, the leadership team, the employees, the volunteers, our families, and I all believed in ourselves and this institution, and that's the kind of leadership that makes an organization a great organization."[31]

Wallace and his team believed that a great organization was capable of even greater accomplishments. This was a proven theory at Texas Children's Hospital in 2004. Following the completion of its $345 million expansion project, the once, three-story, 106 bed main campus of Texas Children's Hospital became a four-building complex connected by walkways and tunnels. Licensed for 639 beds, Texas Children's Hospital became one of the largest freestanding pediatric hospitals in the United States.

Although undetectable to the eye of the beholder, there was something old in the glistening newness of this greatly expanded family-centered environment, with its child-friendly bubble columns, colorful aquariums, and elevators equipped with twinkling lights and funhouse mirrors.

Indelibly ingrained in every aspect of the new facility was something that had been intrinsic to Texas Children's Hospital since its opening five decades earlier. Instilled by the founders and embraced by all who followed, it was the ongoing legacy of loving care.

4

✌ THE FIRST PHYSICIAN-IN-CHIEF ✌

THE ROOTS OF TEXAS CHILDREN'S HOSPITAL were inextricably intertwined with those of the department of pediatrics at Baylor College of Medicine.

The person responsible for planting the seeds of that affiliation, and nourishing its growth, was Dr. Russell J. Blattner.

Nine years before Texas Children's Hospital opened, Blattner was an associate professor of pediatrics at Washington School of Medicine. As one of the pathologists who had isolated the St. Louis encephalitis virus, later proving it to be borne by arthropods, Blattner already was recognized in the medical community in 1945 as a virologist, pathologist, and specialist in infectious diseases. He was about to become a legend in Houston.

It was a future that Blattner had no way of predicting. In fact, he had never even been to Texas before 1945, when he visited to deliver a series of lectures throughout the state. Blattner decided to stop in Houston, where he wanted to see the newly reestablished Baylor College of Medicine. The 37-year-old physician soon discovered that the medical school, which had moved to Houston from Dallas in 1943, was temporarily ensconced in a Sears, Roebuck & Company warehouse.

Blattner's spur-of-the-moment trip to Houston permanently changed his career—and the lives of countless others.

From the moment he arrived in the city, Blattner became intrigued with the possibilities he found in Houston, particularly at Baylor College of Medicine. "I was very much impressed with the fact that they were carrying on classes and even research in this converted warehouse," he said, recalling the tour of the facilities and his favorable observations of Dr. Walter H. Moursund, dean of Baylor College of Medicine, and his "adventuresome" full-time staff of 12.[1]

"I felt a tremendous spirit there," Blattner explained. "Under the most adverse circumstances the faculty had a remarkably effective program. They didn't have any walls, just partitions that ended one foot from the ceiling. So whatever the dean said could be heard throughout and, as students told me, when they heard the duplicating machine going, they knew an exam was coming up."[2]

Blattner was also given a tour of the Texas Medical Center, a large and still undeveloped wooded area adjacent to Hermann Park in Houston, which at that time contained only Hermann Hospital and the Baylor College of Medicine construction site. He was again left with a favorable impression. "The medical school building was half-way up," he remembered. "In just two years they had accomplished this."

In tandem with Blattner's admiration of Baylor College of Medicine was a fascination with the city of Houston. This interest was inspired not only by his brief visit, but also by a gentleman he happened to meet on the train home to St. Louis. The man was a New Yorker who served as financial advisor to several wealthy Houstonians. He and Blattner struck up a conversation that remained memorable decades later. "I discovered Houston wasn't just an oil capital," Blattner said. "It had a lot of ranching. It had a seaport. It had sulfur. It just had every resource which could predict that it was going to be a major metropolis."

That chance conversation in 1945 marked the precise moment that Blattner "began to appreciate the great future that Houston's wealth, vigor, and expansiveness offered." But when he received an offer to become chairman of the department of pediatrics at Baylor College of Medicine, Blattner was hesitant to accept. When he was offered the same position at the University of Kansas, the University of Colorado, and in North Carolina, Blattner could not forget what he had seen in Houston—or his feelings about the exciting possibilities for pediatric medicine in the city's limitless future.

Blattner remained intrigued, but he was not yet convinced that Houston was where he should go. Dr. James A. Greene, Baylor College of Medicine's professor of medicine, went to St. Louis to interview him, but Blattner was still undecided. Dr. George W. Salmon, acting head of the pediatrics department at Baylor College of Medicine and a former colleague of Blattner's at St. Louis Children's Hospital—himself a Texan—encouraged him to accept the offer. Blattner was appreciative, but still unsure. "Dr. Salmon said he wanted to go into private practice, and that he would turn the reins over to me," Blattner recalled. "He just begged me to come."[3]

Another desperate plea came from Dr. James Park, a prominent practicing pediatrician who was chief of pediatrics at Hermann Hospital. To entice Blattner, Park made a personal promise to step down and to convince the board of Hermann Hospital to appoint Blattner in his place—even though the hospital did not have an official affiliation with Baylor College of Medicine.[4] Still Blattner vacillated.

Ultimately, the generous interventions of Salmon and Park, together with Blattner's enthrallment with the school and the city, proved irresistible. He "finally decided to take my chances in Houston."[5]

In September 1947, two years after his first visit, Blattner returned to Houston. Named that year as professor of pediatrics and chairman of the department of pediatrics at Baylor College of Medicine, he was unsure how long he would stay.[6] During his first few years at Baylor, Blattner remained reluctant to embrace his fate completely. According to one of his first faculty members, Dr. Murdina M. Desmond, this lingering tentativeness was visibly evident during her initial job interview with him in 1948.

"Dr. Blattner had two staff members, one resident, one part-time volunteer secretary, and one office in which his books were still in boxes, his pictures on the floor, and his diplomas stacked against the wall," Desmond remembered. "A year later, his pictures and diplomas still were not hung, his books still crated. When Dr. Blattner saw my looking around, he quickly explained, 'I'm not sure if I'm going to stay.'"[7]

The truth be known, he had been just too busy to unpack.

Blattner had bypassed the traditional settling-in period. Instead, he had immediately begun to assess the situation, noting which programs needed to be developed for the near and not-so-distant future. "The department of pediatrics was started with Dr. Florence Heys, who came with me from St. Louis," Blattner explained. "Dr. Joseph Stool, who was at Hermann and completed his training there, Robert Lomas, and Jack McKeemie, who had one year in St. Louis and took his second year with me here in Houston, were the only people we had in the department. Miss Frances Heyck, who was secretary of the Junior League Children's Clinic at Hermann Hospital, served as my half-time secretary and half-time secretary of the Junior League Children's Clinic."[8]

Although understaffed in his department, Blattner was supported by a voluntary faculty—the members of the Houston Pediatric Society. This group of local practicing pediatricians contributed a great deal of time to teach students and house staff and to take ward rounds, as well as give formal lectures.[9]

Joining that voluntary staff was Salmon, who had gone into private practice. As he had promised, Salmon had relinquished his roles as acting head of pediatrics at Baylor College of Medicine and medical director of the Junior League Children's Clinic of the outpatient department at Hermann Hospital. Also true to his word was Park, who stepped down from his position at Hermann Hospital. Soon after, Blattner was appointed chief of pediatrics by the Hermann Hospital board. This de facto relationship between Hermann Hospital and Baylor College of Medicine continued for more than two decades, with Blattner reappointed chief of pediatrics each year.

In addition to his clinical duties at Hermann Hospital, Blattner taught classes at Baylor College of Medicine. Along with every member of the department's faculty—including his research assistant, Heys—Blattner began teaching the first postgraduate course in the partly completed Baylor College of Medicine building in the Texas Medical Center in 1947. With lectures also presented by the practicing doctors from the volunteer staff, the pediatric program was not only a pioneering effort, but also a popular one. "Everybody seemed to think of it as quite courageous of us to do this with very little in the way of facilities," Blattner recalled.[10]

Also inventive was the way in which Blattner and his instructors formed the curriculum in those early years. The process was anything but the lengthy and formal course of action that it was destined to become. In fact, it was just the opposite. One of Blattner's first instructors was Desmond, who recalled how the impromptu planning sessions were held at the Bill Williams restaurant across the street from the Texas Medical Center. There, late in the evening, over hamburgers, Blattner, Heys, and Desmond plotted and planned the year's schedules.[11]

For the purposes of clinical teaching, the only patients available were those from the few pediatric beds at Hermann Hospital and from the Junior League Children's Clinic. Blattner believed that this situation was inadequate. Knowing that the funds necessary to expand his department were marginal, he devised an all-encompassing long-range plan for a well-balanced program that also included financial support. His method was to contact every medical unit in Houston that had anything to do with children, a feat he accomplished in record time.

Within the first few years, Blattner established working relationships with Jefferson Davis Hospital; The Blue Bird Clinic for Children's Neurological Disorders, which Blattner helped found, at The Methodist Hospital; the Southwestern Poliomyelitis Respiratory Center; the March of Dimes; the DePelchin Faith Home, a residence for orphans deemed "unadoptable"; the Pauline Sterne Wolf Memorial Foundation Rheumatic Fever Hospital; and the Florence Crittenden Home for Unwed Mothers. He had not only initiated an extensive resident training program at Baylor College of Medicine, but had also secured financial support.[12]

Another avenue of fiscal support involved consultations with local doctors. Blattner's first consultation in Houston was an auspicious beginning. After seeing a child from a prominent Houston family who was said to have leukemia, a fatal disease, Blattner correctly diagnosed infectious mononucleosis, a condition with an excellent prognosis. With the recovery of the child, Blattner had instantaneously established a sterling reputation for both himself and the department of pediatrics at Baylor College of Medicine. This had happened through "great good luck," he always said.

With an expanding universe of clinical opportunities for pediatric training, Blattner enhanced his teaching capabilities. "When we got residents, we already had a rotation for them," he said. "We had a nucleus of a teaching staff, we had the continuing support of the practicing doctors who did much of the clinical teaching in the early years, and we had community support."[13]

The next challenge for Blattner to tackle was how to attract the most qualified residents to the newly established program. Fortunately, this was not the problem he had expected it to be. It all had to do with timing. With the war over, the vast number of returning veterans in search of residencies found that the quotas for the better-known programs in Texas had already been filled. So, they applied instead to Baylor College of Medicine. From this highly qualified group of individuals, Blattner was able to choose some of his first residents.[14]

"We got excellent people who were eager to get the jobs," he recalled. "I think we couldn't have chosen a better time in history. After the war, there was great euphoria. There was wealth. Everybody was making money. There was also this great advantage of sulfa's being discovered in 1937 and antibiotics in the early 1940s, so the complete complexion of medicine was changing, enabling us to take care of many patients we never could cure before. It was almost fate that this was thrown together."[15]

Recruiting others to the department, however, could not depend on chance or outside influences. It required a strategic plan. "It was necessary for us to make some effort on our own behalf to let people know what was going on in Texas, at Houston," Blattner recalled. "We did this in several ways."

One approach was subtle. It was Blattner's association with the *Journal of Pediatrics,* at that time the official organ of the American Academy of Pediatrics. The journal had branched off on its own and would now be published by the Mosby Company of St. Louis. Asked to serve on the journal's board before he left St. Louis, Blattner had begun writing his "Comments on Current Literature," a

monthly review of newsworthy articles that had appeared in journals published in Europe, Canada, South America, and the United States. The widely
read column was considered one of the publication's main features.

Blattner's first column from Houston was in December 1948.
Reviewing the recent advances in pediatrics, he focused on viral encephalitis. The next column appeared in July 1950 and concerned nitrogen
mustard as a therapeutic agent, which constituted the beginnings of cancer
chemotherapy in tumor work. Then, every month thereafter, from
December 1948 through June 1969, Blattner's columns covered a vast array
of subject matter.

"I had the very strong support of my research assistant, Dr. Florence
M. Heys, who was not only a PhD in biology, but also an English major. Dr.
Heys, and the members of the staff who kept an eye open for interesting
new developments, contributed greatly to my publication of this monthly
'Comments on Current Literature,'" said Blattner. "In a sense, it drew attention to the fact that there was something going on in Houston, and I'm sure
served an important function in attracting young people to this center."[16]

Perhaps even more important was the national recognition that
Blattner garnered over the years as the author of these highly regarded
columns. Such renown no doubt played an integral part in the success of
the pediatric department's nationwide recruitment efforts.

Recruiting residents for the pediatric department was an intensive
enterprise that required a great deal of traveling—not only by Blattner, but
also by his small but growing faculty. The process involved attending
national meetings, making speeches, lecturing at universities and medical
centers, and interviewing medical students. It also included entertaining
promising candidates wherever they were found.

On one occasion, Blattner and members of his faculty were in Seattle.
They had gathered 15 people, including candidates for residency, for dinner at an authentic Japanese restaurant. The guests were seated around a
table recessed into the floor. Blattner had just seen the movie *The Pink
Panther,* starring Peter Sellers, and found it to be terribly funny. One
moment he particularly enjoyed was a line delivered by a character dressed
as Cleopatra, complete with an asp wrapped around her arm. "After we'd
had a couple of highballs, I got the courage to tell this story," he recalled,
admitting that he was never very good at telling stories.

"When I got to the punch line, 'Keep your hand off my asp,' everybody
roared with laughter. I've never told a story where everybody laughed like
that. I looked around and realized the Japanese waitress, leaning over to ask

whether she should serve or not, had put her hand on my back just as I'd said 'Keep your hand off my asp!' Well, as a result of this, we got three residents!"[17]

With an influx of these and other new residents to the program, along with the burgeoning subspecialties that became available in pediatrics during the late 1940s, Blattner soon realized that his department had inadequate resources to train residents sufficiently in certain areas. It was a shortcoming that required both immediate attention and a great deal of money, the latter being something that the department was sorely lacking.

Tackling this seemingly insurmountable problem, Blattner conceived a brilliant solution. With the support of a scholarship fund, he could send his young faculty members and residents to Children's Hospital Boston, Johns Hopkins, and any other medical center with expertise that was not available at Baylor College of Medicine. Blattner believed that this strategy, which would provide Baylor College of Medicine with the best of various departments throughout the country, would result in an up-to-date and well-balanced program.

After Blattner had garnered enthusiastic support for the idea from dean Moursund, the two made an appointment to see Jesse H. Jones, the legendary Houston businessman and philanthropist. The eponymous Jones Foundation seemed a likely source to fund such a unique and educational endeavor. The supposed meeting turned out to be an unusual experience, one that Blattner never forgot.

"As far as we got was to an office where the secretaries and the assistants sat," he recalled. "We never saw Mr. Jones. But Dr. Moursund would write down what we were wanting, and then this was sent upstairs to Jehovah, and Jehovah would send the message back down."[18]

What made the process even more memorable was its conclusion. The unseen Jones approved the request, giving a $50,000 grant. To be spent in yearly $5,000 allotments named Jesse H. Jones and Mary Gibbs Jones Fellowships, the grant enabled Blattner to instigate his "inheritance of excellence" training program, one that would surpass expectations over the next decade.

The successful implementation of this aspect of Blattner's training program was instrumental in changing the medical community's perception of the department of pediatrics at Baylor College of Medicine. "Under no circumstance could it be considered a provincial center, and it certainly was not a one-man center," Blattner recalled. "The inheritance came from many, many excellent places."[19]

In a field where reputations were steeped in decades of history, Blattner's pediatric department at Baylor College of Medicine began to come of age in less than ten years. "The reason our pediatric center evolved so quickly and became world famous so quickly was that we really inherited the best training that was available at the time," he explained. "It was a conscious policy which I pursued. This way we short-circuited the development of a medical school. We had people who had the best training they could get. This is how we planned it. We also set up the stage for their return so they could work with patients within a week of returning here. These people all emerged not because of what I taught them, but what they learned and brought back."[20]

Bringing back not just new techniques, but also new faculty members from other medical centers was a Blattner trait. Appointed to the consulting staff of the Brooke Army Medical Center at Fort Sam Houston in San Antonio, Blattner made monthly rounds with the residents of that institution. He befriended many of them. One such resident was the "versatile, resourceful, and cheerful" Dr. Fred M. Taylor, who joined the faculty at Baylor College of Medicine after completing his military responsibility in 1948 and became "the first full-time person with enough courage to join our department."[21]

Also recruited to join the faculty from Brooke Army Medical Center was Dr. William A. Spencer, a graduate of Johns Hopkins University School of Medicine. Upon arriving in Houston, Spencer immediately began addressing the many problems being encountered with the resuscitation devices utilized during the 1948 outbreak of poliomyelitis in Houston. Ultimately assuming the directorial responsibility for the Southwestern Poliomyelitis Respiratory Center adjoining Jefferson Davis Hospital, Spencer later developed that entity into the Texas Institute for Rehabilitation and Research (TIRR).[22]

Similar accomplishments and career advancements would also be made by other faculty members during Blattner's three decades at Baylor College of Medicine. Each achievement became an integral part of his legendary tenure. "He was building a department with experts in every area of pediatrics, so the patients could receive the best possible management," said Dr. Martha Dukes Yow, Blattner's recruited expert in infectious diseases.[23]

Another area in which Blattner excelled was that of community relations. He had a remarkable ability to encourage and nurture the involvement of Houston's practicing pediatricians in his program. Unlike at other medical schools, where faculty members often clashed with those not in academics—a phenomenon known as "town and gown"—Blattner conscientiously avoided these problems at Baylor College of Medicine. Having witnessed the results of such divisive conflicts elsewhere, he was determined to create an optimal working relationship between academics and private practitioners.

One tactic was a policy that prevented faculty members of the pediatric department from going into private practice. Available for consultations only by referral, the Baylor College of Medicine staff doctors diagnosed the patient, suggested or administered a treatment plan, and sent the child back to the originating pediatrician.

This strictly enforced rule was instrumental in cementing the department's close working relationship with members of the Houston Pediatric Society. With no fear of losing their referred patients, the "town" slowly, but surely, became enamored with the "gown."

With the practicing pediatricians happily involved, the teaching and residency-training program in place, the rotation schedule planned, and the ongoing recruitment process established, Blattner was ready for a new challenge. He turned his attention to Dr. David Greer's dream of a children's hospital in Houston. Blattner's participation in the 1948 national and international inspection tour of hospitals sponsored by the Texas Children's Foundation underscored his belief that "it was ripe to develop a children's hospital."[24]

Blattner's aspirations for the new children's hospital included its affiliation with Baylor College of Medicine as a pediatric center for teaching and research. After returning from the tour with architect Milton Foy Martin, he presented his observations and recommendations to the Texas Children's Foundation board. To his dismay, most of the pediatricians present— including Greer—did not share his vision. Instead, they wanted the hospital to be freestanding and independent in the Texas Medical Center.

This opposition to Blattner's proposed plan for the hospital's affiliation with Baylor College of Medicine was debated often. During the monthly meetings of the Houston Pediatric Society, a seemingly endless series of discussions ensued. At each gathering, Greer and Blattner, seated at opposite ends of the conference table, championed their opposing viewpoints. The lively and lengthy conversations that followed resulted in no definitive conclusions.

Finally, during one such debate, society president Dr. Raymond Cohen, who previously had sided with Greer, made a cogent observation. It was one that subsequently swayed the majority vote to Blattner's proposal—and an affiliation with Baylor College of Medicine in the Texas Medical Center. To at least one faculty member who attended that meeting, it was a truly remarkable event worth remembering.

"I know I've told everybody that will listen about Dr. Cohen, because I think he should be honored," recalled Desmond. "His reasoning was this: We would like to have residents to help us. We would like to have interns and residents. 'Who will teach them?' he asked the Pediatric Society. He said he himself had thought about it and thought about it and figured he did not feel adequate to teach them and practice. So, he was switching his thinking. And that was the key."[25]

The next step for Blattner was to convince the Texas Children's Foundation board of directors. It was a task that required expert help from outside, and he knew exactly whom to ask. Dr. Sidney Farber was the scientific director of the Children's National Cancer Research Foundation and a professor of pathology at Harvard Medical School. He also served as a consultant to the foundation. While visiting Houston in 1949 to address the Baylor College of Medicine faculty and students about challenges and problems in the study of pediatric diseases, Farber met with the Texas Children's Foundation board of directors. At Blattner's request, he explained the benefits of a hospital's associating with a medical school. Farber delivered a convincing presentation and the board approved.[26]

With the foundation's approval and the official Baylor College of Medicine affiliation agreement in hand, Blattner—ever mindful of avoiding any town-and-gown conflicts—concentrated on making the hospital's planning a collaborative effort. Including the society members in every aspect of the process, he went out of his way to make them feel wanted and needed.

These efforts were successful. "This was the pediatricians' hospital and there was never any question that they weren't right in on the ground floor," Dr. Edward B. Singleton recalled. "They helped with the planning, they did everything they could because it was their baby."[27]

In reality, the pediatricians shared custody, but it was Blattner who was to take command. This inevitability was made possible by a pivotal policy agreement made by Blattner with the newly formed board of trustees of Texas Children's Hospital. Effective the day that the hospital opened, and in perpetuity, the chairman of the department of pediatrics of Baylor College of Medicine was to be the physician-in-chief of Texas Children's Hospital. This agreement made Texas Children's Hospital the only hospital in the Texas Medical Center that had a true university affiliation.[28]

Also masterminded by Blattner and approved by the Texas Children's Hospital board of trustees was a policy by which members of the Houston Pediatric Society immediately became members of the new hospital's staff, eligible to serve on the executive medical committee. In addition, the president of the Houston Pediatric Society was designated as the hospital's medical director. Both of these valuable arrangements contributed to the continued close cooperation and to the avoidance of town-and-gown tensions, which was among Blattner's masterstrokes during the early planning period.

During the construction of Texas Children's Hospital, Blattner also gained great respect as chairman of the architectural advisory committee. Forming a close-knit team with members of the Houston Pediatric Society, he devoted countless hours to poring over the plans and, subsequently, the construction site. Traipsing around the girders and cement late at night with blueprints in hand, Blattner explained to society members where everything was going to be when the building was completed, ensuring that all were informed of any changes made—of which there were more than a few.[29]

When alterations met with Blattner's disapproval, he did not shy away from voicing his opinion. "Baylor's interest in research was something that was not very well understood by some of the board members," he recalled. "One saw no reason to provide living space for residents, asserting that all residents were married and live at home, so the top floor was stricken from the plans. Another saw no reason for a laboratory in the new hospital, since the work was to be done by private laboratories, and the plans for the laboratory were deleted."[30]

As Blattner had predicted, both omissions proved imprudent and required rectification after the hospital had been completed. To house residents, a two-story building—which Blattner deemed an "excrescence"—was erected in the parking area adjacent to the hospital. For the much-needed laboratory, space allocated for storage in the hospital's basement was usurped and utilized.[31]

Fortunately, one innovative concept proposed by Blattner was unanimously approved by the board and incorporated into the design of the hospital. Rather than the wards found in most children's hospitals, Blattner had suggested that individual rooms be made large enough to accommodate parents who wished to stay overnight with their child. In so doing, Texas Children's Hospital became the first in the country to provide such facilities.

Blattner's idea was inspired by his time in St. Louis, where he had seen how sick children were separated from their parents for weeks at a time. Fearful of infectious diseases, hospital staffs would place each child in a ward and allow the parents to visit only during certain hours on Sundays. However, with the advent of antibiotics in the early 1940s, Blattner decided that the danger of psychological damage to the child was far greater than that of infectious disease.

He wanted parents to be comfortable when they had to stay overnight at Texas Children's Hospital. "They put Barcaloungers in each room for the mother or father. No more than one at a time could sleep there. We would not allow a congregation," said Blattner. "I remember once, we had a sick child and all the neighbors came in. The first thing I said was, 'You are all going home. This child has to have air to breathe and you're taking up all the oxygen.' I made them all leave except the mother and the father. A good thing can be ruined if it is abused."[32]

Never abused, this groundbreaking service was a great success. The overwhelming positive response of patients' families at Texas Children's Hospital inspired other children's hospitals all over the world to adopt the practice, which eventually became a standard in the quality care of patients and their families.

Another unique service included in the plans and credited to Blattner was the newly named Junior League Diagnostic Clinic, a multidisciplinary outpatient service. Blattner believed that the clinic was a necessary component in providing services for those in the community who were less fortunate. He planted the seed for the idea among volunteers at the Junior League Children's Clinic at Hermann Hospital. Blattner suggested that the league should not abandon the clinic at Hermann Hospital altogether when coming to Texas Children's Hospital, but rather establish a model well baby clinic in its place.

Blattner's close working relationship with the Junior League of Houston and his subtle tactics were successful. When formally invited by the board of directors to join forces at the new hospital in 1953, Junior League president Lida Edmundson not only accepted "with great pride," but also offered $8,000 as a financial gift to the hospital. Committing the league members as volunteers to run the Junior League Diagnostic Clinic of the outpatient department at Texas Children's Hospital, Edmundson also agreed to contribute to the salaries of the pediatrician in charge and the secretary of the clinic.

While continuing to supply volunteers for the newly established well baby clinic at Hermann Hospital, the Junior League immediately began focusing its efforts on Texas Children's Hospital. The organization's goal was to provide "medically indigent parents with special diagnostic care for their sick children and to provide special clinical material for teaching and research purposes."[33]

Music to Blattner's ears was the league's pledged support for his department's fledgling research program. Often stating that "medical research is as essential to the well-being of a hospital and to a medical center as oxygen is to breathing," Blattner was anxious to expand his research program. Having been awarded the first research grant for Baylor College of Medicine by the National Institutes of Health (NIH), Blattner and Heys were eager to progress from small isolated studies conducted by a few individuals to a vast complex of interrelated investigations requiring the cooperation of many disciplines in many different fields of endeavor.[34]

What Blattner envisioned was in concert with what the board of trustees wanted for Texas Children's Hospital. For the hospital to provide the best possible care and treatment of sick children, specialists needed to join "the ranks of those highly trained and specially qualified investigators who seek tirelessly for new means to combat disease, lessen pain and deformity, and prevent death. New knowledge discovered through research will be made available to physicians and child specialists, thus benefiting children everywhere."[35]

To achieve those lofty goals, Blattner knew that he had to develop resources. Once again, the timing was favorable. It was the era in which the federal government began supporting research programs with grants. Admitting that he "didn't know too much about grant writing," Blattner nonetheless was appointed to a national committee charged with the responsibility of reviewing research grants for other people throughout the country. It turned out to be a fortuitous opportunity.

Blattner transformed his valuable learning experience into one that would benefit all staff of the department of pediatrics at Baylor College of Medicine and of Texas Children's Hospital. "With the permission of the committee chairman, I got copies of these various grants and took them back to Houston with me," Blattner recalled. "I had meetings at my house in the evenings with my staff, and together we would read and learn how to get a grant. It's an art which we conscientiously learned by studying how the best people at Harvard and Johns Hopkins presented grants."[36]

Although somewhat unorthodox, this imaginative solution to a perplexing problem proved effective. Members of the department of pediatrics at Baylor College of Medicine, including Blattner himself, soon excelled at grant writing. Within ten years, intensive investigation supported by grants was underway in various scientific fields.[37]

One such grant came from the NIH in 1964. Initially totaling $511,938.85, the grant funded the specially constructed Clinical Research Center on the south wing of the fourth floor of Texas Children's Hospital. The first clinic in the United States to research infectious diseases in children, the six-bed unit had its own laboratory facilities and special equipment, as well as trained investigators. Under the direction of principal investigators Dr. George W. Clayton and Blattner, its services and facilities were available to all investigators who had a significant research problem in specific areas involving children.[38]

The establishment of the Clinical Research Center was a milestone in the history of Texas Children's Hospital and of Baylor College of Medicine's department of pediatrics—one in which Blattner took great pride. "The pioneering work done in this center corrected the notion that little people have little problems," he said. "The center has given Baylor a vital instrument for focusing on the child as a developing individual with different problems at different age levels."[39]

Another grant in 1964, this time for $109,000 a year from the Children's Bureau of the Department of Health, Education, and Welfare, supported the mental evaluation and mental retardation clinic, a division of the Junior League Diagnostic Clinic of the outpatient department at Texas Children's Hospital.

The research fostered by those grants, and the countless others received during Blattner's tenure, benefited untold numbers of patients. Many patients survived when they otherwise would have died. Grant-supported efforts to review and research medical and surgical methods to achieve optimal patient care were quickly accelerated over the following decades, growing tenfold and more. Although there are no contemporaneous records of the euphoria surrounding the receipt of each grant, it is safe to assume that the joy sometimes matched but never surpassed that experienced when the first grants were awarded in 1964.

There was also immense gratification for another type of support made available to Texas Children's Hospital. To create the best possible atmosphere for the loving care and treatment of patients and their families in the hospital, Blattner wholeheartedly endorsed and helped champion the formation of the Women's Auxiliary at Texas Children's Hospital. This grassroots effort by various community organizations and corporations in Houston at first comprised only women volunteers. The Auxiliary was responsible for staffing the information desk, giving directions to visitors and patients, operating a snack bar, and performing non-medical duties and errands when required. Agreeing to keep the organization informed about the hospital's activities, Blattner scheduled monthly meetings in which he presented updates.

Motivating the members of both the Women's Auxiliary and the medical staff was Taylor, Blattner's newest staff member, who was appointed director of the Junior League Diagnostic Clinic by Blattner in 1954. Taylor's approach to patient care was encapsulated in the philosophy of loving care that he often repeated: "It is well to be close to the mind and heart of a child—to know as he knows, to understand as he understands, and to fear as he fears."[40]

Taylor and Blattner shared a belief that Texas Children's Hospital exist-ed to ensure the welfare of the children who were its patients. Blattner challenged his department at Baylor College of Medicine and the medical staff at Texas Children's Hospital never to lose sight of the fact that neither education nor research should take precedence over the quality of the lov-ing care of children.

This insistence on quality care played an integral part in the phenom-enal growth of the hospital. Within 13 years of its opening, Texas Children's Hospital had outgrown its facilities, leading to the announcement of its expansion from four to seven floors in 1967. With 154 patient beds added to the original 106, the hospital had more than doubled in size.

As Texas Children's Hospital grew, so too did Blattner's other responsi-bilities. Appointed pediatrician-in-chief at Houston's Ben Taub General Hospital in 1963, he also began serving on the national level as a member of the perinatal research committee of the National Institute of Neurologic Disease and Blindness of the NIH and as a consultant to the NIH perinatal research branch of the National Institute of Neurologic Disease and Stroke.

During these extracurricular activities, national committee member-ships, and travels to recruit residents, students, and faculty, Blattner inadvertently served as the unofficial goodwill ambassador for Houston. Representing Texas Children's Hospital, the Texas Medical Center, and Baylor College of Medicine, he never missed an opportunity to extol the accomplishments of each. He often spoke about his faculty members and the hospital's voluntary medical staff; explained his well-rounded rotation pro-gram for training residents; announced the formation of subspecialty areas within both the department and the hospital; cited the exciting progress made in clinical research; and illustrated how quality patient care could be enhanced by allowing parents to stay overnight. Complimenting the volun-teer efforts of the Junior League of Houston and the Women's Auxiliary, Blattner told stories of the philanthropic endeavors of Houstonians and praised the unprecedented community support for the children's hospital. His unbridled enthusiasm was contagious, inspiring many to travel to Houston for a closer look at the wonders that were taking place there.

The ability to inspire others was nothing new to Blattner. As a teacher, he garnered the praise and admiration of the Baylor Medical Alumni Association, which presented him with the Outstanding Faculty Award on May 12, 1972. The "richly deserved honor" commended the newly appoint-ed occupant of the J. S. Abercrombie Chair in Pediatrics for his "vision, imagination, and timing, his enthusiasm for excellence, his perception and responsiveness to the problems and needs of his own community, his broad view of pediatrics and its ramifications, and his green thumb for people—a gift for encouraging each person to follow his personal interest in medicine within the framework of his specialty."[41]

Praise for Blattner was not limited by geography. National recognition for his growing number of achievements at Baylor College of Medicine and at Texas Children's Hospital came in June 1974, with the prestigious Abraham Jacobi Award. The award is the highest honor bestowed on a pediatrician by the American Medical Association.

To salute the educational programs Blattner had championed during his three decades at Baylor College of Medicine, faculty members and former students hosted a two-day symposium in his honor in March 1977. Designed to impart the very latest in clinical research and practical pediatrics, the program was chaired by Clayton, the principal investigator of the Clinical Research Center at Texas Children's Hospital. Also a professor of pediatrics and physiology at Baylor College of Medicine, Clayton said: "Very few faculty who've come to join the pediatric department through the years have ever left Baylor and they'll all say it's because of the quiet, inspirational leadership Dr. Blattner provides."[42]

Within four months, the man who 30 years earlier had been hesitant to unpack his belongings began to pack them up again. But instead of moving to another hospital, Blattner was simply moving down the hall. After stepping down from his responsibilities as physician-in-chief of Texas Children's Hospital and chairman of pediatrics at Baylor College of Medicine on July 1, 1977, Blattner became a consultant to Texas Children's Hospital and a professor of pediatrics at Baylor College of Medicine.

The tributes to his career poured in. Labeled a "living legend" in the *Houston Post*, Blattner and his impressive record at Texas Children's Hospital and Baylor College of Medicine were chronicled and lauded. Having begun at Baylor in 1947 with a small faculty, he ended in 1977 with more than 90 full-time and 131 clinical faculty members. The training program included 70 residents and 29 postdoctoral fellows. As the first and only physician-in-chief at Texas Children's Hospital and the first chairman of pediatrics at Baylor College of Medicine, Blattner had trained more than 500 pediatricians.[43]

Blattner had witnessed unprecedented growth during the 23-year existence of Texas Children's Hospital. During its opening year in 1954, there were 4,588 sick and injured patients admitted; 5,492 visits to 11 clinics in the Junior League Diagnostic Clinic of the outpatient department; and approximately 92,000 laboratory tests. By 1977, Texas Children's Hospital had doubled in size and that year the hospital counted 10,020 patients admitted; 25,252 visits to 28 specialty clinics in the Junior League Outpatient Department; and more than 500,000 laboratory tests.[44]

Never one to take credit for his myriad and remarkable accomplishments, Blattner attributed serendipity to the success of his endeavors, saying: "It was a progression of very interesting coincidences that made Texas Children's Hospital, Baylor College of Medicine, and the Texas Medical Center blossom."[45]

Perhaps that was true. But, one fact was irrefutable.

The inextricably intertwined roots of Texas Children's Hospital and the department of pediatrics at Baylor College of Medicine had been securely planted by Dr. Russell J. Blattner, a visionary who turned out to have a green thumb for people.

5

Texas Children's Hospital was on the threshold of a new era in 1976.

This was a certainty to the search committee formed to find a successor to Dr. Russell J. Blattner as chairman of the department of pediatrics at Baylor College of Medicine and physician-in-chief at Texas Children's Hospital.

Chaired by Dr. Bobby R. Alford and comprised of representatives from the Baylor College of Medicine faculty and the Texas Children's Hospital board of trustees, the committee began an extensive national survey of leadership in the specialty of pediatrics. Serving as a guideline for the selection of nominees was an overview of the joint position crafted by the Texas Children's Hospital and Baylor College of Medicine planning committee.

Written to ensure the continuance of optimal care, teaching, and research to meet the health needs of both sick and well children, this 16-page overview was all-encompassing. The dual role included numerous areas of responsibility, ranging from day-to-day operations to financial planning and controls, program and space planning, and the development of common goals, objectives, and policies.

"This position description is presented in a very broad manner to emphasize the physician-in-chief/chairman of pediatrics has a wide variety of crucial roles in the operation and further development of the children's medical center program," the overview stated. "The individual who fills these roles must be sufficiently strong, tolerant, and understanding in order to meld these responsibilities productively."[1]

The definitive goals set by these criteria necessitated a thorough search, leading to recommendations for more than 98 candidates. Over the following months, Alford and the search committee continued to narrow the field. Eventually, the five most-promising applicants were invited to come to Houston for on-site interviews.[2]

One of those five was Dr. Ralph D. Feigin, a 38-year-old specialist in infectious diseases at St. Louis Children's Hospital and a professor of pediatrics at Washington University School of Medicine in St. Louis, Missouri.

Feigin's curriculum vitae chronicled an impressive career path. A native of New York and a 1958 graduate of Columbia College in New York City, Feigin had earned his medical degree from the Boston University School of Medicine in 1962. Following an internship in pediatrics in 1963, he became a resident at Boston City Hospital for one year. In 1964, he was a resident at Massachusetts General Hospital before joining the military in 1965 for two years of service as a researcher at the United States Army Research Institute of Infectious Diseases in Frederick, Maryland. Returning to Boston in 1967, Feigin became a teaching fellow at Harvard Medical School and chief resident of children's services at Massachusetts General Hospital. In 1968, he began his career at Washington University School of Medicine in St. Louis, Missouri, as an associate director of the school's Clinical Research Center and an instructor in pediatrics. He became director of the division of infectious diseases in 1973 and a professor of pediatrics in 1974.

Feigin's active participation in professional organizations was noted favorably by the search committee. A member of the Midwest Society for Pediatric Research since 1969, Feigin had served as its president in 1975. A fellow in the American Academy of Pediatrics, he also held memberships in the American Federation for Clinical Research, the American Association for the Advancement of Science, the American Society of Microbiology, and the Society for Pediatric Research, the Infectious Diseases Society of America, and the American Pediatric Society.

Although the search committee knew a great deal about this candidate, there was something that they did not know. Feigin's stated interest in "looking at" the dual position offered was simply that: wanting a look, and nothing more. "I had been very fortunate in my life, and I had the opportunity to look at a lot of different chairmanships prior to that," he recalled. "I had pretty much determined that I would never take the chairmanship or a physician-in-chief position, unless it was someplace that I thought could become the best place in the world. And if I didn't think it had that potential, or didn't have the commitment of the people there to want to do that, then I wasn't interested. If you are going to move at all, then it better be to somewhere that can be the best."[3]

Rather than being limited by those parameters, Feigin was instead motivated to accept all invitations to "look" at whatever opportunities were made available to him. He knew that eventually his internal compass would point him in the right direction, one filled with possibilities for achieving excellence.

That precise moment came in December 1976, during Feigin's first visit to Texas Children's Hospital and Baylor College of Medicine. At the request of the search committee, he met with not only its members, but also faculty members at Baylor, Texas Children's Hospital executives, and trustees. With each encounter, he learned more about both institutions. Feigin became increasingly intrigued.

"The number of operating inpatient beds at Texas Children's Hospital was 234 and there were approximately 2,800 admissions," Feigin said. "Emergency Room visits numbered a little more than 9,000 per year. The hospital and department of pediatrics at Baylor College of Medicine had less than $1 million per year of extramural grant support."[4]

To Feigin, these were not mere statistics, but opportunities to excel. Bolstered by the evident strengths of both institutions and inspired to find solutions to the weaknesses he perceived, Feigin found himself pondering the possibilities. Instinctively, he knew that both institutions were likely to achieve preeminence in their respective fields.

It was a conclusion that Feigin reached tentatively during his first interview and confirmed during his second, four weeks later. When the search committee asked him to return for this second interview in February 1977, Feigin had a request. Instead of meeting with various individuals, as he had before, he wanted to make rounds on the floors of the hospital to see the patients. Given that opportunity, Feigin found the patients' medical problems to be unexpectedly broad and varied.

"Some were very unusual problems, ones that you wouldn't see frequently, even in larger children's hospitals," he said. "I don't think the people here recognized necessarily what they really had, or what they could have. I realized you could build all those areas, bring the right people together, recruit the right people, and bring the resources."[5]

His interest piqued by such observations, Feigin enthusiastically shared his thoughts and proposed plan with the board of trustees at Texas Children's Hospital. "The only other issue in my mind was whether the board was committed to preeminence," he said. "If the board's committed, fine. I will go out and try to do that, help them, work with them, lead the way, but they had to tell me it was also their vision. If not, they could do anything they wanted and never get there."[6]

The Texas Children's Hospital board members responded to Feigin's proposal with one of their own. In concert with the search committee and the board of Baylor College of Medicine, they agreed that Feigin was the best choice to succeed Blattner. A joint institutional letter of invitation was to be "extended as soon as possible," they collectively and unanimously decided immediately after Feigin's February visit.

"Dr. Feigin made an especially favorable impression on everyone with whom he came in contact," Alford said in his official report. "His extensive academic pediatric background, his outstanding professional achievements, his management capabilities, his capacity for leadership, his enthusiasm, and his vigor were strong features that led us to make this recommendation."[7]

The selection of Feigin also met with Blattner's approval. "I am especially pleased with the physician who was chosen to succeed me," he said. "He is an energetic young man, 39 years of age, from Washington School of Medicine and St. Louis Children's Hospital, with a special interest in infectious diseases. By chance, those were my credentials when I came to Houston 30 years ago."[8]

Feigin did not immediately accept the job offer. The official invitation letter arrived in St. Louis two days after he returned from his February trip to Houston. Determined to be more knowledgeable about certain aspects of both institutions before considering the offer more seriously, Feigin decided to send detailed questionnaires to every member of the pediatric department and to every house officer and fellow. "It was a little different questionnaire for each person, and they were different for section heads and for other faculty members," he explained. "I got back lots of information and condensed it into a summary."[9]

Included in this summation were notes that Feigin made about what he thought the pediatrics chairman and physician-in-chief needed to do. He addressed such issues as those regarding space and staff, funds that were available or that needed to be secured, conferences that needed to be held for teaching purposes, research grants funded and pending, and fellowships. Once he had identified what he thought were the major problems, he noted his recommendations on how to fix them. In essence, the summary indicated what could be accomplished in five years at Texas Children's Hospital and Baylor College of Medicine.

Feigin decided to accept the dual position in March 1977 and assumed his new role the following June. Although influenced by his five-year plan, Feigin's decision was ultimately based on his perception of the Texas Children's Hospital board of trustees. "I thought they had an absolutely total dedication to the future of the hospital, and that they were interested in absolutely having the premier place for the care of children anywhere," he said. "That's what I wanted."[10]

Feigin appreciated the board's recognition of his philosophy regarding Texas Children's Hospital's mission to provide quality teaching, research, and patient care. Instead of regarding each as a separate entity, he believed the three to be equally important parts of a single inclusive mission that would allow the institution to achieve preeminence. "You can't have excellence in patient care without excellence in education and research, they are all integrated," he said. "You can't go after one, you've got to do all three at the same time. And I approached from the very outset that there is only one mission, and I went after everything together."[11]

This viewpoint was known well in advance of Feigin's arrival. His avid interest in simultaneously improving all three components of the hospital's mission was clearly evident to those who read his questionnaire, responded to it, and received the resulting summary. To others, his intentions would become evident in his actions and deeds.

Stepping into his new role, Feigin paid homage to his predecessor and to the accomplishments of the past, but he concentrated his remarks on the future. "Sustaining the excellence instilled by Dr. Blattner during the past 30 years will be a challenge, but a welcomed one," he said. "The opportunities here are phenomenal. At Baylor and Texas Children's, we have one of the finest facilities anywhere. We have virtually unlimited potential for growth that doesn't exist elsewhere in the world and I'm excited to be here."[12]

From the day Feigin arrived, he demonstrated his steadfast commitment to the five-year plan and his dedication to the teamwork required to achieve it. Within nine months, all of the long-range goals of the three-pronged plan had been met.

The rapidity of these accomplishments, and of others during his first few months on the job, was to become one of Feigin's trademark patterns at Texas Children's Hospital and Baylor College of Medicine. For him, such speed was not a newfound trait. Feigin had been tagged "Rocket Ralph" by students at Washington University, who were in awe of his fast pace and his ability to multitask. In Houston, his velocity would only accelerate.

Throughout the complicated process, Feigin maintained clarity of purpose. He was determined to translate his vision of preeminence into reality. Building onto the foundation established by Blattner, he passionately and relentlessly pursued that goal.

Feigin wasted no time in articulating specific methods to achieve his vision. Within three weeks of his arrival at Texas Children's Hospital, he took measures to enhance the quality of day-to-day patient care by ensuring that a full-time faculty member was assigned to every floor of the hospital. "They are literally on each unit, along with the pediatric residents who are MDs in training to become pediatricians, with the patient, 24-hours-a-day, seven days a week," Feigin said. "They are able to respond to the intermittent changes and needs for care that the child has on a minute-to-minute basis."[13]

To serve the immediate needs of patients in the Junior League Outpatient Department, Feigin completely reorganized the department's layout and enhanced its staffing. Consolidating many different ambulatory care services, he concentrated more faculty and more house staff in one area to provide optimal care. In a prescient effort to appropriately position these services for the future, he began searching for a qualified physician who could take over the ambulatory care program.

This was just one of the leadership positions that Feigin planned to fill as soon as possible. Because his blueprint for preeminence called for the building of new programs and for the further development of existing ones, the recruitment of promising candidates in each area became one of his top priorities. Within his first 18 months at Texas Children's Hospital, Feigin was successful in recruiting numerous physicians and scientists for the sub-specialties of immunology, neurology, and infectious diseases, several of whom were former colleagues at Washington University in St. Louis.

That Feigin's search led him back to those he knew and trusted in St. Louis was to be expected. In actuality, his recruitment campaign had begun there—albeit in stealth—shortly after he accepted the position at Texas Children's Hospital and Baylor College of Medicine. Before he left St. Louis, he enthusiastically discussed his vision of preeminence with certain faculty members who were leaders in their individual subspecialties, as well as with several residents and fellows who had demonstrated a potential to achieve greatness. To each, he explained exactly what he planned to do and how he planned to do it. One physician received a specific and detailed invitation.

"Before he left St. Louis, he told me that if I decided to come with him that he would make sure that I had a laboratory, a technician, a secretary, and all the nice things you like to have," recalled Dr. Sheldon L. Kaplan, whose infectious diseases fellowship was with Feigin at that time. "I was interviewing for positions elsewhere, but I came down a few weeks later and took a look. I was very impressed and decided to come."[14]

The successful recruitment of this promising 29-year-old infectious diseases specialist reflected another aspect of Feigin's recruitment plan. He wanted to infuse youthful energy into the existing medical staff. Projecting a minimum of at least ten new full-time faculty members annually, he reasoned that this continual integration of new thoughts and new talents was one method of keeping the staff fresh and current.

Feigin also recruited recognized experts to establish new services. The first of these was noted immunologist Dr. William T. Shearer, a former colleague at Washington University School of Medicine. Shearer embraced Feigin's vision, finding the latter's abundant enthusiasm and will to succeed contagious. "He wants you to succeed, and he gives you everything to help you succeed," he said after accepting his position at Texas Children's Hospital in 1979. "If you don't succeed, it's your fault."[15]

In tandem with this steady influx of external knowledge, Feigin championed the creation of internal knowledge through research. He knew that institutions must seek to create new knowledge, rather than merely utilize old knowledge, in order to become leaders in the field. His aspirations were for Texas Children's Hospital and Baylor College of Medicine to become not only a leader, but the preeminent leader in pediatric research. When Feigin launched the beginnings of an aggressive research program in 1977, his reasoning for how such an aggressive program directly benefited patient care was unassailable: "If you are not doing research fundamentally all the time, with rapidity of change that occurs in medicine, within five years you would be giving people care that is completely outdated, that is not current."[16]

Unless immediate measures to prevent this outcome were taken at Texas Children's Hospital and Baylor College of Medicine, Feigin predicted the eventual obsolescence of existing medical knowledge. He based his opinion on the fact that there were "too few people who were doing state-of-the-art research" in 1977.

"I helped him get their research started at Texas Children's Hospital," said Dr. Martha Dukes Yow, head of the infectious diseases section since its inception under Blattner in the 1950s. One of the nationally recognized experts in the field of infectious diseases at the time, she recalled how "our colleagues around the country watched with glee to see us lock horns. We disappointed them. During the first year of Ralph's tenure, he was a dynamo and I must admit that at times I felt competitive, but he treated me with the utmost respect and consideration, including giving me a big raise. He respected performance."[17]

In turn, Feigin garnered his new colleagues' respect for quickly assessing and solving existing problems at Texas Children's Hospital. Because the existing faculty was "much too few in number" and "stretched to the limit clinically," Feigin understood why staff members were unable to devote more of their time and effort to research. His solution was to recruit a sufficient number of highly trained investigators to supplement the existing research efforts.[18]

It was a well-conceived plan that produced measurable benefits. In addition to their research capabilities, those seasoned investigators knew how to be competitive at the national level for highly coveted federal grant money. At Baylor College of Medicine, this was important new knowledge. Although the competition for public financing had been fierce among medical institutions for decades, Baylor had not been a contender until it became a freestanding institution in 1969. Previously, because of the college's church affiliation through Baylor University, federal funding was not an option. Feigin's recruitments were to make a significant impact on the institution's efforts to secure such funds.

The result was immediate. By 1979, the amount of federal and non-federal research support at Texas Children's Hospital had increased from $1 million to $4 million per fiscal year. Included in these funds was an infectious diseases grant brought to Texas Children's Hospital by Feigin in 1977. Initiated in St. Louis and funded by the National Institutes of Health, the laboratory studies and clinical studies of meningitis were, and continued to be, a combined effort of Feigin and Kaplan, his new recruit.

In addition to these increased research dollars in 1979 was the $1.5 million per year funding of the newly acquired children's nutrition research center (CNRC) at Baylor College of Medicine and Texas Children's Hospital. Made possible through a grant from the United States Department of Agriculture (USDA), the CNRC was the first USDA human research center for children in the United States. The acquisition of this prestigious center in 1978 was the culmination of more than six years of planning, plotting, lobbying, and waiting by Blattner and pediatric nutritionist Dr. Buford L. Nichols. The two were determined to secure the USDA grant.

The delay was noted and acted upon by Feigin. Three weeks after his arrival at Texas Children's Hospital in 1977, he decided that another method was required to achieve the long-awaited grant from the USDA. His approach was bold. Feigin composed a letter stating that Baylor College of Medicine and Texas Children's Hospital were going to establish a children's nutrition research center, whether it was funded by the USDA or not. Signed by Baylor College of Medicine executives at Feigin's insistence, the letter to the USDA was dated July 29, 1977. The first appropriation of funds came in 1978.

Feigin's boldness in this endeavor was indicative of another of his strong beliefs: "If something is worthwhile doing, then you'd better have the courage to do it and then find the resources to make it work."[19]

This conviction became the cornerstone of Feigin's development of new and expanded programs at Texas Children's Hospital and Baylor College of Medicine. Adequate funding was a necessary component, but Feigin knew that outstanding people with great ideas were the pivotal resource required to achieve his vision.

Feigin sought just such an individual to take over the pediatric residency training program at Baylor College of Medicine and to serve as director of house staff training at Texas Children's Hospital. "The education of pediatric residents is of extraordinary importance, since they represent the future of pediatrics," he said. "They are the individuals who will be delivering care to our children and grandchildren for years to come. Many of the residents will become physician scientists and the academic leaders of the future."[20]

A national search to find the best possible individual for the position commenced within weeks of Feigin's arrival at Texas Children's Hospital. That process led him to Dr. Martin I. Lorin, director of house staff training at Columbia University College of Physicians and Surgeons and Babies Hospital in New York City. Known as an innovative teacher who consistently improved training opportunities for residents, Lorin—who could not fathom why he should move to Texas—nonetheless accepted Feigin's invitation to visit.

His skepticism was short-lived. During his initial visit, Lorin found Houston to be "a very cosmopolitan, very eclectic, very sophisticated city and the medicine and the medical center just superb." His opinion of Texas Children's Hospital and Baylor College of Medicine was that "primarily because of Dr. Feigin's vision, it didn't seem to have the constraints that other places had. Most other places, if the department had extra money, they would use it on lab technicians or things like that, rather than be willing to use it on education. His attitude was clearly very different."[21]

Equally enticing to Lorin was Feigin's obvious passion for teaching. As a pediatrics professor at Washington University School of Medicine, Feigin was voted Outstanding Teacher of the Year by the seniors in 1975. At Baylor College of Medicine and Texas Children's Hospital, the mutual respect he shared with his students and residents continued—as did his desire to help each attain his or her goal. To them, he was a "walking encyclopedia" who possessed an uncanny memory for both facts and faces. Known to call each student, resident, and fellow by name within days of their arrival, he also remembered their birthdays and other special occasions. What they never forgot was Feigin's saying that his greatest satisfaction came from watching them achieve.

Feigin believed that the success of his students and residents was dependent on good teaching—not only that which they received, but also that which they eventually were to give themselves. A good teacher, Feigin believed, was one who had an absolute thorough mastery of that area of interest, as well as many others. "The more you know about everything in life, the better teacher you are," he reasoned. "I think the ability to teach is being able to take complex material and being able to present it in terms that are explicable to anyone, regardless of their degree of knowledge or lack thereof. And I think if you couple that with logical thought process and a lot of enthusiasm, you usually have a good teacher."[22]

This opinion was shared by Lorin, as was Feigin's preference for those who taught by example, not simply by word. Together, the two envisioned how to revolutionize educational opportunities in pediatrics at Baylor College of Medicine and Texas Children's Hospital. When challenged by Feigin to develop one of the finest pediatric training programs in the world, Lorin accepted the offer in July 1978 and proceeded to do precisely that. Within ten years of his arrival, Lorin's educational program attracted more than 109 residents and was the largest pediatric residency program in the United States. As a master teacher and mentor, available to the house staff at Texas Children's Hospital for their personal and professional problems 24 hours a day, Lorin had taken Feigin's vision and made it his own.

"I think Dr. Feigin knows what is needed, what he wants to do, what is best for everything—from the hospital as an entity, to individual faculty, to individual residents, etcetera," Lorin said. "He is incredibly effective and efficient about going out and accomplishing that. He also is an incredible human being. He is probably the finest clinician I've met. He is obviously the most knowledgeable. He is also an individual with superb humanistic qualities."[23]

Praise for all of these attributes also came from Feigin's students, who—similarly to those he had taught in St. Louis—voted him Teacher of the Year in 1979. He received that award every subsequent year until 1986, when he was inducted into the medical school's Hall of Fame. Legendary status was also accorded to his nickname, Rocket Ralph, which had followed him from Washington University. Students continued to use the moniker behind his back. To their thinking, it was the appropriate appellation for the boundless energy demonstrated by the physician-in-chief, professor, hospital administrator, pediatrician, infectious diseases expert, and guest lecturer at medical conferences worldwide.

Another title applied to Feigin was that of acclaimed author. Published by the W. B. Saunders Company on March 6, 1981, was the *Textbook of Pediatric Infectious Diseases,* coedited by Feigin and Dr. James D. Cherry, chief of the division of infectious diseases at the University of California at Los Angeles School of Medicine. The lengthy collaboration in compiling this comprehensive and authoritative text began in 1976. Eventually translated into nine languages, the resulting two-volume, 1,858-page manual was recognized as the definitive infectious diseases reference source for pediatricians all over the world. Eventually expanding to its current 3,200 pages, subsequent editions were published in 1987, 1992, 1998, and 2003.

The international recognition garnered by that publication served only to motivate Feigin. While developing techniques for the rapid diagnosis of infectious diseases in children, he also concentrated his efforts to improve the understanding, treatment, and prevention of bacterial meningitis. From the federally funded research conducted in tandem with Kaplan at Texas Children's Hospital, he contributed vital information that led to a reduction in complications for children throughout the world.[24]

Another Feigin accomplishment in the field of pediatric infectious diseases was enhanced in 1981 when Kaplan became chief of the infectious diseases service at Texas Children's Hospital. In so doing, Kaplan became one of the 17 former fellows in infectious diseases who were trained by Feigin in St. Louis and who later became directors of infectious diseases sections elsewhere in the United States.

While helping to build and expand the infectious diseases program into one of the largest and most respected in the United States, Feigin devoted equal energy to all the other existing subspecialties at Texas Children's Hospital. He also began to recruit recognized experts in the newly emerging subspecialties. Although each service's physical space inevitably became stretched to its limits, Feigin's steadfast mantra was to build programs first, and the appropriate space to house the programs was sure to follow.

"I probably said this one thousand times in one thousand different venues," recalled Feigin. "Programs that help patients are what we try and build. And, when I talk about programs, I am talking about the constellation of education, research, and patient care. The only way you build programs is with outstanding people who have great ideas. If you do both of those things, you are forced periodically to create new space, new opportunities, reconfigurations of operations, outlying areas perhaps, and other things of that nature."[25]

What Feigin predicted became a reality in the early 1980s. After the allocation of every available nook and cranny at Texas Children's Hospital, he began to create new spaces for subspecialty services in neighboring buildings adjacent to the medical center. By 1981, the need for additional space for outpatients and laboratory research inspired Feigin to begin campaigning for the building of a new outpatient facility, an ambulatory research building.

"We have to have it," Feigin later recalled telling the joint operating board of Texas Children's Hospital and St. Luke's Episcopal Hospital in 1981. "You can't run an inpatient service without it. The future of medicine, even complex medicine, is going to be more and more ambulatory-care driven. Outpatient work may only be 3 percent of our revenues today, but in the future it's going to be 30 to 40 percent."[26]

The financial officer of the joint operating board informed Feigin that his idea was crazy, unprofitable, and impossible. Feigin was not deterred. Rather, he was inspired to escalate his campaign for board approval. "If you tell me something is impossible, you can be sure I'm going to do it," he explained. "That's how I tend to live my life."[27]

It would take Feigin two years to convince the board of trustees. His approach was twofold, stressing the growing importance of ambulatory care and also the "need to house our research programs, or your faculty in clinical care are going to leave." Since ambulatory care involved every subspecialty that provided clinical care, it was a convincing plea for the new ambulatory and research building. After agreeing to begin construction in the mid-1980s, the board soon found its attention diverted elsewhere—to the possible dissolution of the joint operating agreement with St. Luke's Episcopal Hospital.

While the board's negotiations about the possible separation from St. Luke's Episcopal Hospital continued to be a priority in 1986, the number of outpatient visits at Texas Children's Hospital escalated to more than 148,000. Since 1977, when there were 37,000 visits, the number had more than quadrupled in less than a decade. Feigin once again returned to the board in search of a solution to the problem he had predicted would be inevitable. Scattered in 26 different locations in the Texas Medical Center and throughout Houston, each Texas Children's Hospital outpatient facility already functioned at its capacity. With the construction date of the newly approved ambulatory care and research facility still uncertain, Feigin saw an urgent need to alleviate the overcrowding.

It quickly became evident to Feigin and to the board that the problem required an immediate solution. Another facility for outpatient care had to be found. "We knew we could not just hatch a building, but we literally were out of space for outpatients and for labs," Feigin said. "The economy in Houston was in a ditch, and buildings were being sold at auctions. So, we went down and bought 8080 North Stadium Drive, a shell building on two acres of land, for $2 million at an auction."[28]

The 46,176-square-foot facility had been built to house offices. Because it was not in move-in condition, architects and interior designers were enlisted to create a "warm, cheerful, and appealing" atmosphere, "so children of various ages could relate to it." After undergoing a $6.7 million conversion, the office building became a child-friendly clinical space that also boasted sophisticated research labs. The Texas Children's Hospital Clinical Care Center was the hospital's first off-campus pediatric center. Opened in August 1986, the center offered specialized care for children in nine specific areas, ranging from nutrition to learning disorders.[29]

"It was at that time that the board began to talk seriously about the split from St. Luke's Episcopal Hospital," remembered Feigin. "When the split occurred, it was clear then that we needed operating rooms. So, suddenly the ambulatory building plans ceased to progress until we could figure out the magnitude of what we really were going to do."[30]

Feigin became an integral part of that decision process on June 17, 1987. At the request of the Texas Children's Hospital board of trustees, he assumed the position of executive vice president and interim executive director while the search committee looked for a new chief executive officer. Although it was assumed that Feigin's new job would last for a few months at most, he remained in the position for more than two years.

It was a challenge that Feigin eagerly accepted, knowing it would be an opportunity to work towards his vision. He also knew how difficult it would be for someone new to step into the job, handle the separation difficulties, become familiar with every aspect of the hospital, and make informed decisions.

"I thought I could provide some stability to the situation," Feigin said. "My heart and soul and life are in this hospital and department. I'm very familiar with every aspect of the hospital, whether it be dietary, housekeeping, finance, or you name it. I thought that I would be in a potential position to be able to have a positive impact."[31]

In his combined roles of executive vice president, interim executive director, hospital administrator, physician-in-chief, teacher, researcher, and visionary, Feigin worked 24 hours a day, seven days a week. While sustaining active and enthusiastic participation in all of his previous endeavors, he was also immersed in creating a sturdy foundation for the soon-to-be independent Texas Children's Hospital. Feigin and the board concluded that the hospital would require not just the ambulatory care and research facility that had previously been approved, but also a critical care and surgical facility that would become known as the West Tower. Designed to house operating rooms, an emergency room, and other independent services, the five-story West Tower was built on a foundation that allowed for future expansion.

"We made all the plans and designed the facilities and had groundbreaking for the two new buildings," Feigin recalled of this two-year time period in the late 1980s. "We culminated the separation agreement. We started our own pharmacy department and the whole central supply, and our own operating rooms and everything else, even while we still were in St. Luke's operating rooms."[32]

These were but a few of Feigin's accomplishments during this hectic period of transition and growth. The $149 million expansion project and its priorities were ultimately Feigin's responsibilities, but so were all the areas he oversaw. While the external bricks and mortar were being put into place, Feigin's internal vision of preeminence—and the tripartite mission to enhance patient care, education, and research—remained his predominant motivation.

No matter how demanding his schedule, Feigin always made time for teaching—especially the Tuesday rounds with residents, fellows, and students. Whether it was his trademark pace, consummate knowledge, or loving care and gentleness with patients, Rocket Ralph continued to generate awe among his students. It was an appreciative audience that continued to grow. In 1987, there were more than 109 residents, a tribute to Lorin's success at creating the largest pediatric residency training program in the United States.

In the area of research, Feigin's ongoing efforts to increase both basic and applied clinical research resulted in an increase in annual funding to more than $20 million in 1987, most of which came from the federal government. The amount would continue to grow in future years. The anticipated need for additional laboratory space was to be met by a new $55 million ambulatory and research facility designated for the CNRC, the collaborative research program established in 1979 by Texas Children's Hospital, Baylor College of Medicine, and the USDA. Built adjacent to Texas Children's Hospital and completed in 1988, the facility housed the largest research program of its kind. It was the first federally owned building in the Texas Medical Center.

"Research conducted at this unique facility is leading the world to a better understanding of the effect of nutrients on health and on the prevention of disease and nutritional disorders," Feigin stated. To emphasize the importance of the CNRC and its efforts, he added: "If you're a pediatrician, you'd better be interested in nutrition."[33]

With the CNRC completed and construction plans for the two new buildings at Texas Children's Hospital finalized, Feigin's open-ended tenure as interim executive director came to a close on October 9, 1989. On that day, Mark A. Wallace became executive director and chief executive officer of Texas Children's Hospital. Feigin relinquished his duties and responsibilities in all areas of administration, except one. He explained: "My view is that if it affects patient care, it's my problem."[34]

Such problems were to be expected with the completion of the construction project in 1991. The new buildings with centralized patient services made Texas Children's Hospital one of the largest pediatric hospitals in the United States. With an escalating outpatient population and a marked increase in the severity of inpatient illnesses, Feigin focused on the quality delivery of intensive and intermediate care for these children.

"Technology has advanced to the point that many children or infants who would not have survived several years ago can now be saved," he stated, noting the advances made in neonatology. "Baylor College of Medicine faculty at Texas Children's Hospital were among the first to participate in studies designed to document the efficacy of surfactant therapy of hyaline membrane disease. As a result, neonatal mortality for premature infants has been halved."[35]

The effects of such medical breakthroughs and technical advances were evident in many of the pediatric subspecialties at Texas Children's Hospital in the 1990s. The impact of this new knowledge and the improved ability to treat children resulted in the unbridled growth not only of neonatology, but also of such services as cardiology, cardiovascular surgery, hematology-oncology, immunology, gastroenterology, and infectious diseases, to name only a few. That Texas Children's Hospital boasted many of the recognized leaders in each of these areas—and was also training the future leaders—was directly attributed to Feigin's vision.

It was an accolade Feigin modestly accepted, saying: "Anyone in my position can do only one thing and that's to try to carry out a vision and hope that other people whom you've occasionally nudged along the way will see that vision, participate in it, and follow it."[36]

Many of those participating followers were involved in the planning of a surprise tribute to mark Feigin's fifteen years as physician-in-chief in 1992. After Wallace praised Feigin for his "extraordinary devotion to children and his untiring pursuit of excellence," William K. McGee, Jr., chairman of the board of trustees, said: "The reputation that Texas Children's has attained, both nationally and internationally, in the areas of patient care and research, is a result of his hard work, dedication, and obvious joy in what he does."[37]

As Feigin's reputation continued to grow, both within the organization and beyond, he frequently was offered prestigious positions at other medical institutions throughout the country. He always turned them down, preferring to remain in Houston to nurture his vision at Texas Children's Hospital.

After being appointed senior vice president and dean of medical education of Baylor College of Medicine in 1993, Feigin became an eager participant in Baylor's core management team. His appointment in 1996 as president of Baylor College of Medicine came as no surprise to most observers, but it did to Feigin. Honored to have been offered the job, he was nonetheless unwilling to relinquish his duties as physician-in-chief of Texas Children's Hospital and chairman of the department of pediatrics. When allowed to retain those responsibilities, Feigin accepted the position at Baylor College of Medicine, calling it "an opportunity to continue to mold the future."[38]

The extraordinary skills needed to execute these multiple roles were second nature to Feigin—as were the relentless hard work and dedication required to achieve his preset goals in each area of responsibility.

After moving his base of operations to Baylor College of Medicine, the new president continued his familiar routine as physician-in-chief at Texas Children's Hospital. At work each day by 5:30 a.m., he began his observational tour of the hospital. Starting on the patient floors and ending in the emergency room, he assessed the number of beds available and briefly visited with the patients and families he recognized from previous stays. Feigin often encountered children whom he had originally diagnosed, relying on his remarkable memory to discuss the specifics of each situation. With equal ease, he knew each resident by name, even those who were new to the program. By 10 a.m., Feigin had made the day's administrative decisions before moving on to other responsibilities elsewhere in his domain.

Feigin's Tuesday morning ritual remained sacred to him. As he had every week for 26 years, he made rounds at Texas Children's Hospital with the medical students and residents. "That way I get to meet 100 percent of Baylor students," he said. "It is important that I do that. People will always come first, I can't change my course of 63 years."[39]

What also remained unchangeable were Feigin's will to succeed and his ability to instill that belief in others. It was a quality of his teaching that became legendary. Genuinely interested in the success of his learners, he noted with pride the number of pediatric residents and fellows who had trained in pediatric subspecialties at Baylor College of Medicine and Texas Children's Hospital and then gone on to become leaders in academic medicine.

"During the past 16 years, more than 500 residents have graduated from our Pediatric Residency Program," Feigin announced in 1993. "Of these, 49 percent hold full-time faculty positions with medical schools. Of the 404 fellows who graduated from our subspecialty Fellowship Training Programs, 66 percent hold full-time faculty positions at one of 88 United States medical schools or are in government service. When statistics are combined, our former residents and fellows can be found on the full-time faculty of 114 of the nation's 126 accredited medical schools."[40]

Former residents and fellows also were recruited by Feigin to become full-time faculty at Baylor College of Medicine and Texas Children's Hospital. Feigin's ongoing recruitment program to infuse new learning and new talent never wavered from its original goal of keeping the hospital's collective knowledge entirely up-to-date. On a personal level, Feigin derived immense satisfaction from knowing that some of the recruits who were teaching with him he recently had taught himself.

One former fellow with whom he continued to work closely was Kaplan, chief of the infectious diseases service. From the results of a 1993 survey funded by a grant from the Robert Wood Johnson Foundation, they discovered that fewer than one in five local two-year-olds was fully immunized against preventable childhood diseases. In an effort to ensure the immunization of all infants in Harris County, Feigin and Kaplan developed a system to track compliance countywide. Initially implemented at Texas Children's Hospital as a pilot program, Feigin hoped "to see the system expanded into the offices of private physicians."[41]

It was Feigin's passionate interest in the welfare of all children that influenced his advocacy efforts in the local, state, and federal arenas. Feigin tirelessly campaigned for children's rights to healthcare, insurance, and federal aid. "I have dealt with every health commissioner and every governor in the state over the years, every single one," he said. "And on the national level, I routinely deal with our own senators and many others in the Congress, some of whom are close friends of mine."[42]

These efforts to bring national recognition to Texas Children's Hospital received an enormous boost in the November 1993 issue of *Child* magazine. Honoring Texas Children's Hospital as one of "The 10 Best Children's Hospitals in America," the magazine praised the hospital for its research, cancer care, heart surgery, pediatric AIDS services, and microsurgery. Grateful for the recognition, Feigin envisioned heading that list in the future. In order to achieve that goal, he said, "We are just beginning."[43]

This steadfast adherence to his vision of preeminence was honored in 1997 by the board of trustees of Texas Children's Hospital. In appreciation of the 20 years that Feigin had devoted to improving the health of children all over the world, the Clinical Care Center was renamed the Feigin Center in honor of Feigin and his wife, Dr. Judith Z. Feigin, director of the Learning Support Center at Texas Children's Hospital.

Built to house outpatient clinics and services, as well as research activities, the newly named Feigin Center was only six years old at the time. Yet the overcrowded center was already in urgent need of additional space, due to a marked increase in outpatient visits and the ongoing expansion of subspecialty and research programs. The proposed solution to this problem involved making the Feigin Center a designated research facility and building a new 16-floor outpatient center. Also planned was a new 15-story inpatient building to be constructed atop the five-story surgical and critical care facility known as the West Tower. In 1999, the board decided to embark on both projects. The four-year $345 million expansion would be one of the largest healthcare building projects ever undertaken in the United States.

"This effort touches each part of the hospital's mission of patient care, research, and the training of general pediatricians and pediatric subspecialists," Feigin stated during the press conference announcing the project.

Although the planning for this project had begun during Feigin's tenure as interim executive director of Texas Children's Hospital during the late 1980s, he did not expect it to occur so soon, less than a decade after the 1991 expansion. However, he knew that the statistical numbers dictated new facilities were an immediate necessity. "The number of inpatients exceeds 20,000 per year with more than 145,000 patient days," he explained in 2002. "There are more than 196,000 discreet outpatient visits each year to the various subspecialty pediatric, medical, and surgical services and Emergency Room encounters exceed 88,000 per year."[44]

These numbers reflected more than just the staggering increases in the patient population. During the 25 years of his tenure, Feigin had prodded, promoted, and persuaded approximately 350 full-time faculty members based at Texas Children's Hospital to embrace his vision of preeminence. To him, these statistics indicated that they had all proven themselves to be outstanding leaders with innovative ideas who built excellent programs for children.

Just as Feigin had envisioned during his initial visit to Texas Children's Hospital in 1977, the hospital could boast numerous clinical care centers that were rated among the best in the United States for providing specialized patient care. In addition, there were more than 40 pediatric subspecialties offering treatment for every known pediatric illness and injury.

With more than 130 residents and 121 fellows in training, Feigin established a round-the-clock house staff of outstanding individuals who embraced his passionate pursuit of quality healthcare. "I think you improve healthcare by literally taking care of one child at a time," said Feigin. "But you do that in a way that is, hopefully, always at the cutting edge of knowledge. If you're not trying to expand the frontiers and if you're not trying to apply newly acquired knowledge to the care of individual patients, then you're probably not giving the absolute best that healthcare can provide."[45]

In the process of acquiring knowledge, Baylor College of Medicine faculty members at Texas Children's Hospital reached a milestone in 2003. They collectively became the leading recipient of competitive grant funding for pediatric research through the National Institutes of Health, receiving more than $33 million in funding in just one year. The achievement exemplified Feigin's vision of preeminence.

Of priceless value was the national recognition received from *U.S. News & World Report,* which ranked Texas Children's Hospital as one of the country's top ten pediatric hospitals for three consecutive years, from 2000 to 2003. Texas Children's Hospital had come of age.

The opportunity for Feigin to reflect publicly on these accomplishments came on April 23, 2003, during the re-dedication ceremonies for the newly enlarged research facility now known as the Feigin Center. As he had done so often in the past, Feigin deflected the credit. Instead, he preferred to share the glory with his entire team.

"Judy and I are extremely grateful and humbled by the naming of this building in our honor," he began. "We are deeply grateful to the Texas Children's Hospital board of trustees and to its chairman, Mr. L. E. Simmons, and president of the board, Mr. Gary Rosenthal, the administrative team led by Mr. Mark Wallace, president and chief executive officer, to all of the members of the medical staff, and our colleagues at Texas Children's Hospital and Baylor College of Medicine whose courage, intellect, time and energy, and extraordinary commitment have made all that has been accomplished possible."

"We have had the opportunity to observe repeatedly the application of science and compassion, knowledge, skill, and sympathy by members of this audience in the service of children. We recognize that it is all of you who should be congratulated today."[46]

As Feigin stressed the importance of the past contributions made by physician–scientists at Texas Children's Hospital, he also emphasized that much remained to be done. For many diseases, the cause was still unknown. For others, the cause was known, but an effective diagnostic test or therapeutic modality remained elusive. Feigin predicted that the recent unraveling of the genetic code and the understanding of the gene function, structural biology, and neural networks would lead to advances over the next ten years that would eclipse anything previously seen.

"We intend to participate in these discoveries as we have in the past and we should be able to do so at an ever-accelerated pace," he stated. "This building is an attestation to the fact that research is an integral part of the mission of Texas Children's Hospital. It is a tangible demonstration of our commitment to research as a means of improving the health and welfare of children."

When Feigin stepped down as president of Baylor College of Medicine in March 2003, he packed up his office there one Monday and returned to his original office at Texas Children's Hospital. The following Tuesday morning, Feigin resumed his uninterrupted 26-year-old ritual of Tuesday morning rounds with the residents and fellows.

What also remained unchanged was Feigin's vision for the future. "I predict Texas Children's will continue to be one of the leading hospitals in the nation," he said. "Our goal, of course, is to be absolutely preeminent. I hope to participate in being able to accomplish that with all of the wonderful people who have worked side-by-side with me as colleagues for years to come."[47]

In 2004, 28 years after it had begun with Feigin's arrival, the new era at Texas Children's Hospital continued, its legacy of loving care ongoing and its vision of preeminence intact.

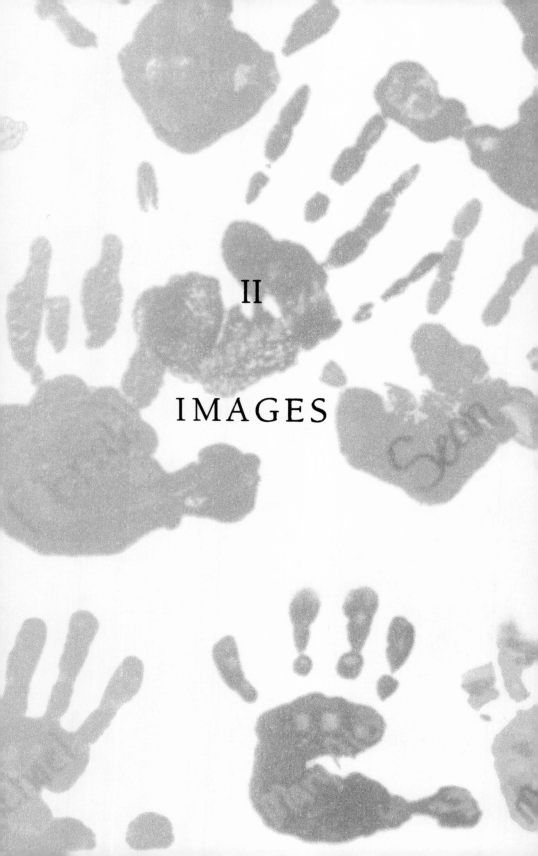

II

IMAGES

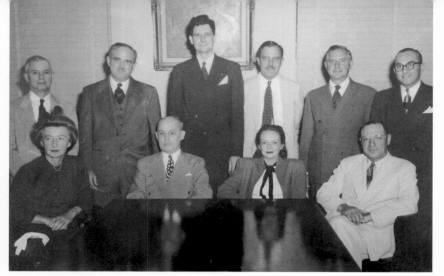

Texas Children's Hospital Foundation forms in 1947

There are ten charter members of the Texas Children's Hospital Foundation board of trustees, established in 1947 to build a hospital for children in Houston, Texas. Standing, left to right, Dr. A. Lane Mitchell, Dr. John K. Glenn, Dr. George W. Salmon, Dr. H. J. Ehlers, George Butler, secretary, and Dr. Raymond Cohen, vice president. Seated, left to right, Miss Nina Cullinan, Dr. David Greer, president, Mrs. H. Malcolm Lovett and Leopold L. Meyer, treasurer.

"Let's Save Our Children" becomes community's mantra in the late 1940s

Enthusiastic community support for the mission of the Texas Children's Hospital Foundation in 1947 includes extensive media coverage in Houston newspapers and weeklies, such as this "Let's Save Our Children" cartoon. Throughout the subsequent planning and construction of Texas Children's Hospital, incremental progress will be reported meticulously and often.

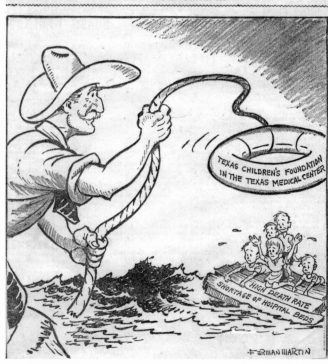

Let's Save Our Children

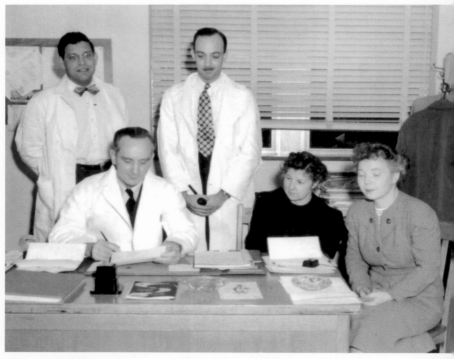

The entire pediatric department at Baylor College of Medicine in 1950

The department of pediatrics at Baylor College of Medicine in 1950 consists of only five faculty members. Standing behind department chairman Dr. Russell J. Blattner are Dr. Joseph Stool and Dr. Fred M. Taylor and seated beside him are Dr. Florence M. Heys and Dr. Murdina M. Desmond. In the following five decades, the department of pediatrics will grow to include more than 535 full-time faculty members in 2006.

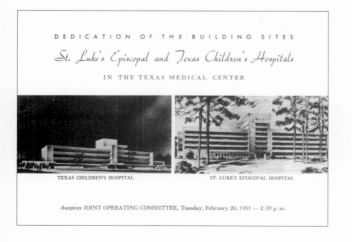

Dedication of Texas Children's Hospital and St. Luke's Episcopal Hospital is February 20, 1951

On October 18, 1950, the boards of trustees of Texas Children's Hospital and St. Luke's Episcopal Hospital signed a commitment contract to construct adjoining buildings in the Texas Medical Center. Less than six months later, the conjoined boards preside over the February 20, 1951, dedication ceremonies for the building sites.

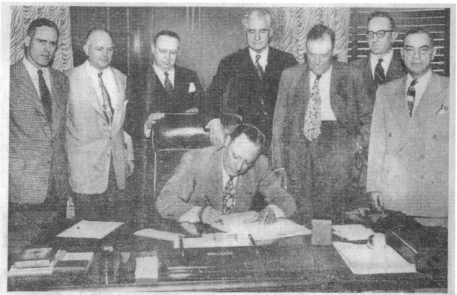

SIGNIFICANT DEVELOPMENT in Houston's hospital history occurred Thursday afternoon when Leopold L. Meyer, seated, signed a contract with the Tellepsen Construction Company for erection of the $2,000,000 Texas Children's Hospital in the Texas Medical Center. Mr. Meyer is president of the hospital board. Grouped around him for the ceremonies are, left to right, Milton Foy Martin, architect; Howard Tellepsen, president of the construction firm; William A. Smith, vice-president of the hospital board; Jesse H. Jones, J. S. Abercrombie, chairman of the hospital board; Lee C. Gammill, hospital administrator, and R. H. Abercrombie.

Children's Hospital Contract Let

Contract to erect Texas Children's Hospital signed May 17, 1951

The Houston Chronicle *documents the signing of the contract with the Tellepsen Construction Company for erection of the $2 million Texas Children's Hospital on May 17, 1951. Standing behind Texas Children's Hospital board of trustees president Leopold L. Meyer are, left to right, Milton Foy Martin, architect; Howard T. Tellepsen, president of the construction firm; William A. Smith, vice president of the hospital board; legendary philanthropist Jesse H. Jones; James S. Abercrombie, chairman of the hospital board; Lee C. Gammill, hospital administrator; and R. H. Abercrombie.*

Texas Children's Hospital ground-breaking ceremony is May 23, 1951

A cadre of nurses, physicians and four children with shovels turn the first earth on the site for Texas Children's Hospital on May 23, 1951. Blessing the occasion was Houston Rabbi Hyman Judah Schachtel, who said, "May all children who come here aching and in pain leave healed; and all those who come in tears leave smiling."

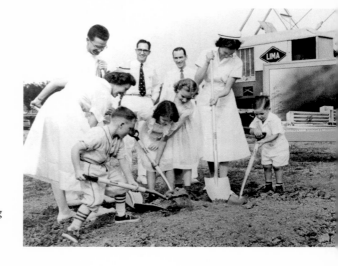

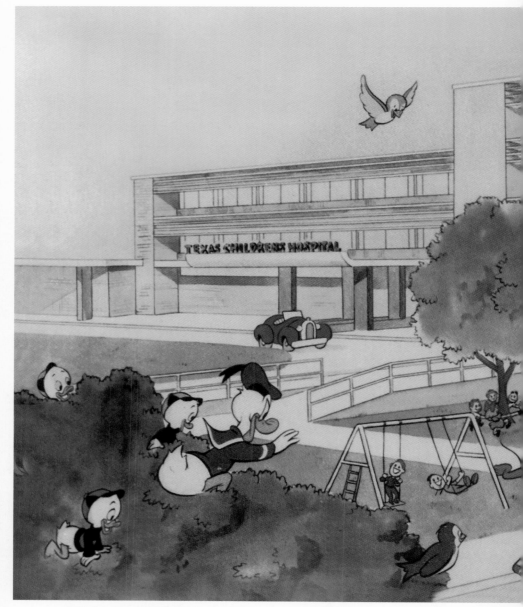

Walt Disney and Walt Disney Productions donate illustration for brochure in 1952

A spectacular fund-raising brochure, illustrated and donated by Walt Disney and Walt Disney Productions, debuted January 21, 1952. Although a swimming pool was never in the construction plans, this fantasy rendering caused a splash in the community. "Texas Children's Hospital Catches Popular Fancy!" states the headlines that accompany a full-page reproduction of the brochure in the Houston Post *on March 16, 1952.*

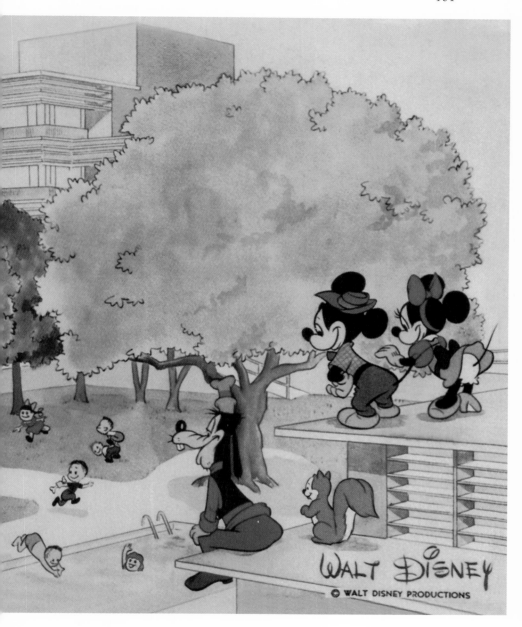

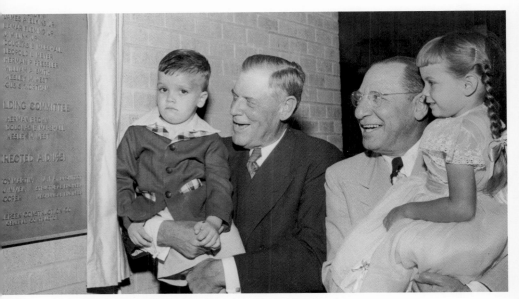

Texas Children's Hospital cornerstone laid May 15, 1953

At the May 15, 1953, ceremony to lay the cornerstone of Texas Children's Hospital, chairman of the board of trustees of Texas Children's Hospital James S. Abercrombie, holding Donald Lynn, and president of the board Leopold L. Meyer, holding Dea Lemke, unveil the commemorative plaque.

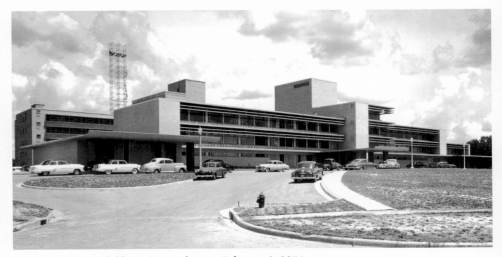

Texas Children's Hospital opens February 1, 1954

The three-story Texas Children's Hospital opens February 1, 1954. With custom-designed medical equipment, child-friendly décor, and colorful furnishings, it also boasts 106 specially designed beds for pediatric patients and loungers for parents' staying overnight in the room. Because of a construction delay, St. Luke's Episcopal Hospital, visible in the background, will not simultaneously open, as originally planned. Its opening is postponed until August 4, 1954.

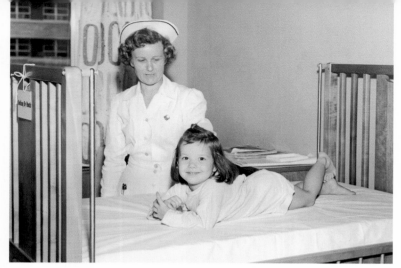

The first patient at Texas Children's Hospital is admitted February 1, 1954

The first patient admitted to Texas Children's Hospital is three-year-old Lamaina Leigh Van Wagner, a kidney patient referred by her pediatrician. Her February 1, 1954 visit in room 411 at Texas Children's Hospital lasted less than 24 hours, but includes posing for this historic photograph with her nurse. Four decades later Van Wagner will fondly recall the loving attention she received at Texas Children's Hospital.

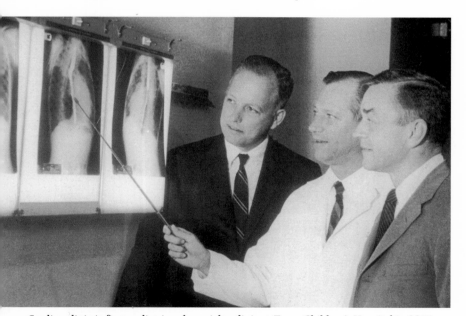

Cardiac clinic is first pediatric subspecialty clinic at Texas Children's Hospital in 1954

The first pediatric subspecialty clinic at Texas Children's Hospital is the cardiac clinic, which opens February 9, 1954. Examining the X-rays of one of the first patients in that clinic are other firsts: the first chief of cardiovascular surgery Dr. Denton A. Cooley, the first physician on staff at the Texas Children's Hospital, pediatric radiologist Dr. Edward B. Singleton, and Dr. Dan G. McNamara, the first trained pediatric cardiologist in Houston.

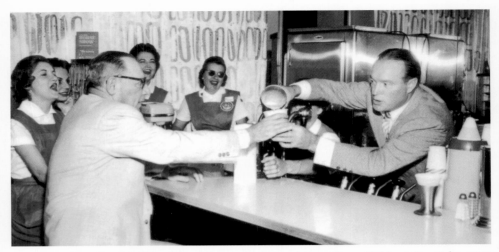

Comedian Bob Hope shakes things up in the Snack Bar at Texas Children's Hospital in 1958

With members of the Women's Auxiliary to Texas Children's Hospital to cheer him on, comedian Bob Hope serves a milkshake to Leopold L. Meyer at the Snack Bar in Texas Children's Hospital in 1958. Located in the main lobby, adjacent to the admitting desk, the glass-enclosed Snack Bar was open 12 hours a day and became a very popular spot with patients' families and hospital staff.

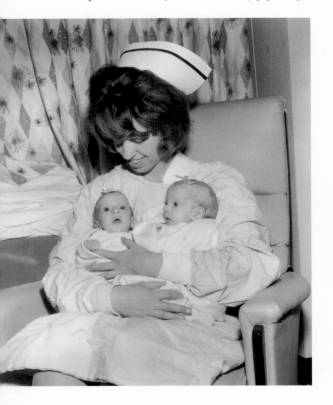

Conjoined Webber twins separated at Texas Children's Hospital in 1965

Seated in one of the Barcalounger reclining chairs standard in each patient's room at Texas Children's Hospital, an unidentified nurse cuddles twins Karen and Kimberly Webber in 1965. Born conjoined in 1964, the twins were separated in a procedure pioneered at Texas Children's Hospital. A medical milestone, it was the first successful separation of twins conjoined at the liver and pericardium.

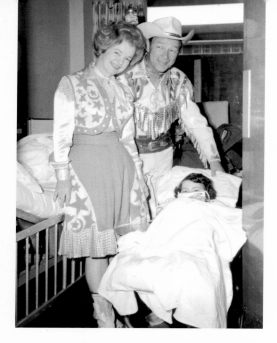

Television and movie stars Roy Rogers and Dale Evans at Texas Children's Hospital in 1968

Dressed in their trademark outfits for stage performances in March 1968, "King of Cowboys" Roy Rogers and "Queen of the West" Dale Evans visit with a Texas Children's Hospital patient. The popular couple was in town to perform at the thirty-sixth annual Houston Livestock Show and Rodeo at the nearby Astrodome.

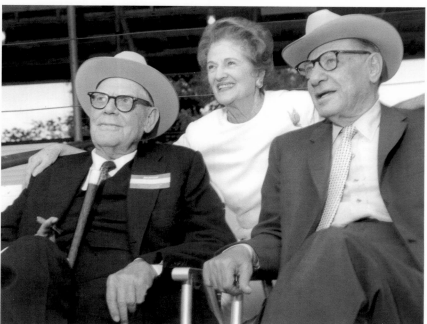

Twenty-first annual Pin Oak Charity Horse Show at Pin Oak Stables in 1968

At the twenty-first annual Pin Oak Charity Horse Show at Pin Oak Stables benefiting Texas Children's Hospital in1968, founders and patrons James S. Abercrombie, "Miss Lillie" Abercrombie and Leopold L. Meyer admire the competition. They are seated in the 10,000-seat stadium the Abercrombies constructed for the first charity horse show in 1947, an event that soon became the annual gathering in which one could see and be seen in Houston society.

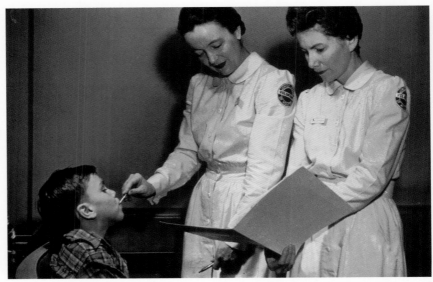

The newly renamed Junior League Outpatient Department at Texas Children's Hospital expands in 1971

Two Junior League of Houston volunteers administer to a patient in the newly expanded Junior League Outpatient Department at Texas Children's Hospital in 1971. Boasting more than 24 specialty clinics and a voluntary staff of more than 100 Junior League volunteers, the expanded clinic occupies more than four times its original space. After it opened as the Junior League Diagnostic Clinic in 1954, it averaged 600 patients a month. In 1971, the monthly average has escalated to 2,000 patients, a trend that will continue.

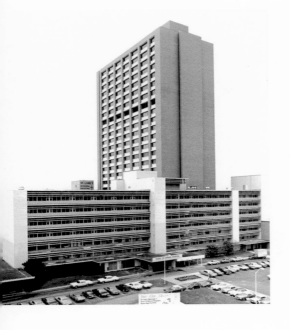

After five years of construction, the newly expanded Texas Children's Hospital opens in 1972

Completed in 1972 following five years of construction, the newly enlarged, seven-story Texas Children's Hospital expands to 331 beds from the original 106. In the background is the additional new 26-story tower with underground facilities constructed for the joint use of Texas Children's Hospital, St. Luke's Episcopal Hospital and Texas Heart Institute.

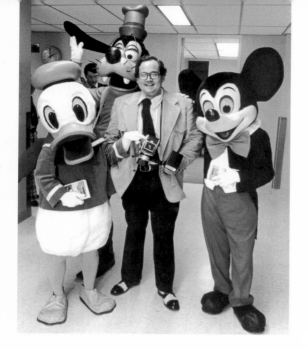

Stars of 1952 Disney brochure visit expanded Texas Children's Hospital in 1972

To celebrate the expansion of Texas Children's Hospital in 1972, the recognizable stars of the hospital's first brochure drop in for a visit. Helping longtime medical photographer at Texas Children's Hospital Jim deLeon make some snap decisions were Disney greats Donald Duck, Goofy and Mickey Mouse.

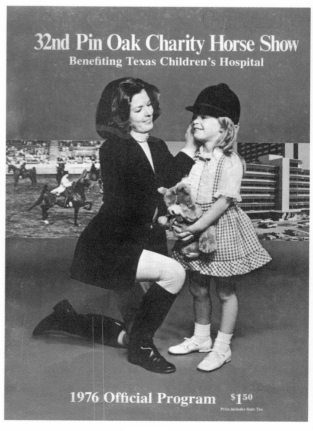

Thirty-second annual Pin Oak Charity Horse Show is at Abercrombie Arena in 1976

Having moved from Pin Oak Stables in 1975, the thirty-second annual Pin Oak Charity Horse Show benefiting Texas Children's Hospital takes place in Abercrombie Arena at the Astrodome complex. It will remain in that space for the following decade, moving to larger facilities in 1986.

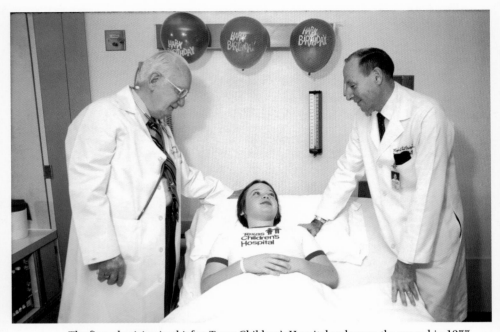

The first physician-in-chief at Texas Children's Hospital welcomes the second in 1977

Dr. Russell J. Blattner, the first physician-in-chief at Texas Children's Hospital, left, welcomes his successor, the hospital's second physician-in-chief Dr. Ralph D. Feigin in 1977. While making rounds together, they also share a birthday celebration with a patient, whose décor is compliments of "The Balloon Ladies" in The Women's Auxiliary to Texas Children's Hospital.

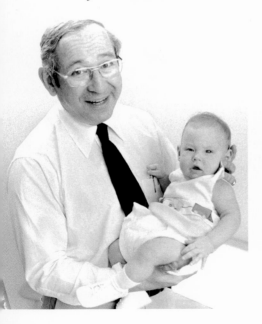

Pediatric surgeon Dr. F. J. "Jim" Harberg with Texas Children's Hospital patient in 1978

Named chief of the general surgery service at Texas Children's Hospital in 1970, Dr. Franklin James "Jim" Harberg is a veteran member of the surgical staff, which comprises 63 surgeons in 1970. After being the first to complete the two-year pediatric surgery residency at Texas Children's Hospital in 1958, he has become recognized as an expert in the surgical correction of birth defects and as an inventor of tools and procedures, including neonatal bedside surgeries.

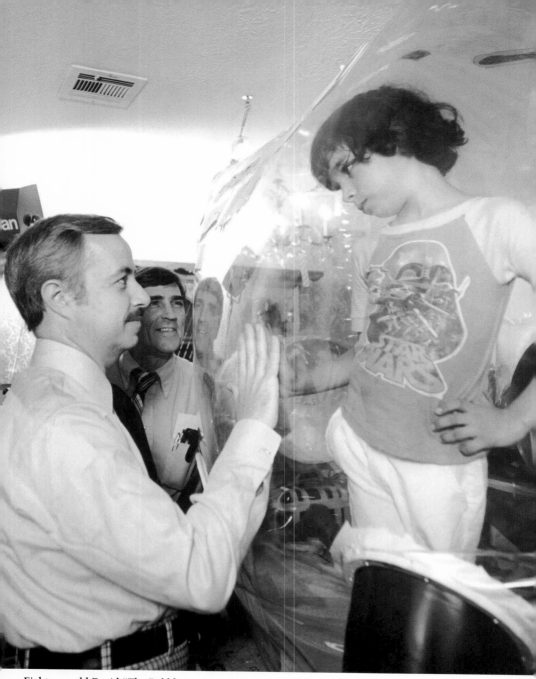

Eight-year-old David "The Bubble Boy" Vetter at Texas Children's Hospital in 1979

From inside the specially designed bubble that was his home at Texas Children's Hospital and in which he had lived since his diagnosis of severe combined immune deficiency at birth in 1971, eight-year-old David "The Bubble Boy" Vetter makes eye and hand contact with the newly arrived pediatric immunologist Dr. William T. Shearer in 1979. Pediatric gastroenterologist Dr. Buford L. Nichols looks on.

A celebration for Dr. Murdina M.
Desmond and Leopold L. Meyer
in 1979

*Five years after the official 1974
naming of the Leopold L. Meyer
Center for Developmental
Pediatrics at Texas Children's
Hospital, director Dr. Murdina M.
Desmond and Leopold L. Meyer
celebrate his namesake center's
becoming one of the largest services
in Texas dedicated to children with
developmental disabilities.*

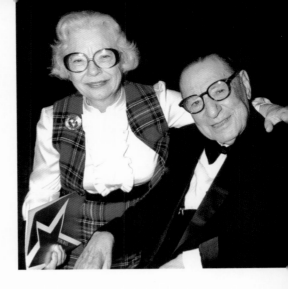

WATCH Magazine marks
twenty-six years of
continuous publication
in 1981

*Titled with the acronym
derived from its creators'
official name, the Women's
Auxiliary of Texas
Children's Hospital,
WATCH Magazine is in its
twenty-sixth year of
publication in 1981.
Published continuously
since its 1955 inception as
a six-page booklet, it has
matured into a slick, multi-
page, four-color quarterly.
In 2004, WATCH
Magazine celebrates its
forty-ninth year of
publishing. Still compiled
and edited by members of
The Auxiliary, it continues
to chronicle the current
events at Texas Children's
Hospital and serves as a
highly visible link between
the past, the present, and,
given its uninterrupted
longevity, the future.*

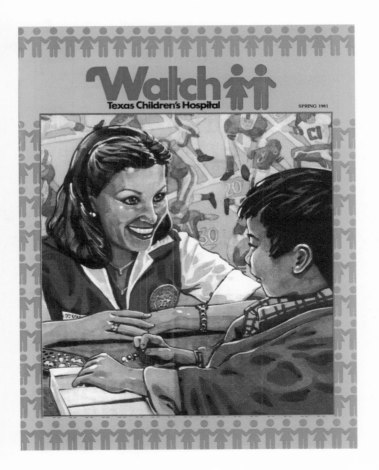

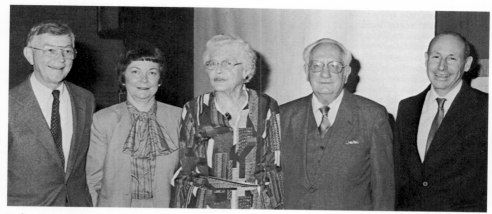

Pediatric cardiologist Dr. Helen B. Taussig makes a return visit to Texas Children's Hospital in 1983

The legendary pediatric cardiologist Dr. Helen B. Taussig is a featured participant in the 1983 Russell J. Blattner Lectureship, given annually since 1978 by the Baylor Pediatric Alumni Association. Welcoming Dr. Taussig to Texas Children's Hospital are, standing left to right, former Taussig fellow and pediatric cardiologist Dr. Dan G. McNamara, neonatologist Dr. Reba Hill, Dr. Taussig, and Texas Children's Hospital's first two physicians-in-chief, Dr. Russell J. Blattner and Dr. Ralph D. Feigin.

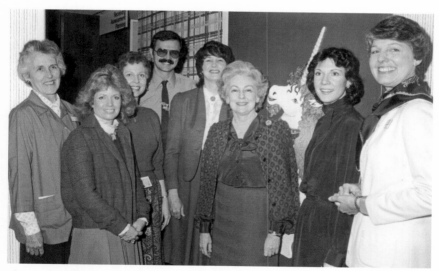

The Pi Beta Phi Patient/Family Library debuts at Texas Children's Hospital in 1984

With funding provided by the Houston Pi Beta Phi Alumnae Club, the 400-book Pi Beta Phi Patient/Family Library at Texas Children's Hospital opens February 18, 1984. Library coordinator Julia D. Allison, right, welcomes Pi Beta Phi alum and Texas Children's Hospital trustee Virginia McFarland, center. By 2004, the library will have expanded to 4,000 books in the West Tower, with additional satellite Pi Beta Phi Book Nooks in the waiting rooms of the Clinical Care Center.

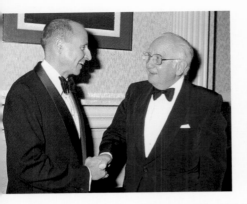

Texas Children's Hospital hosts its thirtieth anniversary celebration in 1984

Proud of the past and hopeful for the future, Texas Children's Hospital's first two physicians-in-chief, Dr. Ralph D. Feigin and Dr. Russell J. Blattner, congratulate each other at the thirtieth anniversary of Texas Children's Hospital in 1984. The unforeseen future includes the separation of the joint services of Texas Children's Hospital and St. Luke's Episcopal Hospital in 1987 and an expansion project that would make Texas Children's Hospital one of the largest freestanding pediatric hospitals in the United States.

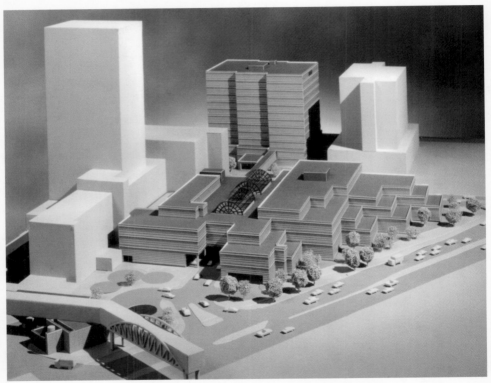

Architect's model of 1987 Texas Children's Hospital expansion project

Following the formal separation of joint services with St. Luke's Episcopal Hospital in 1987, Texas Children's Hospital board of trustees unveil a one-million-square-foot, $149 million expansion project that includes two new buildings. Shown in detail on the architect's model is the 12-story ambulatory care and research facility, later known as the Feigin Center, and the five-story critical care and surgical center, later known as the West Tower. The expansion represents a fourfold increase in size for Texas Children's Hospital, expanding its capacity to 456 licensed beds. Construction begins in 1989 and is complete in 1991.

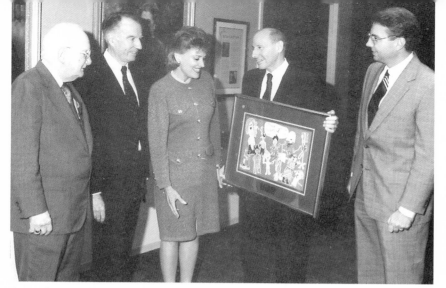

Original Texas Children's Hospital structure renamed the Abercrombie Building in 1990

Josephine E. Abercrombie receives a patient-designed illustration at the December 1990 renaming of the original Texas Children's Hospital structure as the "Abercrombie Building," in honor of her parents, founders James S. Abercrombie and Lillie Abercrombie. Making the presentation are, left to right, former physician-in-chief Dr. Russell J. Blattner, chairman of Texas Children's Hospital board of trustees George A. Peterkin, Jr., physician-in-chief Ralph D. Feigin and Mark A. Wallace, president and CEO of Texas Children's Hospital.

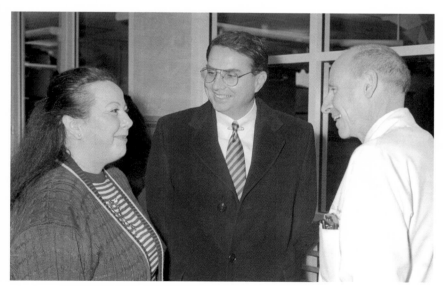

The first patient at Texas Children's Hospital returns in 1991 as honored guest

Thirty-seven years after becoming the first patient at Texas Children's Hospital Lamaina Leigh Van Wagner returns to be one of the first to see the newly completed expansion in 1991. Texas Children's Hospital president and CEO Mark A. Wallace and physician-in-chief Dr. Ralph D. Feigin welcome her back at the formal dedication ceremonies on November 8, 1991.

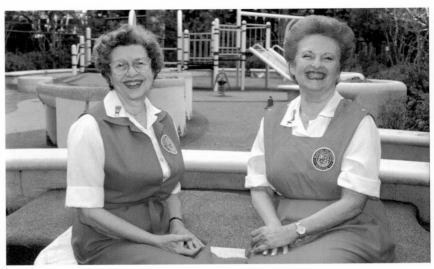

Longtime volunteers at Texas Children's Hospital Elaine Kuper and Helen Blumberg in 1993

Volunteers at Texas Children's Hospital since 1954, Women's Auxiliary to Texas Children's Hospital members Elaine Kuper and Helen Blumberg enjoy a moment of relaxation in the newly constructed "Get Well Playground." Donated by the Women's Auxiliary to Texas Children's Hospital and dedicated November 17, 1991, the protected, outdoor playground is available to any hospitalized patient at Texas Children's Hospital.

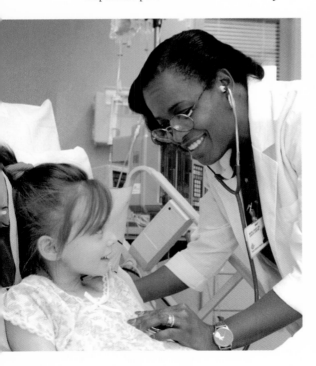

Texas Children's Hospital bone marrow transplant patient in 1997

Texas Children's Hospital bone marrow transplant unit nurse Marie James administers loving care to a patient undergoing treatment in 1997. Established in 1959 by chief of pediatric hematology-oncology Dr. Donald J. Fernbach, the bone marrow transplant program expands under the direction of Dr. David G. Poplack, named chief of hematology-oncology in 1993. By 2001, the greatly enlarged, 15-bed bone marrow transplant unit at Texas Children's Hospital will be the largest of its kind in the Southwest.

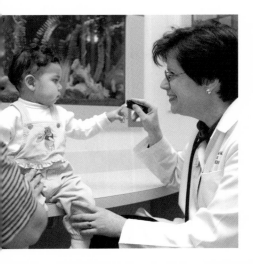

Shedding a little light on emergency care in 1999

With her trademark smile and calming touch, Dr. Joan E. Shook examines one of the more than 63,000 children seen during 1999 in the Meyer and Ida Gordon Emergency Center at Texas Children's Hospital. Named director of the emergency center in 1987, Shook has been a member of the emergency care staff since she was an intern in 1981 and has experienced firsthand its phenomenal expansion of services, staff and space through the years. By 2004, the annual average of emergency center visits will be 80,000.

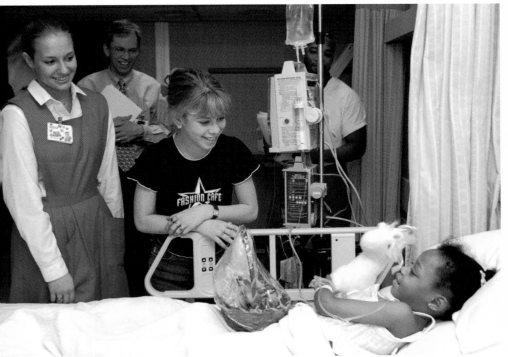

A frequent visitor to Texas Children's Hospital is 1998 Gold Medalist Tara Lipinski

An avid supporter and frequent visitor to Texas Children's Hospital is Sugar Land resident and 1998 Olympic gold medalist Tara Lipinski. Graciously willing to sign autographs and pose for pictures, she and junior volunteer Jennifer Mahar take a few moments to chat with a patient. In honor of this ice skating champ and aspiring actress, Texas Children's Hospital dedicates the Tara Lipinski Exercise Room in the Texas Children's Wellness Center in 2002.

116

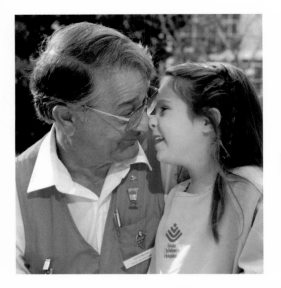

Auxilian and ultimate "Patient Pal" Gene Macey charms another patient

A volunteer at Texas Children's Hospital for more than 25 years, retired second-grade school teacher Gene A. Macey is recognized by both peers and patients as the star of The Auxiliary's Patient Pals program. Able to abandon his grown-up demeanor and act silly at a moment's notice, Macey has the ability to immediately connect with children. A selfless volunteer, he is often seen during the 1990s at Texas Children's Hospital seven days a week, one of which he devotes exclusively to the information desk in the Abercrombie Building. In 2005, that desk will be named posthumously the Gene A. Macey Information Desk as a tribute to his countless contributions to Texas Children's Hospital.

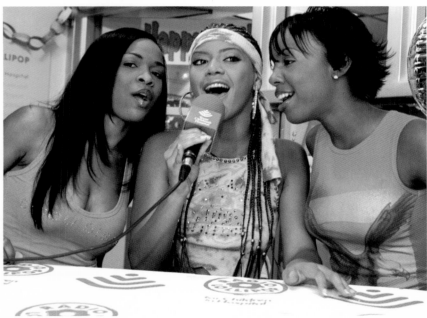

Destiny's Child celebrates first anniversary of Radio Lollipop at Texas Children's Hospital

On the first anniversary of Radio Lollipop at Texas Children's Hospital in 2000, singing its praises during a guest appearance in the studio is the Houston-based, Grammy award-winning Destiny's Child. Shown left to right are Michelle Williams, Beyoncé Knowles and Kelly Rowland. One of 18 Radio Lollipops around the world and the only one in Texas, the fully equipped radio station broadcasts to patients' rooms via closed circuit television and is manned by volunteer, patient and celebrity deejays.

Catching the fancy of pitcher Roger "The Rocket" Clemens

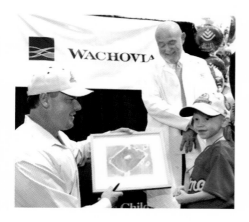

Five-year-old Texas Children's Cancer Center patient Dustin knows how to catch the fancy of seven-time Cy Young Award winner and Houston Astros pitcher Roger "The Rocket" Clemens. When this baseball legend came to Texas Children's Hospital to deliver holiday cheer to patients, Dustin throws him a curve ball by giving him a gift, too. As Clemens accepts Dustin's artwork, a vividly interpreted baseball diamond, Texas Children's Cancer Center director Dr. David G. Poplack umpires the proceedings with an approving smile. (Photo courtesy of Allen Kramer)

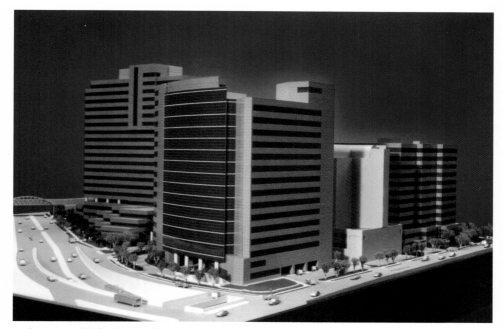

Architect's model for $345 million expansion project at Texas Children's Hospital

Already one of the largest pediatric hospitals in the United States, Texas Children's Hospital unveils an ambitious, $345 million expansion project in 1999 that will nearly double its structural space. In addition to a new 15-story addition to the hospital's existing five-story West Tower for inpatients, shown left, and a new 16-floor Clinical Care Center for outpatients, shown center, construction plans include the renovation of the existing 12-story Feigin Center, far right, into a dedicated research hub. Construction begins in 1999 and is complete in 2003.

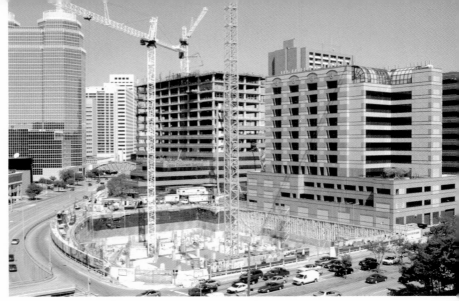

Construction of Texas Children's Hospital expansion progresses in 1999

Adding more than 1.2 million square feet to the existing facilities, the hospital expansion project is one of the largest in United States history. As 15 additional floors are erected on top of the existing West Tower at Texas Children's Hospital, shown in the background, construction progresses on the new 819,280-square-foot, 16-story Clinical Care Center in the foreground. The existing structure to the right of the construction site is the 11-story Children's Nutrition Research Center, the unique cooperative venture between Baylor College of Medicine, Texas Children's Hospital and the U.S. Department of Agriculture/Agricultural Research Service that opened in 1988. To the far right is the 12-story Feigin Center.

The renovated Feigin Center becomes a dedicated pediatric research center in 2002

Following a $40 million renovation of the 12-story Feigin Center in 2002, the reconfigured former outpatient-care facility is a dedicated research center with more than 200,000 square feet of bench laboratory space. In both 2003 and 2004, Baylor College of Medicine and its primary teaching affiliate Texas Children's Hospital are named the No. 1 recipient of pediatric grant funding through the National Institutes of Health, the world's foremost medical research centers and the focal point for federal medical research. Construction of an additional six floors on the Feigin Center is to begin in 2006.

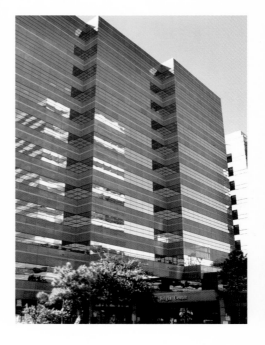

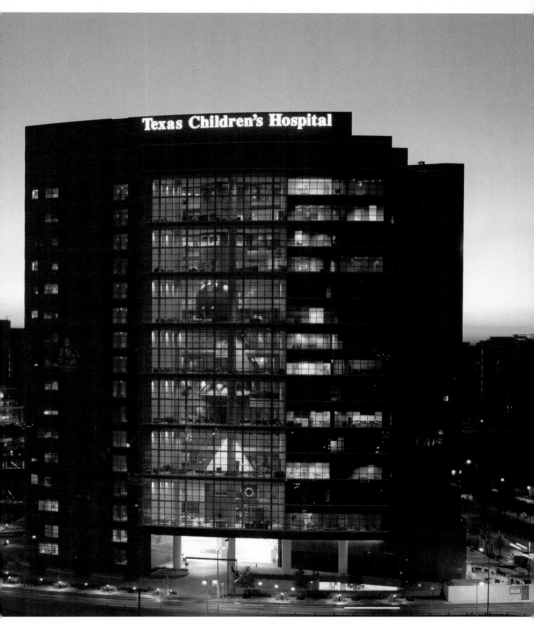

The Clinical Care Center at Texas Children's Hospital at dusk in 2003

The award-winning, colorfully designed two-story waiting rooms of the outpatient clinics in the 16-story Clinical Care Center at Texas Children's Hospital take center stage in this dramatic photo taken at dusk in 2003. Opened in 2001 and designed to accommodate a variety of general medical, surgical, and subspecialty clinics, the $175 million Clinical Care Center boasts twinkle lights in the elevators, bubble columns, aquariums and other visual delights for children and their families.

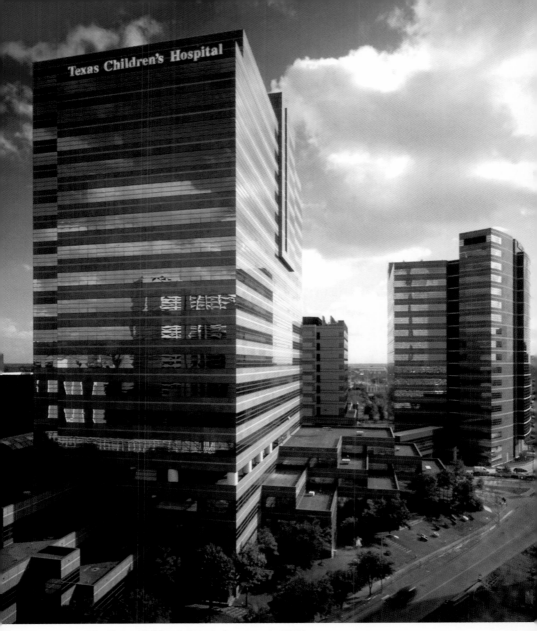

The Texas Children's Hospital campus in 2004

In 2004, the main campus of Texas Children's Hospital comprises four separate structures. The 20-story West Tower, the inpatient facility completed in 2001, is shown above in the foreground with the 16-story Clinical Care Center for outpatients to its rear, right. Not visible are both the 12-story Feigin Center and the Abercrombie Building, the reconfigured seven-story structure that was the original Texas Children's Hospital. For patients and their families, pedestrian sky-bridges allow convenient, climate-controlled access between each of these four buildings, which collectively represent a combined corridor length of more than 11 miles. During its first 50 years, Texas Children's Hospital has become one of the largest freestanding pediatric hospitals in the United States.

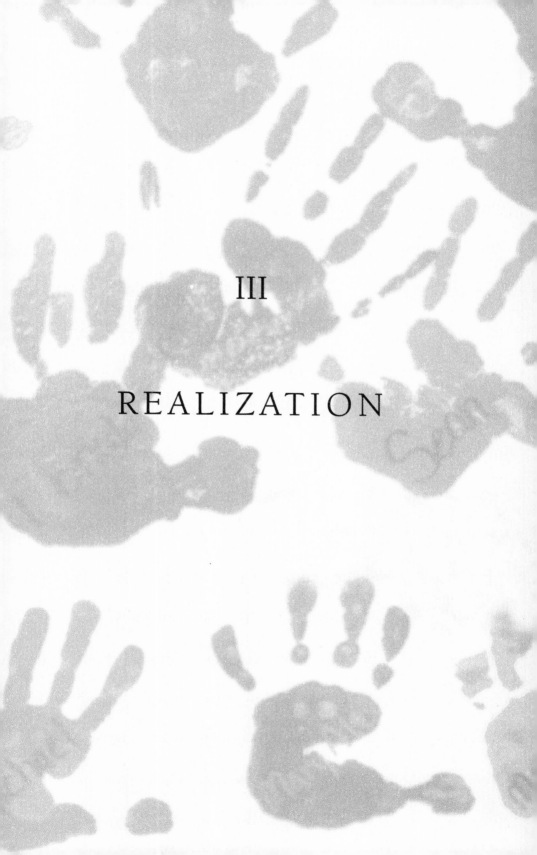

III

REALIZATION

6

✋ ALLERGY AND IMMUNOLOGY ✋

IT WAS A FAMILY SECRET, one that required anonymity.

Born in 1987 with an incurable fatal disease, she was not expected to live more than two years.

She defied that prediction and survived for more than 15 years—and counting.

Except for those who needed to know, no one outside her family was aware that she had the disease. The decision not to tell others was made at the time of her birth by her mother and grandmother. This was not unusual. Other families of similarly infected children also embraced secrecy.

Inspiring such deception was the well-founded fear of being ostracized and discriminated against, the prevalent public reaction to anyone infected with the disease. To protect themselves from this stigma, families felt that any means were justified, including not telling the infected children.

"We didn't tell her about it until she was nine years old," said her grandmother, now her parent. "It then was her decision not to tell others and I have to respect that. Certainly those who need to know do know, but her friends do not know."[1]

Nothing that the seemingly healthy teenager did betrayed her secret. An honor-roll student, she participated on the teen council at school, played basketball, and pursued an avid interest in photography. "She has lots of activities that she is involved in," her grandmother reported. "Medications and the timing of medications are so very important and how to do that privately is a problem for her. But it is something she wants and it's the way she wants it."

At her own request, the pseudonym used here in telling her story is "Amanda Wells."

The disease responsible for Amanda's elaborate charade—and that of so many other infected children and their families—was the human immunodeficiency virus (HIV).

"It's not like cancer. It's not like heart disease. It's not like diabetes. It's not like asthma," explained Theresa Aldape, LMSW, a social worker in the allergy and immunology service at Texas Children's Hospital in 2002. "You can tell someone you have one of those diseases and gain compassion, gain support, and gain a friend. With HIV, that does not happen. Instead of friendship, there is fear, isolation, and discrimination."[2]

At the time of Amanda's birth, the public fear and ignorance associated with HIV-infected children and those with acquired immune deficiency syndrome (AIDS) was clearly evident in the media. Beginning in 1985, there were published accounts about Ryan White, the Indiana teenager who contracted AIDS through a blood transfusion, and his public fights to attend public school. Although White's efforts eventually were successful, there continued to be public apprehension, fueled by persistent myths about contracting the disease through casual contact with someone infected with HIV or suffering from AIDS.

Moreover, misinformation about AIDS and HIV infection was rampant, even in the medical community. In 1987, the nature and extent of these diseases in children was just beginning to emerge. Four years earlier, the first case of pediatric AIDS appeared in a report compiled by the Centers for Disease Control (CDC). In 1987, with more than 471 pediatric AIDS cases reported by the CDC, enlightened pediatricians estimated that there were hundreds more cases that did not meet the strict AIDS identification criteria set by the CDC and therefore went unreported. Also not tracked by the CDC was the number of children like Amanda—those infected with HIV at birth, of which there were thousands.

Justifiably alarmed by these escalating figures, pediatrician and surgeon general Dr. C. Everett Koop instigated a Surgeon General's Workshop on Children with HIV Infection and Their Families at The Children's Hospital of Philadelphia in April 1987. In his keynote address at that workshop, Koop stated: "The nearly 500 cases of AIDS among young children is double the number of cases reported a year ago. Sixty percent of those children have already died. We need guidelines for our communities to bring together local officials, health professionals, educators, religious leaders, and parents to develop an interdisciplinary, moral, and just approach for the battle against AIDS ... and also to the alleviation of some of the burden borne by the children with HIV infection and their families."[3]

To Amanda's family, the workshop offered hope for the future, but their needs were immediate. "She was just two months old and she was exposed to chicken pox," her grandmother recalled. "Her mother was in a panic about her exposure and what it could do to her."[4]

Acutely aware that there were very few doctors—and fewer pediatricians—who had any experience with HIV-infected children, Amanda's mother and grandmother began making phone calls around the country in search of medical help. Within hours they had located a recognized expert who also happened to be one of the major participants in the surgeon general's recent workshop. It was Dr. Gwendolyn B. Scott, head of infectious diseases and immunology at the University of Miami School of Medicine in Florida.

With one call to Scott, the family's frantic search for help was over, but not in the way they had imagined. Rather than having to pack their bags and head to Florida for Amanda to see a doctor, they were given a more geographically convenient alternative. Remembered Amanda's grandmother: "When she asked, 'Where are you?' and we said, 'The Houston area,' she immediately said, 'Go directly to Texas Children's Hospital and talk to Celine Guerra.' That's when we went to Texas Children's Hospital for the first time."

When they arrived at the hospital, Amanda's family was surprised to learn that pediatric immunologists Dr. I. Celine Guerra Hanson and Dr. William T. Shearer, chief of the allergy and immunology service at Texas Children's Hospital, had identified more than 100 children with real or suspected HIV infection in the Houston area since 1983.

Just as finding HIV experts in their own backyard was unexpected, so was the loving care and treatment the family immediately began receiving at Texas Children's Hospital. "It had to be difficult for any doctor to take on the responsibility because the life expectancy of an HIV-infected infant was two years," her grandmother said. "It was just amazing."

It also was the precise moment at which Amanda's never-ending fight for survival officially began.

When Texas Children's Hospital opened in 1954, the subspecialty of allergy and immunology was one of the few existing in pediatrics. Established in 1944, the subspecialty was dedicated to improving the care of children and adolescents with allergic, asthmatic, and immunologic disorders.

"The whole science of current immunology really began with these pediatricians," explained Dr. William T. Shearer, chief of the allergy and immunology service at Texas Children's Hospital in 2002. "They were the doctors who saw these diseases. The internists didn't see them because the children back then didn't live to be adults. So it was the pediatricians who stumbled onto the fact that these children who were dying early in infancy have special problems with their immune system. So, it's been the pediatricians, to a large degree, who have initiated this investigation of the immune system. Some of the real pioneers in this area are pediatricians."[5]

One pioneering endeavor involving a genetic form of immunodeficiency took place at Texas Children's Hospital seven years before the hospital's allergy and immunology service officially began. In 1971, Baylor College of Medicine immunologists Dr. Mary Ann South and Dr. John R. Montgomery, together with experimental biologist Dr. Raphael Wilson, placed a newborn child in a sterile germ-free isolator unit.

Diagnosed at birth with severe combined immune deficiency (SCID), David Philip Vetter lacked lymphocytes, the specialized white blood cells made in the bone marrow that are necessary to fight infections. Without an effective immune system, David's body could not fight off the viruses, bacteria, and fungi that cause infections.

Knowing that other children born with SCID died from infection and disease soon after birth, the doctors concluded that sterile isolation was vital to the baby's survival. David's family agreed, having already lost a son to the disorder. Anticipating that David might also be born with SCID, the Vetters knew of the plan in advance. After receiving approval from Baylor College of Medicine, the doctors applied for and received a federal grant from the National Institutes of Health (NIH) for the care and housing of the baby in the Clinical Research Center at Texas Children's Hospital.

When they placed the newborn in the isolator unit, the three doctors, the medical community at Baylor College of Medicine, the NIH, and David's family all expected that the extraordinary living conditions would be temporary. They were collectively convinced that a medical breakthrough in SCID treatment was eminent—certainly within a year, two years at the most. Unfortunately, this was not the case.

With no viable treatment available, the baby grew into a boy inside his isolator in the Clinical Research Center at Texas Children's Hospital. As the years passed, David garnered intense international media attention—especially during his annual birthday celebrations. He arguably became the most famous of the one in every 100,000 children born each year with

SCID—although he maintained his anonymity. At the request of his family, David's last name was not released to the media while he was alive. So, because of his plastic-enclosed environment—which was continually enlarged as he grew—the media tagged him "David, the Bubble Boy."

By the time David reached his seventh birthday, the three doctors who had placed him in the isolator were no longer at Baylor College of Medicine. Instead, David's care in the Clinical Research Center was the responsibility of Dr. Buford L. Nichols, pediatric gastroenterologist at Texas Children's Hospital; his primary physician; and a multidisciplinary team of pediatric specialists from Texas Children's Hospital, representing disciplines including development, nutrition, and child life. That this team did not include a necessary, if not key, discipline did not go unnoticed—in fact, the omission served as a catalyst for action.

"David's future management requires the leadership of a superb immunologist," physician-in-chief Dr. Ralph D. Feigin stated in 1978, announcing the September arrival of Shearer. "A nationally renowned pediatric immunologist, he comes to us from Washington School of Medicine and St. Louis Children's Hospital. Dr. Shearer brings with him a complete research and training program in pediatric allergy and immunology."[6]

Created by Shearer for the St. Louis Children's Hospital during his pediatric internship and residency there, the research and training program was "small, but nevertheless new at that hospital and I was torn between continuing there and coming to Texas Children's Hospital and starting that whole process over again," Shearer recalled. "But the potential at Texas Children's Hospital was enormous and I recognized that. The responsibilities, particularly those of becoming the primary physician for the 'Bubble Boy,' were daunting. Yet, the encouragement of Dr. Feigin was most important in my decision to come."[7]

The day of Shearer's arrival, September 1, 1978, marked the establishment of the allergy and immunology service at Texas Children's Hospital and the pediatric allergy and immunology section of pediatrics at Baylor College of Medicine. Although the program consisted of only two people— Shearer and Dr. David Tanner, who was also recruited from St. Louis Children's Hospital—it made a big impact. For the allergy clinic at Texas Children's Hospital, the repercussions were enormous.

Founded in 1956 by pediatric allergist Dr. John P. McGovern, the allergy clinic at Texas Children's Hospital offered treatment for patients with allergic rhinitis or asthma, allergic skin manifestations, and some forms of gastrointestinal disturbance. Predominantly consisting of pediatric allergists who cared for patients with chronic and severe asthma, the clinic grew over the next two decades to become one of the largest in the Junior League Outpatient Department at Texas Children's Hospital.[8]

With the arrival of immunologists Shearer and Tanner, the spectrum of illnesses cared for in the allergy clinic increased dramatically. In addition to its existing patients, the clinic began caring for children with immune deficiencies of all kinds, congenital and acquired; immune complex disease; autoimmune disease; and immunology aspects of cancer.

Those changes in procedure took time to implement, but others—one in particular—took immediate effect. Within two days of his arrival, Shearer assumed responsibility as primary physician for the most famous patient at Texas Children's Hospital. "Dr. Buford Nichols, who had been David's physician for years, walked me over to the Clinical Research Center and introduced me to David and handed me his chart," recalled Shearer. "As I glanced at the chart, I noticed an 'off service' note indicating that Dr. Nichols was turning David over to me. I looked around the room and saw this child looking at me from his world inside a bubble and I realized the enormity of the task before me. Needless to say, I will never forget that day."[9]

Also memorable was how this first encounter with David surprised Shearer. As a pediatrician who was accustomed to talking with children on their level, Shearer found himself to be eye-to-eye with eight-year-old David, who was standing on an elevated platform in the isolator. "It was a bit disconcerting at first," recalled Shearer. "In addition, he had at his command a language foreign to most adults, much less children, in the complex medical terminology of those attending him. And in spite of living his life in a bubble, or perhaps, precisely because he lived that way, David demonstrated a maturity and sophistication far beyond his years."[10]

Over time, Shearer found David, the oldest living child with the SCID disorder, to be well-informed about his unique circumstances. He knew that his family and the medical team expected a medical breakthrough in the treatment for SCID. He knew that until that treatment was found, he was confined to his bubble at the hospital and at home. He knew that a bone marrow transplant, the only known treatment to restore his immune system, was not possible because an exhaustive search for an exact match continued to be fruitless. He knew that it was necessary to remain in his germ-free environment. He knew why there were extraordinary precautions taken, constant medical attention given, and seemingly endless laboratory testing of his cells and blood performed. He knew that there were questions about his future. He knew that, along with everyone else, he had to continue to wait for the answers.

During the following four years, as Shearer fervently searched for a solution to David's dilemma, the allergy and immunology service at Texas Children's Hospital began to grow. "Patients started coming," explained Shearer. "Pediatricians would call and say, 'I have this patient and I don't understand what the problem is. I have been treating this sinus infection ten times and it's not getting any better. Can you examine the patient and see what's going on?' And we would examine the patient and call back and say, 'Your patient has an antibody deficiency disease and needs to be on gamma globulin infusions every month for the rest of his life.' So, the referring doctor is, like, 'Wow, this guy needs to see my patients.' And we were getting referral patients from all around the state and South America, Central America, and the Middle East."[11]

While the primary emphasis of the service continued to be on the care and treatment of children with allergic and immunologic diseases, Shearer also concentrated on research. "Strong efforts are being made to unravel the complex regulatory mechanisms of the immune system, abnormalities of which produce clinical problems," he reported in 1982.[12]

To assist in the implementation of his expanding efforts, Shearer applied for grants every time he could. "You know, if you don't apply for the grants, you don't get the money," he explained. "You start little by little. People give you grant money, and you hire a secretary, and you hire a lab tech, and you hire the people who wash the lab equipment, and so on."[13]

The strategy proved invaluable to the growth of the allergy and immunology service. Four years after founding the two-person program, Shearer had expanded it to include four fellows-in-training, five technicians, a research nurse, and a secretary. The workspace for the growing service had also been increased, with more than 4,000 square feet of space allotted for laboratory work and another 1,000 square feet for offices.[14]

Yet it was unimaginable in 1982 that the ever-growing allergy and immunology service at Texas Children's Hospital was already on its way to becoming the largest pediatric service of its kind in a children's hospital in the United States. Also unthinkable was the advent of a new immune-deficient disease in the pediatric population.

Originally designated a "gay disease" by the CDC in 1981, gay-related immune deficiency (GRID) was not expected to affect the pediatric population. When the disease became known to affect other adult populations, Haitians and intravenous drug users, it became known as acquired immune deficiency syndrome, or AIDS. In 1982, the CDC reported 1,600 cases and

619 deaths from the disease in the adult population. Although suspected AIDS cases in children were reported to the CDC in 1982, the strict criteria set by the CDC for the identification of AIDS prohibited it from reporting these cases itself.

The pediatric immunologists at Texas Children's Hospital were intensely aware of this disturbing new threat. "The causative agent was not defined in 1983," remembered Dr. I. Celine Guerra Hanson, who was one of the fellows-in-training that year. "I believe we were classically poised to pick up on the pediatric cases before we identified the causative agent. This was because we were picking up other infections that were so common to children who had a primary disturbance in their immune system."[15]

In 1983, Hanson had her first encounter with a suspected pediatric AIDS patient at Texas Children's Hospital. It was a little boy diagnosed with pneumocystis carini pneumonia (PCP), a disease rarely found in pediatric patients. "We thought he had picked up on an unusual case of primary immune deficiency," she explained. "Primary immune deficiencies are the ones children are born with, not the ones they acquire, which are secondary immune deficiencies. I remember calling the CDC and asking if they would be willing to accept this boy's specimen for testing. The lab director at that time said to me, 'No, we really have not identified any children, so it's not likely to be AIDS.' Of course, in hindsight, it certainly was."

While progress in this aspect of pediatric immunology appeared to be stymied in 1983, technological advances were being made in another area. Of strategic importance were research studies indicating that non-identical bone marrow could be purified of those elements that prevented successful transplantation. With the risk of immunologic rejection minimized, the results looked promising. Although the procedure was still experimental, having been performed only on a few cancer patients, it "might be the key that would open a new door for David," said Shearer.[16] He presented that possibility to the 12-year-old David and his parents, who agreed to attempt the procedure. The bone marrow to be purified and transplanted was to come from David's sister, they decided.

On October 21, 1984, David's sister, Shearer, and a medical team from Texas Children's Hospital flew to Boston, where the recognized experts in the procedure harvested the bone marrow and performed the antibody purification process. Shearer returned to Houston that same day and infused the purified bone marrow into David. The results were not known immediately. After waiting for 12 years for this opportunity, David and his family continued their vigil of hope.

Two months after the transplant, David began to experience fever, abdominal pains, and diarrhea. It was the first time in his life that he had displayed these clinical symptoms, which were thought to be a result of graft-versus-host disease. The reaction seemed to be an indication that David's immune system was beginning to take hold. Unfortunately, this was not the case. Blood tests indicated that there were no signs of an established immune system.

David's health began to deteriorate rapidly during the following months. Shearer decided to remove him from the isolator so that he and other physicians could attempt to remedy the boy's unidentifiable symptoms and to determine their cause. David was finally out of the bubble and in his mother's arms, able to feel human contact for the first time in his life. Riddled with disease and fatally ill after suffering massive blood loss, he died two weeks later, on February 22, 1984. Exactly what caused his death was a mystery—one that Shearer and the medical team at Texas Children's Hospital were determined to solve through study.

What these studies indicated was a medical breakthrough, a lasting legacy of David's short life. Announcing the findings to the media, Shearer said: "David has provided us with the missing link that connects infection with cancer. The studies show definitely and for the first time how a virus can induce a malignancy."[17]

David had died from a form of cancer called immunoblastic sarcoma. The cause was determined to be Epstein-Barr (EB) virus, a common infection that usually lies dormant, which was present in the transplanted bone marrow that David had received from his sister. Since the bone marrow transplant had not stimulated the development of David's immune system, as hoped, his body could not fight off the EB virus. "Tragic as it is, because it happened to David, it is nevertheless very clear that one must have natural immunity to prevent the development and spread of cancer," Shearer told the media. "What has been learned from David may aid in the development of future therapies for cancer as well as treatments for immune deficiencies."

That David's legacy had made an immediate impact was soon evident. Two months after his death, NIH scientists announced that the probable cause of AIDS was a new variant of a human cancer virus. Initially identified as human T-cell leukemia/lymphoma virus (HTLV-III), it later became known as the human immunodeficiency virus (HIV). Also announced were federally funded research efforts to develop a vaccine that would combat the virus.[18]

Such a breakthrough discovery marked the beginning of an explosion of information about the importance of the immune system viruses. "Let's be very clear about this. David did not have AIDS, nor was he HIV-infected. Both are secondary immune deficiencies that are acquired," Shearer explained. "He had a primary immune deficiency, SCID, one that he was born with. But the lessons from his life, and SCID children like him, set the stage for the spectacular advances in the understanding of how the immune system protects us against virus infections and cancer."[19]

Those advances included the development of new techniques in bone marrow transplants for SCID. The progress made in tissue matching and medical therapies to ward off complications like David's saw favorable results at Texas Children's Hospital and around the world. Within two years, the procedure was perfected. It was the only known cure for SCID.

In honor of David's legacy, including the developments yet to come, physician-in-chief Feigin and Shearer created the David Center in his memory in 1984. The center was not a specific area in Texas Children's Hospital, but a concept dedicated to the research, diagnosis, and treatment of immune deficiencies.[20] Although unknown at the time, in the empty space where David had lived in a bubble for 12 years—the NIH-funded Clinical Research Center—a new chapter of David's legacy would begin in 1988.

In the intervening four years, the David Center became what Shearer called "the clinic of last resort" for children whose infections could not be cured by other physicians. "They just tumbled in," he said, recalling the hundreds of patients referred to the allergy and immunology service at Texas Children's Hospital.[21]

All of these children had either primary or secondary immune deficiencies. Seven were SCID patients, five of whom survived successful bone marrow transplants performed by Shearer and his team. Others were found to have a genetic disposition to acquire an immune deficiency later in life. Countless were malnourished, the most prevalent acquired immune deficiency diagnosed in children. Alarmingly, many were HIV-infected or had AIDS.

Whether to assume the responsibility of treating these fatally ill children or simply refer them elsewhere was never a question for Shearer. "I don't know how you could justify taking care of very sick children who had an inherited immune deficiency or a secondary immune deficiency and ignoring the ones with HIV infection or AIDS," he said. "We took care of them."[22]

Since the prognosis for these infected children was dim, only Texas Children's Hospital and a few other centers nationwide offered any forms of significant intervention. Texas Children's Hospital adopted a multidisciplinary approach. In addition to the allergy and immunology service, patients had access to development, infectious diseases, nutrition and gastroenterology, pulmonary, and neurology services.[23]

The first HIV-infected children identified at Texas Children's Hospital were hemophiliacs, as was the case at other children's hospitals across the United States in the early 1980s. "This was before anyone knew HIV was the causative and the blood donations pool had not been screened," explained Hanson. "In 1985, after the national blood screening program began, we continued to evaluate children with hemophilia because we knew they had risks stemming from factor replacement. Then, relatively quickly, we began to see babies who acquired the infection from their mothers."[24] Hanson noted: "I have lost many, many babies to AIDS. It's a hurtful thing to see."[25]

Able to treat only the symptoms of the disease, Shearer applied for a National Institute of Child Health and Human Development (NICHD) grant to study the efficacy of intravenous immunoglobulin (IVIG) treatments to boost the immunity system of children with AIDS and HIV infection. Receiving the $425,000 grant in 1988, the Clinical Research Center at Texas Children's Hospital became the first center in the nation chosen to participate in a federal study of therapy for children with AIDS and HIV infection. The study, expected to take as long as three years, was to be co-directed by Shearer and Hanson. The precise location for the study was of sentimental, if not historical, significance to Shearer and his team.

"Until that study, we saw these children in the allergy and immunology clinic and treated them the very best that we could," explained Shearer. "With the NIH funds for the study, we redesigned the empty space where David lived in the Clinical Research Center and it became the AIDS clinic for all our patients who are on special NIH protocols for AIDS and HIV infection. Basically, David's living quarters remained the place for children with an immune deficiency, but from a different cause."[26]

When more than 100 children in the Houston area were found to be HIV-infected in 1988, Shearer declared that AIDS was "the number one health threat in pediatrics today" and vowed to continue his efforts on these children's behalf.[27] With the number of verified pediatric cases escalating throughout the United States, the National Institute of Allergy and Infectious Diseases announced the formation of the Pediatric AIDS Clinical Trials Group (PACTG). Shearer's group was among the first to apply for and receive the federal grant for PACTG. On behalf of Baylor College of Medicine, Shearer had joined together with physicians from the University of Texas Medical School in Houston, the University of Texas M. D. Anderson Cancer Center, and the University of Houston to request the funding.

With the $4 million grant, infected Houston-area children were among the first to receive experimental medications for AIDS and HIV infection. The grant also enabled the founding of the Texas Children's HIV Center, destined to become one of the leading NIH-funded pediatric HIV/AIDS research centers in the United States.

"One reason for our success in achieving the grant was that we had something up and running already," Shearer said in 1988, referring to the nation's first intravenous gamma globulin study for pediatric AIDS underway at Texas Children's Hospital. "This grant represents hope for families who have children infected with this virus. It's good to have something to offer them."[28]

In particular, Shearer hoped that the research supported by the grant would offer a more optimistic outlook for babies born with the infection and for their families. Studies in New York City in 1988 revealed that more than half of HIV-infected mothers gave birth to infected children. Since expectant mothers in Texas were only rarely tested, Shearer and Hanson worried about the potential number of babies born with the infection. Already at Texas Children's Hospital there were eight babies who had been infected by their mothers, and the number was expected to increase. How to solve this emerging problem of perinatal infection, designated "vertical transmission," was to be a major focus of the PACTG protocol 076, one in which Shearer's group was a major participant. "It was a shot in the dark," Shearer said. "And it was a spectacular success."

"We were one of the largest centers that contributed patients to that study," he explained. "And Dr. Hunter Hammill is the person who really made it possible. He was the obstetrician at Baylor who has made it his mission, frankly, to see those mothers. Even after his going into private practice, his dedication to them has not budged. He continues to see these patients in his private practice."[29]

Six years later, the results of PACTG protocol 076, released in February 1994, provided the first major breakthrough in the prevention of HIV vertical transmission. Described in medical journals as "a clinical trial that would change the face of the pediatric HIV epidemic in the United States," protocol 076 "demonstrated that a zidovudine regimen given to HIV-infected women during pregnancy and labor and to the neonate for the first six weeks of life could reduce the risk of perinatal transmission by two thirds."[30] By August 1994, the United States Public Health Service had published guidelines following this protocol. Since then, vertical transmission in the United States has continued to decline substantially.

"It was a milestone," said Shearer, justifiably proud of his group's involvement in the PACTG protocol 076 breakthrough. "The next step was to identify those expectant mothers who were infected. It is a law in Texas now. But you know, it was a battle back then and Celine Hanson played a major role in getting the Texas legislature to adapt that."[31]

"I was involved in testimony and in lobbying to get the bill passed in Austin," said Hanson. "When the data from protocol 076 proved you could reduce transmission, then that gave us far more impetus. We felt we could keep the kids from even getting infected at all. The bill encouraging pregnant patients to be tested for AIDS virus during regular prenatal visits passed in 1995. It became effective in 1996. We were one of the first four states to pass that type of law, so it was very exciting."[32]

Hanson's efforts were praised by physician-in-chief Feigin, who noted that "her total dedication to these children goes far beyond the traditional efforts of most physicians. She has served as the clinical coordinator for all the pediatric AIDS research projects and has made herself available to the news media in an attempt to educate the public about this disease in children. We applaud her for her tireless efforts on behalf of Texas Children's Hospital and, particularly, for her devotion to children with AIDS."[33]

An integral part of the allergy and immunology service since 1983, Hanson briefly left Texas Children's Hospital in 1990. She worked for two years in pediatric HIV and AIDS surveillance at the CDC in Atlanta before returning to Houston in 1992. During that interval and afterwards, Dr. Mark Kline assumed Hanson's responsibilities as coordinator of the pediatric AIDS research, diagnostic, and treatment efforts in the allergy and immunology service at Texas Children's Hospital.

While the number of pediatric cases in the United States began to stabilize in the thousands during the late 1990s, it was estimated that millions of children in the world were HIV-infected. These devastating developments influenced Kline's decision to leave the allergy and immunology service in 1997. The AIDS specialist decided to branch out into retrovirology and maintain his own section at Baylor College of Medicine.

"His main interest is international work, an area of growing importance to the NIH in 2002," explained Shearer. "He anticipated that need years ago. I am dealing with domestic HIV infection. However, our NIH grant, which has recently been renewed, is now turning toward more international studies, but not completely. We are not abandoning the children of this country by any means, not as long as I can have anything to do with it. But more attention has to be paid through working with sites like ours, the 18 or 20 sites that make up the PACTG coalition, we want to start working in international studies with maybe 20 percent of our effort. That's up from about 5 percent right now."[34]

From 1997, Kline was devoting most of his efforts to international studies. He became director of the Baylor International Pediatric AIDS Initiative (BIPAI) at Baylor College of Medicine and Texas Children's Hospital. BIPAI provided comprehensive medical and social services to HIV-infected infants and children in programs conducted in Romania, Mexico, Panama, southern Africa, and Houston. In 2000, BIPAI received a $1.4 million grant from the NIH to create a new AIDS international training and research program. Upon announcing the grant, Kline described it as being "essential to building research capacity and answering important research questions in parts of the world hit hardest by the HIV/AIDS epidemic."[35]

For those affected by the epidemic in Houston, the allergy and immunology service at Texas Children's Hospital continued its efforts to offer specialized care and management of the infection. With more than $60 million in peer-reviewed grant awards and NIH-funded clinical trials in two decades, the Texas Children's HIV Center provided a variety of research and treatment options for infants, children, adolescents, and pregnant women with HIV infection. The center offered the most up-to-date anti-retroviral treatments, including protease inhibitors and immunotherapy. Many of the perinatally infected children originally diagnosed during the 1980s, such as Amanda Wells, benefited from these efforts and continued to survive as adolescents.

The children at Texas Children's Hospital who did not survive the infection nonetheless made immeasurable contributions to our understanding of the disease. "I think it's of some comfort to parents of these special children that their child really taught us how to deal with the epidemic," said Shearer. "They helped open the door to our understanding the whole spectrum of the failure of the immune system."[36]

Children with genetic forms of immunodeficiency have taught us much about normal immunity—David being an outstanding example. For those children throughout the world born with SCID, the impact of his short life had enduring value. Not only did David draw widespread attention to the disorder, but also "the very cells that we maintained, his lymphocytes, are maintained in perpetuity in our laboratory," explained Shearer. "They are growing today. Those cells actually contributed to the molecular definition of SCID and are of enormous benefit to all of the babies who have had that disease since."[37]

From the scientific study of David's DNA came a breakthrough nine years after his death: the discovery of the gene responsible for SCID. When the NIH announced this finding in 1993, David's mother, Carol Ann Vetter, said: "We are so proud. David's legacy continues. This helps somewhat with the sorrow."[38]

The discovery led to a medical milestone in 2000, one that Shearer defined as "something you dream about." In France, one year following experimental gene therapy, two infants born with SCID had "complete restoration of immune system function." Of historical importance, it was the first successful gene therapy to correct inborn genetic errors.[39]

The legacy of David and of all the other children continued to be felt at the David Center, the Texas Children's HIV Center, and the allergy and immunology service at Texas Children's Hospital. By 2002, the service that Shearer had launched in 1978 with that one special patient and just two physicians had grown to include thousands of patients and more than 60 full-time physicians, nurses, social workers, and laboratory, administrative, and clerical personnel.

With its expanding spectrum of complex allergic and immunologic diseases, the service continued to make myriad contributions to advance the care and treatment of afflicted children. In 2002, the allergy and immunology service at Texas Children's Hospital boasted specialists in allergic rhinitis, asthma, genetic immunodeficiencies, and acquired immunodeficiencies. The service also offered diagnosis and treatment of hypersensitivity diseases, severe asthma, antibody deficiencies, and cellular immune defects requiring immune reconstitution.

"We specialize in immunoreconstitution of these illnesses with allergen-specific immunotherapy, intravenous immunoglobulin replacement therapy, highly active antiretroviral therapy (HAART), immunomodulatory therapy with fusion proteins, and bone marrow stem cell transplantations," said Shearer. "We actually did the transplants ourselves back in the early days. But now that Texas Children's Hospital has such a wonderful transplant team, we ask them to do the transplants. But we follow our patients because we know what we are looking for in terms of grafting. It's a great arrangement. It couldn't be better. They have a beautiful transplant unit in the cancer center."

While working closely with bone marrow transplant specialists in the hematology-oncology service at Texas Children's Hospital, the allergy and immunology service also joined forces with the pulmonary service to diagnose and treat children in the Texas Children's Asthma Center in 1993. "We share patients," explained Shearer. "We look at it as a synergy. We look at it as the expertise they need, and vice versa. We think asthma is a genetic disease, especially the allergy component, and an allergy is actually the result of an excess of the immune system. We work very closely with Dr. Seilheimer and his team to find out which of his patients have an allergic problem as well as the asthma."[40]

To Shearer, the implementation of these inter-disciplinary relationships exemplified the mission of Texas Children's Hospital to create a better world for children with whatever mechanism worked. The allergy and immunology service steadfastly pursued that goal throughout its existence, changing directions and methodology whenever circumstances dictated.

"In pediatrics, we adapt to change," said Shearer. "A child changes every single day, and people who specialize in pediatrics are very used to change. They must adapt to change, and I think that's healthy."[41]

I n 1988, Amanda Wells participated in the nation's first federal study of intravenous immunoglobulin therapy for HIV-infected children and children with AIDS.

For one-and-a-half-year-old Amanda, the treatments administered by Drs. Shearer and Hanson at Texas Children's Hospital also included a treat. Arriving in the Clinical Research Center at the appointed time, she was always greeted with a small bowl of steamed broccoli.

"She was a vegetarian, even at that age, and the dietitian, Mrs. Potts, knew she was coming and would make it for her," Amanda's grandmother said. "Amanda had the IV in her arm and an IV pole and we would put her in a wagon and walk around the hospital and she would eat her broccoli."

Nourishment of another variety, one for their own well-being, awaited Amanda's family. As one of the participants in this protocol, they gained the services and support of the newly hired social worker, Theresa Aldape. Joining the staff of the allergy and immunology service at Texas Children's Hospital to assist the children and families in this first clinical trial, Aldape had previously worked for five years at Houston's Ben Taub General Hospital.

"I was in general pediatrics at Ben Taub," said Aldape. "We started seeing children who were infected with HIV in 1984 and 1985. At that time,

Dr. Shearer said, 'We are the department that is going to take care of these kids with HIV.' He applied for funding for clinical trials and part of those funds were for hiring a social worker. Dr. Shearer and Dr. Hanson asked me if I were willing to come over to Texas Children's Hospital. I knew it was going to be difficult, knowing that the children were not doing well and knowing how sick they would get. At that time, we did not know how to prevent opportunistic infections and serious infections that cause disabilities. We could only treat the symptoms then, we had nothing to help them survive."[42]

To alleviate the consequences of that reality, Aldape began to develop and implement social services and programs exclusively for children infected or affected by HIV/AIDS and for their families.

For patients like Amanda and her family, Aldape offered information about the services available in the community and at Texas Children's Hospital. She helped them find community agencies that offered assistance; directed them to resources for housing, transportation, and healthcare information; and, most importantly, became their trusted friend, always there in times of need.

"We do a psychosocial assessment when they first come in for a clinical trial," Aldape explained. "We find out what their support systems are, what services they are accessing, and what it is we have to get done for them. Ninety-five percent of our patients are on Medicaid, so we know it is very important to request federal and state assistance for their parking while they are here. Since it sometimes takes two or three hours for treatments and to get the lab work done, we know we have to help them with food to eat. Since we want to see all of our HIV-infected children in homes that are comfortable, we cannot have them go without electricity, so we help with the payment of those bills. Whatever it is, parents know if they have a need that they can call us and that we will try and help them."

While fulfilling these needs over the following 12 years, Aldape rejoiced at the inauguration of each new medication introduced and each new treatment perfected. These breakthroughs led to the miraculous survival of Amanda and other such perinatally infected HIV children, who had previously been doomed. "It was unbelievable to see how much better they did just on AZT," Aldape recalled. "And then there was the study conducted for Bactrim, which also produced amazing results in the children. Then came the protease inhibitors and the so-called 'cocktails.' It was all miraculous, and it continues to be so."

For those less fortunate than Amanda, the children who did not survive, Aldape mourned their loss with the families. Often assisting with funeral arrangements and the patient's last wishes, she eventually lost count of the number of dead but never forgot the memory of each child.

She also learned never to abandon hope for those who are very sick. "We have had some children who were dying who made it through," Aldape said. "I met one little boy in ICU who was dying. We had talked to his family about invoking a 'Do Not Resuscitate' order and they refused that, preferring to hold on. And you know what? That little boy kept getting better and better. He's now six years old and he is beautiful."

Whether diligently monitoring Amanda's progress, helping a dying child create a memory book for his family, issuing McDonald's vouchers for hungry families, or quietly listening as a sick child voiced concerns, Aldape followed her personal motto: "Try to do the best I can do every day."

In turn, she endeared herself to patients and their families—especially Amanda, who knew her from the day she began work at Texas Children's Hospital. "She is like family," said the 15-year-old. "Everyone there is like family."[43]

As Amanda's extended family at Texas Children's Hospital began to grow, it went through many changes but somehow always remained the same. Having made monthly trips to the allergy and immunology service since 1987, Amanda had a unique perspective on the growth of the service. She encapsulated her history over the past 15 years by listing the succession of doctors she had seen from the beginning: "First I saw Dr. Hanson, then Dr. Kline, then Dr. Hanson again, then Dr. Kline again, then Dr. Hanson again, and now Dr. Paul, but always Dr. Shearer."

Amanda was thus measuring her life by naming the doctors who had helped to extend it. Her grandmother reflected on this lifelong struggle. While praising Amanda's conscientious approach to living with HIV, she said: "I just cry sometimes when I think of how hard a burden it is for this child to carry."[44]

"To maintain our health is a job as we get older, not when we are a small child," she continued. "Health is the farthest thing from your mind as a child. I think Amanda was born old. Although she was not told of her infection until she was nine, her mom taught her the universal precautions. Even when she was in kindergarten and fell and scraped her knee, she was careful about her blood. She would say, 'I will get a Band-Aid. That's all right. I got it.' Today she is a grown-up person and has been a marvel since she was old enough to be in charge of her life."

In awe of her granddaughter's achievements, she reveled in the facts that Amanda survived past two years of age to become 15 years old; that she excelled in school, making straight A's; that she was learning how to drive; that she was planning for college; and that she was thinking about what she wanted to do with her life.

"What a reward it must be for the doctors who took on the task of HIV-infected infants," she exclaimed. "It just has to be so rewarding for them. Every time I see Dr. Shearer at Texas Children's Hospital, I try to pat him on the back. Because, it's a miracle."

It also was a family secret.

7

✋ AUXILIARY ✋

WHEN TEXAS CHILDREN'S HOSPITAL opened its doors on February 1, 1954, the population of metropolitan Houston was nearing the million mark.

In the eight years since Dr. David Greer had first proposed a children's hospital to the Houston Pediatric Society, the population had more than doubled. With such unprecedented growth, Houston was quickly becoming the seventh-largest city in the United States, an astonishing ascent from its 27th-place ranking in 1940.[1]

Characterized as "an ambitious small city" before World War II, Houston suddenly became the focus of the national and international media. In 1953, *Holiday* magazine's "The 12 Most Exciting Cities of North America" touted that Houston, as one of the dozen cities selected, possessed "that rare combination of qualities which has always spelled greatness," and the *London Times* predicted that America might "eventually be based on a quadrilateral of great cities—New York, Chicago, Los Angeles, and Houston."[2]

However, along with such flattering predictions about Houston's future came stories about the city's residents that would soon become legendary. This attention was predominantly due to the worldwide media coverage of the opening on March 17, 1949, of a Houston millionaire's hotel. With the world's largest swimming pool and a lobby the size of a football field, the Shamrock Hotel epitomized the adjective "Texas-sized."

"The King of the Wildcatters and his hotel titillated the American imagination with tales of huge pools of black gold, mountains of money, and beautiful women," remembered *Houston Post* columnist Bill Roberts. "The opening of Glenn McCarthy's Shamrock Hotel in 1949 changed all our lives and changed Houston forever."[3]

This was not an understatement. More than 50,000 Houstonians had driven or walked past the hotel on its opening day, and tall tales of the Texas-sized fiasco that took place were not easily forgotten and were often retold. Stories about the 30 Hollywood stars—including Ginger Rogers, Sonja Henie, and Maureen O'Hara—who were elbow-to-elbow with hundreds of well-dressed Houstonians paled in comparison to those about Dorothy Lamour's live national radio broadcast from the hotel. Sprinkled with drunken obscenities uttered by the boisterous crowd, the show was yanked off the air in mid-broadcast by network executives in New York.

Not only did the Shamrock's colorful opening garner international media coverage, it also inspired author Edna Ferber to create the flamboyant McCarthyesque character of Jett Rink in her novel *Giant* and the disaster-filled scene surrounding the opening of his hotel.

Therefore, in the early 1950s, a mixture of fiction and fact characterized perceptions of Houston and its citizens. After journalist Gerald Ashford wrote in 1951 that many "think of Houston as a cluster of mud huts around the Shamrock Hotel, in the cellars of which people hide from the sticky climate, emerging at long intervals to scatter $1000 bills to the far winds," the *Houston Post's* George Fuermann observed that such a myth, "though arresting to the world, was a liability to Houston. For one thing, it obscured the city's reality, which was itself exceptional enough."[4]

Indeed, the Houston of the 1950s was not a city filled with wildcatters and millionaires, although there were more than a few of each. There was no question that Houston's economy was oil-driven, but several other factors figured into the substantial postwar growth: the Houston ship channel's linking of the city to the outside world; the vast resources of not only oil, but also natural gas, sulfur, lime salt, and water; and the proliferation of chemical plants dependent on the process of crude oil refinement, thereby creating one of the greatest concentrations of petrochemical industries in the world.

With its newfound recognition as a prosperous international city, Houston also displayed a transformation in personality. Although founded only in 1836, the young city had outgrown its primitive ways. No longer rough and ragged, like a typical outpost of the Wild West (as fictionalized in *Giant*), or relaxed and easygoing (like other Southern and Texas towns), Houston had evolved into something completely different. It had emerged after World War II to "become not so much a Texan town but an Americanized one," wrote the *Houston Post's* Hubert Mewhinney.[5]

And, as in most cities in America, it wasn't just the millionaires—like Houston's James S. Abercrombie, who had made his fortune in the oil industry and was making his dream of a children's hospital come true—who were rich in generosity. The desire to help others soon became contagious. Countless Houstonians of every income, age, denomination, and race donated their time and service to worthy causes. Many of these people were elevated to legendary status for their selfless contributions to the community over the years.

One such legend was Elaine Kuper at Texas Children's Hospital.

Kuper, a 31-year-old wife and mother of two, lived not in a mythological mud hut with a cellar full of cash on the prairie near the Shamrock, but in a recently built house in the nearby neighborhood of Bellaire. On the morning of February 18, 1954, she officially donned a cherry-red pinafore, white blouse, and white shoes for the first time.

Leaving her three-year-old daughter in the care of her housekeeper, and with her nine-year-old son already at school, Kuper got into her car and drove the few short blocks to the recently opened Texas Children's Hospital in the Texas Medical Center, located directly across the street from the famous Shamrock Hotel.

As one of the charter members of the Women's Auxiliary to Texas Children's Hospital, Kuper had already gone through an orientation program, received her uniform, and been asked in which area of Texas Children's Hospital she wished to work. With two small children at home, she preferred not to interact with patients. Instead, Kuper wanted to be of service to the patients' families and to Texas Children's Hospital's staff. After agreeing to volunteer three hours a week as a worker in the snack bar, which served sandwiches and drinks prepared by The Auxiliary, she underwent training for the job.

"They taught us how to make sandwiches and drinks," Kuper recalled. "It was very simple. The snack bar was very small, one counter and only about five bar stools and a few tables. The rest of it was toys and gifts. We would wrap gifts, ring them up on the cash register, and then make a sandwich or something. We were doing everything. I loved it."

Located in Texas Children's Hospital's main lobby, adjacent to the admitting desk, the glass-enclosed snack bar was a very popular spot with patients' families and hospital staff. Supervised by an Auxilian "chairman of the day" and open 12 hours a day, the facility was staffed by volunteers who worked four three-hour shifts. And the volunteers did indeed do everything. Glasses and dishes were washed by hand and then professionally sterilized. Not only did the volunteers make and sell all the food and drinks, Auxilians—including "Miss Lillie" Abercrombie, wife of "Mr. Jim" Abercrombie—also mopped the floor.

"It was very amusing to see all those ladies in the dishpan," remembered Dr. Russell J. Blattner, the first physician-in-chief at Texas Children's Hospital. "It was extremely popular and good. When you wanted a really good sandwich in the Texas Medical Center, you would go to the Snack Bar at Texas Children's."[6]

Amused by the doctors who regularly came to the snack bar and ordered the same sandwich every time, Kuper began calling them by the name of their sandwich. And, upon seeing the doctors enter the snack bar, she would prepare their favorite food before they had time to sit down and order it.

"Mr. Tuna Fish, Mr. Grilled Cheese, and Mr. Roast Beef, that was Dr. Jim Carter, Dr. Morton Blum, and Dr. Jim Cody," Kuper said. "I don't know why we didn't call them Dr. Tuna Fish, Dr. Grilled Cheese, and Dr. Roast Beef. We should have."[7]

Nonetheless, since their "Mr." nicknames soon were well-known throughout The Auxiliary, the doctors never complained. Once, when Auxilian Helen Blumberg had surgery at St. Luke's, she thought she recognized a voice in the operating room. Sure enough, it was Mr. Tuna Fish, anesthesiologist Dr. Jim Carter, whom she remembers saying to the others, "This lady makes great tuna fish sandwiches."[8]

When Kuper's daughter was ill, she took the child to see Dr. Blum. "He was examining her and she was tugging on my dress and I said, 'What is it, Laurie?' and she said, 'Is that Mr. Tuna Fish?' and he said, 'No, honey. I'm Mr. Grilled Cheese.' We still laugh about it," recalled Kuper.

Also humorous to Kuper was how she first came to volunteer at Texas Children's Hospital. Weeks before her first day on the job, neighbor Helen Blumberg had asked her if she would join the newly formed Auxiliary and volunteer at Texas Children's Hospital. Kuper had replied, "Sure, why not? I have Tuesday mornings open. I didn't know a thing about what I was getting into."[9]

Kuper wasn't kidding. At that time, she didn't even know that a children's hospital had been built. And, having retired from her office job after giving birth to her first child in 1945, she preferred to keep a busy schedule. Every Saturday, and sometimes Sundays as well, she had volunteered her services as a teacher at Beth Israel, where she also was the voluntary librarian of the children's library, buying, categorizing, and maintaining the inventory. At her son's school, she volunteered in the library and served as a room mother, Scout leader, and volunteer at various school festivities. When not involved with her children or the synagogue, Kuper joined a group of friends who played cards once or twice a week. Her husband, Harry Kuper, an executive at the Sakowitz specialty store, also traveled extensively and often asked his wife to join him, an invitation she eagerly accepted.

Looking forward to her daughter's entering school in a few years, Kuper knew she would repeat the efforts expended on her son's behalf as a school volunteer. However, at the time Blumberg asked her, she did have three hours a week to volunteer at the new children's hospital and was willing to commit herself to that obligation—at least for a year or two, she thought at the time.

Undoubtedly, during that first year in The Auxiliary, Kuper never imagined that her career as a Texas Children's Hospital volunteer would last longer than did the Shamrock Hotel.

But it would.

The formation of a women's volunteer organization at Texas Children's Hospital officially began with an offer from an unexpected source.

"Could you possibly use me and maybe some of my friends?" wrote secretary Freda Magnuson in a letter to hospital director Lee C. Gammill on November 3, 1953.[10]

Working just across the street at the new Southwestern Home Office of Prudential Insurance Company of America, Magnuson had been watching the construction of Texas Children's Hospital progress since 1952. A 19-year-old babysitter whose mother had died the previous June, she had firsthand knowledge of how valuable hospital volunteers were. And, realizing how much she enjoyed working with children, Magnuson decided to offer her services—and those of other Prudential workers, if possible.

Because they worked during the day, Magnuson suggested that their volunteer duties take place in the evenings or on weekends. However, before asking others if they wanted to volunteer with her, she wanted to know if Texas Children's Hospital was interested.

"I hasten to accept," came the quick and ecstatic reply from Gammill, genuinely surprised by the offer. And when the 179 coworkers whom Magnuson recruited to join her arrived for their first meeting at Texas Children's Hospital in late November, Gammill was astounded and "more than very happy" to see them.

"It's extraordinary to have volunteers of this age group (the majority are 19 to 21), vivacious young adults who respond to the ways of children," he said. "And they want night duty, the time when we need them the most, when doctors are making rounds, when we are getting ready for the next day's work and the children are restless and have to be gotten ready for bed."[11]

Gammill did not know exactly how these working women would participate in the activities of the soon-to-be-formed volunteer group, but he was determined to include them in the planning process.

So, several weeks later, on December 9, 1953, at Gammill's invitation, Magnuson joined representatives of various women's organizations who previously had expressed interest in volunteering at Texas Children's Hospital. Gathered by Gammill to discuss the formation of the Women's Auxiliary to Texas Children's Hospital, the women represented Delta Phi Epsilon, Kappa Kappa Gamma, Sigma Delta Tau, Pin Oak Charity Horse Show, the National Council of Jewish Women, the Junior League, and the Sisterhood of Temple Beth Israel. To this list of venerable community organizations, 19-year-old Magnuson added another name, the newly formed "Prudential Girls."

Also introduced at that meeting was Nancy Bateman, a past chairman of the Junior League Children's Clinic at Hermann Hospital, who had been asked by the trustees of Texas Children's Hospital to organize efforts to form a women's group. Bateman, striving to create a concordant union, advised everyone at the meeting to go back to their respective organizations and explain that anyone who joined The Auxiliary would lose her identity with the other group and become an Auxilian.[12]

Next, Bateman asked that each organization send an official representative to the next meeting, on January 18, 1954, to become members of the first board of the Women's Auxiliary to Texas Children's Hospital. Also scheduled to be presented at that meeting was the constitution and by-laws, presented for approval by Mabel Parks and Virginia Noel.

In subsequent planning meetings, with the guidance of older auxiliaries in Houston and with information garnered from the American Hospital Association's *Manual of Women's Auxiliaries,* Bateman and her committee decided that the mission of the Women's Auxiliary to Texas Children's Hospital would be threefold: to provide a service, to raise funds, and to serve as a public relations outlet in the community. The commitment to undertake both service and fund-raising was not the norm for hospital auxiliaries, but Bateman and her committee were convinced that both could be done successfully and they confidently scheduled the first general meeting for February 18, 1954, 17 days after Texas Children's Hospital opened.

On the morning of the meeting, charter members such as Elaine

Kuper in the snack bar and Helen Blumberg at the information desk were already dressed in the approved cherry-red uniforms and were at work as usual when 300 women gathered in the auditorium, adopted the constitution, and made the commitment to join The Auxiliary. Each paid the $1 membership dues and pledged three hours of service per week.

To accomplish the seemingly unwieldy task of coordinating the scheduling and placement of more than 300 volunteers, who collectively had pledged to work 46,800 hours in the first year, Bateman—who was named president of The Auxiliary in March—depended on Lillian Newman, Texas Children's Hospital's newly appointed director of volunteers.

First on Newman's agenda was the requirement that all volunteers attend at least four of the six orientation programs in the auditorium. Featuring a variety of doctors and administration executives, the six programs addressed such topics as "Getting to Know Your Hospital," "What an Auxiliary Can Mean to a Hospital," and "How Texas Children's Hospital Fits into the Pediatric Program at Baylor," presented by Texas Children's Hospital physician-in-chief Blattner.

Also open to volunteers, but not required of them, was a weekly meeting with Blattner and the nursing staff. These meetings featured discussions of general medical topics, as well as the specific medical advancements being made at Texas Children's Hospital and at Baylor.[13]

"One of the features of these activities was the very intimate contact between the medical staff and The Auxiliary," recalled Blattner. "Because of The Auxiliary's interest in the educational programs there was an awful lot of person-to-person contact and mutual discussion and understanding."[14]

Even with all the planned activities, Newman's placement of volunteers into service was a slow process at first. In the early days, she assigned only a few to the most important jobs. But, with the activities of Texas Children's Hospital escalating after the first few months of operation, Newman increased her assignments, placing more than 260 volunteers in six general areas of service: receptionists or floor hostesses, recreation, sewing, clerical work, patient welfare, and snack bar.

Because she had the volunteer support of the Prudential Girls in the evenings, Newman was able to staff the key areas from 8 a.m. to 8 p.m. by instituting four three-hour shifts.

The end result made quite an impression. Everywhere you looked, there were women dressed in cherry-red uniforms. They were answering the phones, directing visitors, running errands for nurses, distributing mail, delivering flowers, accompanying admitted patients to their rooms, interacting with patients' families, delivering specimens to the lab, holding and rocking babies, playing with patients, leading tours, and always being smiling and cheerful.

Behind the scenes, Auxilians were blatantly visible to Texas Children's Hospital staff. Volunteers worked in medical records, filing, indexing, and photostating. They posted requisitions in central service, helped with files and purchase orders in the diet kitchen, and served as ushers at all functions in the auditorium.

Although the value of such Herculean efforts in the first year of The Auxiliary was hard to measure in dollars and cents, there was one area of service that was tallied on a daily basis. It was the strictly bottom-line-oriented snack bar.

Managed and operated completely by Auxilians, who prepared and served reasonably priced sandwiches, salads, cakes and beverages from 8 a.m. to 8 p.m., seven days a week, the small snack bar did big business. Its popularity with visitors, doctors, and employees was clearly evident in its gross revenue for the first fiscal year: $25,139.50.

"The amount of food served during a day was a real surprise to everyone," recalled charter member Julie Finger. "A group of housewives, most of whom had done only weekly household grocery shopping and meal preparation, embarked on what was to become a very successful business venture."[15]

Believing that the snack bar's revenue-producing potential was limited by its size, The Auxiliary asked for and received permission from the board of Texas Children's Hospital to enlarge the facility in 1955. The $4,000 renovation, paid for by The Auxiliary, was completed in November. The results confirmed the hunch. By the end of fiscal year 1957, gross revenue for the enlarged area had increased dramatically to $54,700.11, netting $27,978.36.[16]

With fund-raising activities spearheaded by the successful snack bar, Mabel Parks, elected president of The Auxiliary in 1955, turned her attention to the area of public relations. This was another of The Auxiliary's missions. Parks, who held a degree in journalism from Sam Houston State University, wanted to inform others about Texas Children's Hospital and about the past and future achievements of The Auxiliary. She used the acronym from the Women's Auxiliary of Texas Children's Hospital as the title for a new quarterly publication, *WATCH Magazine*.

Edited by Lee Malcolmson and chronicling the day-to-day activities at Texas Children's Hospital in pictures and words, *WATCH Magazine* debuted in 1955. With a first issue of six pages and an initial print run of 500 copies, Parks had created more than just a vehicle of communication. Published continuously since 1955, WATCH Magazine provided an ongoing history of The Auxiliary and of Texas Children's Hospital.

The first issue contained stories about the founding of The Auxiliary and the creation of its Welfare Fund, which was in need of donations; the history of Pin Oak Charity Horse Show's support of Texas Children's Hospital, written by Dr. David Greer; and a progress report by the newly appointed hospital director, Dr. Maynard W. Martin.

Also included, under the title of "WATCHING" and stylistically resembling a three-dot newspaper gossip column, were snippets of social news about Auxilians and the medical staff. One such item, under the headline "Seen Around About," was the following: "Lillian Newman, Volunteer Director, paying us a visit last week, after her siege with a misplaced disc… We've missed you so, Lillian, and hope you'll be back soon."[17]

Unfortunately, after serving as volunteer director for one year, Newman returned after her absence and announced that she wanted to retire. The administration of Texas Children's Hospital planned to implement an extensive search to replace her, but this proved unnecessary. A patient in the newly opened St. Luke's Episcopal Hospital, Mary Elizabeth "Bess" Patton, heard about the job opening and the work of the volunteers from a visiting friend who was an Auxilian at Texas Children's Hospital. After being discharged from the hospital, she decided to apply for the position. It was a decision that led to a 21-year career at Texas Children's Hospital.

Serving more than two decades as staff director of volunteer services, Patton guided The Auxiliary from infancy to maturity. Instrumental in forming the Texas Association of Staff Directors of Volunteer Services, an affiliate of the Texas Hospital Association, Patton instigated the exchange of ideas and strategies between volunteer programs across the state. Such interaction, together with Patton's innovative ideas, resulted in countless new Auxiliary programs and services at Texas Children's Hospital.

One of the first was the recreation department, organized in 1956 by Auxilians Mrs. Andrew Delaney, a former pediatric nurse, and Mrs. James Harrop, trained in arts and crafts at Peabody College. "The primary purpose of the new recreation program is to meet the basic needs of growing children in a temporary abnormal environment," they told WATCH Magazine in January 1957. "To accomplish this purpose, all effort will be made to create an environment which is as child-centered as possible."[18]

After attending training sessions and demonstrations on how to use arts and crafts with the children, volunteers also attended monthly evening meetings to discuss new ideas and solve problems that had been encountered in their activities with patients. A third-floor play area was staffed for those patients who were not confined to their beds and a cart of age-appropriate projects and toys was wheeled around to those confined to their rooms.

In time, magazines and books for adults also were added to the cart for stressed parents of patients and for other family members. Early each morning, a Prudential Girl stopped by on her way to work and replenished the book cart. During the holiday season, needlepoint kits for tree ornaments were passed out to mothers of patients and an instruction class was offered in The Auxiliary office, where a small tree awaited their finished products.

The product most associated with the recreation department at Texas Children's Hospital was, however, balloons. In 1976, more than 300 gross had been distributed by the always-cheerful volunteers in red uniforms whom the children called the "balloon ladies." The nickname remained long after latex balloons were banned from Texas Children's Hospital in 1990, after being designated as a possible choking hazard. With or without balloons, the volunteers always were a welcome sight to the children.

Also spreading cheer to the patients at Texas Children's Hospital was a program devised by Parks in 1955. Officially named "Patient Pals" in the 1970s, Parks' idea was for volunteers to serve as surrogate family members and friends. Advised by the nursing station when parents needed a short break from caregiving, a volunteer would visit the patient with a book to read or a game to play, freeing parents from the guilt of leaving their child alone.

When Patient Pals became a recognized program in the 1970s, there were playrooms available for patients on each floor. Staffed by volunteers who had been trained by professional child life and play therapists, the playrooms—stocked with games and supplies for arts-and-crafts projects—opened in 1976 and soon became one of the favorite placements for Auxilians.[19]

Also experiencing an increase in popularity was the snack bar. By the late 1950s, it had achieved a glamorous reputation—thanks not only to its reputation for "outrageous" food at "reasonable prices," but also to the photographs taken of the visiting Hollywood stars, European royalty, and heads of state who stopped by during their tours of Texas Children's Hospital.

If not the most famous photograph, certainly the most memorable one captured the moment when comedian Bob Hope stepped behind the counter and made a milkshake for hospital board chairman Leopold L. Meyer in May 1958. After Meyer generously tipped him $100 for the drink, Hope immediately donated the money back to Texas Children's Hospital.[20]

Also being returned to Texas Children's Hospital from the snack bar was more and more revenue from its continually growing business. Renovated again in 1959 to accommodate the crowds, it doubled its original size and capacity by incorporating part of the lobby. Recognizing the need for continuity in service and operation, The Auxiliary hired three paid employees to work alongside the four shifts of volunteers in the expanded snack bar. Giving the operation continuous coverage, the paid staff answered to the volunteer chairman and improved the organization, records reflect, as the volume continued to grow.[21]

Other fund-raising projects in Texas Children's Hospital also flourished. The toy shop grew rapidly over the years, moving from a shelf in the snack bar where it began in 1954 to a cart and then to a closet in an empty elevator shaft. Staffed solely by volunteers and netting more than $35,000 in 1976,[22] the toy shop later evolved into three different shops that were managed by a paid staff supplemented by volunteers. This turned out to be a very profitable venture.

Another profit center for The Auxiliary was the rental of television sets to hospital rooms. Although revenues from this service were modest in the 1950s and 60s, demand increased in the 1970s and 80s. As a way of comparison, rental income in 1964 was $4,554; by 1977, it had jumped to $54,750. When a television set became an integral part of every hospital room in 1987, the rental service was discontinued.[23]

What did continue were the contributions to the Welfare Fund—individual donations made as memorial gifts, profits from vending machines around Texas Children's Hospital, and proceeds from many other different events and projects. Spearheaded by one group of Auxilians were the annual ticket sales to the Pin Oak Charity Horse Show benefiting Texas Children's Hospital. For several years, another group staffed a resale shop, located off site. Others devoted tireless efforts to selling everything from Christmas cards, baked goods, postcards, calendars, matchbook covers, and napkins to raffle tickets for "Fan Harriet" dolls. Named for the late daughter of Adelena and Leopold L. Meyer, each of the dolls was dressed in a design created and donated by Adelena Meyer, who also was a member of The Auxiliary.

With a portion of these collective funds, The Auxiliary participated in the creation of the J. S. Abercrombie Chair in Pediatrics at Baylor College of Medicine in the 1970s. Helping to provide funds for the support of the chairman of pediatrics at Baylor, who also served as the physician-in-chief of Texas Children's Hospital, The Auxiliary honored hospital founder and benefactor Abercrombie.[24]

Ironically, it was Miss Lillie Abercrombie, the honoree's wife, who initiated one of the most popular fund-raising events for The Auxiliary. Named the Silver Tea, this annual gathering was sponsored by The Auxiliary and attended by hundreds of Houstonians. After Miss Lillie hosted the premier effort in her River Oaks Boulevard mansion in 1959, the tradition continued until the early 1990s. Described by an Auxilian as "one of the social highlights in Houston during the winter months," the affair, held at some of Houston's most beautiful homes, became more of a public relations event than a fund-raiser. The Auxiliary decided to discontinue the Silver Tea, but did not falter in fulfilling its mission to provide financial support to Texas Children's Hospital. Instead, the organization generated funds successfully through various efforts within the hospital.

One such effort was a seized opportunity in 1971, when Texas Children's Hospital expanded to 254 beds and St. Luke's Episcopal Hospital was enlarged, adding a towering 26 floors to its building. When asked to oversee the day-to-day operation of the newly constructed 100-seat coffee shop in the reconfigured admitting area for both hospitals, The Auxiliary decided to close the snack bar and accept the challenge.

It was a fortuitous decision. Within a few years, the gross revenue produced each month in the coffee shop exceeded that of the entire first year of the snack bar's operation. Out of necessity, more and more paid employees were hired, resulting in fewer and fewer Auxilians on duty in the coffee shop. However, the management of operations, including staffing, payroll, inventory, and supplies, remained in the hands of The Auxiliary—as did the net proceeds, which were substantial.

And, with its suddenly healthy bank account, in 1977 The Auxiliary began a new phase of service to Texas Children's Hospital. In a tribute to Bess Patton, who had retired as director of volunteer services the previous year, The Auxiliary established the Mary Elizabeth Patton Fellowship in Pediatric Subspecialties. The first recipient was Dr. Virginia Michels, who later became the professor and chairman of medical genetics at the Mayo Clinic.

The Auxiliary established a second fellowship in 1979, the WATCH Fellowship, which was awarded to Dr. Robert Shulman and Dr. Carlos Lifschitz. The two shared both the fellowship and their futures as professors of pediatrics at Baylor College of Medicine.

With a contribution of $100,000 from Mr. and Mrs. Frank P. Horlock in 1981, The Auxiliary established its third fellowship, the Frank Prescott Horlock III Fellowship, in tribute to the Horlocks' late son. The first recipient, Dr. Michael Brady, went on to become a professor of pediatrics and preventative medicine at Ohio State University of Medicine.

Renaming the WATCH Fellowship in 1985 to honor Dr. Russell J. Blattner, the first physician-in-chief at Texas Children's Hospital, The Auxiliary presented the Russell J. Blattner, M.D., Fellowship to Dr. Michele Mariscalco, who later became director of the Leukocyte Function Laboratory at Baylor and Texas Children's Hospital.

Also renamed in 1985 was the Patton Fellowship, which became the Adeline B. Landa Fellowship and was presented to Dr. Mark Kline, who continued at Baylor and became an associate professor of pediatrics.

The Auxiliary's fourth fellowship was established in 1996 to honor the appointment of Dr. Ralph D. Feigin as president of Baylor College of Medicine. First awarded to Dr. Alison A. Bertuch in 1996, the Ralph D. Feigin, M.D., Fellowship was presented to her again in 1997, 1998, and 1999.

With the awarding of the 1999 fellowships, The Auxiliary had invested more than $1.5 million in the pediatric subspecialty training of 40 pediatricians. An investment praised by Feigin as one that "benefits hundreds of thousands of children across the country as a direct result not only of the clinical care, but also the research advances the former fellows have achieved."[25]

But it wasn't just fellowships to which The Auxiliary allocated its funds. The organization converted the abandoned snack bar into a teen room in 1971. And in 1986, when plans for an ambitious building program were announced by Texas Children's Hospital, The Auxiliary pledged $1.5 million to the Building for Children Campaign, payable over a five-year period. After requesting that the contribution be applied to the building of a protected outdoor playground for the hospitalized children—a long-held dream for the Patient Pals program—The Auxiliary was not disappointed. In a sheltered corner near the Abercrombie Building, on the specially reinforced roof of an underground parking lot, an area specifically designed for hospital patients was built.

Dedicated on November 17, 1991, the Get Well Playground featured special slides and swings that were accessible for wheelchair-bound children, large sandboxes, and a boat-like structure containing support services for those who were playing there. Call systems to the nursing floors, oxygen, and emergency buttons were strategically placed close by and the emergency center was only a short distance away. Best of all, the sophisticated design was not intimidating to the children, a fact confirmed by observing the patients who happily played there immediately following the dedication ceremonies. The Auxiliary again had made a wise investment.[26]

With funds seriously depleted after fulfilling the $1.5 million pledge for the Get Well Playground, as well as supporting the ongoing fellowship programs, the Abercrombie Chair and numerous other disbursements for patient needs, special projects, nurses' wish lists, and medical equipment, The Auxiliary had to replenish its bank account.

Dependence on proceeds from the coffee shop was no longer an option in the early 1980s. Gen McClelland, the director of volunteer services since 1976, had decided that the coffee shop was both an enormous responsibility and a huge worry. Because of the ever-increasing volume of business, only one volunteer was working there as a cashier while the rest were paid employees. The hiring, firing, and managing of the coffee shop's paid personnel, not to mention the accounts payable and receivable, were time-consuming tasks from which McClelland wished to be freed. "We were so successful, we put ourselves out of business," recalled Mary Liz Grose, Auxiliary historian.[27]

However, knowing that the loss of the coffee shop's revenues could severely impact The Auxiliary's services, and not wishing to proverbially kill the goose who laid the golden egg, McClelland had a suggestion: Why not research the possibility of having a restaurant operation lease and operate the space?

This idea was embraced enthusiastically by the hospital's administration. McDonald's Corporation was contacted to determine if the company wanted to become involved. With its franchises already operating in other hospitals, McDonald's was indeed interested. "They said they would come in, gut the old coffee shop, and pay for all of the remodeling costs," McClelland recalled. "They also said The Auxiliary would get a percentage of their business and a guarantee."

Other restaurants also expressed interest, offering similar financial arrangements. However, because of the hospital's association with the Ronald McDonald House, the McDonald's bid was accepted. An independently conducted nutritional study of foods to be served in the restaurant allayed all worries about quality control, and the new McDonald's at Texas Children's Hospital opened in 1987.

Ever since the first Big Mac off the McDonald's grill was served to McClelland, The Auxiliary's bank account has been richly enhanced by golden arches instead of golden eggs. "It's one of the biggest moneymakers in their operation and the largest in Houston," McClelland said. "It has the highest volume and costs us nothing. Because of this, we were able to build up The Auxiliary's bank account again after giving $1.5 million to the building fund."[28]

McClelland also was responsible for the opening of other new vistas for the Texas Children's Auxiliary. Affectionately tagged "Sarge" by a volunteer's husband, she had the ability to muster her troops effectively. In one such effort, McClelland organized and led a two-week trip to Ecuador so that six Auxilians could visit Boca Ortiz Hospital, the only children's hospital in Quito. As part of an exchange program, the Auxilians served as consultants to the women who volunteered at that hospital, sharing their expertise and ideas. They also visited more than five general hospitals, schools, and treatment centers in Quito and the surrounding area. It was an eye-opening experience for all.

After returning home, Joan Reuther, one of the Auxilians in the group, spearheaded a campaign to gather sorely needed clothes, appliances, medical equipment, and supplies for the Quito hospitals. Her one-woman campaign, wholeheartedly supported by The Auxiliary and Texas Children's Hospital, resulted in a warehouse full of not only the needed medical items and equipment, but also bed linens, pillows, children's clothes and pajamas, kitchen utensils, stoves, dishwashers, clothes washers and dryers, fans, heaters, and air conditioners. The Ecuadorian consul in Houston shipped the collected supplies to Boca Ortiz Hospital.

Such a caring and giving attitude was second nature to members of The Auxiliary, who ranged in age from teenagers in the junior program to grandmothers. During McClelland's tenure as director of volunteer services, the membership consisted mainly of women in their thirties and forties. Feeling it was beneficial for all the volunteers, regardless of age, to establish close friendships, McClelland encouraged them to eat together in The Auxiliary's boardroom whenever they could. As a former volunteer, "Sarge" knew that such camaraderie was good not only for the morale of the troop, but also for that of the children in Texas Children's Hospital and their families.

It was this commitment to the health, education, and welfare of patients that led to McClelland's focusing her energies on legislative action that affected children's hospitals. With her guidance, the Texas Children's Auxiliary became active in both state and national legislative issues. McClelland also was responsible for inspiring the establishment of The Auxiliary's first fellowship programs for pediatric subspecialties.

Also during McClelland's era, The Auxiliary's many other programs flourished and its traditions of decorating Texas Children's Hospital for holidays, hosting birthday parties for patients, organizing special events in the lobby, and leading celebrities on tours of Texas Children's Hospital continued without interruption. "Those were the golden years," recalled charter life member Elaine Kuper. "Everybody knew everybody. If, for some reason, you didn't join the group for lunch one day, someone would call and say 'Are you all right?' We really were a close group when Gen was here. But it's all changed, now."[29]

Changes in The Auxiliary were inevitable. Over the years, as the former 106-bed hospital grew to become one of the largest pediatric care facilities in the world, the services performed by Auxilians expanded in some areas and diminished in others. By the early 1990s, instead of volunteering in only one building, the Texas Children's Auxilians found themselves assigned to various areas in the hospital's multiple structures, both on and off the main campus. In some cases, such as the multiple information desks, their services no longer were required and their jobs were assigned to paid personnel.

Also changing was the constituency of The Auxiliary. Although varying in number from year to year, it was not the average age of members that was different. It was their gender. In 1986, men officially were enlisted as members, necessitating a change in nomenclature. The word "Women's" was dropped and the organization became The Auxiliary to Texas Children's Hospital. So welcomed was male participation in The Auxiliary that in 1996 a man was elected as the group's president.

The program instigated by the Prudential Girls in 1954 continued to benefit the patients at Texas Children's Hospital. With the increased use of flextime options and four-day workweeks offered by employers, more and more working women and men began volunteering. Some participated in one-time events, while others continued the pattern set by the first "professional" volunteers and worked in shifts at night and during the weekends.

As the number of volunteers grew, The Auxiliary's office needed to expand. From its original location on the fifth floor of Texas Children's Hospital, the office was moved from one location to another, finally landing on the first floor of the Abercrombie Building, close to where the original snack bar had been located in 1954.

By 2004, there were more than 1,700 members of The Auxiliary to Texas Children's Hospital. Identified as individual, corporate, and organization volunteers and placed in 60 different areas, they collectively contributed more than 75,000 hours of service in 2003. Individual volunteers automatically became members of The Auxiliary and were the responsibility of Pat Dolan, director of volunteer services and patient relations, who operated the department like a well-oiled machine.

"To be considered a current Auxiliary member, you're supposed to volunteer six hours a month to keep your active status," Dolan said. "If you work less than that for a consistent number of months, you get a letter that asks: 'Are you unhappy in your placement? Can we help you? Do you need a leave of absence?' We feel if you are not here six hours a month, there's a reason why, so let's figure it out and fix it. We'd rather you be happy than upset. Because Texas Children's Hospital is open 24 hours a day, there is always something to do. We can find you a job that you will like."[30]

By the late 1990s, Dolan could offer more than 100 volunteer placement opportunities at Texas Children's Hospital. Volunteers staffed the sno-cone cart, art cart, book cart, humor cart, and recreation cart. They escorted patients to waiting rooms and clinics, ran errands, tutored patients, organized craft sessions, and played with children. They could be found interacting with patients in the playrooms, teen room, pre-teen room, Get Well Playground, and Patient Pals programs. They assisted the patients who ran the in-house radio station broadcasts on Radio Lollipop. They offered educational assistance as teachers aides, worked in the Pi Beta Phi Patient/Family Library, and hosted bingo games, movies, and various weekend activities. Or, like Kuper, they performed office and clerical duties in departments throughout Texas Children's Hospital.

Since 1954, Auxiliary members had served more than one million volunteer hours and raised more than $3 million to help support pediatric patient care, education, and research at Texas Children's Hospital. With proceeds from sales at its three toy and gift shops, income from the McDonald's restaurant at Texas Children's Hospital, and donations from individuals and organizations in the community, The Auxiliary donated more than $1 million to underwrite fellowships for outstanding young doctors in more than 40 pediatric subspecialties. In addition to the $1.5 million donated to build a special playground accessible to all children, Auxiliary funds were utilized for the purchase of the little extras that make a young patient's stay more pleasant, such as rocking chairs, games, puzzles, and toys. Through its Wish List, The Auxiliary also assisted departments throughout Texas Children's Hospital with special grants for specific equipment and program needs. But its contribution in kindness to patients and their parents was incalculable.

"There are many warm fuzzies that go along with this business," Dolan said. "Often it's the little things patients and parents remember— the man who played cards, the teen who pushed the sno-cone cart, the tutor who helped with algebra. Many of their positive comments just can't be measured."[31]

What could be counted was the growing number of male volunteers of every age at Texas Children's Hospital. Men represented more than one-third of The Auxiliary in 2004 and Dolan expected their numbers to increase, particularly among young adults. "It's not unusual today to see a 38-year-old man here after work in the evenings," she said. "He takes off his business coat, puts on a red vest, and works. Or you might see a young medical student who comes in at 8 p.m. to work in the emergency center until midnight."

Such nighttime volunteering had become the norm in the late 1990s for most Auxilians at Texas Children's Hospital. Reflecting a major evolution from the beginning decades when volunteers donated their time on weekdays, nearly 60 percent of the 1,700 volunteers in 2004 could be found at Texas Children's Hospital at nights and on weekends.

With all of these developments, one thing remained unchanged since the beginning. Dressed in their distinctively colored vests, jackets, or pinafores—the original cherry red having evolved into a brilliant red—Texas Children's Auxilians excelled in providing loving care and service to the children and their families in Texas Children's Hospital, raising much-needed funds and serving as public relations representatives to the community.

This was the mission that had been established in 1954 at the inception of The Auxiliary and it was destined to continue in perpetuity at Texas Children's Hospital. "People often question why someone would want to volunteer at a children's hospital," Dolan said. "I guess they think it must be sad or depressing. Actually, nothing could be further than the truth. These kids are hurting and a volunteer has the opportunity to make them feel better. One person can make a difference in a child's life. There's a lot of joy here."[32]

As of February 18, 2000, Elaine Kuper had volunteered at Texas Children's Hospital continuously every Tuesday morning for more than 46 years. In addition, she had volunteered on Fridays for more than 32 years.

Helen Blumberg, the neighbor who invited her to join the Texas Children's Auxiliary in 1954, and Kuper were the two remaining charter members at Texas Children's Hospital. Their lengthy association with Texas Children's Hospital had outlasted the life of the legendary Shamrock Hotel by eight years—and counting. After surviving for less than 38 years, the hotel was demolished in 1987.

In appreciation for her service, the 77-year-old Kuper has been awarded with honorary lifetime membership in The Auxiliary, as well as legendary status. Both are mantles she has worn with modesty.

This was not surprising. From the beginning, Kuper's reasons for volunteering were not for personal recognition, but rather to satisfy her desire to help others selflessly and cheerfully. So strong was that desire that Kuper doubled her original commitment from working three hours a week to six.

"When the kids were in high school, I wanted to work two days a week and asked if I could work at the information desk," Kuper—dressed in her red vest, white shirt, and black slacks—recently recalled. "After 14 years, I gave up the snack bar because by then it had turned into the coffee shop and there were few jobs for volunteers. I loved it at the front desk and worked there two days a week."[33]

"We tried to do anything we could do to help. Every day was an experience. It really was fun," recalled Kuper. "We always said 'Keep a smile on your face' and 'Be positive,' because that's what patients and their families expected."

"We had all the records from St. Luke's, so we could help the patients from both hospitals. It was like being a detective. We did all the work for the admitting office. All the paperwork, all the lab reports, we did everything. We took the children up to their rooms. Ran errands. Delivered the mail. Led tours. Helped the visiting ministers. We knew every patient and family by name. We knew every doctor. And they knew us. I absolutely adored the front desk."

Such a recognizable fixture at that desk on Friday mornings over the years, Kuper said that many doctors used to come in the door, stop, and say, "Oh, it must be Friday."

Although her Friday assignment remained the same for years, Kuper never found herself bored with the routine. In fact, there was no routine. Each day at the desk was unpredictable, at best. And she always tried to learn something new rather than be complacent with the old.

For instance, Kuper knew she could help some of the non-English-speaking patients and their families more than she already had. Although she had taken Spanish in high school, she felt inadequate in her conversation skills and enrolled in a course at Houston Community College to learn more. Afterwards, she said, "I was able to at least understand a little of what they were saying and could direct them to the right place. There was someone in the toy shop who could speak Spanish, so I could take them there, if need be. We just did the best we could. It's a blessing to be able to speak Spanish. I loved the challenge and helping people."

With such a generous spirit, Kuper easily befriended patients and their families, Texas Children's Hospital staff, and her fellow Auxilians at the front desk. Many of these relationships became long-lasting friendships, especially those involving members of The Auxiliary.

"Julie Finger, a former president of The Auxiliary and a charter member, and I worked together at the front desk for years. She was my superior and so knowledgeable. She taught me so much about the hospital and insisted I get on the board for just one year," Kuper recalled. "What has it been? Thirty-something years now? Once you're on the board, you find you are president and chairman of everything. I held every office except treasurer."

Kuper's involvement with the board represented a dramatic change. She admitted that while working at the snack bar for fourteen years, she really hadn't known anything about what was going on in Texas Children's Hospital. It was not her priority. What was important to her, she did know: sandwiches were 25 cents apiece, coffee was a nickel, and milkshakes were a dime.

What soon attracted Kuper's attention as a member of the board were the inner workings of The Auxiliary, its interaction with the administration of Texas Children's Hospital, and its fund-raising activities. Elected president in 1977, she found herself involved with every aspect of the operation from 1977 to 1978.

But, if the truth were known, it was working at the front desk that had captured Kuper's heart and fueled her energy to be of service. Helping patients and their families is what she always wanted to do, first and foremost. "It's so wonderful to do something for people because you want to do it, not to be paid for it," she said. "When I am here, I don't worry about anything larger than what I am doing. I have loved every day of it. I can't wait; I count every hour until I can come. I love it so. I love whatever they ask me to do. I'm glad to do it. I feel like it is my family."

When asked about her amazing accumulation of 17,000 hours of service, Kuper replied with a shrug: "Two days a week for more than 40 years adds up, you know."

Adding to her hours for the past ten years, Kuper has worked as a "gofer" in The Auxiliary office. It was a job she created for herself in the late 1980s, when it temporarily was decided that paid employees and security personnel were going to work at the front desk and volunteers no longer were needed there.

Leaving her beloved Tuesday and Friday job was not easy for Kuper, but she understood why changes had to be made. Although she missed the interaction with patients, their families, and hospital staff, she knew she could be of service in the office. After all, she had worked professionally for five years in an office in the early 1940s, and what she didn't know, she could learn, she told herself.

Although Kuper remained "computer illiterate" and therefore unable to work full-time at the information desk in the Abercrombie Building, she was able to substitute for others there, when needed. Having taught herself how to run the fax machine and the photocopier, she was hesitant to tell others of her typing skills, fearing ponderous assignments. But realizing how much she could contribute, she quickly confessed. And, as predicted, Kuper soon found herself doing all the typing, as well as the mailing and filing.

"Whatever they ask me to do, I'll do," Kuper explained, unnecessarily. For more than 49 years at Texas Children's Hospital, she always had done exactly that: whatever was asked of her. Helping countless children and their families and inspiring multitudes in the process, Kuper was honored with the Mayor's Award in 1998 as the outstanding volunteer in Houston's health community.

Five decades after coming to Texas Children's Hospital as a volunteer, "I am now computer literate and am still volunteering and still love it," Kuper said in 2004.

Even though the expression was used to describe all Houstonians in 1954, it was Elaine Kuper at Texas Children's Hospital who truly turned out to be "one in a million."

8

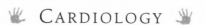

❧ CARDIOLOGY ❧

I<small>T BEGAN WITH A MURMUR.</small>

A little heart murmur was detected with a pediatrician's stethoscope. It happened hours after identical twins Karly and Kestly Tinklepaugh were delivered by cesarean section on October 24, 1994, at Northwest Medical Center in Houston. Pediatrician Dr. Bin Sung advised parents Jill and Scott Tinklepaugh that both of their newborn daughters, who also looked a little jaundiced, should see a cardiologist about the murmurs. "We had no idea it was anything to worry about," Jill remembered, thinking of that exact moment.[1]

But soon after the couple returned home from the hospital with the twins, they received a telephone call from Sung's office. An appointment had been made for them with a pediatric cardiologist, they were told. "What's the hurry?" Jill asked.

That question was soon answered. The identical twins had identical congenital heart defects, according to the pediatric cardiologist. "That doctor was the first person who diagnosed them with what they have," Scott recalled. "They had all sorts of tests. We were there four or five hours. It was a very long day. And finally they took us into a room and explained to us and it just ... walls went up! He was very gentle and very professional in telling us, but I thought 'not my babies.'"[2]

The diagnosis was tetralogy of Fallot, a combination of four different heart defects: narrowed and underdeveloped pulmonary arteries, a ventricular septal defect, a misplaced aorta overriding the ventricular septum, and an enlarged right ventricle. The most common form of cyanotic congenital heart defects, or "blue heart" disease, tetralogy of Fallot might require palliative surgery to increase the levels of circulating oxygen in the blood, the doctor told them. The Tinklepaughs were dumbfounded.

The twins, although small in size—Karly was 4 pounds and Kestly was 5.3 pounds—did not look blue, the telltale physical sign of cyanosis. To their parents, they looked and acted like normal one-month-old babies. "He told us we could go home, and gave us his home phone, cell phone, and pager, and told us we needed, in a week or two, to make an appointment at Texas Children's Hospital with the pediatric cardiologist, Dr. Bricker," said Scott. "And this all happened on Thursday."

The following Saturday night, Jill awakened to find that Karly was gasping for air and had turned blue. Scott immediately called 911. "When the ambulance came, the emergency medical service personnel checked her out and said, 'She's fine' and 'Don't worry about it,' but we called the cardiologist and he said, 'You had better bring them to the Texas Children's Hospital,'" Jill remembered.

"We found out later it's what they call a 'tet spell,'" Scott interjected. "We didn't know that because they had not forewarned us about the tet spell."

"But if we hadn't called the doctor, she would have died," Jill continued. "Karly stopped breathing on the way to the hospital. Completely stopped breathing. We were riding along in the ambulance and I looked down at her and said, 'She looks funny. Doesn't she look a funny color? Sort of gray?' And the ambulance crew says, 'Oh, my God!' and then they put oxygen on her and all that stuff. And then we started going real fast."

Closely following Karly and Jill in a second ambulance that night were Scott and Kestly. As soon as they arrived at Texas Children's Hospital, both babies were examined and admitted as patients. "They checked us in and then it must have been the next morning, Sunday, when Dr. Bricker came in and talked to us," Scott said.

Doctor J. Timothy Bricker, chief of pediatric cardiology at Texas Children's Hospital and professor and chief of the Lillie Frank Abercrombie Section of Cardiology in the department of pediatrics at Baylor College of Medicine, first met the Tinklepaughs in the twins' room at Texas Children's Hospital. Bricker explained tetralogy of Fallot to them again, advised them that the twins would have to be tested, and assured them that there was a palliative, or temporary repair, surgical procedure—the Blalock-Taussig shunt—that could be performed should the tests indicate such heart surgery was absolutely necessary.

It was. After complete clinical examinations, full blood counts, chest X-rays, electrocardiograms, cardiac catheterizations, and echocardiograms, doctors confirmed that Karly and Kestly had identical severe cases of tetralogy of Fallot, the four-part disorder named after the French doctor who first described the condition in 1888. Bricker told Jill and Scott that it was possible their babies would not live more than a few months without immediate palliative surgery.

Once again, the Tinklepaughs were speechless. "I spent four years in the U.S. Marine Corps. Usually any problems we have I can take care of and straighten out, but this was something that was out of my hands," Scott remembered. "The possibility of losing two babies was there."

Bricker understood their feelings of apprehension. To help calm their fears, he explained the history of the Blalock-Taussig shunt procedure, an operation first performed in 1944 on a "blue baby" at Johns Hopkins in Baltimore, Maryland. The surgery, which creates increased blood flow to the lungs, involves the insertion of a shunt between the aorta, or a branch artery and one of the branch pulmonary arteries.

"When the surgery was first being done in Houston in the late 50s and early 60s, it was really quite a remarkable thing," Bricker told them. After pointing out the recent medical and surgical advances in the treatment of tetralogy of Fallot, he reassured them that "now the long-term prognosis is good."[3]

Scott remembered the exact conversation: "Dr. Bricker gave us the complete history. He brought pictures in, and we have them now all over the house in boxes and stuff. We got an education. He told us medical details, pictures, everything."[4]

Bricker called in cardiac surgeon Dr. David A. Ott and the surgeries were scheduled for Tuesday, two days before Thanksgiving. "It took two and a half hours for each operation, plus a 30-minute break for Dr. Ott. After a matter of about six hours, we walked into the pediatric intensive care unit at Texas Children's Hospital. There they were. Two babies, 5 pounds and 6 pounds each, and out of the main artery is a tube to keep the blood flowing, to allow more blood circulation and flow, catheters, respirators to keep their lungs going and breathing for them. They would be in the pediatric intensive care unit for two days," Scott vividly recalled.[5]

"I slept in the pediatric intensive care unit," said Scott. "The nurses even let me, because I had two of them there. They brought a chair out to me in the pediatric intensive care unit and let me sit in the corner there for the first night they were in there. I could stay there all night. Whenever I woke up and wanted to go back and look, instead of standing there for 20 minutes, I could sit down and look through the window and watch them. And watch the nurses."

Knowing one of them would have to remain there, the Tinklepaughs had decided that Scott would stay with the twins at the hospital and Jill would go home to look after their other two daughters, five-year-old Taylor and three-and-a-half-year-old Shelby. For Thanksgiving dinner, Jill and the two older girls went to the home of Jill's parents, Jo Anne and John Bruskotter. Alone at the hospital, Scott shared a covered-dish, holiday supper with other families who had children in the pediatric intensive care unit. "That was the hardest part," said Jill. "You know, most people want to be with their kids, but sometimes you just can't. I mean, you've got a life at home. You've got a life at the hospital. My parents were very helpful. People who don't have anybody to help them, I don't know what they do."

After Karly and Kestly had been moved to a room, the twins were so tiny that they were placed in a single bassinet. Scott was amazed by how quickly the twins were healing and how they were crying. He later commented that babies don't know they're supposed to lie still when they're recovering from an operation. And because they don't do that, he reasoned, they heal faster.

Regardless, Scott had decided that the twins were too loud and he should keep them quiet. So he sat close by their bed, and each time one of the babies would cry, he would put a bottle in her mouth and the crying would stop. He was very proud of his accomplishment. However, when one of the nurses questioned Scott's overfeeding of the twins, he replied defensively: "They would only drink an eighth of an ounce, you couldn't even measure it."

"Dad, you're fired," the nurse smiled. "You don't feed babies no more." And from that moment on the former Marine was "at ease." Each 12-hour shift, a nurse fed the babies. Whenever Scott wanted to take a break or get a breath of fresh air, the nurses placed the twins in a safe area behind their station so that they could keep an eye on them. The nurses also watched the babies at night, so that Scott could sleep. "Everyone at Texas Children's was just wonderful," Jill said. "Every department we were in. They're all wonderful people."

Karly and Kestly and Scott stayed in the hospital for eight days. "And it was right on the money as to what Dr. Bricker had told us they were going to be in. He hit it right on the nose," Scott declared.

Told by Bricker to return for a checkup in a month or two, the Tinklepaughs celebrated a joyous Christmas at home and returned to Texas Children's Hospital with the twins in January 1995. It was then that Bricker told the parents that both girls would have to have another surgery to correct the four defects in tetralogy of Fallot. The ideal age for the open-heart procedure, he said, would be when they were two years old.

"He said they wanted to wait until they were two to do the corrective procedure because at two, they're still baby enough but they're growing so quickly that they'll heal so quick," Scott said. "Dr. Bricker told us to take them home and love them and if we needed anything, he gave me all of his phone numbers. He said, 'Not just medical, anything. You got any questions, call me.' He was very open with us."

So the Tinklepaugh family did what they were told. They took Karly and Kestly home. And loved them. And waited.

During the late 1940s, the methods physicians used to identify tetralogy of Fallot and other congenital heart defects were strictly by the book.

One book, to be precise—titled *Congenital Malformations of the Heart*, written by Dr. Helen B. Taussig, and published in 1947. Upon its publication, the author soon became the recognized expert on the subject. But her name was well-known in the medical community even before the book was published, mostly because Taussig's simple and brilliant concept of surgical palliation of tetralogy of Fallot had been proven valid. In November 1944, Johns Hopkins surgeon Dr. Alfred Blalock successfully performed the Blalock-Taussig shunt procedure on a fourteen-month-old girl with cyanotic congenital heart disease. The immediate improvement in color and mobility of the former blue baby was visibly noticeable to all, doctors and family alike. And the resulting media coverage of this startling medical breakthrough gave the first tangible hope of survival for a child with cyanotic congenital heart disease. The word "incurable" no longer would precede the words "blue baby."[6]

The other good news was that *Congenital Malformations of the Heart* was easy to read and understand. Written in Taussig's clear and precise language and presented in a simple style, the book offered an explanation of systemic blood flow in the different complex anomalies. Such simplifications of the complexities made it possible for physicians who studied the pages to understand the features necessary to diagnose various congenital cardiac defects.[7]

One such physician was Houston pediatrician Dr. George W. Salmon, the acknowledged authority on congenital heart disease in the Houston area in the 1940s. With no formal training in pediatric cardiology, Salmon admitted that he had been self-taught by the book: "... in those days, I held cardiac clinic with a stethoscope in one hand and Dr. Taussig's book in the other."[8]

His was not a singular experience. The book had widespread appeal and became not only a vital tool for physicians throughout the United States and abroad, but also the "Bible" on which the discipline of pediatric cardiology was built. And to many of those who chose to enter that newly developed field, it was the primary stimulus.

One, in particular, was Dr. Dan Goodrich McNamara, a 1946 graduate of Baylor College of Medicine in Houston. As a pediatric resident at Houston's Hermann Hospital, McNamara had borrowed Salmon's "dog-eared" book. He was so intrigued with what he had read and learned about congenital heart defects that he decided to travel to Baltimore and apply for a fellowship with Taussig at Johns Hopkins.[9]

It was a pivotal decision—one that shaped not only McNamara's career, but also that of countless other medical professionals.[10] And therein lies the story of the 50-year history and limitless future of the pediatric cardiology service at Texas Children's Hospital. It was, is, and will be an endless chain of noteworthy events—a chain in which McNamara always was, and always will be, inextricably linked.

Planning for the pediatric cardiology service began in the early 1950s, several years before the opening of the hospital. Dr. Russell J. Blattner, physician-in-chief at Texas Children's Hospital and chief of the department of pediatrics at Houston's Baylor College of Medicine, was looking for a dedicated clinician to help build Houston's heart program for children. He also needed a trained pediatric cardiologist to head the cardiac clinic at the new Texas Children's Hospital, scheduled to open in 1954. Blattner found exactly who he was looking for at Johns Hopkins in 1952—a Taussig fellow by the name of McNamara.

After being successfully recruited by Blattner, McNamara continued his two-year training with Taussig. He began making plans for his return to Houston in 1953. As Houston's first pediatric cardiologist, he knew that he would be the lone pioneer in a vast frontier. Even with his responsibilities as an instructor in pediatrics at Baylor College of Medicine and as the head of the cardiac clinic at Texas Children's Hospital, McNamara was worried. What if there were not enough patients to keep him busy? An alternate plan was devised.

He decided that he also would go into private pediatric practice. In a letter to Blattner dated November 9, 1952, McNamara stated: "I plan to have a private general pediatric practice in addition to my work at the clinic. I should like to ask if you can estimate now the amount of time that I would be spending a week at the cardiac clinic. The catheterizations would require about half a day—a work-up on a new patient may take 2 hours."

McNamara also addressed his projected needs for the clinic: "As you might imagine I have formed some rather definite notions about the equipment needed in a heart clinic. The expense of a catheterization lab will at least equal that of the radiology unit. I will be glad to make a list of the needs of such a lab at your direction."[11]

Later, McNamara learned that already in 1952 Blattner had contacted the Houston Chapter of the Texas Heart Association and requested "diagnostic equipment" for the "pediatric-cardio-respitory center" at Texas Children's Hospital. In February 1953, Blattner received a $20,000 grant for the equipment. Orders were placed to McNamara's specifications and the requested equipment arrived in Houston shortly before he returned from Johns Hopkins.

When Houston's first pediatric cardiologist arrived on the scene, the occasion generated news coverage. "Hospital Services for Children Expand Rapidly," a story in the *Houston Chronicle* announced on September 27, 1953: "For children with heart disease it is good news that a pediatric cardiologist with two years special training at Johns Hopkins Children's cardiac clinic begins work at the Texas Children's Hospital."

Even with the media attention and the community excitement about the opening of the new hospital and its state-of-the-art cardiac clinic, McNamara remained anxious about his future and the possible insufficient workload. He worried whether he "would ever see enough children with heart disease to justify getting up each day."

To address this imagined predicament, McNamara ordered 1,000 announcements, which he intended to send all over the state of Texas. The printed cards listed the address and phone numbers of the cardiac clinic at Texas Children's Hospital and McNamara's private practice on Montrose Boulevard. He figured that it would only take an hour or two to address and mail them—something he would do in his spare time, which was something he would have plenty of, he figured. He was wrong. After six months, there were so many patients in the cardiac clinic that McNamara closed the office on Montrose and moved full-time to his office at Texas Children's Hospital.

Twenty-five years later, McNamara confessed: "I got so busy, my secretary would say, 'When are you going to send out those announcement cards?' And I said, 'Well, I don't have time. Let's do it next month.' To this day, April 30, 1979, I still have those cards. All 1,000 of them. But they make wonderful notepads, you know. I'm serious. Excellent quality paper, and you can write notes. I'm serious."[12]

The success of the cardiac clinic at Texas Children's Hospital was evident from day one. One reason for the immediate and hectic pace can be attributed to the self-taught pediatric cardiologist and pediatrician who had lent McNamara the book that had changed his career. The day the clinic opened—February 9, 1954—McNamara received a phone call. "We have 60 patients for you here," Dr. George Salmon told him. "How do you want them? One at a time? Two at a time? Just how?"[13]

Another influential factor in the clinic's initial success was the policy of a Dallas pediatrician, Dr. Gladys Fashena, who founded a specialty clinic for children with heart murmurs at the Children's Medical Center of Dallas in 1939. In those days, there was little that could be done for babies with congenital heart defects, so Fashena's policy was not to see infants in the clinic. She told the parents, "When the child is two years old, come back." But many of these babies did not live to become two years of age. Some did not live past the age of one and a great number died during the first three months of their lives. Because of this, instead of sending their infant patients to Fashena, who would tell them to come back later, referring physicians contacted McNamara, who said, "Send them down, we will see them immediately." So the parents bundled up their babies and headed for Houston and Texas Children's Hospital.

In retrospect, McNamara opined, "I think it was this policy of Dallas that really got us started. I believe Dr. Fashena unwittingly gave us a great boost because all the infants would end up coming here. Of course, 90 percent of the mortality of congenital heart patients is in the first year of life. We tried to concentrate on early diagnosis and early treatment of these very small children. Plus the fact George Salmon referred all his consultations to us."

Over the first few years, the number of patients dramatically increased and, consequently, so did the space allotted to the cardiac clinic. Where all these patients came from was one thing; where they all went was another. It was to the Junior League Diagnostic Clinic of the outpatient department at Texas Children's Hospital. For Frances M. Heyck, longtime executive secretary of the Junior League clinic, the sudden influx of heart patients was memorable. "I used to kid Dr. Dan McNamara all the time," she recalled. "One of the first things they did not foresee—nobody foresaw—the tremendous immediate growth of the cardiology service. There were no plans in the hospital for a cardiology suite of offices and cath labs and so forth, so guess whom they took them from. It was the clinic. So his first office was part of our immediate office space for the clinic, Junior League clinic, right quick.

I used to kid him, saying 'creeping cardiology,' and he would take more and more and more. Because it just exploded. The technology became available and Dr. Denton Cooley came about that time and the whole cardiology experience kind of exploded! I mean it was just an immediate need for larger quarters. Nobody had foreseen it."[14]

Heyck's "creeping cardiology" also applied to the cardiac clinic's staff. McNamara had been its part-time, one-person occupant when the clinic opened in 1954. Two years later, the cardiac clinic staff consisted of a full-time director, a National Heart Institute research fellow, a consultant for the diagnostic clinic, a consultant for cardiac catheterization, two nurses, a nurse's aide, three technicians, and a secretary. The radiologist, thoracic surgeon, and staff pediatrician were available for consultation when needed.

From the day the clinic opened, the fact that McNamara had an office at all was noteworthy, no matter the size. He often credited Blattner with the idea of establishing a full-time office in the hospital for the pediatric cardiologist. At the time, it was an unheard of luxury for such a clinician to have a private office on the premises. Blattner's reasoning for such an innovative setup was sound, McNamara said. Patients with congenital malformations were often acutely ill, requiring a clinician to be close by them at all times. In addition, the diagnostic work-up on these patients required hospital facilities and special equipment that were not available elsewhere. McNamara's office was one of the first of its kind, not only in Houston hospitals, but also across the state.

Although small and cramped, McNamara's original office was the envy of radiologist Dr. Edward B. Singleton, the first physician on staff at the hospital. He always could be found there in the early morning, reading the newspaper and drinking coffee. But it wasn't just the office he coveted—it was the private bathroom adjoining it. But "creeping cardiology" took its toll on that singular luxury. Remembered Singleton: "One of the greatest disappointments of my life in my friend McNamara was the fact that he turned his private bathroom into a library."[15] It was "a long narrow library, the only green tile library in Houston," McNamara responded.[16]

The first catheterization laboratory also was minuscule. At the time, Blattner said that when the team of doctors and technicians were in it, they almost had to breathe in unison to survive. "This was not an exaggeration," he said.[17] Regardless of its size, the cath lab soon became one of the most active centers in the cardiac clinic. "We did our first heart catheterization in September of 1955," McNamara recalled. "So, the hospital opened in February of 1954 and we did our first catheterization about 18 months later.

A young man, I still remember him very well. He had an atrial septal defect and went on to have surgery. Dr. Earl Beard had had catheterization experience at the Mayo Clinic with Dr. Earl Wood. And Dr. Beard is an adult cardiologist, and a very fine one, but he had not had much experience with children, but he had really had more experience with catheterization than I had had, although I had had some exposure at Hopkins. Dr. Beard had had a lot more in setting up the equipment of the laboratory itself and he was a tremendous help to me. And I'll never forget it."[18]

Cardiac catheterization—the threading of a specialized catheter up through the large blood vessels and into the heart under X-ray guidance—was one of the limited number of sophisticated methods for diagnosing heart disease available in the early 1950s. Since all of the X-ray equipment in the Texas Children's Hospital's catheterization laboratory had been designed for use with adults, not children, McNamara challenged two pediatric cardiology fellows, Dr. Joseph R. Latson and Dr. Robert D. Leachman, to design and customize the facility for pediatric use.

By the late 1950s, Latson and Leachman had established a diagnostic cardiac catheterization laboratory that greatly improved the accurate diagnosing of heart problems in children. Latson began working with the first image-intensifying fluoroscope to improve its application to angiographic study of congenital defects. Finding that the placement of the X-ray tube four-to-six feet beneath the patient minimized the distortion present in the pictures taken of the heart, he created the new mounting, thereby allowing the entire heart to be shown on the film. Next, he developed a hydraulic support system for monitoring two intensifying fluoroscopes to record biplane cineangiograms. Latson's innovations, improvisations, and designs for new apparatus soon were recognized and replicated worldwide.[19]

Reminiscing in 1979 about the first catheterization laboratory, McNamara said: "I suspected then that the cath lab equipment all together would have cost maybe $25,000–$30,000. Now, these days, to set up a cath lab takes about half a million dollars. So, the point is, within this period of time, in this 25 years that the equipment has changed so much, we can do a better job. We can do a better catheterization. But that's how the equipment has changed. So, there's a lot more to it than you would think. It takes people and it takes your equipment but it takes testing the equipment first to make sure it's absolutely correct. You know, if you have a new automobile and it goes out of order, it does nothing but stop or maybe backfire or something. And that's no problem. You can get out and get another one or have it repaired. But, in the cath lab, if the equipment goes out, you have a sick patient with a catheter in their heart, which is some risk to the patient. So, you have to make absolutely certain that it's safe for the patient."

Although the catheterization laboratory saw its first patient in 1955, the first cardiac surgery at Texas Children's Hospital took place on June 21, 1954. Performed by surgeon Dr. Luke W. Able and assisted by McNamara, the surgery was the first of its kind in the region. The patient, a blue baby, had pulmonary stenosis and heart failure and was treated with a right ventriculotomy and a Potts pulmonary valvulotomy. The results were gratifying, producing a vast improvement in the infant's heart condition.

Afterwards, McNamara made a decision: it would be his first and last assisting effort in a surgical procedure at Texas Children's Hospital. At Johns Hopkins, where he had trained, pediatric cardiologists provided assistance to surgeons in the operating room. But at Texas Children's Hospital, neither McNamara nor any pediatric cardiologist he trained would perform such a function again.

Rather than assisting surgeons during surgical procedures, pediatric cardiologists were to be involved in the diagnosis and treatment of patients with cardiac problems—those who either will have surgery or have already had surgery, as well as those for whom surgery is not required. Patients would be seen from a medical standpoint only. As McNamara explained: "Pediatric cardiology is one of the few specialties where the surgeon is not his own diagnostician. The field is complicated enough that the surgeons' training is all involved in the technical aspect, in the technique. And the diagnosis and medical treatment is complex enough that it requires all of your time spent in training in that. A team approach is necessary."

McNamara believed that a cardiovascular surgeon was not trained to perform diagnostic studies, nor is a cardiologist trained to do surgery. So, the two specialists must work together for the total benefit of the patient. "It's kind of a marriage," he explained. "It has to be. Many of the cases that we see don't require a surgeon, so we don't call them. And when we see a patient that does require surgery, we make the diagnosis and we make recommendation for surgical treatment. And most of the time that the patient goes to surgery and there's really no particular need or any occasion for any extensive consultation. When the problem is very clear and the type of surgical treatment is very clear, it really requires no discussion. In other cases, there may be a difference of opinion whether a child requires operation or not, and then we'll discuss it with the surgeon. 'Do you think surgery can be done? Is it feasible?' And then we have a consultation on that. But, you see, about half the patients with congenital heart malformations really don't require an operation. Either the condition cannot be corrected surgically or it is too benign to require an operation. Many of the congenital heart malformations are compatible with a perfectly normal, long, active life that doesn't require any surgical treatment. So, that's part of our job, really, is to decide the ones that do and the ones that don't."[20]

When McNamara diagnosed a patient with tetralogy of Fallot at Texas Children's Hospital, he discussed the optimal surgical correction with Dr. Denton A. Cooley, who was a veteran at performing the preferred Blalock-Taussig shunt procedure. Before becoming the first chief of cardiovascular surgery at Texas Children's Hospital, Cooley was a surgical intern at Johns Hopkins where he assisted Blalock in that landmark 1944 operation. During his subsequent surgical residency with Blalock, Cooley assisted or independently performed more than 200 Blalock-Taussig shunt procedures at Johns Hopkins.

The fortuitous pairing of the Blalock-trained Cooley and the Taussig-trained McNamara had immediate repercussions that would shape the future of the pediatric cardiology service at Texas Children's Hospital. The two doctors also became lifelong friends. From the beginning of their association, they shared not only a mutual background, but also admiration and respect.

Recollecting one of the first patients he had diagnosed and referred to Cooley, McNamara said: "In 1954, shortly after the cardiac clinic opened, all these infants that were sent in, some of them had terrible problems that we could do nothing about. Some of them had transposition of the great arteries. And, since the natural mortality in these babies is at least 90 percent in the first year of life, one out of ten is still living at the end of the year. I thought, gee, we don't have a lot to lose, let's give it a try. Dr. Cooley had never done that operation. He knew it was being done. He knew the concept of it. The first patient he did breezed through surgery. You'd think he'd done 50 of them because it was so smooth."[21]

Years after they first had met, Cooley reflected on their professional association: "Dr. Dan McNamara and I became very close friends immediately. He, to me, was the real ray of hope which I had, to have a trained pediatric cardiologist in the Texas Medical Center. One of the things that encouraged me, too, was that Dr. McNamara had received his training in the same institution where I had received mine. The cardiology service at Texas Children's Hospital began to flourish soon after the hospital opened in 1954. Dr. McNamara, being the well-dedicated, heavily dedicated type of person with the only real formal training in congenital heart disease in this area, became known as the authority in these diseases and, because of that, he developed his clinic very rapidly."[22]

The rapid development of one area in the clinic was spurred by an August 1955 trip that McNamara and Cooley took to Minnesota. The purpose of the trip was to visit Dr. C. Walton Lillehei of the University of Minnesota and Dr. John W. Kirklin of the Mayo Clinic, the two surgical pioneers who had developed a heart–lung machine, the external apparatus designed to assume the functions of the heart and lungs during intra-cardiac surgery. Each had successfully utilized their inventions to perform medical milestones in 1955, the first open-heart surgeries.[23]

Inspired by what they had observed, McNamara and Cooley returned to Houston with plans to create their own heart–lung machine. Within less than a year, Cooley and his team had fashioned such a machine, allowing Cooley to perform his first open-heart surgery on an adult patient at St. Luke's Episcopal Hospital on April 5, 1956. That procedure marked the beginning of the era of curative open-heart surgery at St. Luke's Episcopal Hospital and Texas Children's Hospital. By the end of 1956, Cooley had performed 95 open-heart operations on adults at St. Luke's Episcopal Hospital and on children at Texas Children's Hospital.

The advent of open-heart procedures at Texas Children's Hospital brought about constant changes within the cardiology service. "In those days, I did not have pediatric cardiology fellows, or staff to help," McNamara remembered. "So, I had to do the work of the resident. And we were learning a lot of new things. You know, heart surgery was still in its infancy. And a lot of operations, we didn't know what was going to happen to the patient and we had to watch them one minute to the next. So, Dr. Cooley and Dr. Arthur Keats, the anesthesiologist, and I all acted virtually as doctor and nurse. We had good nurses, but we were all learning how to watch these patients after the operations. And we had a lot to learn."

That learning process was to be an escalated one throughout the following 16 years. By September 22, 1972, Cooley had performed 10,000 open-heart surgeries on children and adults. Having chartered the Texas Heart Institute in 1962 to study and treat diseases of the heart and blood vessels, he began performing adult procedures in the newly built operating suites of the Texas Heart Institute at St. Luke's Episcopal Hospital in January 1972. Cardiac procedures performed on children by Texas Heart Institute surgeons continued in the institute's original location, the operating suite shared by Texas Children's Hospital and St. Luke's Episcopal Hospital. Fulfilling two roles simultaneously, the Texas Children's Hospital team of pediatric cardiologists also served as staff members of the pediatric department of the Texas Heart Institute.

"The structure and establishment of the Texas Heart Institute does not in any way affect the structure of the cardiology service at Texas Children's Hospital," McNamara explained. "We believe that the Texas Heart Institute will provide an unusual stimulus for certain joint projects and will thus increase the productivity of the individuals involved as well as the institutions and we look forward to a close and fruitful relationship toward this effort."[24]

With Cooley's surgical advances, as well as the emergence of new medical treatments, early diagnoses and patient referrals became essential to the pediatric cardiology service. And, to achieve optimal results, clinical research was of paramount importance. As one of the functions of physicians attached to academic institutions, medical schools, and teaching hospitals, research was a key factor in the exponentially expanding pediatric cardiology service at Texas Children's Hospital.

In 1979, McNamara reported that deaths from heart defects in infants and children had decreased "from about 90 percent in the 1940s to 15 percent in the late 1970s." Crediting curative surgery, experimentation, and clinical research, McNamara stated: "Despite the vastly improved outlook for the infant born with a birth defect of the heart, there remain many conditions for which treatment is lacking and other problems for which treatment is lacking and other problems for which the value of current management is unproved or controversial. Methods used by one center may be in disrepute in others. Aware of these needs, the 11 full-time staff of pediatric cardiologists and the 14 trainees at Texas Children's Hospital are involved in several categories of investigation aimed at improving patient care."[25]

"Creeping cardiology" had grown again. In 1979, the staff of 25 was involved in two categories of research: basic science research, sponsored by the National Heart, Lung, and Blood Institute and titled "developmental cardiac pharmacology and physiology"; and clinical investigation, directed by Dr. George W. Clayton in the Clinical Research Center, where meticulous attention was given to patient care as well as to the scientific recording of data in patients with all types of problems.

Also being investigated at that time were methods to improve the safety and accuracy of cardiac catheterization. Pediatric cardiologist Dr. Charles E. Mullins "had perfected a safe method for entering the left side of the heart, a formidable problem in the small infant." Regarding the investigation of arrhythmias, the irregularity of the heartbeat, McNamara reported that Dr. Paul Gillette "has distinguished himself and the Cardiology Section of Texas Children's Hospital by publishing studies concerning the diagnosis and treatment of arrhythmias in infants and children."[26]

Also praised in that 1979 McNamara report was Dr. Howard Gutgesell, who had set up "the first ultrasound laboratory in the area for echocardiography in infants and children." Echocardiography allowed for rapid non-invasive diagnosis of postoperative patients, improving the speed of medical management. Gutgesell, it was noted, "was the first to recognize the nature of the heart problem sometimes associated with the infant of the diabetic mother."[27]

The noteworthy achievements and continuing growth of McNamara's service at Texas Children's Hospital mirrored the entire subspecialty of pediatric cardiology. Before the Blalock-Taussig shunt procedure in 1944, there was no recognized subspecialty of pediatric cardiology. In 1972, there were 300 individuals certified as specialists in pediatric cardiology. In 1991, there were 884. By the late 1990s, the number had surpassed 1,500.[28]

McNamara addressed this rapid growth in a 1983 review titled *Twenty-five Years of Progress in the Medical Treatment of Pediatric and Congenital Heart Disease,* published by the American College of Cardiology. Stating eight major contributions that "are merely examples of the many developments that have occurred in the past 25 years," he listed the organization of pediatric cardiology and the contribution of volunteer health organizations; continuing medical education aimed at promoting early diagnosis of congenital heart disease and prompt referral to a cardiac center; advances in the technology of cardiac catheterization; Rashkind's balloon atrial septostomy and other catheter manipulative procedures; pharmacological manipulation of the ductus; Beta-adrenergic blockade for control of a variety of problems, including paroxysmal hypoxemic attacks, certain arrhythmias, and symptoms in hypertrophic cardiomyopathy; echocardiograph; and advances in arrhythmias, electrophysiologic studies, and the use of pacemakers.

Most of these advances could be attributed to the research instigated and completed by the pediatric cardiology service at Texas Children's Hospital, a fact not stated by McNamara in his published review. Such modesty was characteristic. Praised and quoted by peers in the field as "a valuable resource of references and analytic thinking," McNamara rarely, if ever, boasted of his personal accomplishments.[29]

A prime example of McNamara's remarkable unselfishness occurred when Josephine E. Abercrombie, daughter of Texas Children's Hospital founders Lillie Frank and James S. Abercrombie, offered to present him with a $1 million grant in memory of her mother. Instead of using the funds for a named professorship—something that would have given him an even higher profile in the pediatric cardiology community—McNamara earmarked the funds for research. That grant opened a variety of research opportunities and tremendously expanded the clinic's scope.

In appreciation of Abercrombie's grant, on February 24, 1978, the cardiac clinic was named the Lillie Frank Abercrombie Section of Pediatric Cardiology of the Baylor College of Medicine and Texas Children's Hospital. At the dedication ceremony, applauding the efforts of McNamara and his team was the person who was credited with being the reason they all were there—the "original pediatric cardiologist," Dr. Helen B. Taussig.

It was not Taussig's first visit to Texas Children's Hospital. In 1966, she had stopped in to visit with former trainee McNamara and take a tour of the cardiac clinic. The guest register reflects that Dr. Paul Dudley White, the founder of the American Heart Association and the recognized "father of cardiology," toured the clinic on the same day. The reputation of McNamara and his service attracted such well-known pillars of the medical community.

Unknowns came, too. In 1977, these included Dr. J. Timothy Bricker, a graduate of the Ohio State University medical school. The reason for Bricker's arrival, he explained, was simple: "The cardiologists and the surgeons at Columbus Children's Hospital would always make rounds together on Saturdays, and we'd end up in the coffee shop over coffee and donuts. There usually would be a contentious issue in pediatric cardiology or cardiac surgery under discussion by that point in time. The discussion got as far as, 'Well, Dan McNamara says and therefore ...'. That carried such a high level of authority with everyone there that, even though I didn't know Dr. McNamara, this was the first place that I looked for residency with the intent of being one of the fellows in Dr. McNamara's program."[30]

Unlike the clinic, the pediatric cardiology training program had a slow start. In the late 1950s and in the 1960s, McNamara trained no more than a dozen doctors in total. However, in the 1970s and 1980s, eager-to-learn young doctors such as Bricker flocked to McNamara's fellowship program in exactly the way that McNamara and others had been drawn to Taussig's in the early 1950s. According to Bricker, some features of McNamara's fellowship training program have since been incorporated into many other training programs throughout the country and abroad. In addition, faculty members from Texas Children's Hospital have served on the sub-board of cardiology of the American Board of Pediatrics.

The strength and popularity of the training program were directly related both to McNamara's leadership skills and to the pioneering advances made in the field of pediatric cardiology at Texas Children's Hospital that occurred during his tenure there. In electrophysiology, some of the earliest studies recording the intracardiac electrocardiogram were completed at Texas Children's Hospital; Mullins and Gillette pioneered the use of artificial pacing in children; and Dr. Richard A. Friedman developed laser applications for electrophysiology. In cardiac imaging, Gutgesell—who had been told by McNamara in the mid 1970s to go into the echocardiography room and not come out until he knew all he could about that unknown ultrasound apparatus—published his *Atlas of Pediatric Echocardiography* in the 1980s. The book, which included precise descriptions of cardiac conditions, heralded the era of surgery without catheterization.

In the cardiac catheterization laboratory at Texas Children's Hospital, diagnostic precision was advanced by the development of specialized angiographic techniques by Dr. Michael R. Nihill and the introduction of the framework for laboratory calculations and specialized procedures prepared by Dr. Thomas A. Vargo. Provided with Mullins' anatomically descriptive information about children with heart disease, former trainees disseminated these catheterization diagrams throughout the United States. Pediatric cardiac catheterization labs throughout the country began using Mullins' concepts.

Mullins also worked with the Children's Hospital of Philadelphia's Dr. William Rashkind, the "father of interventional cardiology," on the development and refinement of the ductus occlusion device that enables doctors to close the patent ductus arteriosus without surgery. With his coworker, Mullins has led the field in innovations for the application of endovascular stents in pediatrics. Under Mullins' supervision, pediatric cardiology fellow Dr. Ronald G. Grifka developed the Grifka-Gianturco vascular occlusion device as a research project. Approved by the Food and Drug Administration in 1995, the transcatheter device has been used to treat various vascular abnormalities in cardiac catheterization labs around the world.

Along with the introduction of this and other such innovative advances in the field of cardiology, the birth of a new era in cardiovascular medicine also occurred during the last decade of McNamara's tenure at Texas Children's Hospital. Although molecular genetics was in its infancy in the 1980s, one of the first efforts dedicated to the application of the techniques of molecular biology to cardiovascular research in adults took place at Baylor College of Medicine in 1982. Four years later, acceleration of these efforts occurred when the American Heart Association and the Burgher Foundation formed a partnership in 1986 to create and administer centers for molecular biology in the cardiovascular system at various institutions. Baylor College of Medicine was one of the six sites selected. It was there that Dr. Jeffrey A. Towbin—a fellow in pediatric cardiology and molecular cardiology at Baylor College of Medicine and Texas Children's Hospital—became the first pediatric cardiology trainee in the world to be funded for this pioneering research.

While Towbin was a trainee in 1986, McNamara encouraged him to use his prior research background to develop a new scientific research arena for pediatric cardiology worldwide—that of pediatric cardiac molecular genetics. "The focus on research was strengthened by Dr. McNamara's vision of the future," Towbin said. "Before I joined McNamara's staff, I worked for three years in the laboratory of Dr. Edward McCabe at Baylor College of Medicine."[31]

After joining Texas Children's Hospital in 1989, Towbin established and served as the medical director of the Phoebe Willingham Muzzy Pediatric Molecular Cardiology Laboratory at Texas Children's Hospital, named for a young girl with severe congenital heart disease and supported by her family. "The goal of this laboratory is to understand the molecular basis of sudden cardiac death with emphasis on disorders of cardiac rhythm and heart muscle diseases, as well as congenital heart disease and cardiac inflammation," Towbin explained.[32] "Our focus has been a combination of understanding the underlying genetic mechanisms of these diseases, generating good diagnoses, and tailoring our therapy, which may be based on genetic defects."[33]

In addition to mapping, isolating, and characterizing genes responsible for familiar cardiomyopathies in humans and in animal modules, research in the Phoebe Willingham Muzzy Pediatric Molecular Cardiology Laboratory at Texas Children's Hospital led to the discovery of facts relating to the gene for X-linked dilated cardiomyopathy. Also discovered was evidence that a mumps virus infection had been the cause of most cases of endocardial fibroelastosis. After studying the genetic and acquired causes of heart disease and sudden cardiac death, Towbin developed novel diagnostic tests and therapies for children and adults.

Towbin also joined Bricker's pediatric heart transplantation program at Texas Children's Hospital and Texas Heart Institute. Established in 1984, the program remained small in 1989, with only four or five transplants annually. However, achievements had become routinely successful following the availability of cyclosporine in the 1980s. Research conducted by Towbin and Bricker in this area included neonatal biopsies; work to understand neurologic complications; progress in pediatric left ventricular assist; studies related to pulmonary resistance and suitability for transplantation; and electrophysiologic assessment of transplantation candidates.[34]

With these and countless other achievements made in the field of pediatric cardiology at Texas Children's Hospital, by the late 1980s the cardiac program had gained a reputation as one of the best in the country. "When I look for reasons why, I could provide several answers," said Bricker. "The support of Josephine Abercrombie is something that has been essential to the development of the section. Another is Dr. McNamara's leadership and judgment. The other is the people that he trained, recruited, and kept in the department. If you look at the track record of Texas Children's cardiology, it includes having trained the current cardiology chiefs at the University at Arkansas, the Children's Hospital in San Diego, the Mayo Clinic, the Cleveland Clinic, the University of Virginia, Eastern Virginia Medical College, the University of Alabama in Birmingham, and the University of Pittsburgh. We can just go down the list of what our trainees are doing and where they have gone. That really has been the mission of this section; not just training people for pediatric cardiology, but training people who will contribute to the field and to advance the field of pediatric cardiology."[35]

One of those early former trainees reunited with McNamara at an awards ceremony decades later. "You look the same, Dan," he remarked. "You haven't changed at all."

McNamara smiled and shyly replied, "Well, thank you. I've been working out and trying not to work those 24-hour shifts at the hospital like we used to do."

"Oh, no. That's not what I meant," replied the former trainee. "I meant same suit, same tie, same shoes."[36] It was a conversation that McNamara often recalled with great amusement.

When McNamara stepped down as chief of pediatric cardiology at Texas Children's Hospital in 1988, Dr. Arthur Garson, Jr., another one of his trainees, succeeded him. In the more than three decades of McNamara's leadership, numerous advances in the field of pediatric cardiology had been attributed to the pioneering efforts of his team at Texas Children's Hospital. These developments ranged from heart transplantation techniques and methods of nonsurgical catheterization to the use of echocardiogram as a definitive tool in pediatric cardiac diagnosis. Under McNamara's guidance, Texas Children's Hospital had become renowned for its expertise in the care of children with heart disease and was recognized as one of the major centers of pediatric cardiology in the United States.

It was that emerging reputation that enticed Garson to spend the summer at Texas Children's Hospital between his second and third years at the Duke University medical school in the late 1960s. "When I left Houston and entered my third year of medical school, Dan McNamara said, 'You have a spot here if you want it,'" remembered Garson, who returned in 1976 for a three-year fellowship in pediatric cardiology.[37] After completing his training, Garson remained at Texas Children's Hospital and on the faculty of Baylor College of Medicine, where in six years he rose to the rank of professor of pediatrics and professor of medicine. "Dan McNamara was my true mentor," Garson said. "He was gentle, smart, had a good sense of humor and great values."[38]

Before assuming McNamara's position in 1988, Garson served as director of the pediatric cardiology training program, the electrocardiography laboratory, the pacemaker clinic, and the electrophysiology laboratory during his thirteen years at Texas Children's Hospital. He had worked with Gillette to develop pediatric cardiac electrophysiology as a distinct subspecialty of pediatric cardiology, and to develop treatments for children with heart rhythm problems. Garson also cowrote a book on ways to analyze pediatric arrhythmias. He was a prolific author, writing more than 257 scientific papers and four books. He also served with McNamara and Bricker as one of the coeditors of a pediatric cardiology textbook, *The Science and Practice of Pediatric Cardiology*. Comprised of 154 chapters contributed by faculty members of Baylor College of Medicine, including many former McNamara trainees, the three-volume first edition was published in 1990.[39]

During Garson's first year as chief of pediatric cardiology at Texas Children's Hospital, he had breakfast every week with McNamara, who remained active in the service. "It was a wonderful transition time," he said. "I learned I could honor him by continuing some of his initiatives and at the same time bring a little something different."[40] What Garson brought to the service was the knowledge of how to run a business, something he knew from working in the international business concern owned by his family. Another interest emerged while Garson continued his work in heart rhythm problems. When he began studying these problems in adults with congenital heart disease, he discovered that there was an alarming lack of healthcare funding. His desire to develop a policy for providing healthcare coverage for these patients prompted him to earn a master's degree in public health at the University of Texas in Houston.

What became Garson's passion was a failure brought on by success.

Because of the research and progress made in the field of pediatric cardiology, children with complex congenital heart disease who previously had not survived childhood were growing up to become adults. "The young adults who have been treated for congenital cardiac malformations at Texas Children's Hospital in childhood are still followed here in most cases," Garson explained. "And their concerns are very important to Texas Children's physicians and staff."[41]

Garson's own abiding concern never wavered. When two collapsed disks necessitated neck surgery for him in 1990, he came out of the operating room paralyzed. Unable to move his arms, he was allowed to complete his master's degree by independent study in courses that included macroeconomics, microeconomics, strategic planning, and health policy. After being awarded his degree, he "really felt that I wanted to do something different." In 1992, Garson accepted an offer to become vice chancellor of Duke University in Durham, North Carolina.[42]

Named chief of pediatric cardiology at Texas Children's Hospital in July 1992 was another McNamara trainee, Bricker. After arriving in 1977, Bricker became chief resident in 1979–80 and was one of a number of academic pediatricians whose postdoctoral training was funded by the Auxiliary to Texas Children's Hospital. Awarded the Patton Fellowship in 1980–81, the WATCH Fellowship in 1981–82, and the Frank Prescott Horlock III Fellowship in 1982–83, Bricker was an associate professor of pediatrics at Baylor College of Medicine. Actively involved in the pediatric heart transplantation program, he also displayed strong interests in exercise physiology, preventative cardiology, and epidemiology. Upon assuming his new position, Bricker stated: "My role and my goal, in many ways, is what I saw Dr. McNamara doing in the 1970s, which was to provide a supportive environment. We are extremely productive as a team and I am less concerned about what I am specifically doing myself than what I am able to facilitate to be done by the department."[43]

Bricker's dedicated efforts produced a continuance of the trademark growth in the Lillie Frank Abercrombie Section of Cardiology at Baylor College of Medicine and Texas Children's Hospital. Within three years of his tenure as chief, outpatient visits escalated to more than 8,000. Departmental statistics for 1995 also indicated more than 21,000 echocardiograms, 15,000 electrocardiograms, 744 pacemaker evaluations, and 803 cardiac catheterizations.

In that same year, Texas Heart Institute surgeons performed more than 440 pediatric cardiac procedures on patients at Texas Children's Hospital. As originally planned by McNamara and Cooley in the late 1960s, the pediatric cardiology service at Texas Children's Hospital continued its intertwined relationship with the Texas Heart Institute in the 1990s. According to Bricker, this successful coexistence for more than two decades was based not only on a singular purpose, but also on mutual need and respect. "Surgeons are interested in diagnostic issues and the cardiologists are interested in therapeutic issues," explained Bricker. "We are very much a team. A pediatric cardiologist without a good surgical program is in difficult shape, as is a congenital heart surgeon without a good cardiology department. It's like a PT boat. The PT boats had two engines and there were two propellers on the back of the PT boats in World War II. If either engine got knocked out, all the boat could do is go around in circles."[44]

A new direction for the pediatric cardiology service at Texas Children's Hospital had its beginnings with the 1995 arrival of Dr. Charles D. Fraser, Jr., as chief of congenital heart surgery at Texas Children's Hospital. While also serving in that capacity at the Texas Heart Institute, Fraser laid the groundwork for a separate surgical service devoted exclusively to pediatric cardiac surgery at Texas Children's Hospital.

Also undergoing a transformation was the cardiac transplant program at Texas Children's Hospital. Serving as the medical director of heart transplantation since 1992, Towbin expanded the program by introducing weekly heart transplant and cardiomyopathy clinics, as well as inpatient consultation and care. Within a decade, Towbin's team was to gain international recognition and become the largest pediatric cardiomyopathy and heart failure service in North America.

Fraser's efforts to establish a separate surgical service were evident five years after his arrival at Texas Children's Hospital. By 2000, there was a new team of pediatric surgeons, pediatric perfusionists, pediatric anesthesiologists, pediatric cardiac nurses, and pediatric operating room technicians. The establishment of pediatric cardiac surgery at Texas Children's Hospital was an integral aspect of the long-range plan developed by McNamara, Bricker, and physician-in-chief Dr. Ralph D. Feigin. The next goal was to centralize the medical and surgical services of pediatric cardiology in a specifically designed physical space.

The location for the envisioned Texas Children's Heart Center was in the soon-to-be-constructed West Tower, scheduled for completion in 2001. Planned to encompass four floors of that building, the heart center would offer extensive medical and surgical services to children with heart disease, including fetal echocardiography, arrhythmia surveillance, diagnostic and interventional catheterization, pacemaker follow-up, electrocardiography, cardiovascular genetic testing and research, pediatric cardiovascular anesthesiology, and congenital heart surgery.

Offering valuable input for these future plans was someone from the past, Garson, who returned to Baylor College of Medicine and Texas Children's Hospital in 1995. "Ralph Feigin, the chairman of pediatrics at Baylor, recruited me back as vice chairman of pediatrics and vice president of Texas Children's Hospital for quality and outcomes," he said. "The next year he became the president of Baylor College of Medicine and he asked me to take the lead in developing a new strategy for the medical school. At the end of that year he asked me to become the dean for academic operations, and to direct the strategic planning process for the medical school."[45]

Garson also returned to the pediatric cardiology service at Texas Children's Hospital, where he lectured fellows and participated in the cardiac clinic. "His role at Baylor was much more related to big-picture issues and other departments, but it was a huge advantage for me that the dean was one of the names on our letterhead," Bricker said. "I remember one afternoon when the three guys in clinic were Dr. Garson, Dr. McNamara, and me, and Tim said, 'The only guys in clinic are the only three guys who have ever been chief here.' And then he paused for a moment and said, 'That is either really good or really bad prognosis for you, depending on how you look at clinic.'"[46]

Bricker and Garson also collaborated as editors of the second edition of their 1990 textbook, *The Science and Practice of Pediatric Cardiology*. Coedited with Dr. David J. Fisher and Dr. Steven R. Neish and published in 1998, the new 2,959-page, two-volume textbook included extensively updated information, as well as new chapters devoted to the latest advances in pediatric cardiology. Upon publication, it was lauded by the *Journal of the American Medical Association* as one of the "authoritative, 'must-have' books in the field." The chapters of the book are described by the *JAMA* reviewers as being clearly written and sensibly organized "to educate both the clinician who may be unfamiliar with molecular biology and the basic science teacher who is looking for a comprehensive review of a topic presented with a clinical bias."[47]

Crediting McNamara with developing the environment, tradition, and value system that inspired the book's first edition, the new editors dedicated the second edition to him. Speaking for the more than 107 other trainees listed in the textbook, the editors wrote: "He was a father figure to several generations of pediatric cardiologists trained in Houston. Dr. McNamara supplied wisdom, guidance, support, encouragement, enthusiasm, resources, and boundaries to those of us who had the opportunity to begin our pediatric cardiac training and careers as part of 'McNamara's band.' Our field is truly fortunate that Dr. Dan McNamara's career had been dedicated to the science and practice of pediatric cardiology."[48]

Shortly after this dedication was published, McNamara's sudden death on September 9, 1998, cut short his highly praised career. After devoting more than four decades to the care of children with heart disease at Texas Children's Hospital, McNamara ended his career the way it had begun, with a clearly written book about pediatric cardiology.

The author of that first book was McNamara's mentor, Dr. Helen B. Taussig. Although she had a dream that the "great day will come when we learn how to prevent these birth defects rather than only to treat them," it did not happen in her lifetime, nor in his. "I remember Dr. Taussig talking about McNamara and her other Taussig fellows," Bricker recalled. "She said that she had been privileged to see the first 21 flames of the field of pediatric cardiology and she hoped to be privileged to see its dying embers."[49]

Instead of being extinguished, McNamara's flame ignited an eternal torch carried by his trainees in the pediatric cardiology service at Texas Children's Hospital. "We look forward to the day pediatric cardiology will not be needed and we can move on to something else," Bricker stated. "We want to be able to move from the level of high tech treatment of congenital heart disease to understanding the causes of congenital heart disease, both at the cellular and molecular level as well as at the population and epidemiological level. We want to be able to eliminate pediatric cardiac disease."[50]

Emphasis continued to be placed on the longitudinal follow-up of patients treated at Texas Children's Hospital for congenital heart disease. Instigated by McNamara and attributed to Taussig's influence, the continuous observation of young patients as they grew to adulthood remained a steadfast commitment, as did the pediatric cardiology service's commitment to research.

"On the molecular level, we're increasingly being able to understand the cause of disease at the very basic level, which helps us evaluate our therapies better," Bricker said. "We know what we are really treating. This will lead to our doing more directed interventions and less invasive surgery. Cardiac molecular biology is becoming an everyday part of what we do. The cardiac research program is the better part of one floor in the Feigin Center, which is amazing. This is by far the best research department of pediatric cardiology in the country. That is largely due to Jeff Towbin himself, and due to the support he has gotten from Dr. Feigin, donors, and Texas Children's Hospital over the years and to the great people he has trained and hired. He has been the driving force for Texas Children's Hospital's being in a very key position with regard to pediatric cardiovascular research."[51]

Since joining Texas Children's Hospital in 1989, Towbin had developed various innovative programs in pediatric cardiology. In addition to the Phoebe Willingham Muzzy Pediatric Molecular Cardiology Laboratory, Towbin collaborated with Drs. John Belmont and William Craigen from the department of molecular and human genetics at Baylor College of Medicine to establish the cardiovascular genetics clinic at Texas Children's Hospital in 1997. With the recruitment of nurse/genetic counselor Susan Fernbach in 1998, the clinic played an important role in the care of children with genetic-based disorders and syndromes and grew to become the largest of its kind in the United States. Towbin and his colleague also developed important molecular-based and clinical research projects that "will hopefully lead to new paradigms for caring for these patients."[52]

Also established by Towbin was the John Welsh Cardiovascular Diagnostic Laboratory, founded in 2002. "Named in honor of a significant supporter of our studies of pediatric heart disease, the laboratory is focused on the molecular diagnosis of the causes of myocarditis, fetal hydrops and other inflammatory/viral diseases, as well as the genetic causes of cardiac disease," Towbin said. "Currently, the laboratory offers diagnostic genetic testing for infantile cardiomyopathies, as well as acquired viral heart disease."[53]

As one of the recipients of the 2003 Michael E. DeBakey, M.D., Excellence in Research Award at Baylor College of Medicine, Towbin was recognized for his significant published contributions to clinical research. "In the last five years or so, we have made important discoveries about the underlying causes of heart disease in kids and adults," Towbin said. "Understanding the gene defect helps in choosing a more effective medicine to treat the functioning of a particular protein, instead of simply treating the symptoms."[54]

With more than 300 publications, 50 book chapters, and two books, Towbin exemplified his determination to lead Texas Children's Heart Center to new heights. His prolific studies of acquired heart disease, the genetic causes of cardiac disease, and sudden cardiac death in children garnered much praise. "Jeff's research efforts have advanced the treatment and cures for many pediatric heart conditions," Feigin said. "The hard work and dedication shown by Jeff sets an example for other physicians."[55]

Towbin's exemplary career in pediatric cardiology at Texas Children's Hospital began a new phase in 2003. When Bricker stepped down to pursue other interests, Towbin was named chief of pediatric cardiology. It was a career move of historic importance. Having served as associate chief of pediatric cardiology since the early 1990s, he became the fourth chief of the pediatric cardiology service in 50 years and the third to have received his training under McNamara.

By 2004, much had changed since McNamara arrived at Texas Children's Hospital in 1954. What began as a one-person, one-clinic, pediatric cardiology service evolved to become the four-floor Texas Children's Heart Center, one of the three leading children's heart centers in the United States. Offering the full spectrum of cardiac care, it was one of the few such centers exclusively dedicated to the treatment of children with congenital and acquired heart disease. "We are greatly indebted to our legacy at Texas Children's Hospital," Bricker said. "Those who have provided the advances that have lessened suffering and death from childhood heart disease are the inspiration for us to push forward with enthusiasm."[56]

An enthusiastic Towbin agreed, noting the promising future of pediatric cardiology at Texas Children's Hospital in 2004. "We are about to learn the secrets of heart disease that afflicts children and adults," he said. "Once these secrets are unraveled, new diagnostic methods and therapies are in the offing. Stories of survival thought impossible a few short years ago are likely to become common events."[57]

Whatever lay ahead, the past would not be forgotten. The flame in the torch passed by pediatric cardiology founder Taussig to McNamara and then, in turn, to Garson, Bricker, and Towbin had not diminished during more than five decades. Rather, the torch had flourished. It also was destined to illuminate the path of pediatric cardiology at Texas Children's Hospital well into the twenty-first century.

For almost two years, Jill and Scott Tinklepaugh had kept more than a watchful eye on twins Karly and Kestly. The girls were never out of sight.

Acutely aware that there was a possibility one or both girls may have a "tet spell," turn blue, or be unable to breathe, the Tinklepaughs and Jill's parents, the Bruskotters, constantly watched over them. Luckily, what they were afraid might happen did not.

But everything else did. Or so it seemed. Routine trips to the pediatrician's office always ended up being frantic situations, Jill recalls. The doctor would look at one baby and say "You call an ambulance for this baby." Then the doctor would look at the other baby and say "You call an ambulance for this baby."[58]

Three times the twins contracted viral pneumonia. Three times they went to see the pediatrician. Three times they were rushed to the hospital. Jill remembered one time when "Mom went with Karly to the hospital and stayed 11 days. Never came home one day."

"That was probably one month after the shunt procedure," Scott said. Then came the ear infections. Jill couldn't find an ear, nose, and throat doctor in her community, so she called Texas Children's and took them there to have tubes inserted.

But it wasn't just the children who needed immediate care and attention.

One day Scott complained of a pain in his chest. He thought he was having a heart attack like the one that had killed his father at an early age. Jill assured him that it was only gas and told him to go and mow the lawn. So that's what he did. However, three days later, when the pain became unbearable, Scott was taken to the hospital by Jill's father. There, he was diagnosed and treated by a cardiologist who performed angioplasty to clear his clogged arteries.

Finally, in September 1996, the time came for Kestly, the bigger of the two girls, to undergo the corrective procedure. So, back to Texas Children's Hospital they went. "Before the procedure Dr. Nihill did an angiogram," Scott said. "He tested pressures and so forth because they wanted to get an idea what was going on in the heart and they can actually measure, I believe, what pressures are in each chamber of the heart and where it's flowing out and all this and that. They each had this done."[59]

Kestly's surgery, performed by Dr. Charles D. Fraser, Jr., chief of the congenital heart surgery service at Texas Children's, lasted eight hours. Before the operation, Fraser explained to the Tinklepaughs exactly what he was planning to do. The open-heart surgery included multiple steps to correct the four defects comprising tetralogy of Fallot: closing the hole between the two ventricles in the heart, opening up the artery from the right ventricle into the lungs by removing muscle that was obstructing it, and enlarging the pulmonary arteries.

As Jill and Scott and other family members waited outside the operating room, a hospital representative periodically updated Fraser's progress with intermittent messages from the doctor, such as "I've got another two hours" and "Kestly is doing just fine." The anxious parents and family were grateful for such words of encouragement.

Afterwards, when Fraser came to report the completion of the corrective procedure, Scott saw the effects of an eight-hour operation on the doctor's face: "He had grooves around his face around his eyes. I could measure it in depth. Just from having those goggles on for eight hours. One of the operating room nurses said that he could sew like no machine that she had ever seen. No sewing machine. Small, close-together stitches that you look at and it doesn't even look like it's stitched."

Following the operation and her stay in the recovery room, Kestly once again became Dr. Bricker's responsibility. As before, the team of pediatric cardiologists at Texas Children's Hospital monitored the twins as they recuperated in the hospital, as well as during their long-term follow-up over the years. Jill and Scott recalled the many visits Bricker and the other doctors made to the room. "It was never just one person. When they'd make their rounds in the hospital, there was always the lead doctor and there were always all these interns and fellows. They'd all come in the room with everyone asking questions like 'What is the best way to go about this? And correct this? And what steps should we take?' It was fascinating."[60]

As Bricker and his team of pediatric cardiologists predicted, Kestly soon was able to leave the hospital and return home. Seven months later, in April 1997, it was Karly's turn to have the same open-heart surgery. Also performed by Fraser, hers would take seven and a half hours. She, too, was the center of the pediatric cardiologists' attention and, shortly after the procedure, Karly was back home.

The identical twins with the identical congenital heart defects now had identical scars, each almost invisible because of Fraser's signature tiny stitches. And each had the identical prognosis. "We haven't made their hearts normal, but we've made them function normally," Fraser said. "In our experience, less than 5 percent of patients with this type of repair will need subsequent surgeries."[61] Added Bricker, "For this type of heart defect, we expect a good long-term result. We've had individuals with tetralogy of Fallot repair who are now medical students, residents, and nurses."[62]

As to whether the twins will make those kinds of career choices in the future, only time will tell. For now, for Jill and Scott Tinklepaugh, just knowing they will have the opportunity over the coming years to be able to ask Kestly and Karly, "What do you want to be when you grow up?" is the best short-term result possible. And for that they will be forever grateful. "I've always said, if I become independently wealthy, that a lot of that wealth would go back to that hospital. Just as payment. I know my insurance paid and so forth like that. But I would pool all my wealth and give it back to Texas Children's Hospital," Scott declared.

With that thought, the Tinklepaugh's story ended with a bang.

It had begun with a murmur.

9

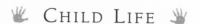

✋ CHILD LIFE ✋

WHILE AT TEXAS CHILDREN'S HOSPITAL, child life specialist Loree Smith learned to expect the unexpected.

After working for ten years as a full-time child life specialist in the child life department of Texas Children's Hospital, Smith began working two weekends a month on a per-diem basis. She soon found that her clearly defined duties on Saturdays and Sundays were never routine. Rather than being responsible for one specific area of the hospital, where the needs for child life's unique services were somewhat predictable during the week, the weekend child life specialist was on call in areas throughout the hospital.

Available to respond to any and every request, Smith arrived one Saturday morning at her usual time of 7 a.m. She immediately logged on to the computer to access the list of patients admitted since 5 p.m. on Friday. After noting the new arrivals, Smith retrieved all of the telephone messages recorded during the night. "This provides a starting point to prioritize the day," she said. "Some days I will check with the charge nurse or staff on each unit."[1]

Sometimes the phone started ringing the minute she arrived, as was the case on this particular Saturday morning. A nurse concerned about an "upset and angry" patient called the child life office for assistance. "She has a sign on her dry erase board that she hates Dr. So-and-so," the nurse explained. "She is so mad. You have got to go see her."[2]

Grabbing her beeper, Smith locked her office, attached the key to her identification badge on her denim blouse, and headed for the nurses' station on the fourth floor. She quickly looked at the patient's chart, discovering that the 15-year-old was a cystic fibrosis patient who had recently been placed in isolation. After receiving more detailed information from the nurse, Smith headed down the hall to the reportedly irate patient's room.

Upon finding a handwritten sign on the closed door, Smith did not enter. "Only these people are allowed in my room," the teenager's directive declared, listing six specific names and "my pulmonary doctor." Noticeably absent was the allegedly maligned Dr. So-and-so, Smith noted without commenting. As a child life specialist, she instinctively knew to obey the sign. "She's 15 years old and I want to respect that that's how she feels," she later explained. "She doesn't want anybody else in there. I have to respect a teen's issues."

Although advised to ignore the sign by the nurses on the floor, Smith took a different approach. After gently knocking on the door and hearing "Yes?" from the patient, she tentatively stuck her head in and said, "My name is Loree Smith from child life, but my name is not on your sign."

Cheerfully told that she could come in, Smith entered to find that the patient was not the petulant teenager she expected to find curled up in bed in a dark and dreary room. Not only were the blinds open, but the smiling and talkative patient was fully dressed and sitting in a chair. Already familiar with the child life specialist who worked on that floor during the week and who had contacted her on Friday, the teenager asked, "What happened to Leslie? You know what? I'm going to add you and her and child life to my sign on the door."

As she added the names to the sign, Smith determined that hers was the behavior of a normal, chatty teen who was coping appropriately. "She's smiling. She let me come in. She's willing to talk to me. She's easy to talk with," Smith said. "While she is expressing everything, I am looking at all the visual cues in her room. Her blinds are open. She's got crafts and things to do in her room. She has a VCR."

While visually surveying the room, Smith noted that the vitriolic message no longer was on the dry erase board. Having found the teenager so easy to converse with, Smith decided to bring up the subject and said, "Well, the nurse mentioned that you had a note here, something about hating a certain doctor?" To which the teen replied, "Oh, yeah. He just knows nothing. He said this and this and this. I'm waiting for my pulmonary doctor to come. I have lots of questions."

After encouraging the teenager to write down the questions so that she wouldn't forget anything, Smith asked if she and her stepsister wanted any more crafts or activities. Given an enthusiastic reply, Smith went back to her office and soon returned with the requested items. Although she saw that the handwritten sign was no longer on the door, she did not mention it.

"Did you notice I took my sign down?" the excited teenager asked when Smith re-entered the room. "Aren't you proud of me?"

"If you want to leave the sign on the outside of your door, that is OK," replied Smith. "You can put up any sign that you want."

"Oh, I don't need it any more," the teenager replied with a smile.

This immediate positive outcome did not come as a surprise to the child life specialist. Afterwards, Smith summarized her intervention in the patient's chart and made the following assessment: "Typical, normal teen development. She's a teenager. She was mad at the doctor. She wrote that note on the dry erase board and stuck up that sign on the door because she was mad. We have to allow the patient that control in her environment."

Moving right along, Smith's next few phone calls concerned newly admitted patients who were thought to be eligible for the Houston Independent School District (HISD) Hospital School Program. Making a quick stop in the child life department to pick up the medical consent forms necessary for each chart, she stopped in each patient's room, explained that the program required written consent from the doctor, and advised that someone from HISD would visit on Monday to answer any questions.

More phone calls for her services followed. Referred by nurses to three more patients who were thought to require the attention of a child life specialist, Smith visited the children and assessed their situations. Deciding that what each patient needed was the kind of lengthy, loving, one-on-one attention offered by members of The Auxiliary through the Patient Pals program, she called the Auxiliary office to place their names on that list.

When nurses advised her of the seven-year-old child who was awaiting surgery for a fractured femur, Smith began her efforts to learn more about the patient. First, she read the child's chart and discussed it with the nurse. Smith learned that the injury was from a bicycle accident and that the child had been transported from another hospital to the emergency center at Texas Children's Hospital in the middle of the night. Since it was Saturday, Smith knew that there was going to be a long wait for an operating room and an anesthesiologist. With this in mind, she was concerned about the child's anxiety level.

"I want to look at the background information before I go into the room and introduce myself," Smith explained. "I know she is seven, but the chart might give me information about whether she is developmentally seven years old or has a developmental delay. I know she came in the middle of the night and did not get much sleep, so I do not anticipate her being awake."

Smith entered the room and introduced herself to the obviously exhausted mother. After explaining how the mother could help prepare her daughter for surgery and alleviate the child's fears through therapeutic play activities, she was told by the mother: "You want to do that? I don't care. You know what? She just wants to get it over with. She's in a lot of pain. They've given her morphine and she's asleep right now."

"Well, I'll be back to check on her later and we'll decide what to do then," Smith advised, knowing that she also wanted to get the child's permission before proceeding with her surgery preparation.

In the meantime, she had another call. It was from the nurse in the pediatric intensive care unit, who said that the patient in bed 19 needed more bubbles to blow. "The bubbles were for incentive spirometry to help keep the child's lungs clear," Smith said. "I also will take a pinwheel to help encourage the patient to do deep breathing exercises."

Knowing that she might be needed to supervise unexpected visits to the unit from siblings under the age of 14, Smith was quick to respond to the call. "Whenever I get a call from ICU, I usually need to drop everything and go," she explained as she scurried down the hall with the pinwheel and a bottle of liquid bubbles in her hand.

I n 1975, Texas Children's Hospital was the first hospital in Houston and one of the first in Texas to offer the unique services of a child life specialist.

The innovative idea behind the child life service was to meet the psychosocial needs of hospitalized children through preparation, therapeutic play, crafts, and activities was unique at the time. However, caring for the emotional well-being of patients had been a priority at Texas Children's Hospital since its inception. Efforts to alleviate the traumatic experience of hospitalization for children and their families were an integral part of the hospital's planning. The results were evident on opening day in 1954.

"We have a beautiful, well-equipped play room on both patient floors," stated a welcome letter to parents of the first patients admitted. "When the child is free of fever and is convalescent, ask the nurse in charge if it will be all right for you to take your child there."[3]

For those patients who were unable to leave their rooms, Auxiliary volunteers began visiting with toys, games, and books. With the addition of handcrafts in 1956, The Auxiliary officially formed its recreation program and assumed responsibility for the third-floor play area. "The primary purpose of the recreation program is to meet the basic needs of growing children in a temporary abnormal environment," stated an article in

WATCH Magazine. "To accomplish this purpose, all effort will be made to create an environment which is as child-centered as possible."[4]

Staffed at first entirely by volunteers, who were required to attend a short training session and lectures given by the chief pediatric resident and the nursing director, the program flourished. With weekly conferences to reiterate the rules, regulations, and philosophy, the volunteers shared their experiences with patients, introduced new ideas, and observed arts and crafts demonstrations. As the program rapidly grew, so did its success and the need for a paid director.

The first director of recreation at Texas Children's Hospital was Margaret Ward, a British citizen who previously trained with the Nursery Nurses' Association in London. Ward's credentials were impressive. A former governess to the grandson of Sheik Bashar El Khoury, the president of Beirut, she also boasted ten years' experience working with children in South Africa, Egypt, Cyprus, Turkey, and Lebanon.[5]

Under Ward's direction, the recreation department introduced an organized play-therapy program in 1957. With her staff of 30 volunteers, Ward championed the idea of offering each child the ingredients to create bejeweled mailboxes from paper plates, dolls from colorful yarns, and other such age-appropriate crafts.

The overwhelming success of these creative efforts garnered enthusiastic praise not only from patients, families, nurses, doctors, and onlookers in the hospital, but also from the local media. "Child's play is more than a phrase at Texas Children's Hospital. It's a way of life," extolled one newspaper's account of the recreation program's activities.[6]

To a reporter who questioned whether play therapy worked, Ward replied, "We use everything but the kitchen sink. Toilet paper, string, tongue presses, glue, glitter, and goop are the backbone of our program. These darling youngsters will do anything to get to our play carts. They'll gladly take their shots, medicine, anything."[7]

With such accomplishments, and having effectively established a close working relationship with the nursing staff, the recreation program continued to thrive—not only under Ward's leadership, but also after her departure. Rather than replacing Ward, The Auxiliary volunteers once again assumed full responsibility for the recreation program in 1959. It was a decision that was to remain unchanged for 16 years.

Throughout the 1960s and early 1970s, Auxiliary volunteers on the recreation committee devoted their efforts to arranging seasonal activities, organizing entertainment programs, introducing new craft projects, and delivering toys, games, books, and balloons from a recreation toy cart. When no longer afforded the luxury of designated play areas on the patient floors due to the necessary expansion of medical services, the volunteers devised group play activities for the patients in other areas of the hospital.

"When I first came in 1975, there were no playrooms," remembered Jacqueline Vogel, Texas Children's Hospital's first director of recreational therapy. "The playrooms where they are right now used to be smoking areas. The volunteers had to rope off the area. I got them some clothesline rope and they would loop it around chairs and tell the smokers to all get on the other side so that they could get the toys from the cupboards and play with the kids."[8]

Hired to direct the play-therapy activities in the four new playrooms planned for the expanding Texas Children's Hospital, Vogel arrived before construction had been completed. Trained in child development at the University of Wisconsin, she joined the staff of Dr. Barry L. Bowser, chief of the physical medicine service at Texas Children's Hospital and St. Luke's Episcopal Hospital.

"For the child in the hospital, play is not merely a diversionary activity," explained Vogel. "Play is used to assess children's individual needs. It meets emotional and developmental needs and it provides information to other members of the healthcare team. My primary function is to help interpret the healthcare setting to the child, and in turn to interpret the child to other healthcare professionals."[9]

Since such a formalized play program at Texas Children's Hospital was completely different from the existing recreation efforts put forth by The Auxiliary, Vogel was prepared for the consequences of introducing something new. Of her initial efforts, she recalled: "You had to earn your wings. You certainly had to win people's respect. You had to demonstrate you had some kind of knowledge and some sort of expertise that would be helpful to them."[10]

Instead of instigating her program with less seriously ill children in the playrooms as planned, Vogel began to work with the critically ill patients in the pediatric intensive care unit (PICU) at Texas Children's Hospital. Depending on the child's age and physical capabilities, she tailored individual therapies for each patient.

"With 12 beds in ICU, it was basically a triage system. I took referrals on the ones who were most in need, had the fewest family resources, and were long-stay," Vogel explained. "If you have a child who is on a ventilator and can't move, your options are very limited. You can do creative puppet play at bedside. You can read to them. You can show them pictures. You are very limited if they cannot actively engage in play. You have to create opportunities to play and provide stimulation for them at bedside."

As the playrooms became available in 1976 and 1977, Vogel began training volunteers from The Auxiliary and the Junior League as supervisors of the therapeutic play program. In her training classes, she stressed the difference between simply offering diversional activities and focusing on the emotional and developmental status of the patients. She explained how the alleviation of emotional stress was possible through techniques of art, modeling clay, dolls, puppets, or whatever else was suited to the age and temperament of the child. With the opening of the teen playroom in 1977, Vogel advocated unstructured play and minimal supervision.

Her department's efforts received the enthusiastic support of the nursing staff, physicians, volunteers, and hospital administrators. Considered an integral part of medical treatment at Texas Children's Hospital, Vogel's therapeutic play activities provided the patient with a sense of normalcy and also eased the fears generated in a hospital environment. For the patients and families who were unable to go to a playroom, Vogel's bedside activities achieved similarly favorable results.[11]

As the recreation therapy department's area of responsibility expanded, Vogel began using another title. Rather than continuing as a recreation therapist, she identified herself as a child developmentalist. Changing once again in 1978, she began calling herself a child life specialist, renaming her department child life/play therapy.

This inability to settle on a definitive title for her professional work was not unique to Vogel and Texas Children's Hospital. Throughout the United States in the 1960s and 70s, other child developmentalists working with children in hospitals experienced the same identity crisis. During the 1965 "Patient Recreation in Pediatric Settings" conference, which later became known as the Association for the Care of Children's Health (ACCH), the child development participants were called "recreation workers." Although many preferred "child-care worker" instead of "recreational therapist," "play therapist," "teacher," or "play lady," the term "child life" eventually emerged 14 years later in 1979 as the newly established profession's agreed-upon name.[12]

With the 1982 founding of their own professional organization, the Child Life Council, child life specialists began to define the specific requirements for the profession. In addition to minimal academic preparation at the bachelor's-degree level with supervised care in the healthcare setting, the child life specialist had to have a demonstrated ability to work with individuals and groups of children. Also required was a demonstrated understanding of growth and development, family dynamics, play and activities, interpersonal communication, developmental assessment, the learning process, group process, behavior management, the reactions of children and their families to illness and healthcare encounters, interventions to support coping, collaboration with other healthcare professionals, basic understanding of children's illnesses, and medical terminology and supervisory skills.[13]

Next for the Child Life Council came the ratification of standards for clinical practice in 1986, followed by the establishment of a Child Life Certifying Commission with the authority to regulate who became a certified child life specialist (CCCL).[14]

Available by examination only, the child life certification was for individuals who met the criteria established by the commission. "These criteria include having completed (1) a Bachelor's degree, (2) a minimum of 10 courses in child life, child development, child and family studies, or closely related areas and (3) 480 hours of child life clinical experience (through internships, practicums, fellowships, and/or paid work experience), supervised by a certified child life specialist. Once certified, an individual may become recertified after five years either by examination or by accruing 50 professional development hours. To maintain certification, however, one must pass the Child Life Professional Certification Examination at least once every 10 years."[15]

At Texas Children's Hospital, such clearly defined standards helped Vogel not only to reinforce the identity of the child life/play therapy department, but also to expand its size and services. Included in the growing list of inpatient responsibilities in 1978 was the renal dialysis unit. From 1979 to 1984, the department grew to include four additional members, each a child life specialist.

"Child life specialists are basically child development specialists who are particularly trained for the healthcare setting," Vogel explained. "Our focus is both the emotional and the developmental status of children while they are in the hospital. We certainly use play as a tool, but we also do a lot of preparation for procedures and consultation with parents about children's reaction to hospitalization. Not just the child that's in the hospital, but also the siblings who are having a difficult time with the fact that they have a brother or sister in the hospital. Child life focuses more on emotional issues and issues of preparation and explaining the healthcare experience to children and their families. And so, the concept of child life is really a good bit broader than just trying to divert children through play."[16]

Such a distinction became obvious in the 1984 planning and opening of the Pi Beta Phi Patient/Family Library at Texas Children's Hospital. Vogel and a child life specialist from her department, Julie Branson, helped select the 400 age-appropriate books for children and parents, activated the operating system, trained the Pi Beta Phi and Auxiliary volunteers, and planned the details necessary to establish a well-coordinated children's library. The subsequent operation of the library became a continuing responsibility of the child life/play therapy department.[17]

After the 1987 separation agreement between Texas Children's Hospital and St. Luke's Episcopal Hospital, Vogel was no longer affiliated with the previously combined and now separated physical medicine service. Instead, the newly named and independent child life department at Texas Children's Hospital came into existence. The transformation marked the beginning of what was to become the department's meteoric rise in stature.

Having already expanded her staff in 1985 to include one child life specialist to work with adolescents and another to work with outpatients, Vogel also began offering semester-long child life internships. From 1989 to 1995, the child life department grew to include a staff of 17. Along with clerical workers, the Pi Beta Phi Patient/Family Library coordinator, and part-time assistants, the staff included two child life specialists in the emergency center, two in the outpatient clinics, one in the surgery area, one in renal dialysis, one in pulmonary, one in hematology-oncology, one in general medicine, one in the pediatric ICU and the progressive care unit, one in neurology, and one in cardiology.

In each assigned area of responsibility, the child life specialist not only supervised group and individual play activities, but also prepared children for their scheduled medical procedures. Utilizing anatomically correct dolls, medical equipment, photographs, and various other props, the specialist explained in age-appropriate and comprehensible terms the experience that the child was about to encounter.

"You used to tell a child going into the hospital that he would get a lot of ice cream," Vogel said. "Now you prepare him for the injections, pain, anesthesia, and separation from his parents. You tell them the truth in simple terms. We include parents as part of the treatment team and encourage them to participate. One of the best things a child life specialist can experience is seeing a child master a difficult situation. To see a child and a family come through successfully—not only medically, but also emotionally—is very rewarding."[18]

Such positive outcomes also resulted from the patient and family support programs supervised by child life specialists in each area. Involved in the patient support camps and the school re-entry services, child life specialists formed and developed lasting relationships with patients and their families. For those less fortunate families in the bereavement support groups, child life specialists offered continuing comfort and encouragement.

In the early 1990s, with this multiplicity of programs to administer and an ever-increasing child life staff to supervise, Vogel began developing another area of service. In her spare time, she concentrated her efforts in the neonatal intensive care unit (NICU), working with neonates referred by the nursing staff. For those infants with working or absent parents, she offered daily stimulation to help develop their social skills. Vogel also worked with parents who were getting ready for their babies to be discharged, giving them special techniques for handling their premature infant or advice about the development stages to expect. In *The Magic of Play: A Guide for Parents of Babies and Children in the Hospital,* the book published by the child life department of Texas Children's Hospital in 1991, Vogel included activities expressly for those in NICU, showing the importance of a parent's interaction and ability to understand what's going on with a very fragile neonate.

"I'm very interested in early development, and so infants have become of particular interest to me," Vogel explained in 1992. "As my workload has gotten greater with more and more people to supervise and the program's sort of burgeoning, it's been easier for me to manage the timing of it. It would be very hard for me to be tied to a playroom that has to run at a specific time because I have too many other things to do. It's much easier to fit the babies into my schedule."

Fitting something into her busy schedule was nothing new to Vogel. In the two decades she spent building the child life department at Texas Children's Hospital from a one-person staff in 1975 to a team of more than 20 in 1995, she always found time to respond to a call for her services. "If a physician said to me, 'I have a patient in such and such unit and they really need you,' I had a terribly hard time saying no," she recalled. "And so I would just manically run around trying to do all of these things. And I think in retrospect, perhaps, had I concentrated in one area, maybe the development of the department might have had a little bit different pattern. I will never know that. But I do think that's probably a valid argument."[19]

Because of Vogel's myriad accomplishments, the positive impact of the child life specialists in every medical service area and the increasing emphasis on family-centered care throughout Texas Children's Hospital, there was an organizational change in the child life department in 1995. In order to integrate the individual child life specialists more fully into a medical service team, the assistant director of nursing for each area's unit assumed the supervisory responsibilities for the child life specialist. Instead of having a full-time director, the child life department became self-directed. Although offered another position, that of child life specialist in the NICU, Vogel resigned in 1995.

In order to fulfill the administrative duties of a self-directed department, the child life specialists formed various committees for scheduling, hiring, and education. As for their specific day-to-day duties, the different roles became works in progress. Finding themselves accountable to the unit in which each worked, the child life specialists began finding more freedom to expand to different programs, ones based on the individual needs of their units. With this expansion, acquiring more child life specialists became a necessity.

The establishment of goals for the child life department came in 1998, when the department's overall direction became the responsibility of Dana Nicholson, MS, MBA, RN, director of nursing for special care areas. To strengthen relationships in each unit, Nicholson stressed the importance of involving the child life specialist in the unit's leadership team, meeting with the assistant directors regularly, and becoming more involved in the unit.

"My philosophy is that child life really should be the expert on family-centered care," said Nicholson. "I think that they have the responsibility to continually educate the nursing staff as well as the other clinical professionals to be sensitive and to continually refine their practice towards family-centered care. I believe child life should be at the center of that development. I think that we have worked very hard to put our child life program there."[20]

Nicholson also wanted to broaden the scope of the child life department. In 1999, she created two new positions, hiring additional child life specialists to serve as outreach coordinators for inpatient program development and ambulatory program development. "People need to understand what we do and recognize it. If we want funding, we need big, visible programs to be recognized within the hospital," she explained. "We decided to bring Radio Lollipop in and I said, 'Here's our first initiative.' So we started to look at very non-traditional roles."

The launch of Radio Lollipop at Texas Children's Hospital was announced at a news conference on May 18, 1999. An international non-profit organization with locations throughout the world, Radio Lollipop was a fully equipped on-site radio station that was broadcasted to patients' rooms via the hospital's television system. The station began operating at Texas Children's Hospital in October 1999, becoming the first Radio Lollipop in Texas and only the second in the United States.

A volunteer-driven program dedicated to stimulating the imaginations of hospitalized children by providing care, comfort, play, and entertainment, Radio Lollipop featured interactive games, art projects, and contests.

On the air two nights a week—Terrific Tuesdays and Thrilling Thursdays—the volunteer deejays took patients' call-in requests and put children on the air, either from their bedsides or in the studio. It was an immediate success, exactly the type of "big, visible" initiatives that Nicholson had wanted for the child life department.

"Sarah Fallon, the child life specialist who is our outreach coordinator on inpatient programs, coordinated the startup of the Radio Lollipop program," Nicholson explained. "She works with the volunteers on their programs to make sure that they are developmentally appropriate. She helps the volunteers deal with the different children's reactions and emotions. She does their training and she does their budgeting, signing off on their supplies and expenses."

Along with instigating new programs, Nicholson expanded existing ones. When child life specialists and social workers at Texas Children's Hospital saw the need to provide aid to grieving families in age-appropriate support groups, an association with Bo's Place began. Named in memory of Laurence Bosworth Neuhaus, Jr., a Texas Children's Hospital patient who had died of liver cancer in 1985 at the age of 12, Bo's Place was founded in 1990. A nonprofit organization, Bo's Place was dedicated to helping grieving children and families.[21]

"We have two nights a week where our families are at Bo's Place. Texas Children's Hospital's social workers and child life specialists run the support groups," Nicholson said. "It's fabulous because these people usually, not always, already have a relationship with these children and families so they can help them talk about their siblings. We've gotten really favorable reviews from the program."

Also receiving compliments from patients and their families was Nicholson's decision to offer the services of child life specialists seven days a week. "I am very proud of that accomplishment," she stated. "If we believe, as we do, that the services of a child life specialist are critical and important in helping children cope and normalize their environment, then we should not be offering it only Monday through Friday from 8 a.m. to 5 p.m. So, in 1999, we put in evening hours and weekend coverage. I was just very, very excited about that."

Also enthusiastic about the extended coverage were the child life specialists, who rearranged their weekly schedules to take turns with the duty. During weekends, rather than working in an assigned unit, the child life specialist on duty was on call in every area of Texas Children's Hospital—except for the emergency center, which already had seven-day-a-week coverage. From its inception, the weekend coverage received positive reactions from patients, their families, and the medical staff.

"I think throughout the country there are many areas where child life struggles to be recognized and to be part of a team," Nicholson said. "Philosophically, I believe that the child life specialists in our program will tell you that they are highly valued and respected members of the health-care team. Child life is at the heart of our family-centered care philosophy. They help us stay focused on delivering developmentally appropriate care that involves the family."[22]

As an integral part of the Texas Children's Hospital family in 2004, the staff of the child life department comprised more than 30 certified child life specialists, child life partners, interns, fellows, and the Pi Beta Phi Patient/Family Library coordinator. Each a professional who had studied normal child development and the reactions of children to healthcare settings, child life specialists provided emotional and psychosocial interventions with hospitalized children based on their individual needs.

Serving all areas of Texas Children's Hospital, child life specialists worked on inpatient floors and in outpatient clinics, neonatal units, renal dialysis, and the emergency center. Child life specialists were also involved in patient and family support groups, community outreach, patient camps, school re-entry services, and bereavement support.

With its constantly expanding responsibilities, the child life department at Texas Children's Hospital seemed destined for future growth, the possibilities limited only by available funding. Were an unlimited budget suddenly available to Nicholson, she knew exactly what she would do: "I would follow Child Life Council's recommended ratio and have one child life specialist for every 15 patients at Texas Children's Hospital. We would just have them tripping over each other."[23]

Nicholson's dream for the child life department at Texas Children's Hospital was ambitious—but so was the one that Jackie Vogel had 25 years earlier, and that proved to be achievable. Having introduced one of the first child life departments in Texas in 1975, Vogel planted the seed of a service that eventually blossomed into one of the largest and best of its kind in the United States.

C hild life specialist Loree Smith gathered the props needed to prepare the seven-year-old patient with the fractured femur for surgery.

It was late Saturday afternoon and, "since she cannot leave her room,

I will not be able to walk her over to the surgery suite like I normally do with patients," Smith explained. "Instead of walking her through the experience from the moment she leaves her room, goes to surgery, and then to the recovery room, I will have to explain verbally what happens. Why she cannot eat or drink anything, what she can take with her, how she will be taken there on a bed, and all of the other issues will be explained."[24]

In a large plastic box, Smith placed a blood-pressure cuff, a stethoscope, EKG leads, a pulse oximeter, bubble-gum-flavored extract, and a child-sized anesthesia mask. Along with these props she planned to take a stuffed doll to illustrate how each of the items was used and a book with pictures of the holding room, operating room, recovery room, and monitoring equipment.

Having prepared children for surgical procedures for more than ten years as a child life specialist at Texas Children's Hospital, Smith was confident about the specific age-appropriate preparation she expected to give the seven-year-old. "I try to go from the non-invasive to the little more scary stuff," she explained. "I usually do the blood-pressure cuff first. With the blood-pressure cuff, I keep in mind the developmental age of the child. Most of them have seen a blood-pressure cuff. I say, 'Do you know what this is? Do you know what it is called?' I let them put it on the doll and I explain, 'It gives your arm a little hug or a little squeeze. It just measures how the blood pumps in and out of your heart. The heart pumps blood through your whole body. Your heart takes a beat and it pumps the blood in and out through your whole body and back to your heart.' Then I show them the stethoscope and say, 'Do you know what a stethoscope is? Do you know what it is for? That's how the doctor checks your heart and checks your breathing.' I give really simple explanations."

As she often did with other seven-year-olds, Smith planned to define the pulse oximeter as "a Band-Aid with a little red light." Illustrating how it would be plugged into a monitor, she always said, "I know it sounds really silly, but it can tell if you are breathing good clean air, even in your finger."

With the EKG leads, which she called "heart stickers," the doll was used to illustrate where the "stickers with the snaps" were placed to measure the heartbeat. To explain their purpose, Smith would say, "It does the same thing as the stethoscope. Except, instead of putting it in their ears, like this, they plug the wires into a monitor and the doctors can look up there and see how fast your heart is beating."

Smith planned to introduce the anesthesiology mask, showing the tubing and how it hooked into a "sleep machine" and explaining how the "sleep doctor" would be in the operating room with her. "You are going to have a doctor who is going to do the operation and you are going to have another doctor whose whole job is to make sure you get enough sleeping medicine," she would explain to the child. "He's the 'sleep doctor,' who is also known as an anesthesiologist."

Armed with a few samples of the strawberry, tutti-frutti, bubble gum, root beer, cotton candy, cherries, banana, coconut, peppermint, and raspberry flavors that were available for the anesthesia, Smith would tell the child she could pick her favorite flavor in advance. She also would explain how the anesthesia was administered, saying, "You know the pink medicine you drink? Well this medicine is different. This is medicine that you don't drink or swallow. This is medicine that you smell. And the way you smell it is through this mask."

Then she would place the child-sized mask on the doll to illustrate where it was placed and how it worked, offering a sample sniff from her bottle of the bubble-gum-flavored smell. Always quick to assure the child that the extract was not the medicine, she would promise it would not put the child to sleep during this demonstration. She would explain how the "sleep doctor" made sure she would sleep through the operation so that she did not feel any pain.

She would tell her about waking up after surgery in the recovery room and how she probably would still have the "heart stickers" and the "Band-Aid with the little red light." She would tell her that her parents would be with her when she woke up after surgery. "That last bit of information is as much for the parents as for the child," Smith said. "It can be overwhelming for these parents when they walk in the recovery room and see their child immediately after surgery. Sometimes I say to the mom, 'There will be a tube of oxygen there, too. Sometimes it makes a hissing sound, so you may hear it when you walk up to your child.' So, I try to let them know."

Prepared to make this finely honed presentation to the child with the broken femur and her parents, Smith gently knocked on the patient's door late on Saturday afternoon. Greeted by the child's visibly anxious father, who explained how his child was still in terrible pain, she entered the room with her plastic box packed with props and the stuffed doll under her arm.

In an effort to ascertain the patient's anxiety level, Smith first asked for and received the child's permission to begin her presentation. From the onset, Smith maintained eye contact and closely measured the child's verbal and non-verbal responses. She noted that the child visibly winced when told of being moved from her room to the operating room. As Smith was explaining each of the props in her plastic box, the child slowly became more tearful and anxious. At the mention of the words "sleep doctor," the child suddenly cried out to her father, "I don't want to go to sleep!"

Masterfully changing the subject, Smith asked, "Do you like to play with beads?" Instantly, the child stopped crying, nodded her head affirmatively, and almost smiled.

"Well, let me go get you some," Smith replied, closing her plastic box full of props and placing the doll under her arm. "Do you like to play games with your dad? I'll bring some games for you to play, too."

After briefly leaving the child's room, Smith returned with a bag full of beads, pipe cleaners, and string, as well as several board games from the fourth floor playroom area. Talking with the child's parents in the hallway, she advised that her presentation seemed to be making the child more anxious instead of less so, and that she was not going to continue at that time. Instead, she believed that distracting the child's attention away from the pain and to the craft activities was the best approach. The child's distraught parents agreed.

Several hours later, Smith gathered her prop box and doll and returned to find both the child and her parents much calmer. Now able to continue her presentation, she discovered "after quick rapport building and probing questions that the child was most scared of moving to the transport bed to go to surgery because of her pain."

To remedy this fear, Smith had a solution. She spoke with the child's nurse and together they worked with surgery transport to take the child to surgery in her current bed. "Since this child was given time to lower her anxiety, she could better learn about her situation and seize an opportunity to take some control by not moving to another bed," Smith explained.

It was the type of outcome child life specialists at Texas Children's Hospital were trained to achieve. "It is rewarding to prepare a child completely for surgery and see that child come out of a very scary and potentially frightening experience with a positive, healthy attitude," said Smith. "It is just as important for me not to induce more anxiety than is necessary and to make sure the child and her parents can cope with the hospital environment."[25]

Child life specialist Loree Smith knew that she had to expect the unexpected moments at Texas Children's Hospital. She was confident that she had the necessary training to transform them into positive experiences for patients and their families.

10

 CONGENITAL HEART SURGERY

Excited first-time parents Jean and Scott Parrish were about to be blindsided.

The Houstonians were at the gynecologist's office for Jean's routine prenatal ultrasound exam at 22 weeks. They had just learned that their baby was a girl. As they gazed with wonder at the flickering sonogram, they could see that the baby had rosebud lips, just like her dad's. The Parrishes were happily discussing each newly discovered nuance in their child's snowy image with the equally talkative ultrasound technician, when she suddenly became quiet. Then she excused herself, saying that she needed to see if the doctor wanted to speak with them. Jean and Scott were not alarmed.

"We did not know anything was wrong," Jean said. "While she was gone, we just looked at the sonogram and discussed names for our daughter. By the time the doctor and the tech came back into the room, we had named her Rachel. And that's when the doctor said something was wrong with her heart, but they didn't know at that point what it was."[1]

The previously ecstatic couple was stunned silent when the doctor told them that they needed to see an obstetrical subspecialist for a precise diagnosis as soon as possible. "This was on a Friday, and they got us in to see a perinatologist three days later, apologizing that they were unable to get us in any sooner," Jean recalled. "I thought that was pretty quick, so all weekend long we were wondering what it could be."

The elusive answer came during an advanced ultrasound exam at the perinatologist's office the following Tuesday. The Parrishes were told that Rachel had a congenital heart defect known as hypoplastic left heart syndrome (HLHS). The left side of her heart had not developed normally and would not function effectively to supply her body's needed blood flow once she was born. Told that babies born with HLHS did not survive long, the Parrishes were given four choices by the perinatologist: terminate the pregnancy; try to get on a waiting list for a heart transplantation for the baby; undergo experimental surgical intervention that had not proven successful; or do nothing but give compassionate care to the baby and let nature take its course.

"The perinatologist basically gave us four options that all led to Rachel's dying, and we got to choose which one," Jean said. "She said the medical community would support whatever we decided. She said the operation had such low survival rates—zero survival rates—and that it was something we should not even try, because it put the baby through such turmoil and you just couldn't do that. She said the odds of getting a transplant were slim, even if you moved to Loma Linda, California, and were on that hospital's wait list. Without stepping over the line, she told us to think long and hard about terminating the pregnancy. She suggested we think about all the options for a very, very long time."

At the conclusion of Jean and Scott's visit, the perinatologist suggested that they talk to a pediatric cardiologist at Texas Children's Hospital. "It was the one good thing that came out of that appointment," Jean declared. "We were just devastated. We didn't know what we were going to do. All of the options sounded like roads to nowhere. We went home and cried for a long time."

Later that night, Scott searched the Internet for information about HLHS. What he learned conflicted with what the perinatologist had said about zero outcomes from the surgical option. Scott told his wife about the positive outcomes reported by surgeons at The Children's Hospital of Philadelphia and other institutions. "We might have to go somewhere to have the surgery," he said. "I am willing to go with you to Philadelphia and live there and have the surgery, if the doctors here think she is a good candidate. So, let's go talk to them." Jean thought the idea was premature and remained extremely depressed.

Undaunted, Scott was inspired by what he had just discovered about HLHS. He undertook further research in preparation for the family's appointment at Texas Children's Hospital. Scott learned that the first operation in the three-stage surgical treatment was called the Norwood procedure and had been introduced in 1980. That surgery was performed when the baby was a newborn. The following two surgeries, named the Glenn and the Fontan, were performed separately and before the age of three. Scott also found details of the success rates of the various hospitals in which the three surgeries were being performed.

Equipped with this and other information about the hospitals and surgeons who performed the procedures, Scott planned to ask the pediatric cardiologist at Texas Children's Hospital for advice as to where they should take Rachel. Less optimistic was Jean, who could think only about the zero survival outcomes that the perinatologist had spoken about.

"We went to see Dr. John Kovalchin at Texas Children's Hospital," Jean said. "After he did a fetal echocardiogram, he told us Rachel had a textbook case of HLHS. He then answered all our questions. When he said she was a pretty good candidate for surgery, we showed him the downloaded Internet information and asked him where we should go."

Kovalchin's answer totally surprised them. "He told us about Dr. Charles Fraser, who had come to Texas Children's Hospital two years earlier in 1995," Jean recalled. "He told us a little bit about his background, how long he had been doing the Norwood procedure, and his success rate. He said, 'I am sorry you were told that it was zero outcome for the procedure, because it is a 70 percent favorable outcome here.' All of a sudden, we had gone from zero to 70 and we had hope. It was really something, and we were very excited. He told us to think about it."

To decide what would be best for Rachel, Jean and Scott found themselves in a quandary. As first-time parents, they considered themselves both inexperienced and clueless. They did not even know how to change diapers, much less care for a baby who had undergone openheart surgery. "We didn't know what to expect," Jean said. "We met more and more people at Texas Children's Hospital, and I am sure we asked millions of questions. They were all so patient with us. No one tried to tell us what to do; they let us make the decision."

Their first decisive move was to find a new perinatologist, one knowledgeable about HLHS, to closely monitor the remainder of the pregnancy. Whatever the treatment option chosen, arrangements were also made for neonatologists at Texas Children's Hospital to be in the delivery room when Rachel was born at St. Luke's Episcopal Hospital. Immediately after her birth, Rachel would be taken to the neonatology intensive care unit. There, she would be closely monitored. If surgery were to be performed, it would occur within days of her birth.

"When we met with Dr. Fraser to discuss the possibility of Rachel's surgery, he laid it all out for us," said Jean. "He told us about complications of stroke, problems with anesthesia, and the perils of being on the heart–lung bypass. He doesn't say a lot of things offhand; he thinks care-fully and then says it. He did not push us in one direction or the other, and he made it clear from the beginning that surgery would correct Rachel's problem, not eliminate it. This is your whole world spinning on this and I appreciated knowing the scope of what could happen. We had been blindsided with this news about Rachel's HLHS, and we didn't want to get blindsided again."

For the remaining three months of her pregnancy, Jean and Scott weighed their options, discussed all that could possibly go wrong, and came to the conclusion that their choice for Rachel's future was the best one possible.

The newly opened Texas Children's Hospital played one of the pioneer-ing roles in the rapidly emerging field of congenital heart surgery during the 1950s.

However fast this surgical specialty grew, its beginning was slow in coming. For most of history, the human heart was a special organ thought to be too fragile for surgery. Consequently, up until the 1940s, the progno-sis for children born with complex malformations of the heart was either fatal or a severe disability. Among the 32,000 infants born each year in the United States who were afflicted with congenital heart disease, the death rate for those with severe defects was a staggering 90 percent. Because ther-apeutic options for treatment were limited and surgical procedures for the heart were nonexistent, the future seemed likely to offer a bleak reflection of the past.

This pessimism about heart surgery had been rampant for centuries. Even after the first successful heart operation, a fencing injury laceration repaired by German surgeon Ludwig Rehn and reported in 1895, the naysay-ers remained persistent. The long-established notion that the heart could not be manipulated surgically remained steadfast. Reflecting current opinion in the 1896 medical community was the published observation of eloquent British surgeon Sir James Paget: "Surgery of the heart has probably reached the limits set by nature to all surgery: no new method and no discovery can overcome the natural difficulties that attend a wound of the heart."[2]

Although many shared this belief, others were determined to prove oth-erwise. Four decades later, that goal was accomplished. During the six-year period from 1938 to 1944, the injured hearts of various adult patients were surgically repaired and several congenital cardiovascular defects in children were also successfully treated with surgery.

The first event occurred on August 16, 1938, at Children's Hospital Boston. Performed by Dr. Robert E. Gross, it was the surgical treatment of the sixth-most-common congenital heart defect, the patent ductus arteriosus (PDA). An open blood vessel between the aorta and the pulmonary artery that normally closes shortly after birth, a defective PDA remained open, causing an excessive amount of blood to flow into the lungs. After Gross had achieved the first successful closure, news of this medical milestone spread rapidly throughout the world—as did word of the first repair of another congenital heart defect, a coarctation of the aorta. Performed in Stockholm by Dr. Clarence Crafoord, the resectioning took place on October 19, 1944. In London during this period, Sir Russell Brock was in the process of developing procedures for the treatment of pulmonary valve stenosis and for palliation of tetralogy of Fallot.

However, the events that unquestionably paved the way for the future of not just heart surgery, but all surgery, were those that occurred on the battlefields during World War II. Facing injuries and suffering on a massive scale in Europe, military doctors pioneered advances in antibiotics, anesthesia, and blood transfusions. One particular physician performed surgical procedures previously deemed impossible. While an Army captain in the medical corps between 1943 and 1944, Dr. Dwight Harken successfully removed foreign bodies from in and around the hearts of more than 100 wounded soldiers. This accomplishment was pivotal.

"Harken's work helped overcome the notion that the heart could not be surgically manipulated," said Dr. Denton A. Cooley, the first chief of cardiovascular surgery at Texas Children's Hospital. "It was a catalyst for the creation of the first Blalock-Taussig shunt for treating tetralogy of Fallot, performed at Johns Hopkins Hospital on November 29, 1944. The striking results from this procedure, which increased the circulation through the pulmonary arterial system, caused much excitement in the surgical community."[3]

The breakthrough also had a dramatic impact on the career of Cooley, who had the good fortune to assist Dr. Alfred Blalock in the operation. At the time, Cooley was a 24-year-old first-year surgical intern at Johns Hopkins Hospital. He often recalled that memorable experience by saying, "I witnessed the dawn of heart surgery."[4]

Soon after that dawning, Cooley found himself in what was probably the busiest referral center for congenital heart cases in the country. Over the next several years at Johns Hopkins, he assisted or independently performed more than 200 Blalock-Taussig shunts, as well as countless other procedures. As he continued his surgical training with Blalock and cardiology consultant Dr. Helen B. Taussig, Cooley learned the benefits of a medical–surgical coalition of managing patients with congenital heart disease. In addition to the valuable experience gained at Johns Hopkins, Cooley trained with Brock for a year at London's Brompton Hospital.

With Blalock and Brock as his mentors, Cooley learned his skills from two of the recognized pioneers of cardiovascular surgery for congenital heart defects. During his years training with both surgeons, he was an eager participant in the emerging era of heart surgery. During that time, a total of four congenital heart defects—patent ductus arteriosus, coarctation of the aorta, pulmonary stenosis, and tetralogy of Fallot—became operable for the first time. Cooley became proficient in each of these surgical innovations.[5]

When Cooley returned to his hometown of Houston in 1951, it was as a full-time faculty member of the department of surgery at Baylor College of Medicine. With more formal training in cardiac surgery than any other surgeon in Houston, he began performing heart surgery at The Methodist Hospital, Jefferson Davis Hospital, and Hermann Hospital. "Our methods of diagnosis were extremely crude by today's standards, because most were made on physical findings rather than using the more sophisticated diagnostic techniques available today," Cooley recalled in 1979. "When Dr. Dan McNamara arrived at Texas Children's Hospital, he was to me the real ray of hope which I had, to have a trained pediatric cardiologist in the Texas Medical Center."[6]

In the two years before McNamara's arrival, Cooley had already become known for his skills, his unparalleled training and experience, and his innate talent for speedy surgical procedures. "Denton's reputation as a fast surgeon had spread throughout the Texas Medical Center, and in fact throughout the Southwest," said McNamara. "Operations that I had seen take two to three hours in other centers were taking Denton one half to one third the time."[7]

McNamara had received his cardiology training at Johns Hopkins with Taussig and Blalock, and he knew from experience that most Hopkins-trained surgeons were meticulously slow and methodical. Although Cooley's "expeditious surgical manipulation" was astounding to him, it was justifiable because it made operations on critically ill patients, especially infants and children, feasible and successful. "He believed that the infant and young child with critical heart disease could tolerate no more than a brief period of anesthesia and minimal dissection and manipulation in order to survive the procedure and benefit from it," McNamara said. "Aside from that, it was never his manner to dawdle over anything."[8]

Because McNamara shared this sense of immediacy in treating children with heart defects, rapid response to recent developments in the fields of cardiology and congenital heart surgery became the norm. One example was the creation of a cardiac catheterization laboratory at Texas Children's Hospital. A major breakthrough in the diagnosis of congenital heart defects, catheterization in children was first considered in the late 1940s. Embracing this diagnostic potential, in 1954 McNamara, Dr. Joseph R. Latson and Dr. Robert D. Leachman established an innovative laboratory capable of providing imaging of the heart.[9]

With enhanced diagnostic potential afforded by catheterization, Texas Children's Hospital began to amass a growing population of children and infants with intracardiac congenital heart defects in need of repair. Because most existing surgical operations were palliative extracardiac procedures performed on the heart's exterior, the challenge was to find a way to operate safely inside the heart.

"What was needed was a method for interrupting blood flow during an intracardiac operation," Cooley explained. "Hypothermia was one of the early methods tried, either by placing patients in a tub of ice water or by cooling them with ice packs. Once the patient's temperature was lowered to 26 degrees Fahrenheit, blood flow to the heart could be interrupted. If the repair could be accomplished within eight to ten minutes, the patient was spared cerebral complications. Unfortunately, this technique had some serious drawbacks, including air embolism, which was one of the greatest problems encountered by the developers of open heart techniques."[10]

One technique, introduced in 1937, was an artificial heart and lung developed by Dr. John Heysham Gibbon at Philadelphia's Jefferson Medical College. Although Gibbon proved that life could be maintained by this apparatus during cardiac surgery on animals, all the animals died a few hours later. For more than a decade, Gibbon worked to perfect his method of providing oxygenation and circulation of blood outside of the body. Finally, in 1953, he tested this cardiopulmonary technique during operations inside the hearts of four children with congenital heart defects. When only one patient survived the operation, Gibbon called a personal halt to the clinical use of this technique.

Although unsuccessful, Gibbon's efforts inspired other techniques and the terminology "cardiopulmonary bypass" and "open heart surgery" became synonymous. In the mid-1950s, Dr. C. Walton Lillehei at the University of Minnesota experimented with the technique of cross-circulation, using the patient's parent as the donor oxygenator. Utilizing this method in a 1954 surgical procedure on a child with a congenital heart defect, Lillehei performed the first successful open-heart operation.

Another pioneer, Dr. John W. Kirklin at the Mayo Clinic, began the successful use of a complicated Gibbon-like pump-oxygenator in March 1955. When Dr. Richard DeWall at the University of Minnesota devised a less complicated "bubble oxygenator" for Lillehei in 1955, Cooley and McNamara decided to visit both institutions in Minnesota for a firsthand look at the accomplishments of these pioneers. "I recall that when we returned, Dr. McNamara stated that before I could do an 'open heart' operation on one of his patients, we'd have to duplicate the equipment and the program at the Mayo Clinic," said Cooley. "That was rather discouraging to me, because even today I don't believe we could duplicate the complex type of methodology that they were using at the Mayo Clinic. But I was able to convince Dr. McNamara that we could do it on a much simpler basis."[11]

Cooley moved with trademark speed to accomplish this mission. Within months, Texas Children's Hospital and St. Luke's Episcopal Hospital had a bubble oxygenator similar to the De Wall–Lillehei invention. Inspired by Cooley's motto of "Modify, simplify, and apply," Houston's Dr. Benjamin Belmonte, Dr. Joseph R. Latson, and Dr. Robert D. Leachman developed this first bubble oxygenator, as well as a subsequent vertical stainless steel unit that could be easily assembled.

The concept of a heart–lung machine intrigued Latson and Leachman, who began researching the possibilities of creating one in 1954. "Dr. Latson and I spent much time visiting various oil industry laboratories, where the best technology was available, talking with the technologists who were experts in glassblowing," recalled Leachman of their formidable undertaking. "We had them make many different types and shapes of glass bubble dispersers in an effort to get small, uniform oxygen bubbles through the incoming blood. When this did not work, we decided to try to pass oxygen through porous rock. We had one of the largest collections of pumice-stone bubble dispersers in the Houston area, but our efforts to use them for passing oxygen through, or into, a blood column were futile. We finally found that we could obtain optimal-sized bubbles by making multiple holes in a Teflon disk with a 28-gauge needle."[12]

After extensive testing, refinements, and modifications, the resulting simplified bubble oxygenator was deemed functional. Cooley successfully performed his first open-heart surgery on April 5, 1956. By year's end, after further refinements to the apparatus were made, Cooley's team had performed more open-heart procedures than any other group in the world, on more than 95 adults and children.

One member of this legendary surgical team for open-heart surgeries was nurse technician Mary Martin, who operated the bubble oxygenator. It was her responsibility to control and support cardiac and pulmonary function during open-heart surgery, a method known as cardiopulmonary perfusion. Although Martin continued in that position for five years, her technical role eventually evolved into the healthcare specialty of cardiovascular perfusion during the early 1960s.[13]

Another rapidly evolving field of specialization was the administration of anesthesia for infants with cardiovascular disease. Instrumental in establishing and implementing safe and effective anesthesia techniques for infants at Texas Children's Hospital in 1955 was Dr. Arthur Keats, who arrived that year as head of the department of anesthesiology at Baylor College of Medicine. Before Keats, "there was great concern that it would not be possible to anesthetize these young patients safely and to see them through an operation," explained Cooley. "In the earliest days, nurse anesthetists usually administered anesthesia with great trepidation in very young patients."[14]

Such apprehension was not unusual. Despite the startling advances that had been made in congenital heart surgery, many pediatricians believed that successful cardiac surgery could not be undertaken in infants. Even at Johns Hopkins, "Taussig believed that one should not try to operate on a child younger than four years with tetralogy of Fallot or a child younger than eight years with an aortic coarctation," said Cooley.[15]

This prevailing sentiment did not deter Cooley and McNamara. Both strongly believed that surgical intervention for congenital heart defects was warranted in the first year of life. Their conviction came from knowing that 64 percent of the children with congenital heart defects died within a year of birth, a researched conclusion first published by McNamara in the late 1950s. At that time, most institutions with the capability to offer congenital heart surgery had experience with only a handful of such patients. At Texas Children's Hospital, however, 120 infants with congenital heart defects underwent surgical procedures between 1954 and 1959. "Although many had been in severe cardiac failure at the time of their operation, more than 70 percent survived," Cooley reported.[16]

Among the malformations treated in these infants were tetralogy of Fallot, patent ductus arteriosus, coarctation of the aorta, atrial septal defect, and total anomalous venous return. Although many of the procedures were previously available in the field of congenital surgery, Cooley introduced several new techniques and modifications. To surgically treat cyanotic infants in this group, he performed procedures that included not only the Blalock-Taussig shunt, but also two other aorta-to-pulmonary artery shunts. The first shunt was Cooley's modification to eliminate the difficulties experienced with the shunt that had been introduced in 1946 by Dr. Willis Potts in Chicago. The second was one that Cooley developed for tetralogy of Fallot, an extracardiac shunt to connect the posterior ascending aorta to the underlying right pulmonary artery. That procedure, later named the Waterston-Cooley shunt, became the standard throughout the world.[17]

Sixteen of the babies in that group of 120 were born to mothers infected with measles. Each infant had patent ductus arteriosus and suffered from congestive heart failure in the first few weeks of life. Proper diagnosis and prompt surgical procedures enabled all of these babies to survive. For those infants with coarctation of the aorta, Cooley established a precedent in the field of congenital heart surgery. His surgical results indicated an operative mortality rate of less than 25 percent, thereby confirming surgery as a more effective treatment than medical therapy for coarctation of the aorta.[18]

Another precedent was set with four infants under the age of four months who were suffering from total anomalous venous return, an extremely rare congenital heart defect associated with atrial septal defect. The first correction of this defect while utilizing cardiopulmonary bypass took place at Texas Children's Hospital in 1957.[19]

All of these open-heart operations on infants, as well as countless other congenital heart surgeries on children, took place in the five-year period following the opening in June 1954 of the surgical suites at Texas Children's Hospital. Simultaneously, Cooley continued to perform adult cardiovascular procedures at both The Methodist Hospital and St. Luke's Episcopal Hospital. "In those days, I would schedule operations in all three on the same day," Cooley later recalled. "I had to race across the parking lot between operations. And it would seem that just about the time I would get over to Texas Children's Hospital to do an operation, they would call me from Methodist to say there was some complication that needed immediate attention."[20]

Cooley's parking-lot sprints did not go unnoticed. Often trailed by his assistants, anesthesiologist, and technicians, the often-in-transit Cooley was a memorable sight to passersby in the Texas Medical Center. What many did not see was how that first invaluable bubble oxygenator was transported. In the early months, the only device available was loaded into the back of a car that was driven from hospital to hospital. Pressed into service as the driver of that car was Cooley's wife, Louise Cooley.[21]

With that logistical problem solved, another one emerged. Demand threatened to exceed supply. By 1958, more than 310 open-heart operations had been performed at Texas Children's Hospital and St. Luke's Episcopal Hospital—more than at any other hospital in the United States, except the University of Minnesota.[22] "We had almost a monopoly on open-heart surgeries at that time," said Cooley. "We attracted patients not only from around the state and around the country, but all over the world."[23]

The number of heart patients in need of surgery continued to multiply when Cooley's expertise became increasingly well known and McNamara's pediatric cardiology service began to flourish. Because only one operating room at Texas Children's Hospital was available for congenital heart surgery, Cooley often scheduled multiple procedures, one after another. "When more than one surgery was to be done there was an exasperating wait while the room was cleaned and restocked," remembered McNamara. "Once, impatient with the nurses' progress in cleaning the room, Denton grabbed a wet mop and began swabbing the floor himself. An irritated and somewhat embarrassed nurse said, 'Dr. Cooley, you are the most aggressive man I've ever known.' His reply: 'Look, I know you think you're insulting me, but I consider that a high compliment.'"[24]

McNamara attributed this amusing incident to Cooley's determination to excel, no matter the obstacles. Known to operate for ten hours during the day, make recovery rounds during the evening, be on call for emergencies during the night, and be at his desk at daybreak the following morning to write manuscripts for publication, Cooley displayed a seemingly endless fund of mental and physical energy. His schedule continuously baffled his associates and confounded his competitors.[25]

Cooley's zealousness produced medical milestones that provided fundamental improvements in surgical treatments of congenital heart disease, as well as acquired heart disease. Within the first three decades of Cooley's career at Texas Children's Hospital, there were countless other "different, small, technical procedures that we have developed here to correct congenital heart defects, the types of procedures that have lasting value," said Cooley. "I think everyone recognizes our contribution toward the progress of surgery of congenital heart disease."[26]

One technique introduced to the world in 1962 by Cooley and his team was bloodless heart surgery. This was the first surgery of its kind to use plastic disposable oxygenators with low priming values and to use glucose solutions instead of blood. The innovative concept, applicable to both children and adults, was a major influence on the rapid proliferation of open-heart surgical procedures worldwide.[27] Another technical procedure introduced by Cooley's team in the early 1960s was the use of hyperthermia and extracorporeal bypass for the first surgical closure of the congenital heart malformation known as aortapulmonary fistula, or "aorticopulmonary window." The approach became the optimal surgical treatment for that condition.[28]

The achievements of Cooley and other pioneers in congenital heart surgery fueled rapid growth in the field of cardiovascular surgery for acquired heart disease in adults. These advances, together with the simplified techniques of open-heart surgery and emerging diagnostic abilities, led to a striking increase in the number of surgeries performed by Cooley's team. "After congenital heart disease yielded to surgical correction, progress in cardiac surgery became unstoppable," Cooley said.[29]

In 1961, most open-heart surgeries at Texas Children's Hospital and St. Luke's Episcopal Hospital were for congenital heart defects and were performed at Texas Children's Hospital. Five years later, in 1966, 68 percent of Cooley's 652 open-heart surgeries at the two hospitals were for acquired heart disease in adults and were performed at St. Luke's Episcopal Hospital.[30]

Anticipating this trend, Cooley foresaw the need for an institute in the Texas Medical Center that would be devoted solely to the clinical treatment, teaching, and research of cardiovascular disease in both children and adults. He believed that this program should ideally be affiliated with both Texas Children's Hospital and St. Luke's Episcopal Hospital, where 90 percent of the heart surgeries in Houston were performed and multidisciplinary support services were available. "With the permission of both institutions, at least with their sanction and not necessarily with their whole-hearted support, I incorporated the Texas Heart Institute in 1962," said Cooley. "I had the charter drawn up at my own expense, and organized it with a board of trustees to make it a freestanding program."[31]

Moving at his trademark speed, Cooley oversaw the creation of architectural plans for the construction of a new wing devoted to the newly chartered Texas Heart Institute. Armed with these drawings, in July 1962 Cooley proposed his elaborate concept to the joint board of Texas Children's Hospital and St. Luke's Episcopal Hospital. Hoping that his entire project would be included in the future expansion of the hospitals, Cooley received only tentative approval. Undeterred, he remained enthusiastic, continuing to pursue the possibilities. Eventually, the joint boards incorporated a modified plan for the Texas Heart Institute—including eight new operating suites—into the 1967 expansion plans.

What expanded immediately in 1962 was the Texas Heart Institute itself. One of the first to join the staff was Dr. Grady L. Hallman, a cardio-vascular surgeon with newly acquired interest in congenital heart surgery. Hallman's fascination with the field began during his recently completed surgical training at hospitals affiliated with Baylor College of Medicine. Within four years, he was recognized as one of the preeminent congenital heart surgeons in the country. In 1966, Hallman and Cooley cowrote the first comprehensive textbook in the field, *Surgical Treatment of Congenital Heart Disease*. It was to become a standard text.

The two surgeons also collaborated on countless articles for publica-tion in peer-reviewed journals throughout the late 1960s. Among these accounts of their congenital heart surgery procedures at Texas Children's Hospital were significant reports concerning the treatment of anomalous coronary arteries, vascular rings, prosthetic arterial conduits, valve dysfunc-tion, complete transposition of the great vessels, tetralogy of Fallot, and ventricular septal defects associated with pulmonary hypertension.

One particular procedure performed by Cooley and Hallman in 1963 made a significant impact, both in congenital heart surgery and in cardiac surgery for adults with acquired disease. It was the first successful coronary artery bypass for a congenital heart defect ever performed and its ramifica-tions were measurable. As stated by both surgeons in the 1975 preface to the second edition of their seminal textbook, the "successful insertion of a graft in the coronary artery system of a child in 1963 led to the use of graft-ing techniques for treatment of coronary artery anomalies and to extensive employment of coronary bypass in adults with acquired disease."[32]

This operation garnered international attention, but it was another procedure that made history for the Texas Heart Institute and its founder. On May 3, 1968, Cooley and his team were responsible for the first suc-cessful heart transplant ever performed in the United States. It was the first of 21 heart transplants performed in a single year at the Texas Heart Institute. When the lack of medications to fight organ rejection resulted in the eventual deaths of all 21 patients, the cardiac transplantation program at Texas Heart Institute came to a temporary halt in 1969. "I have done all I can as a surgeon," said Cooley at the time. "It remains for the immunolo-gists and biologists to unravel the mysteries that have limited our work."[33]

As the cardiac transplantation program faded from the spotlight, anoth-er cardiovascular procedure began to command center stage, producing a startling number of patients. The influx resulted from the introduction of coronary bypass procedures for adults with acquired heart disease. A direct byproduct of expertise gained during congenital heart surgery in children, the procedure revolutionized adult heart surgery.

After refining the bypass technique initially developed in 1963 for children with congenital heart disease, Cooley and Hallman introduced this new procedure in 1968. Within two years, Texas Heart Institute attributed 60 percent of its open-heart operations performed at St. Luke's Hospital to the technique. Once established, the popularity of the procedure never waned and bypasses continuously eclipsed other open-heart procedures performed at that hospital throughout the next three decades.

Equally newsworthy events occurred simultaneously in the field of congenital heart surgery during the 1960s and 1970s. The advances made in the surgical treatment of congenital heart disease provided the stimulus for vast improvements in diagnostic instruments and methods. When the resulting sophisticated technology and refined methods increased the accuracy of diagnoses, more surgical milestones were reached.

The most accurate diagnosis of congenital heart defects took place in the catheterization laboratory in the late 1960s. Advances made in equipment and techniques resulted in sophisticated and complex diagnostic procedures, some lasting more than two or three hours. With the newer diagnostic procedures, pediatric cardiologists were able to give a more defined anatomic and physiologic diagnosis of each defect. Some of these new techniques for infants and children were designed and developed at Texas Children's Hospital by Dr. Charles E. Mullins, a pediatric cardiologist who joined the hospital in 1969. One involved the employment of the Mullins sheath for left heart catheterization, an innovation that later became the accepted standard worldwide.

"As progress was made, a new era was born," said Cooley. "Surgeons were easily able to correct septal defects and pulmonary and aortic valve stenoses. They began to dismantle earlier palliative shunts to proceed with more definitive correction. These breakthroughs permitted surgical triumphs well beyond what had been envisioned in the early years."[34]

One such breakthrough occurred not in the operating suite, but in the laboratory of Dr. William Rashkind at Children's Hospital of Philadelphia. Rashkind's introduction of the balloon atrial septostomy in 1966 marked the beginning of manipulative or interventional procedures in catheterization. Participating with Rashkind on an investigational protocol of this device, Mullins successfully closed a patient's patent ductus arteriosus in the catheterization lab at Texas Children's Hospital. Rashkind's pioneering effort was the first of a succession of innovative techniques introduced during the following two decades, including several developed at Texas Children's

Hospital by Mullins. In 1982, Mullins reported that "there are currently procedures in use and under investigation for treating, and in some case curing, the congenital heart defect during catheterization."[35]

These non-surgical procedures to cure heart defects, particularly the patent ductus arteriosus first operated on by Gross in 1938, dramatically mirrored the rapid advances made in the field. Reflecting on the amazing growth of congenital heart surgery during his career, Mullins remembered when "closing hearts was a big deal. Since then surgeons have reached the point where they tackle any and everything."[36]

In the 1970s, a growing number of surgeons from the Texas Heart Institute were tackling the more complex congenital heart defects at Texas Children's Hospital. One such malformation was complete transposition of the great arteries, a condition in which the arteries and veins to and from the heart were switched and linked to the wrong heart chambers. Recent developments in the field of congenital heart surgery enabled the surgical repair of that inborn error in children one year of age or older. A procedure introduced in 1959 by Swedish thoracic surgeon Dr. Ake Senning was the first attempt to switch the arteries and change the fate of a severely cyanotic child. Another technique, introduced in 1963 by Dr. William Thornton Mustard in Canada, incorporated a different approach. Mustard's was an inflow switch operation, one that utilized the lining around the heart to function as a baffle that would create two upper altered chambers. Known as the Mustard operation, it was a physiologic repair that essentially made the repaired heart function backwards. Within a decade, Texas Heart Institute surgeons at Texas Children's Hospital and cardiovascular surgeons around the world had adopted this procedure for the surgical treatment of children over the age of one with complete transposition of the great arteries.

These and other breakthroughs had a huge impact on Texas Children's Hospital. Beginning in the early 1960s, there were more than 100 diagnostic procedures performed each month by pediatric cardiologists at Texas Children's Hospital. The number of candidates for congenital heart surgery began to multiply. With an increasing demand for cardiovascular surgical treatment for both children and adults, Cooley's team of surgeons grew proportionately. By 1972, more than 10,000 open-heart surgeries had been performed collectively at Texas Children's Hospital and St. Luke's Episcopal Hospital. Although astounding at the time, the number was to pale in comparison to the 5,000 or more completed in each of the following years.

This increased volume reflected several circumstances. The first was the completed construction of the Texas Heart Institute facilities in 1972. Located in the newly built tower of St. Luke's Episcopal Hospital, the spacious facilities included the eight operating rooms designed expressly for cardiac surgery. While adult cardiovascular procedures took place in the new facilities, those performed on children continued in the originally allocated space—that hospital's shared operating room with Texas Children's Hospital.

The second circumstance profoundly affecting the Texas Heart Institute was Cooley's severance in 1969 of his relationship with Baylor College of Medicine, thereby ending his participation in The Methodist Hospital's cardiac program. Deeming it "the best decision ever made," Cooley subsequently confined himself to Texas Children's Hospital and St. Luke's Episcopal Hospital. When the increasing number of both child and adult patients at the Texas Heart Institute warranted the undivided attention of more than two cardiovascular surgeons, Cooley began to recruit more. Within ten years, the number of board-certified cardiac surgeons at the Texas Heart Institute numbered six, including Cooley and Hallman, and all performed procedures on both pediatric and adult heart patients. "We call ourselves the 'Cardiovascular Associates' and there is a large staff of other support personnel," Cooley said while describing the ever-expanding Texas Heart Institute in 1979. "There is something like 18 secretaries and goodness knows how many technicians. We have 25 surgeons on fellowship, physicians in training, and four chest residents."[37]

One of the first surgeons recruited was Dr. George J. Reul in 1973. Reul pioneered work with aortic conduits and bypass in congenital heart surgery patients at Texas Children's Hospital. Another surgeon new to the team was Dr. David A. Ott, who came on board following his residency at the Texas Heart Institute in 1978. In tandem with Texas Children's Hospital's pediatric cardiologist Dr. Arthur Garson, Jr., Ott introduced advanced techniques in the late 1970s for the treatment of cardiac tumors and arrhythmia ablation in children.

Arriving in 1974 was Dr. O. Howard Frazier, named head of the Cullen Cardiovascular Surgical Research Laboratories at the Texas Heart Institute. Nine years later, after the anti-rejection medication cyclosporine became available in 1983, Frazier became director of the reinstated cardiac transplant program at Texas Heart Institute. It was a program in which he immediately excelled, making groundbreaking achievements within the first four years. Of the more than 200 transplants performed through 1987 by Frazier and Cooley at the Texas Heart Institute, 80 percent survived for one year or more.

In this group of survivors were several children, an anomaly at that time. Between 1983 and 1987, when lifesaving immunosuppressant medications were first used, only a few of the more than 1,200 heart transplants performed internationally were on pediatric patients. One of these patients was Sara Remington, an eight-month-old girl whose procedure took place at Texas Children's Hospital in November 1984. Frazier fondly called Sara "our baby" because at the time she was the youngest patient ever to undergo the procedure. Sara was to garner another singular recognition 13 years later, when she became the world's longest-surviving pediatric heart transplant recipient.[38]

Although heart transplantation worldwide continued to be reserved predominantly for adults in the 1980s, it began to emerge as a treatment for children with complex anomalies or end-stage congenital heart disease. When advances made in diagnostic techniques and equipment enabled pediatric cardiologists to diagnose such heart malformations with echocardiographic imaging in unborn infants, heart transplantation, as well as other surgical treatment, began to be performed on newborns. Within 15 years of the introduction of cyclosporine in 1983, one-tenth of the total number of heart transplantation recipients worldwide were children. Of those 2,000 pediatric transplantations, Texas Heart Institute surgeons at Texas Children's Hospital performed 83.[39]

"Leonard Bailey of Loma Linda, California, pioneered heart transplantation in infants and children," Cooley said in 1997, noting the excellent survival rates achieved by that cardiovascular surgeon. "Our results corroborate those of Bailey. In our 83 pediatric heart transplant patients, survival rates have been similar to that of adult transplant patients at one year and better than those of adults at five years. Pediatric five-year survival rate was about 78 percent."[40]

Bailey's initial efforts introduced "cardiac replacement" as a palliative treatment for infants born with hypoplastic left heart syndrome, a severe malformation of the heart detected before birth with the utilization of fetal echocardiography. In the mid-1980s, children born with this severe congenital heart defect rarely survived infancy. Bailey believed that immediate treatment was required. The recipient of his first successful heart transplant was just four days old when that breakthrough procedure took place in 1985.[41]

That congenital heart surgery was not the first to be performed on an infant less than six months old. Since the early 1970s, surgeons at Children's Hospital Boston had advocated primary repair of some defects during infancy, including ventricular septal defect, tetralogy of Fallot, and interruption of the aortic arch. Cardiovascular surgeons there also began to operate on infants under the age of one with transposition of the great arteries. For neonates with that condition, Boston's Dr. Aldo R. Castañeda advocated an immediate repair with an arterial switch procedure, rather than waiting a year to perform a palliative procedure. When this concept was adopted at the Texas Heart Institute in the late 1980s, it marked the dawning of the era of neonatal heart surgery at Texas Children's Hospital.[42]

Hailing the advent was McNamara, whose long-time theories about the necessity of early treatment were legendary in the field. "While only one infant out of 140 live births have some form of heart disease, one out of every 20 deaths in infants under one year of age is caused by a congenital malformation of the heart," he said. "It is in infancy rather than childhood or in adolescence that the greatest number of potentially lethal problems are seen, but the great majority of these seriously ill patients can be helped by proper treatment. Since the early 1940s, deaths from heart defects in infants and children have decreased from about 90 percent to 15 percent."[43]

These significant advances reflected the astonishing 50-year growth of the field of heart surgery in both children and adults. By the late 1980s, there were more than 40 procedures available for the surgical treatment of congenital heart defects. "More than 95 percent of significant congenital heart conditions can be corrected or alleviated by surgical intervention," Cooley explained. "Success with these anomalies encouraged surgeons to attempt other extracardiac and intracardiac repairs. These attempts resulted in a steady flow of advances."[44]

Many of those breakthroughs resulted in the rapid development of surgical treatment for adults with acquired heart disease, the major cause of death in adults. By 1987, more than 14,000 patients were benefiting annually from treatments available at the Texas Heart Institute, but the numbers of surgically treated adults and children vastly differed. In the more than 67,000 open-heart operations that had been performed by Texas Heart Institute surgeons by 1987, less than 10,000 involved pediatric patients.

It was a proportionate disparity not singular to the Texas Heart Institute and Texas Children's Hospital. Evidenced nationwide since the 1960s, the predominance of adult heart surgeries over that of children fueled the eventual development of pediatric cardiac surgery as a separate subspecialty, one devoted entirely to the treatment of neonates, infants, and children with congenital heart defects and acquired heart disease. This was a concept continuously championed since the early 1970s by Castañeda at Children's Hospital Boston and by other pioneers in the field. These proponents also argued for the centralization of all services involved in the diagnosis and treatment of children with congenital heart defects and acquired heart disease. They believed that subspecialization and centralization were necessitated by the complexities and varied nature of congenital heart defects and by the increasingly specialized management required for patients who differed in size, weight, and age.[45]

These ideas began to gain universal acceptance in the pediatric medical community during the late 1980s and early 1990s, and their eventual implementation in select institutions throughout the world heralded a turning point in the care and treatment of pediatric heart patients. Because subspecialization would ideally require the construction of a designated centralized space, the timing could not have been better at Texas Children's Hospital, where both immediate and future expansion plans were already on the drawing board. Necessitated by the 1987 physical separation of the joint services offered by Texas Children's Hospital and St. Luke's Episcopal Hospital, the plans included ten pediatric operating rooms in a new and separate building. Later named the West Tower, the building was constructed to be five stories high initially, but its foundation was designed for vertical expansion in the future.

Throughout the construction of the West Tower and for several months after its completion in 1991, Texas Heart Institute surgeons continued to perform procedures on Texas Children's Hospital patients in the operating rooms at St. Luke's Episcopal Hospital. When the new cardiovascular operating rooms in the West Tower were completed in 1992, the first procedure performed there was of historical significance. "Dr. Cooley wasn't doing many surgeries on children at that point," recalled Dr. J. Timothy Bricker, named chief of pediatric cardiology in 1992. "By that time, most pediatric heart procedures were being performed by Dr. Reul and Dr. Ott. I specifically arranged for Dr. Cooley to do the first case in tribute to his pioneering efforts in congenital heart surgery at Texas Children's Hospital."[46]

Since Cooley's initial surgery on a Texas Children's Hospital heart patient in 1954, the number of pediatric procedures performed either by him or by one of the other Texas Heart Institute surgeons had grown to more than 400 cases a year by the early 1990s. Although the location of the operating room had changed, the surgical team remained the same. Comprised of Texas Heart Institute surgeons, anesthesiologists, and perfusionists, the team continued to be involved in both adult and pediatric heart surgeries. Because the operating suites for each patient population were now situated in two different hospital buildings across the street from each other, the team migrated back and forth as needed, evoking memories of Cooley's legendary sprints through the parking lot during the 1950s.

The situation was not what Bricker and Texas Children's Hospital physician-in-chief, Dr. Ralph D. Feigin, envisioned for the future. "By the early 1990s, we had technically superb surgeons, but they were surgeons who were unable to be 100 percent committed to the care of children," said Bricker. "With the way things have changed, technically superb just really was not good enough. We really needed technically superb and dedicated to children—which, frankly, Texas Heart Institute recognized as well as we did. While there was certainly some tension involved with our decision to go out and recruit a congenital heart surgeon for Texas Children's Hospital, much of the tension was more related to whether it was to be under the umbrella of the Texas Heart Institute as opposed to under the umbrella of Baylor College of Medicine. In fact, we had investigated several possibilities of who that was going to be. I had no question that who we wanted for the long run was Chuck Fraser."[47]

This primary candidate was 37-year-old Dr. Charles D. Fraser, Jr., chief resident in cardiovascular surgery at Johns Hopkins Hospital in 1992. Fraser's designation as favored candidate by both Feigin and Bricker reflected the skills he had perfected during his previous nine years of surgical training. "Everybody who had ever worked with him said he was the best surgeon they had ever worked with," Bricker noted. "That included David Ott, who knew him as a medical student. That included George Reul and Bud Frazier, who knew him as a medical student. That included the people I talked with at Johns Hopkins. So it was clear that this guy was really special."[48]

Fraser's journey to becoming such a well-respected surgeon had begun during his internship at Johns Hopkins in 1984, where extenuating circumstances shaped his career choice. A native Texan, he had graduated from the University of Texas Medical Branch in Galveston. While there, he happened to fall in love with and marry Houstonian Helen Cooley, the daughter of the famous former Johns Hopkins surgical resident who founded the Texas Heart Institute. "I went to Johns Hopkins as a young man thinking of myself as trying to cut my own swath, and I did not want to be viewed as being from Dr. Cooley's lineage," Fraser said. "That is not meant to be anything disparaging about Dr. Cooley; that's just the way I felt."[49]

In order to achieve such independence, Fraser's original goal was to become a general pediatric surgeon. While rotating among the various services, he became intrigued with the heart surgery service and, in particular, the exciting and progressive work of pediatric heart surgeons Dr. Bruce Reitz, Dr. Bill Baumgartner, and Dr. Timothy J. Gardner. It soon became a mutual admiration society, with those surgeons recognizing Fraser's exceptional skills during the early years of his surgical training. "You really have an aptitude for this," the mentors told Fraser. "We realize that you don't want to labor under Dr. Cooley's shadow, but don't cut your nose off to spite your face. This is something that you are good at and something you are interested in. Consider the idea that you can not only be a pediatric surgeon, but you can also be a pediatric heart surgeon."[50]

"So that's how this all started to develop," Fraser explained. "In my third year there, I decided to change tracks a little bit. Instead of general surgery, I was going to do heart surgery and, specifically, pediatric heart surgery." This altered career path necessitated more years in training at Johns Hopkins, a challenge Fraser enthusiastically embraced. In the following seven years there, including a fellowship at the Texas Heart Institute in 1988, he devoted himself to learning exactly what cardiac surgery entailed and what was required to do it well. "When you are at Hopkins, a lot is expected of you and you come to expect a lot of yourself after spending time there," Fraser said. "Having said that, we Hopkins trainees are very confident by the time we have finished there. We are very, very confident. A quote that is used, and I don't know if it is unique to Hopkins, but certainly it is applied to us trainees, is, 'Seldom wrong, never in doubt.' And that's true. By the time you are finished there, you feel that you can pretty much take on anybody, anywhere, any time."[51]

What Fraser wanted to take on following his fellowship in cardiothoracic surgery at Hopkins was a fellowship in pediatric cardiac surgery, but where he would do that was in question. At the time, the most fully established program was Castañeda's service at Children's Hospital Boston. Fraser thought that was where he needed to go, but one of his mentors thought otherwise. "If you are going to do it, I know the sort of person you are. You need to go about it full bore, and what you really want is quality," Gardner told him. "You don't want the name, you want quality. You need to go to Melbourne. There's no question about it. The best guy in the world and the best unit in the world is in Melbourne."[52]

Fraser discovered that the recipient of such high praise was Dr. Roger B. B. Mee, a 45-year-old New Zealander. Mee was at Melbourne's Royal Children's Hospital, which, with 460 beds, was the largest children's hospital in the southern hemisphere. Before his 1980 appointment as that hospital's director of cardiac surgery, Mee trained for six months with Castañeda at Children's Hospital Boston during his three-year adult cardiothoracic surgery fellowship at the Peter Bent Brigham Hospital. Within eight years in Melbourne, Mee had established a comprehensive children's heart center that emulated Castañeda's. Believing that the best results in congenital heart surgery could only be achieved in high-volume centers, he actively sought and received referrals, personally performing more than 600 heart surgeries with superlative results. By 1990, Mee had lowered neonatal mortalities to 2 percent and his congenital heart surgical outcomes not only surpassed Castañeda's, but were reportedly the best in the world.

These unequaled outcomes garnered skepticism within the medical community. No matter the reported facts, many congenital heart surgeons simply chose not to believe what Mee had claimed in published and peer-reviewed medical journals. "He did 25 simple transpositions, his first, without losing one and nobody believed it," recalled Fraser.[53] The consensus of opinion among skeptics was that no one was as good as Mee claimed to be, and therefore the data must be fabricated. Consequently, Fraser's decision to go to Melbourne for his 1991 fellowship generated dubious remarks, including one from a member of his immediate family. "Dr. Cooley sure said I was crazy to go," Fraser said. "But Dr. Cooley also said I was crazy to stay at Johns Hopkins to train in cardiac surgery."[54]

Undaunted by the differing opinions about his fellowship choice, Fraser nonetheless arrived in Melbourne with expectations of learning little, if anything, new. By his own admission, he envisioned himself as "the big guy from Hopkins" who was simply there to "see what these little guys are doing in Australia, and maybe pick up a pointer or two. Well, completely wrong. It was like I had to start all over."[55]

Fraser's attitude readjustment came within the first few months of his fellowship. As a direct observer, he quickly knew that the skeptics were wrong to question Mee's technical expertise in anatomic correction with an arterial switch, neonatal cardiac transplantation, stage palliation for hypoplastic left heart syndrome, and various other neonatal complete repairs. Far from being fabrications, Mee's superlative outcomes were verifiable by observing the skillful surgeon in action, both in the operating room and outside of it. Through observation and participation, Fraser determined that Mee's success in areas where others failed was directly attributable to that surgeon's seemingly simple philosophy: "Outcomes in congenital heart surgery are optimized by surrounding the patient with the greatest expertise possible during all times of the surgical and postoperative period."[56]

Fraser experienced this philosophy firsthand. He continually found himself surrounded by Mee's team of experts, both in the operating room and afterwards with postoperative patients. Each surgeon, anesthesiologist, perfusionist, nurse, and operating room technician was a specialist who worked only with pediatric heart patients and no others. Mee worked extremely well with this team—although he could be tyrannical at times, Fraser discovered. However, having worked with tyrants before, Fraser was not deterred by this. Instead, he began to admire Mee's work ethic increasingly. He found Mee to be a meticulous surgeon, one who analyzed and perfected the component parts of each procedure, and a very sound physiologist, one who easily assembled the elements of physiology. Fraser also discovered that Mee continued to exceed expectations in the field of congenital heart surgery. "What I got the most from Roger was setting the bar very high and not settling for anything less," Fraser said. "It's just this tenacious determination to stay at it until you get it right."[57]

Fraser embraced Mee's attitude wholeheartedly. He was at the hospital morning, noon, and night, whether he was on call or not. After or before treating his own patients in the operating room or in the hospital, he devoured other patients' medical charts, peppering Mee with questions at every given opportunity. At a precise moment, one he remembered with clarity a decade later, a bell went off in his head. "The truth is, I can remember the day, where we were and what the environment was, when I told Helen, 'This is it. Either I am going to do it this way or I am not doing it at all.' It was an epiphany for me. It's like you have seen the other side, and you can't go back."[58]

Totally converted to Mee's philosophy, Fraser returned to Johns Hopkins Hospital in 1992 to continue his training as chief resident of cardiovascular surgery. Uncertain about his future, he contemplated offers of permanent positions at Johns Hopkins, Stanford, and various other institutions— including one from Feigin and Bricker at Texas Children's Hospital. "They started talking to me about my coming to Texas Children's Hospital in 1992," Fraser recalled. "But, for a variety of reasons, it wasn't the right thing for me to do at the time. Roger Mee, who had just left Melbourne to join the Cleveland Clinic Foundation, asked us to join him there in 1993 and we did."[59]

Fraser's refusal of their offer did not dissuade Feigin and Bricker. As they proceeded to search for an alternative candidate, Fraser continued to remain their top choice. "After he joined Roger in Cleveland, I kept in close touch with him," Bricker said. "Periodically, I would say, 'Are you ready to come to Houston, yet?' And at one point, that was something that worked. He joined Texas Children's Hospital in 1995 as chief of the congenital heart surgery service and cardiac surgeon-in-charge."[60]

The timing of Fraser's decision was propitious. Within months of his arrival at Texas Children's Hospital, the vertical expansion of the West Tower was in the final stages of discussion. Although construction plans were indefinite at the time, one certainty existed: the expansion was to include a centralized area for the care and treatment of pediatric heart patients. Fraser found that his vision—one that he openly admitted plagiarizing largely from Mee—dovetailed into what Feigin and Bricker wanted for this new heart center. To assemble the individual members required for a focused surgical team in such a center, Fraser immediately instigated a search for highly skilled clinicians in the areas of pediatric cardiac anesthesia and pediatric cardiac perfusion, and for another pediatric cardiac surgeon.

"The concept of a unified team is something Chuck and I talked about from the beginning," said Bricker. "The unified team is based on a commitment to the best care of children and a commitment to improving the lives and health of children with heart disease, and to an optimistic future for their families. That was the mission we all shared for the Texas Children's Heart Center, and it preceded the actual planning of its physical space."[61]

The mission inspired Bricker and Feigin's "hospital within a hospital" concept for Texas Children's Heart Center, scheduled for completion in 2001. Designed to encompass four floors of the West Tower expansion, the center included an entire floor devoted to cardiac surgery operating rooms, a recovery room, a catheterization lab, a family waiting room, and family services. Also planned for that floor was a cardiovascular ICU, affording the surgical team a new way to follow pediatric cardiac patients postoperatively at Texas Children's Hospital. "Originally, they were followed in one of our regular ICUs here on our third floor, where we had one of three pods devoted to cardiovascular surgery," Feigin explained.[62] Another complete floor housed the diagnostic laboratories, cardiac medical records, and outpatient clinics. For cardiology inpatients, there was another floor where all cardiac services were located.

There was also a floor totally devoted to the academic and scholarly component of the Texas Children's Heart Center. Comprising offices, conference rooms, and a "living room" reception area, this unique arrangement epitomized the shared mission of a unified team effort. "It's very uncommon in children's hospitals for the surgeons, the anesthesiologists, and the cardiologists to interact so routinely," Bricker said. "In the Heart Center they are all officed together, and it was more than a symbolic gesture on our part. It was a functional decision that we would all be one team in one location."[63]

Togetherness was an integral part of the unique design of the Texas Children's Heart Center. Its ability to offer examinations, echocardiography, heart catheterization, congenital heart surgery, and intensive care in one specific area was specifically designed to provide enhanced delivery of care for patients and their families.

To meet the surgical aspect of that goal as construction progressed over the following five years, Fraser succeeded in reorganizing the pediatric cardiac surgery service at Texas Children's Hospital. Appointed chief of the division of congenital heart surgery in the Michael E. DeBakey Department of Surgery at Baylor College of Medicine in 2000, he had already established the nucleus of his surgical team. "We now have two full-time surgeons, myself and Dr. Dean McKenzie, who joined us in 1998," he reported in 2000. "But I emphasize we are only a small part of a very outstanding group of individuals, all of whom are completely dedicated to our service. There are now 12 full-time operating room nurses, 20 ICU nurses, and four perioperative nurse clinicians. We have focused our intensive care unit and it is now a full-time, dedicated, postoperative cardiac unit with four cardiac intensivists. We have three full-time pediatric anesthesiologists, under the direction of Dr. Dean B. Andropoulos, whom we were lucky enough to steal from Oakland Children's Hospital in San Francisco in 1998."[64]

Once established, Andropoulos' service in the Texas Children's Heart Center became one of the nation's few programs dedicated exclusively to clinical care, education, and research in pediatric cardiac anesthesia. While monitoring more than 20 different functions in a patient's body before, during, and after surgery, Andropoulos' team watched "every heartbeat and every breath," he explained. "Because we specialize in surgery of pediatric patients with congenital heart disease, we are very, very familiar with the problems that can occur and we can better anticipate and treat the problems because we see them so often."[65]

For the perfusion support of a child during open-heart surgery, Fraser recruited dedicated pediatric cardiac perfusionists. With that team of specialists, he introduced concentrated efforts to incorporate smaller oxygenators more appropriate for neonates and infants. "Using novel approaches, we monitor cerebral blood flow and brain oxygenation during bypass to precisely regulate perfusion during the entire operation," he explained.[66] Fraser also maintained an increased focus on accuracy in the operating room. Each of the pediatric perfusionists had not only their own physiologic monitors, but also separate monitors to observe the operative field made visible by Fraser's use of a headlight camera. "Our perfusionists customize the perfusion to each child's unique needs," Fraser said. "This customized care allows for a predictable level of perfusion support and children have optimal physiology to help them withstand even the most complex cardiac repair."[67]

The aggressive monitoring of children in the operating room and post-operatively in the cardiovascular ICU also included transesophageal echocardiography, a diagnostic tool that Fraser had grown up with in congenital heart care and without which he felt naked. "It allows us to get a very accurate anatomic view of the patient before surgery, but probably more importantly in the immediate postoperative period," he explained. "What we know is if we can re-intervene on residual problems early in the perioperative period, we have a much greater chance of a successful outcome."[68]

One particular surgical procedure in which successful outcomes became the norm for Fraser's surgical team was the arterial switch operation for children born with transposition of the great arteries. Until the advent of the neonatal arterial switch in the 1970s, the vast majority of these infants did not survive the first few weeks or months of life. By 2001, more than 100 consecutive neonatal arterial switches were performed by Fraser's team without a single patient's death, a unique accomplishment in cardiac medicine at that time. According to Fraser, "No other institution has published success rates better than ours on this procedure."[69]

In 2001, the American Heart Association published a report stating that the national rate of death for patients who underwent congenital heart surgery had declined from 30 percent to 5 percent in the previous two decades.[70] At Texas Children's Heart Center in 2001, Fraser's team performed dramatically above that average. In addition to the 100 percent survival of neonatal arterial switch patients, the team achieved a 98 percent success rate in all congenital heart surgery procedures performed. The caseload of more than 650 cardiac surgeries a year encompassed a variety of complex congenital open-heart repairs, including correction in the smallest neonates with hypoplastic left-heart syndrome, interrupted aortic arch, transposition of the great arteries, and single ventricles.

"I have spent a lot of time focusing on how to support these tiny babies during the operation," Fraser said. "It means having very accurate anesthesia, in our case, a pediatric cardiac anesthesiologist, a very refined subspecialty. We have focused our perfusion on being very accurate and gentle. I think we are among the best at doing this. With the arrival of pediatric cardiovascular surgeon Dr. Jeffrey S. Heinle in 2002, we have assembled a group of specialists, highly talented, dedicated people who do nothing but care for children with heart disease. This includes our nursing staff, perfusionists, anesthesiologists, technicians, and surgeons. There are only a few centers in the world that can make that claim."[71]

With this highly focused team's expertise established, Fraser believed that Texas Children's Hospital afforded each heart patient as good an opportunity for a positive outcome as any place in the world. Collectively, every member of the team took pride in their ability to meet each patient's needs with highly specialized procedures for complex congenital cardiac maladies. Those procedures included the Blalock-Taussig shunt, Glenn shunt, Fontan procedure, patent ductus arteriosus ligation, atrial septal defect and ventricular septal defect closures, coarctation repair, tetralogy of Fallot repair, Rastelli procedure, Ross procedure, aortic arch advancement, and aforementioned arterial switch.

For those infants and children with end-stage heart disease or inoperable congenital structural abnormalities, the only surgical intervention available was heart transplantation. Refined immunosuppression and improved individualization of treatment enabled surgeons Fraser, McKenzie, and Heinle to establish and maintain a favorable long-term survival rate for all pediatric heart transplantations. Noting that the first pediatric cardiac transplant in the world took place at Texas Children's Hospital, Fraser said: "We have a very large body of experience with this therapy."[72]

Fraser and McKenzie also instigated a dedicated pediatric lung transplant program, one of only six such programs in the United States, to treat children with lung disease. The first pediatric lung transplant at Texas Children's Hospital took place on October 3, 2002. Performed on an 11-year-old patient diagnosed with primary pulmonary hypertension, the successful procedure included a bilateral lung transplant and simultaneous closure of an atrial septal defect.

Other new surgical procedures were introduced at the Texas Children's Heart Center at the beginning of the twenty-first century. In certain circumstances, the surgeons began to employ minimally invasive techniques to repair a defect inside the heart of an infant or child. In an open-heart procedure, this technique involved a smaller incision and therefore less discomfort for the patient. "With standard surgery, the child would be left with a six-inch scar that goes from the top of the breast bone to below the bottom of the breast bone," Heinle explained. "With the minimally invasive approach, the scar measures only about 2.5 inches and is just over the lower part of the bone. The scar does not show when a child is wearing regular clothing."[73]

Often performed in concert with a surgical procedure to help make the operation more directed and effective was interventional cardiac catheterization. In certain congenital heart defects, such as patent ductus arteriosus and atrial septal defect, therapeutic catheterization alone could achieve the same results as surgery. When the Texas Children's Heart Center opened in 2001, its highly sophisticated catheterization laboratories became the only facility in the Houston area to offer both diagnostic and therapeutic procedures for infants, children, and adults. "In the last five years, we have had an explosion in the number of ideas and equipment that we can use to improve the care of children with heart defects," reported pediatric cardiologist Dr. Ronald G. Grifka, director of cardiac catheterization.[74] Of the more than 350 procedures performed annually in the catheterization laboratories at Texas Children's Hospital, over half were therapeutic.

While many of the simple defects became correctible with catheter-based interventional approaches, the more complex and rare congenital heart defects continued to require surgical treatment. Traditionally, in the United States and abroad, pediatric surgical facilities with high volumes had the occasion to treat rare heart defects more frequently, thus allowing the surgical team to refine its techniques.[75] Such was the case at the Texas Children's Heart Center. "We have children coming to us from our community, other states, and the rest of the world," said Fraser. "In many instances, they have been evaluated at other centers and turned down for surgery. We take these children at Texas Children's Hospital, regardless of how complex."[76]

Of the more than 10,000 infants and children seen each year by the pediatric cardiologists at Texas Children's Hospital, most suffered from heart defects. As the Heart Center's reputation for excellence grew, the number of referred heart patients continued to increase. When surgical procedures escalated to average more than 750 per year in 2003, the refinement of surgical techniques for complex congenital heart defects was an ongoing process. The result was technical expertise applicable to more than just children with congenital heart disease. Reported Fraser in 2003: "It is becoming increasingly clear that adults with congenital heart disease requiring surgery often should be treated at a children's hospital."[77]

With this divergent and ever-increasing caseload, the surgical team succeeded in building a world-renowned congenital heart surgery program at Texas Children's Hospital. As the field of pediatric and congenital heart surgery continued to develop into a separate super-subspecialty, Fraser and his team offered future pediatric cardiothoracic surgeons the opportunity for concentrated training by establishing a two-year fellowship program. An integral facet of the program was research, fueled by the three surgeons' interests in neurodevelopment, artificial organs, pediatric mechanical circulatory systems, and compliment inhibition during cardiopulmonary bypass and transplantation. Echoing his own fellowship with Mee a decade earlier, Fraser clearly demonstrated his philosophy to fellows at the Texas Children's

Heart Center: "Optimal surgical results are only achieved in highly dedicated, specialized centers with focused specialists attending to the medical necessities of these very ill children."[78]

Also reminiscent of Mee's training was Fraser's bedside manner with patients and their families. Since most surgical procedures performed in the Texas Children's Heart Center involved variable degrees of risk, Fraser believed that the truth should not be sugarcoated when he spoke with a patient's family. "It's something else I plagiarized from Roger Mee. I am very, very frank," he said. "Most people appreciate that, but there are some who are put off by it, including some of the referring doctors. Some of my own colleagues in cardiology would prefer that I pat the kids on the head and smile at the parents and say it's all going to be all right. That's not what I would want for me or for my children. I don't think that is the proper approach. We are very, very direct about it."[79]

Fraser's compassionate frankness was rooted in his years of experience in pediatric and congenital heart surgery. Realizing how difficult it must be to learn that your child has a serious heart defect, Fraser also knew what uncertainties the future held for that child and what a tremendous responsibility it was going to be for the family. "Unfortunately, some children will not have just one operation and be 'fixed,'" Fraser explained. "A few will require another operation. Many of these children are going to require longitudinal management. There will be frequent doctor visits. There will be medications. It will be a different level of surveillance than for children with normal hearts. We think it's very important to provide the family with as much information as we can."[80]

Aware of the increasing number of parents of children with congenital heart disease who accessed the Internet for information in the late 1990s, Fraser and his team conducted the world's first survey to document usage patterns among families whose children required congenital heart surgery. The results, published in *Pediatrics* magazine in 2002, confirmed that Internet use by this patient population was on the increase and concluded that "our vigilance in providing accurate Internet references, as well as identifying inaccurate Internet information available to our patients and their parents, is of paramount importance."[81]

Such dedicated efforts were not singular to Fraser and the surgical team. Rather, they were evident throughout the Texas Children's Heart Center. Families of patients found themselves surrounded by compassionate experts committed to caring for children. "Not only are the people here dedicated professionals, they are drawn here because of a love for the children,"

McKenzie said. "Every day I witness nurses, physicians, child life specialists, social workers, and others giving time and effort above and beyond the call of duty because of the compassion they feel for these children and their families. It's a very special place."[82]

It was this all-encompassing dedication to the loving care of children and their families that helped create optimal outcomes at the Texas Children's Heart Center, Fraser believed. "It can't just be a slick surgeon or a slick cardiologist, or whatever, to achieve optimal results," he said. "You have to have the whole package. That's why we can say, quite boldly, that we can do it better here at Texas Children's Hospital than just about every other center in Texas and probably in the southern part of the United States. Not just because of one individual, but because of all of us."[83]

Fraser and his colleagues were not alone in their assessment. National and international affirmation of their achievements came with the published results of a national children's hospital survey conducted by *Child* magazine in 2003. Listed as one of the top three heart centers in the United States was the Texas Children's Heart Center, which shared the honor with The Children's Hospital of Philadelphia and Children's Hospital Boston, where Gross had performed the first surgical procedure on a child's heart in 1937.

In the more than six decades since that initial congenital heart procedure and the subsequent Taussig-Blalock shunt procedure in 1944, the overall mortality rate of children born with malformations of the heart had significantly declined. Having experienced not only the dawning of the era, but also its maturation, Cooley reflected: "Advances in the treatment of congenital heart disease have dramatically changed not only the lives of the patients involved, but also the lives of the pioneering investigators in this field. As we grapple to overcome today's obstacles to innovative therapeutic breakthroughs, we must not forget the struggles and the contributions of the pioneers whose improvisation, cooperation, perseverance, and vision made the treatment of congenital heart disease a reality."[84]

As one of the pioneering hospitals in the field of congenital heart surgery, Texas Children's Hospital experienced multiple medical milestones in its first five decades. The high standards for the surgical treatment of congenital heart disease established by Cooley and the surgeons of the Texas Heart Institute continued with Fraser and his team. Lesions historically associated with near-ly uniform mortality in the 1940s now were treated with an ever-improving success rate at the Texas Children's Heart Center. Its 2003, surgical survival rates approached 100 percent for many of these previously fatal cardiac malformations, including transposition of the great arteries, interrupted aortic arch, total anomalous pulmonary venous return, and truncus arteriosus.

What remained one of the most difficult congenital heart conditions to treat was hypoplastic left heart syndrome, the most common condition in newborns with congenital heart disease involving a single ventricle. As Fraser and his team refined techniques and concentrated efforts to deliver optimal outcomes with these patients, measurable progress followed. "Using a multidisciplinary approach, the operative mortality for surgical palliation of this difficult and common problem has steadily declined at Texas Children's Hospital," Fraser explained in 2003. "The operative survival for children undergoing first stage surgical palliation for hypoplastic left heart syndrome has been greater than 90 percent during the last three years."[85]

These improved survival rates for surgical patients in the Texas Children's Heart Center completely altered the formerly dismal prognoses for children born with hypoplastic left heart syndrome and other such complex congenital defects. With a combination of tenacious determination, extensive experience, institutional commitment, and dedicated personnel, Fraser's team at the Texas Children's Heart Center delivered optimum care and every possibility of a quality outcome for each of these patients.

Such positive outcomes indicated a certainty for the future. As it had from its inception in 1954, Texas Children's Hospital was to play a pioneering role in the highly specialized field of congenital heart surgery in the twenty-first century.

"You go follow that baby," Jean told husband Scott, as ten neonatologists wheeled newborn Rachel Parrish out of the delivery room at St. Luke's Episcopal Hospital to take her to Texas Children's Hospital.[86]

Moments before, the calm, perfectly pink, eight-pound baby girl had cooed and looked around at the audience gathered for her arrival. In addition to the crowd of doctors in the delivery room, her grandparents and aunts were waiting to greet her in the waiting room. "The neonatologist said Scott could take her out there to meet everybody, so he did," Jean said. "Then they put her in a warming bed and took her down the hall to Texas Children's Hospital, and Scott was following that baby."

Three days after her debut, Rachel underwent open-heart surgery at Texas Children's Hospital. The lifesaving procedure, the first part of a three-stage treatment designed to "replumb" her damaged heart, making it pump blood with one chamber instead of two, was considered the riskiest stage and lasted more than eight hours. Afterwards, Rachel was taken to the pediatric intensive care unit (PICU), where a problem developed.

"She started bleeding and they had to go back in, but a little bit later she was stable," Jean recalled. "The next morning, Dr. Fraser told us Rachel was not coming out of anesthesia. When we asked him what that meant, he told us everything that it could be, including the fact that she might not come out of it."

Distraught that their daughter might never wake up, Jean and Scott began to question their decision to put her through this surgery. After two long hours of introspection while waiting and praying for better news, the parents received word that Rachel was awake. When they visited her in the PICU, they found her on a respirator with unidentifiable tubes and wires coming out of her feet, arms, chest, and nose. Rachel was surrounded by beeping monitors. The incision in her chest was clearly visible and, although she was a painful sight to behold, they were relieved to learn that she was not in pain.

What Rachel's parents also found in the PICU at Texas Children's Hospital was that "everyone respectfully and patiently addressed our concerns," Jean said. "They were very conscious that Rachel was a person, not just a patient. They really made us feel like we were important and that Rachel was important."

The PICU nursing staff also made Jean feel that she was contributing to her daughter's recovery. Encouraged to personalize the sign over Rachel's bed, Jean began fabricating one from pink construction paper during the hours she spent in the waiting room between visits to the PICU. It was a welcome relief to have something she could do. "When you are going through this, you can't do anything for your child," she said. "You are feeling a little bit hopeless because you don't know what is going on. The PICU nurses recognize that you are the parent, and I think they sympathize about how much control we were giving up with our baby. They even gave us the opportunity to moisturize her lips and her hands. They were very helpful to make us feel like we were important and necessary."

What also impressed Jean and Scott was the vast number of pediatric specialists at Texas Children's Hospital. Having never experienced childhood illnesses when she was growing up, Jean had gone to a family doctor. She was unaware of physicians who specialized in distinct areas. "For instance, I didn't know there were perfusionists and all they did was operate the heart–lung bypass machine, a very complicated job," she said. "Dr. Fraser recruited his whole team, and I was amazed at the depth of their knowledge."

The Parrishes were constantly updated on Rachel's progress by Fraser, who often displayed cautious optimism. Two weeks after her birth, they were told that Rachel was well enough to go home for the first time. Armed with detailed information about how to take care of her wounds, administer medications, and watch over her, Jean and Scott officially began to fulfill their roles as mother and father. For the next seven months, Rachel continued to heal, seeing pediatric cardiologist Dr. Louis I. Bezold at Texas Children's Hospital on a regular basis for checkups.

With the exception of a few minor infections that caused major scares to her parents, Rachel continued to thrive. She returned to Texas Children's Hospital for her second surgical procedure when she was eight months old and her third when she was three and a half. As they had done during her first procedure, Jean and Scott sat in the waiting room, anxious to hear a report from the surgeon about Rachel's progress. Both times, the word they received was positive. "I think when Dr. Fraser comes out of surgery to talk to you, or when he is standing by your child's bed with a little smile and says, 'I think we're doing well,' I think he's really pleased how all the pieces fit together and the benefit is to the child," Jean said. "With something that is as damaging as HLHS, Dr. Fraser can bring the child to a point where we have got control. We have not fixed it, but we have repaired it."

After both procedures, Rachel continued her regularly scheduled appointments with pediatric cardiologist Bezold at Texas Children's Hospital. "We were going every day, then every week, and then every two months," Jean said. "When the appointments first got spaced out to two months, I was like, 'Oh, my gosh, I can't believe it.' And then it got to the point where he didn't need to see her for a year. And I loved it when the doctor said, 'No physical restrictions.'"

To follow his advice, Jean had to adapt her new mothering skills. Instead of being overprotective of Rachel on the playground, rushing to her side whenever she stumbled or fell, she learned to practice restraint. Eventually, Rachel began to have a deceptively normal childhood. Other than the several medications she had to take orally every day, her routine became varied. Although the scar from her surgeries was visible, she was not self-conscious about it. She took dancing lessons and learned how to swim at the age of four. In 2003, at the age of six, Rachel began school. "I was a little nervous about school just because her scar comes above her collar, and I wondered whether they would treat her differently because of it," Jean said. "I asked Dr. Bezold what I should tell them at school and, although Rachel never has had an emergency, I talked to the teacher about the possibility. You have to look for little reminders that things aren't exactly typical with Rachel."

With little or no memory of her surgical procedures, the little girl with the telltale scar continued to blossom in school and at home. While playing with her friends or her baby twin brothers, she exhibited no signs of frailty. "It's very easy to forget about her heart," Scott said. "We have every reason to be optimistic. We don't know what the future brings, but no parent does."[87]

Rachel's future, like that of other children with HLHS who underwent the Norwood procedure in the 1980s and 90s, remained unknown. Although many continued to survive at five years of age, just how much longer they could live was uncertain. For Jean and Scott, optimism prevailed. When one long-term survivor was featured on an NBC news broadcast about HLHS in 2003, Jean's mother called to see if she was watching. She was. And, to her delight, the healthy-looking survivor was a very active teenage girl who played soccer.

As for the past, Jean and Scott Parrish were certain that they had made the right decision about Rachel's undergoing the Norwood procedure at Texas Children's Hospital. Just like all parents blindsided with the news that their baby had HLHS, they had devoted hours to weighing all of the options available before reaching a conclusion.

"You have to decide if you can live with yourself knowing you didn't try, didn't take the risk," Jean said. "I can't imagine what it is like to lose a child. It has never happened to us. We looked down that road, but we didn't have to go there."

11

✋ CRITICAL CARE ✋

"**M**OM, I DON'T FEEL WELL," eight-year-old Leslie Meigs reported early one morning.

Knowing that her daughter had been perfectly healthy the day before; Wendy Meigs thought that perhaps she had the flu. She took Leslie's temperature, found it to be 101, and gave her a Tylenol.

An hour later, when Leslie's temperature had climbed to 102, her mother gave her Ibuprofen. When Leslie's temperature reached 103 shortly thereafter, Wendy called the doctor, saying that her daughter had some sort of illness. Told to bring her in, she bundled Leslie up and drove to the doctor's office at 11:30 a.m.

"By then her fever had gone down to 101. Her regular physician wasn't on duty, so we saw another one there. He sat down, checked her out, and said, 'I don't see anything,'" Wendy recalled. "The doctor said: 'Go on home. Something is bound to pop up. Call us when it pops up.' So I took her home."[1]

Still not overly concerned, Wendy stopped at McDonald's when Leslie requested a "Happy Meal." Thinking her hunger signified that the illness was waning, Wendy was surprised when her daughter immediately became nauseated in the car.

When they returned home, Leslie's nausea not only continued, but increased. At one point, she talked about "seeing angels." While comforting, hugging, and patting her daughter late that afternoon, Wendy discovered that Leslie's temperature was 105 and an odd-looking rash was appearing on her arm.

"It was little purple dots, like little blood blisters under your skin," said Leslie's father, Jody Meigs.

"It was weird," Wendy recalled. "So I called the doctor's office and they said, 'Don't worry about the rash. It's not a big deal. It's either viral or bacterial, and just don't worry about it. Just put her in the tub to cool her down and give her some Ibuprofen.'"

After the bath, Leslie's temperature decreased. However, as the evening progressed, the rash continued to worsen. Phoning the doctor's office again and again, Wendy repeatedly was told not to worry about the rash. During her call at 8 p.m., she received instructions to call the triage nurse on duty later at the office only if Leslie's temperature increased.

"At about 10 o'clock, the rash was just unbelievable," Wendy said. "I called the triage nurse and told her about the rash and she said the same thing, 'Don't worry about it.' And I said, 'Look, maybe I've been watching way too many of these biological warfare movies where the CDC accidentally has released something in the air, because this rash really, really doesn't look right. They are irregular in shape. Some are the size of quarters and they're purple.' That's when the triage nurse freaked and said, 'Oh, my God. Oh, my God. Take her to the closest hospital you can find.' It was amazing. After five hours of 'no big deal,' all of a sudden I get these instructions from an antsy nurse?"

After Leslie was taken to a neighborhood hospital, her parents were not the only ones to notice that the strange rash was spreading rapidly. Other people waiting to see a doctor in the emergency room kept their distance, walking way around Leslie to avoid contact. "It was all over her face by then," Wendy said, remembering exactly what she thought at the time. "I was thinking they would give her some antibiotics or something in the emergency room, and we'll go home."

When finally admitted to the ER after a long wait, Leslie was given an IV. Without entering the room when he arrived, the doctor stood at the entryway. From across the room, the nurse showed him the rash on Leslie's stomach and leg. Soon after, he walked away, going behind a nearby curtain. Wendy misinterpreted his behavior.

"I'm thinking the IV fluids is all she needed, and then I hear him say, 'She's critical. We need to rush her into isolation.' And I'm thinking, 'Oh, man, that poor family on the other side of the curtain. Gosh, I feel sorry for them. The mother must be freaking out over there.' And it was us! They immediately came, grabbed her bed, and rushed her into isolation."

What the doctor suspected was that Leslie had meningococcal meningitis, a rare bacterial disease that causes inflammation of the tissues that cover the brain and spinal cord. Upon hearing this, both parents remained confident that their child was to be treated and sent home. They quickly learned otherwise. After a spinal tap was performed, the diagnosis was confirmed and they were told that their daughter was to be transported immediately by helicopter to the hospital of their choice in the Texas Medical Center. "Texas Children's Hospital has such a good reputation, and the ER nurses, I think, were prone to Texas Children's, too," Wendy said, recalling their hasty decision about a hospital choice.

Although somewhat baffled by this sudden turn of events, the Meigses did not believe that their daughter was in harm's way as they waited for the helicopter. That belief was shattered when an ER nurse calmly stated: "I don't think you understand. An employee's daughter came down with the same thing, and presented the exact same way that Leslie did, and died in three hours."

"That's all I needed to hear," remembered Wendy. "As Leslie was flying off, we realized we didn't have any gas in the car. We didn't have anything. We didn't know where our insurance was. We were not prepared."

While everything seemed to be happening so fast for their daughter, the parents fretted that they were too slow to catch up with her. "She got to Texas Children's in about five minutes, and we had to drive," said Jody. "We were in like a daze the whole way there. We met her in the pediatric intensive care unit (pediatric ICU, or PICU) at 3:30 a.m. They already had her in a room. She was conscious. She was able to recognize us. She still was hallucinating and delirious, but she could talk."

Encouraged by what they saw, the Meigses soon realized that they did not comprehend the full extent of their daughter's highly critical condition. "It was explained by several pediatric ICU doctors." Jody recalled. "They were just incredible. We were completely informed. They sat down and explained the chain of events expected to take place. 'She's going to go into respiratory failure. We're going to put her on a ventilator. Her body is going to basically shut down. She's going to be on life support. It's going to be critical. We're going to pump her full of fluids. The first thing we are going to do is try to save her life.' It wasn't until we heard that that we realized her chances were poor. She only had a 10 percent chance of living."

Devastated by these facts, Wendy and Jody called in both of their families and arranged for a priest to administer last rites to Leslie in PICU. Undaunted by this finality, the parents steadfastly refused to abandon hope for their daughter's survival.

Thus began what was to become a two-month bedside vigil.

A ccording to pediatric cardiologist Dr. Charles E. Mullins, the reason for establishing the pediatric intensive care unit at Texas Children's Hospital was perfectly obvious in 1973.

"There was a need," Mullins said. "I couldn't get a bed for my patients."[2]

"We had a joint facility at St. Luke's Episcopal Hospital. I don't know what it was called. Recovery? ICU? Adult coronaries went in there. Adult post-ops went in there. Kids went in there, post-op or meningitis or whatever. And the few neonates who were being worked on to resuscitate would go to the same bedlam area. It was intolerable to have our patients and be fighting for beds versus coronaries."

It was an overcrowded situation that was destined to intensify. With a steadily growing number of pediatric cardiac surgery and pediatric catheterization patients in the early 1970s, the competition for beds began to escalate—as did Mullins' efforts to find a solution to the problem.

He proposed "a specialized unit where critically ill infants and children receive intense, and if necessary, individualized care from personnel with special training and experience in the anticipation and prevention of physiologic catastrophes. Obviously, when these catastrophes do occur, the personnel and equipment must be equally capable of treating them."[3]

In order to gain approval for this proposal, Mullins emphasized the fact that, although there were numerous adult intensive care units and coronary care units in Texas, there were no pediatric intensive care units. Along with other detailed facts and figures about predicted improvements in patient care, morbidity, and outcome, the cardiologist's one-person campaign convinced the board of trustees of Texas Children's Hospital.

"There wasn't a subspecialty of pediatric intensive care or critical care at the time," Mullins explained. "Cardiology had the most patients, and we had the biggest need for it. My interest has always been the cath lab, but out of necessity it became intensive care."[4]

Named medical director of the ICU he championed, Mullins opened the new and fully equipped four-bed facility in July 1973. Created in one of the existing patient rooms on the second floor, it contained two beds allocated for PICU and two for neonatology, each with monitors for individual bedside viewing.

"When we opened the ICU, I was very proud of what we had done and selfishly thought it was opened for cardiology. But soon we got gastrointestinal patients who were bleeding, and lots of neo patients and post-ops. Of course, doing 15 surgeries a week, that wasn't enough beds even then," Mullins said, recalling the unexpected volume of demand.

With more than 300 patients admitted in the first three months, Mullins realized that the PICU was to be more multidisciplinary in scope than he had imagined. Critically ill children from almost every pediatric discipline at Texas Children's Hospital were admitted. Although the number of cardiology patients remained predominant, as he had predicted, he found that there was a surprisingly large number of neonatal patients.

"Very quickly, we got a second room with four beds, and neo got another room with four beds," Mullins said. "It just kept metastasizing down that ward until we filled it. It was like quicksand. As soon as we opened something, it was full and we needed another one. As it grew, we began to separate from neo more and more."[5]

Growing with the PICU was its reputation. Impressed with the volume of patients seen in the PICU at Texas Children Hospital, Dr. Larry S. Jefferson decided to go to Baylor College of Medicine in 1975. Intrigued with the new field of pediatric critical care, he became the first medical student to arrange an elective in pediatric critical care at Baylor.

"He rotated through our ICU," remembered Mullins. "He was very interested and seemed to have pointed his career towards that then. Since there were no fellowships in pediatric critical care at the time, the nearest thing was a pulmonary fellowship, which he later went on to do. Pulmonary was a logical training ground, because certainly one of the most complicated parts of ICU was the respirator and ventilator functions and the management of that area."[6]

Another complicated aspect of managing the PICU was learning how to handle parent participation. At first, parents were allowed to visit only during scheduled ten-minute periods, five times a day.[7] As the unit grew in size and volume, so too did the realization that the presence of parents at the bedside was reassuring to critically ill children, immeasurably contributing to each child's well-being. In 1978, five years after its inception, the PICU abandoned its limited visitation rule, openly encouraging parents to participate in the care of their critically ill child.[8]

Joining the one or more nurses assigned to their child, depending on the severity of the case, along with the physicians, residents, interns, and medical students, the parents soon became an integral part of day-to-day operations in the combined intensive care unit.

In 1979, to alleviate overcrowding, the two units physically separated. After neonatal care moved into a completely new 20-bed neonatal ICU (NICU) on another floor, Mullins and his staff seized the opportunity to reconfigure the haphazardly enlarged PICU. Rather than a series of converted patient rooms along a hallway, they wanted an open concept. To accomplish this, the entire area was gutted to accommodate ten regular patient beds, six recovery beds for heart catheterization and special procedures, and two isolation rooms.[9]

Reflecting the technological advances recently introduced in the field of pediatric critical care, a wall unit behind each bed contained specially designed oxygen outlets, tracheotomy, and gastric suction. An EKG monitor produced a central readout at the strategically placed nurses' station in the middle of the unit.

The physical surroundings were not the only dramatic difference. What had begun six years earlier as Mullins' four-bed unit with a nurse supervisor and head nurse boasted a nursing staff of 26 RNs, two LVNs, and three unit clerks. In addition to the unit's originating cardiologists, interns, and medical students, the PICU medical team consisted of virtually every physician on staff at Texas Children's Hospital.

There was to be yet another change in 1979. With the completion of the renovation, Mullins decided to step down as part-time medical director of the PICU to devote all his attention to his "first love, the catheterization lab," he said. "I figured I couldn't be an expert in both, so I would stick to trying to be an expert in one."[10]

Replacing Mullins was cardiologist Dr. Thomas A. Vargo, who became the first full-time medical director of the PICU. Vargo also was named by physician-in-chief Dr. Ralph D. Feigin to become chief of the newly created pediatric critical care service at Texas Children's Hospital, as well as head of the newly formed pediatric critical care section at Baylor College of Medicine.

Vargo's appointments reflected the rapidly expanding field of pediatric critical care. The opening of pediatric intensive care units in other major pediatric centers occurred during the late 1970s and early 1980s. Suddenly, there was an increased pool of clinical knowledge about the specialized care of critically ill children and the technical applications available. However, even with this foundation for the new subspecialty firmly in place, the establishment of sub-boards in critical care medicine and the offering of certifying exams did not occur until 1987.[11]

Therefore, as was the case with medical directors in other pediatric ICU facilities across the country at the time, Vargo developed his own content and style of pediatric care practice, education, and research. He also introduced a one-year fellowship program in the pediatric ICU at Texas Children's Hospital.

"Since the subspecialty of pediatric critical care wasn't recognized in 1979, they weren't sure whether the director of a pediatric ICU should be a cardiologist, pulmonologist, anesthesiologist, or surgeon," recalled Vargo. "Directors and critical care specialists today have training in all those areas because those are the four areas from which sick patients would come. I was a cardiologist, but now there are intensivist cardiologists."[12]

Whatever kind of cardiologist Vargo was, he was a busy one. Whether the patient had cardiovascular, neurological, respiratory, or infectious disease problems, he was the one who supervised and directed the critical care. Being the only physician who was an in-house presence in PICU, he was on call every night, practically living in his small office.

"I would throw a mat on the floor and sleep when I could. I would spend two nights in a row here frequently," he remembered. "We had these Reyes syndrome patients, where we would constantly be there for three to five days. It became very easy to become dedicated to your work, but I did not see my family as much as I probably should have. Back then, it was very, very easy to just be in love with your work, watching sick patients get better. And those patients who didn't get better, you had this strong sense of duty to make it better for the family."[13]

Realizing that he and his PICU team saw patients at crisis points in their lives, Vargo stressed that the focal point of the drama was the patient and then the family. In addition to their medical responsibilities, the team maintained an atmosphere of open communication, strictly adhering to Vargo's mantra: "We do not give false encouragement, only the facts in the friendliest manner possible."[14]

An encouraging development for the over-stretched Vargo was the arrival of his first fellow, Dr. Fernando Stein. Returning to Baylor and Texas Children's Hospital after a brief sojourn in private practice, Stein was an enthusiastic trainee whose tireless dedication to patients and families in the PICU quickly became evident. "I got into critical care because it is a great opportunity to serve," Stein said. "There is constant action and maintaining an almost permanent state of alertness is a very full way of living."[15]

Capitalizing on his new fellow's unbridled enthusiasm and eagerness to learn, Vargo began sharing his nightly on-call duties with Stein. Together, the two doctors shared not only sleepless nights and medical emergencies, but also some of the moments of sheer joy in the PICU. To Stein, this became a sacred privilege. "You realize that for the families who have been in a critical care unit with their child something as seemingly simple as a step will never be just an every day event," he said. "It will be a little miracle."[16]

For the less fortunate families, those in grief for a dying child, the doctors offered compassion and tenderness. "Surely the most painful thing parents can experience is the death of a child," said Stein. "What they know and feel when their child is dying are pain and grief. I see that it is very much a part of my job to hold their hands, to encourage them, to protect them in whatever way I can, and to try to offer whatever comfort and support I can."

Unwavering emotional support also came from the nursing staff, the core of the round-the-clock care in the PICU. "The acuteness of the child's condition in ICU can be truly heartbreaking," said Roxanna Krafka, RN, supervisor of the unit in 1979. "The nurses support the family as well as each other during the continued crisis situation. In spite of all the new equipment, and we have the best, it is up to the nurses to give each child or infant the special care and attention needed."[17]

Into this highly specialized environment of patient and family care came Vargo's second fellow in 1981. It was Dr. Larry S. Jefferson, the former Baylor College of Medicine student who had elected to rotate through Mullins' first ICU six years earlier. Before becoming a pediatric ICU fellow, Jefferson completed his pediatric residency and internship at Baylor and a two-year pediatric pulmonary fellowship with Baylor's Dr. Gunyon M. Harrison at the Institute for Rehabilitation and Research and Texas Children's Hospital.

"What Dr. Jefferson added to the critical care section was a good understanding of pulmonary medicine and, hopefully, I taught him a little about cardiology, which was my area of expertise," Vargo said.[18]

At the completion of Jefferson's fellowship in 1982, Vargo decided to leave critical care medicine. It was not because he disliked his three years in the PICU, but just the opposite. "I liked it too much!" he declared. "The patients were the most important thing at the time you were taking care of them. But, because of that, I realized I wasn't seeing my family, so I decided to go back to cardiology."

Although he did not foresee the rapid expansion of Texas Children's Hospital, Vargo did envision the limitless future of pediatric critical care. "It was obvious that it would become massive, that every sick child would be taken care of by people who specialized in critical care," he said. "There was no doubt about how big it was to become. And that was part of the reason for my decision, to have some time to do other things."[19]

Vargo's decision to leave the PICU did not surprise Jefferson, who recalled: "He did it all by himself. It was a one-man operation with, usually, one fellow. You know, after you give three or four years of 100 percent, he said, 'I've had it, I'm going back to cardiology.' That was the case around the country. Everybody in that first generation of pediatric critical care just sort of got burned out and went on to do something else."[20]

As a member of the specially trained second generation of pediatric critical care physicians, Jefferson planned to remain in the demanding profession. It was his chosen career path, one that began in medical school and eventually led him not only to a fellowship, but also to a permanent position in the PICU. When Vargo stepped down in 1982, Jefferson was named medical director of the PICU and chief of the critical care service at Texas Children's Hospital, as well as head of pediatric critical care at Baylor College of Medicine. "I was here and Vargo was ready to give it up," Jefferson modestly said. "There just weren't that many prospects around in those years."[21]

Also limited was the number of people trained to be members of the PICU team, should any of Jefferson's dedicated and experienced staff develop burn-out. To address this concern and its future ramifications, Jefferson developed innovative approaches to education, patient care, staff support, and research. To programs already instigated by his predecessors, Jefferson contributed some fine-tuning.

"Vargo really sort of set it up so the residents would all rotate," he said. "Their desire to learn challenges the medical, nursing, and respiratory therapy staff to be as up-to-date and knowledgeable as possible. In addition, medical students and residents from anesthesia, surgery, and family practice began rotating on an elective basis through the pediatric ICU."[22]

To keep the residents, students, and staff constantly stimulated, Jefferson introduced a biweekly lecture series on topics such as cardiopulmonary resuscitation, ventilators, brain resuscitation, and post-op cardiac care. To keep informed about the latest medical and technological advances, the nursing staff began inviting physicians to be guest speakers at their monthly nursing journal club meetings in private homes.

Jefferson emphasized the importance of patients' rights and other ethical concerns. He arranged for residents and staff members to meet on a regular basis with medical ethicist Dr. Earl Shelp.

As part of an effort to boost morale and avoid conflicts among the staff, a psychiatric liaison physician and nurse made regularly scheduled visits to the PICU. According to Jefferson, "In a unit that must deal with death and troubled situations so frequently, and in addition must meet the demands of long hours and large amounts of stress, they provide the chance to air our concerns."

To meet the individual needs of patients and their families, the psychiatric liaison physician and nurse joined the regular rounds made in the unit by representatives from child life, social service, patient relations, and chaplaincy. Also available to parents was a staff-produced film that explained PICU procedures, rules, and services.

With these multiple programs in place, research studies continued. Concentrating on maximizing brain recovery, preventing diseases and accidents that require admission to the PICU, and curtailing costs in the unit, Jefferson worked virtually round-the-clock. Describing that first year in retrospect, he stated unequivocally: "It was brutal."

It also was measurably successful in terms of patient care. With the new programs, procedures, medications, and equipment, the survival of children in the PICU vastly improved. Because of these positive outcomes, there was a growing number of children with technological dependency and chronic morbidity. Although too sick to be moved to the general inpatient area of Texas Children's Hospital, these children required a higher level of attention but did not require the PICU.

"We already had created an 'intermediate care' area in 1979," recalled Jefferson. "We put four young kids in cribs in a semi-private room staffed by a nurse and LVN. It was on a different floor, the fourth floor, of Texas Children's Hospital and it was used for kids with tracheostomies and long-term care on a ventilator. And then, I believe in 1980 or 1981, the new unit opened as a 16-bed unit. It was full-blown by 1982."

Because of its growing and diversified population, intermediate care soon required a medical director and Jefferson filled that position out of necessity in 1984. He continued in the role until the appointment of Dr. Fernando Stein in 1988. Under Stein's direction, the 16-bed intermediate care area, later known as the progressive care unit, expanded to 24 beds and moved to the second floor.

"The progressive care unit at Texas Children's Hospital is the 'swing unit,' where children who are getting sicker can be moved from the general inpatient care area into this unit for more intense observation. It also is for children who are getting better, those who are getting out of the pediatric ICU and not quite ready for the general floor," explained Stein. "It is a higher level of care and observation than they would receive in the general inpatient area."[23]

Into the progressive care unit came several distinctive groups of patients with varying needs. One group consisted of multiply disabled, technologically dependent children, who tended to remain in the unit for long periods of time. Another group comprised acute patients from the emergency center who required a day or two of stabilization before being moved to the general inpatient care area. The third group included children who had progressed from the PICU and whose length of stay always varied.

"You know the inventor of Coca Cola said, 'Create a need and fill it?' We know there is a need and we fill it," Stein said. "We didn't create it, but with the concentration of staff, personnel, and the resources we have here, we cannot turn a deaf ear to a call for service."[24]

One such call came in the early 1980s. It was from Houston-area pediatricians who were concerned with the inadequate method of transporting their critically ill patients from the emergency rooms in other hospitals to the one at Texas Children's Hospital. Knowing the city ambulance service only responded to emergencies, the pediatricians were not comfortable with the alternative.

"Since the private pediatrician goes to the ER and tries to stabilize the child, he could not shut down his office for the day to transport the child to Texas Children's Hospital," explained Jefferson. "So in 1986 we decided what we were going to do was only go by ground and to a 60-mile radius. We will help stabilize the child, but we're only a transport unit. Although other hospitals' transport units at the time, at best, had an intern or a resident, we always send a physician, a pediatric ICU nurse, and, if needed, a pediatric ICU nurse practitioner and respiratory therapist. We really set the national standards, to which very few institutions have reached, of having a physician trained in critical care on each transport."[25]

Community response to the mobile pediatric intensive care unit was immediate, resulting at first in between ten and 15 transports each month. As time passed, the number of transports increased before eventually flattening out. "We were full all the time," Jefferson explained. "We had to turn patients down."[26]

The opportunity to alleviate overpopulation in the PICU came with the expansion plans for Texas Children's Hospital that were announced in the late 1980s. "By that time, I had a pretty good feel how to run an ICU and what was needed," Jefferson said. "And Dr. Feigin basically said that the directors of any particular area had to sign off on the plans before they went forward. We just would not sign them until we were happy with them. And there were those of us who would walk around with architectural tracing paper and architectural scales and monkeying with plans a lot. We had meetings with nurses, respiratory therapists, and physicians. We drew up more and more detailed rooms, planned each head wall and the placement of necessary equipment and strategic support services, like a pharmacy, directly in the unit. It was a team effort, but most of the plans for the new pediatric ICU were drawn on my kitchen table."[27]

Opened in 1991 in the newly built West Tower, the 30-bed PICU was arranged in four separate 'pods,' a visually descriptive word coined by Jefferson at his kitchen table. One pod was for infectious diseases, one for neuro-compromised patients, one for cardiovascular, and one for research. Within each pod was a centralized nurses' station that offered instant access to printed monitor reports and a clear view of each patient area.

Acutely aware of projected needs for the future, Jefferson and his team made sure that each pod had the ability to expand its patient capacity. With its isolable rooms and moveable walls, the delivery of expert care was enhanced and a greater sense of privacy, when needed, was given to patients and their families.

For those parents who never left Texas Children's Hospital during their child's stay in the PICU, there was a large waiting room with sleeper chairs, spacious washroom facilities, a snack area, and lockers for their belongings. In addition, two private family rooms were available for crucial consultations with members of the medical team.[28]

For those physicians, fellows, residents, and nurse practitioners involved in vital research activities, an area expressly designed for that purpose was in the research pod. Located behind the wall of two beds was a discreet nurses' station with monitors and machines for the measurement of nitric oxide and oxygen consumption. Linked by conduits, monitors produced the data required for analysis. Also tabulated were the results from the testing of pharmaceuticals, the measuring of nutritional needs of patients on ventilators, cost containment studies, and myriad research activities.

"At the heart of our commitment to delivering state-of-the-art pediatric critical care is a dedication to research," Jefferson explained. "Our research focuses on preventing ICU-associated morbidity and decreasing patients' lengths of stay, as well as costs to the family and hospital. We insist that all of our fellows are trained in research that strives to meet these goals. More than half of the three-year training program is devoted to research."[29]

One such research project evolved into the creation of a critical care follow-up clinic, one of the first in the United States. "The reality of aggressive, technological support of critically ill children is a certain number of survivors with significant morbidity," Jefferson said. "And some of that morbidity requires continued technological support. At the same time you're minimizing morbidity, you have got a responsibility to the children who develop morbidity under your care."[30]

PICU fellows were assigned to follow a technologically dependent patient through the progressive care unit and for three years in the critical care follow-up clinic. Jefferson wanted the fellows to learn what living with that morbidity was like for patients and their families. "It's important to see what it takes, that fellows or anybody who gets into the critical care area understand all the ramifications," he said. "You can't just take care of a child in ICU, you have to know the long-term outcome. I think that is an important position for us to take."

Another important lesson that Jefferson expected fellows to learn was the ability to communicate with patients and their families. "As they go into a faculty position, I want them to be able to sit down with a family and say, 'You know we are going to work and do everything we can to take care of your child. I don't know what the outcome will be, but I will be with you as part of your physician team for as long as your child needs me or you want me to,'" he said. "That's what we say. We say we don't know if the child will get off the ventilator. Or we don't know if the child will require a tracheostomy. You can't say those lightly if you don't know what it's like."

Hearing about patients' insurance requirements and hassles, arrangements for high-priority power lines, additional equipment needs, home-nursing schedules, and other areas of concern, the fellows gathered valuable information for their future careers as intensivists.

The critical care follow-up clinic also provided a valuable learning experience for the already-established pediatric critical care physicians at Texas Children's Hospital. "When I look up and see a child who was in the progressive care unit years ago and who has now recovered and is growing up, then, all of a sudden, it all makes sense—the endless nights with no sleep, the efforts not only against horrendous disease, but against the attitude of those who want to give up," Stein said. "And it's worth every minute, every hour, every sleepless night."[31]

By 1999, sharing those sleepless nights in the PICU and pediatric progressive care was an ever-expanding staff. Having begun two decades earlier with one full-time physician, the critical care service at Texas Children's Hospital now had eight critical care physicians, ten fellows, and a growing number of nurse practitioners, nurses, respiratory therapists, and other vital members of the medical team.

Also experiencing rapid growth was the transport service. With the introduction of fixed-wing service in 1999, the 24-hours-a-day, seven-days-a-week service became known as the "Kangaroo Crew." Offering greater access to the pediatric critical care units at Texas Children's Hospital, it served all of southeast Texas and an expanded ground radius of 85 miles. Within weeks, the specially equipped airplane and ambulance began transporting more and more patients to the PICU and progressive care unit. As a result, both units were consistently filled beyond capacity.

This recurring predicament did not escape the attention of the pediatric cardiologist who founded the PICU at Texas Children's Hospital in 1973. Although the dramatic advances made in the field of pediatric critical care in the intervening three decades were clearly evident at Texas Children's Hospital in 2004, Mullins lamented there was one aspect of the PICU that remained unchanged.

"I still can't get a bed for my patients," Mullins complained.[32]

From the moment Leslie Meigs entered the PICU at Texas Children's Hospital, Wendy and Jody Meigs felt that they belonged—not only because they gave their permission for Leslie's participation in a double-blind investigational drug study for meningococcal meningitis, but also because they found their constant presence at Leslie's bedside welcomed.

"They allow you to stay there," Wendy said. "Not many hospitals allow you to do that. When your child is dying and this might be all the time you have left, it means a great deal to stay there. And they told us we could be with her at all times."[33]

"They will tell you right away if you are in the way, but they are very understanding," interjected Jody Meigs. "You can tell they make it part of their job to include the parents in a crucial situation like that."

Both parents felt they were an integral part of the medical team responsible for their daughter. "The doctors didn't mind our looking over their shoulders," said Wendy. "They came in and told us what was going to happen. We were completely informed. We saw every medical discipline in Texas Children's Hospital. Everyone was very proactive, always anticipating the next step. Every time a new discipline came in we would say, 'What is this? What are you doing?' They would always go into as much detail as we wanted. Because we are both pharmacists, we wanted all the detailed information and usually got it."[34]

Taking charge of Leslie's case was Dr. Fernando Stein, the medical director of the progressive care unit at Texas Children's Hospital, who happened to be on duty in the PICU when she was admitted.

"We were very, very fortunate that he was there," Wendy said. "He was absolutely fantastic. He's the one who got her stable when she was really critical. He would come in every day and say, 'Here's our goal for today. Here's what we are going to do today. Here's what we're going to try to achieve.' Actually, even throughout everything, all the physicians she had were just absolutely incredible. What sets Texas Children's apart is its ability to take care of the parents, as well as children."

When the predicted chain of events began to unfold rapidly, Wendy and Jody watched in awe as the experts in the PICU multidisciplinary medical team responded. "They move extremely quickly and with incredible precision," Jody said. "Her kidneys failed. She was on constant dialysis the whole time. She went into congestive heart failure. They worried about her heart. They were worried about her lungs. She had respiratory failure. She was on a ventilator. Just everything failed. She was on total life support."

The intermediate result was a frightening sight to behold. Connected to four intravenous feeding lines, a ventilator, and a dialysis machine, Leslie became so bloated and puffy that her features were distorted beyond recognition. Where the rash had been, thick black scabs were beginning to form. While doctors struggled to maintain her blood pressure, Leslie could not be touched or moved. "You couldn't even lift up her arm or just move it slightly, because the blood pressure would start dropping," recalled Wendy.

With two round-the-clock nurses constantly at her side, the comatose Leslie remained critically ill for two weeks in the PICU. "It was touch and go," her mother recalled. "She'd get a little bit better, and then go right back down. Her blood pressure would drop and they would increase her drugs."

"Once we got past all of that, Dr. Stein came in and said: 'I think she's going to live. I don't know about her kidneys, if they are going to come back, but I think she's going to live," remembered Jody. "Then there was the heart thing that we had to worry about, and then the brain thing. Then she had the rash in her eye, and we were worried about her eyesight, then her hearing. We were told that a lot of times this disease will make you go deaf. And then the last thing that we worried about was the scars and potential amputations that could take place because of the necrosis caused by the bacteria. The scabs forming on her knee and thumb were really black."

Advised by "every single doctor" that Leslie "was going to lose her thumb," both parents said, "We were quite content. We can deal with amputations and prosthetics, if she just lives."

Although both parents remained calm about their daughter's possible amputations, others did not share their passivity. "One of our nurses, Randy, was really freaked on that," recalled Wendy. "Every day he would say to the doctors, 'You warned them, didn't you?' And the doctors would say, 'Yes, we warned them.' Even the plastic surgeon was positive she was going to lose her thumb. He even had prepared to do the biopsies when he took her into surgery to take the scars off. But when he took the scab off, her thumb was still there. He just had to remove a small portion from the top part of her thumb."

There was more unexpected good news. After one month in the PICU, Leslie was eligible to move to the progressive care unit. Unable to hold up her head or sit up or walk, she immediately began undergoing physical therapy. "She was so frustrated she couldn't walk. That made her so angry," Wendy recalled. "Of course, she had feet to walk! And she had fingers! And she had toes! We were thrilled!"

With the continuation of daily visits with the ever attentive Stein, Leslie began not only to recover, but also to smile again, thanks to his famous impromptu turns as a magician.

"He was funny," Leslie recalled two years later, unable to remember exactly which card tricks he had performed for her. "He taught me to do one, but I forgot."[35]

What turned out to be even more magical was the fact that Leslie remembered little of her lengthy stay at Texas Children's Hospital. The vivid and often excruciating memories of her critical month in the PICU, two weeks in the progressive care unit, and two weeks in the regular hospital remained the sole possession of her parents and caregivers.

"She remembers the good things, like Dr. Stein's magic tricks, her colorful wheelchair, and the people who did the special things for her, like the nurses, and that's what is good," Wendy said.

After those two now-forgotten months, Leslie was allowed to go home. Her recuperation was just beginning. She returned to Texas Children's Hospital three times a week for dialysis treatment until doctors determined that her kidneys were working properly again and a kidney transplant was not needed. With her alert mind and weak body, Leslie underwent extensive physical therapy and received homebound schooling, enabling her to maintain her grade level and keep up with her friends.

Two years later, Leslie was a healthy ten-year-old who had actively resumed her lessons in ice-skating, ballet, and gymnastics. Back 100 percent and feeling great, she still had scars from the rash, but planned to have plastic surgery to correct those minor problems. As a fourth-grader, she was not concerned about the past, only the future, in which she yearned to be "a famous ice-skater or a famous gymnast."

For her parents, a few cartwheels of their own were in order.

"I'd stand on a hill and shout for Texas Children's," her ecstatic mother said. "Without Texas Children's, Leslie would not be here."

Concluded her equally overjoyed father: "Texas Children's Hospital is the greatest place in the whole world!"

12

✋ DIABETES CARE CENTER ✋

SEVEN-YEAR-OLD CLAIRE CONROY had not been herself since Thanksgiving.

"Claire has always been bright-eyed and bushy-tailed, and she was just off her game," recalled her mother, Liz Conroy.[1]

Uncharacteristically listless, the second-grader also had noticeable weight loss, a constant thirst, and an uncontrollable need to go to the bathroom constantly. Although Liz had at first thought that Claire was just going through a growing spell, she changed her mind when her daughter became lethargic. Concerned, she took Claire to the pediatrician's office.

"It was cold-and-flu season, and we did not see our regular pediatrician because she was busy," Liz recalled. "The doctor whom we saw was not familiar with Claire and what he saw before him was a child who was coming down with something. He prescribed an antibiotic and said she was probably coming down with a bug."

"I have been blessed with three very healthy children, and I can count on one hand the number of times when anybody has been on an antibiotic," Liz said. "But even with that limited experience, I knew within a day or two you see a turnaround. And in a day or two, if anything, she was more lethargic."

For Claire, her weakened condition was not only mysterious, but frustrating as well. "I wanted to do stuff, but I really couldn't because I was so weak," she said. "I wanted to go play with my friends, but I just didn't have the energy."

Determined to participate in the holiday celebrations planned for the last week of class before Christmas, Claire continued going to school. On the following Saturday, she went to a party at a friend's home. Too exhausted to participate in the fun, she lay down on a couch and watched her friends play.

When Claire's father, Tim Conroy, arrived to pick her up from the party, she was still lying on the couch. Alarmed by this abnormal behavior and anxious to find out exactly what was causing it, the Conroys decided to call the pediatrician first thing on Monday morning.

Once again told that Claire's doctor was "booked" and could not see her, Liz was insistent upon it. She remembered stating emphatically on the phone: "I really need to see somebody who knows Claire because something is not right with Claire and we need to get some answers to this."

"They fit us in that afternoon, it was December 23," Liz recalled. "We went into the office and they took a urine sample and from that it was determined that her glucose levels were sky high."

Added Claire, "It was so high they couldn't even tell the number."

The results indicated that Claire was possibly in the onset stage of Type I diabetes, a debilitating disease affecting every organ system. Also known as juvenile diabetes and usually striking in childhood but lasting a lifetime, the disease was caused by an autoimmune destruction of the insulin-producing cells in the pancreas. Insulin is the hormone crucial to converting sugar into energy for the body, which possibly explained Claire's lethargy. To confirm this diagnosis, the doctor advised the Conroys to take their daughter immediately to the emergency room at Texas Children's Hospital.

In the emergency room, the doctor's suspicions were confirmed after further tests. Claire was admitted to the pediatric intensive care unit. "For the possible side-effects on the initial reintroduction of insulin into her body, she needed to be in an environment where she was monitored very closely," her mother recalled. "When she showed no reaction to the insulin, we were then put in a regular room, where we stayed for five days."

Overwhelmed, the Conroys tried not to pass their concerns on to Claire. "You are dealing with so many emotions," Liz said. "You are all over the emotional meter. I spent the night every night with Claire. One night, it was Christmas night, after she had gone to sleep, I went out into the hallway and just cried. It was just kind of getting it out because I had not had any time to do that."

Sitting on the floor at the end of the Texas Children's Hospital hall, the distraught mother faced her fears with seemingly endless tears. She did not know that much about Claire's disease, but she knew enough to be frightened. Consumed with worries about the unknown future, she began to feel sorry for her daughter, for herself, and for her family. Not knowing how Claire's diabetes would affect all of their lives, she wallowed in pity for them all.

"I got through that pretty quickly," she said. "Immediately, you go from one side of the pendulum where you are feeling sorry for yourself, till it swings over."

This particular mood swing occurred when Liz looked down the hall at Texas Children's Hospital that night. "I thought, 'You know, there are a lot of people down here who are dealing with issues where that's not the case. What we have here, even though I may not know much about it at this point, it's going to be doable. We're going to go out there and we're going to handle it. It's just not going to be something that slows us down. It's not going to slow Claire down or slow us down as a family. We'll deal with it. We'll incorporate it in our lives and go on.'"

Already adjusting favorably to her predicament was Claire, who found that spending Christmas at Texas Children's Hospital was to her liking. "There was nothing I did not like," she said. "The doctors were all very nice. They knew what to do and they explained it to us really well. The nurses brought me a doll and Boy Scouts and Girl Scouts brought me little baseball cards."

Such niceties also impressed her mother, who noted how those in the hospital went out of their way to make her daughter feel special. "They were very caring and sensitive to the fact that you were a child in the hospital on Christmas Day," she recalled. "It showed to me a tremendous amount of caring for the patient."

Unquestionably, the best Christmas gift the Conroys received at Texas Children's Hospital was when Claire began to feel like herself again.

A common disease with no known cure in 2001, diabetes affected between 500,000 and one million children in the United States. As in the past, the risk of developing diabetes in childhood remained higher than that of virtually all other severe chronic diseases.[2]

An ancient disease, diabetes had the documentation to prove its longevity. A prescription for one of its symptoms, frequent urination, appeared on an Egyptian papyrus dating back to 1500 B.C.[3]

Before the discovery of insulin by Banting and Best in 1921 and its first published use in children in 1923, few diseases had a prognosis worse than that of juvenile-onset diabetes mellitus. Medical records from the early 1900s indicate that most diabetic children died of diabetic coma within months of diagnosis. With no known cause, treatment, or cure, the disease struck countless thousands of children each year and remained an enigma.

Relegated to the last page of a general pediatrics textbook published in 1911 was this bleak overview: "Diabetes in children is hopeless and all treatment is useless. That patients will live more than three months is highly improbable."[4]

By the early 1920s, the outlook remained bleak. Children diagnosed with juvenile diabetes continued to share their common and irreversible fate. Remembering those days in Houston, pediatrician Dr. Edward O. Fitch talked about his frustrations and how he often went home in despair, wishing he could do more for these sick children.[5]

For Fitch and other frustrated pediatricians throughout the country, the possibility of doing more for diabetic children than write their death certificates came in the mid- to late 1920s, with a medical breakthrough at St. Louis Children's Hospital. Under the leadership of Dr. Alexis F. Hartmann at the Washington University School of Medicine, that hospital became the first pediatric institution in the United States to use insulin in the treatment of children with diabetes mellitus.

Although not hailed as a cure, these revolutionary insulin injections represented a life-support mechanism. Helping to keep the level of sugar in the blood at a normal level, insulin enabled the diabetic child to eat a normal diet, gain weight, and survive. Because only fast-acting insulin was available at the time, multiple doses had to be given each day, sometimes exceeding six or seven injections, and the need for long-acting insulins became a priority.

As the research for long-acting insulins took place during the 1930s, 40s, and 50s, Hartmann continued his renowned efforts to advance the treatment and care of children with juvenile-onset diabetes mellitus at St. Louis Children's Hospital. Named head of pediatrics at Washington University School of Medicine and chief of pediatric services at the hospital in 1936, Hartmann remained at the forefront of metabolic and diabetes research until he stepped down in 1964.[6]

These noted accomplishments, as well Hartmann's reputation as a brilliant teacher, inspired the head of pediatrics at Baylor College of Medicine, Dr. George W. Salmon, to contact him following World War II. In search of a resident position for one of his former interns, Salmon was successful.

The recipient of Salmon's largesse was Dr. Charles William Daeschner, Jr., a fellow Houstonian who had wanted to be a surgeon—until he had a rotating internship with Salmon at Hermann Hospital in the mid 1940s. "My last rotation as an intern was on pediatrics, and it was extremely stimulating," Daeschner recalled. "It opened my eyes to opportunities in research and teaching, which I already felt that I wanted to do, that I couldn't find when

I was in various surgical rotations."[7]

"Dr. Salmon was a tough guy to work for, he demanded a lot," Daeschner said. "We worked every day and every night. He might come in at 2 a.m. in the morning, worried about a child, and get us all up to make rounds with him, look at the child, and maybe even do some procedures, or some studies, or some treatment on that child. Something about the determination and the commitment he had to what he was doing was really contagious. Just about all of us who had experience with him ended up in pediatrics. He is one of those special people who had the charisma that made you want to follow him."

The determination to do just that came to Daeschner while serving in the Air Force after his internship. Writing to Salmon that he wanted to return to the pediatric program at Baylor College of Medicine following his military service, Daeschner received a surprising reply. Instead of accepting him as a resident, Salmon turned him down, explaining, "the Baylor program isn't well enough developed for you. I'll get you a job."[8]

"That's all he said," remembered Daeschner. "About a month later, I heard from Dr. Alexis Hartmann. He said he would accept me on the basis of Dr. Salmon's recommendation and that he looked forward to getting to know me. I was delighted. I had no idea that's what Dr. Salmon was going to do, but that's typical of him. He did what he thought was best for you."

In this particular case, Salmon also did something else. Inadvertently, while masterminding this direction for Daeschner's career path, he established the first link in a chain of events that eventually led to the beginning of the Diabetes Care Center at Texas Children's Hospital.

For Daeschner, the future looked uncertain after his two-year residency at St. Louis Children's Hospital. "Dr. Hartmann asked me to stay on as chief resident a third year," he recalls. "I was pondering that possibility when Dr. Blattner came to St. Louis and asked what I would think about coming back to Houston."

Having replaced Salmon as head of pediatrics at Houston's Baylor College of Medicine in 1947, Dr. Russell J. Blattner was in the process of recruiting instructors for his new pediatric department. Also trained at St. Louis Children's Hospital, Blattner quickly made a job offer to Daeschner. It was for a teaching and clinical position, one that Daeschner accepted with one caveat. He requested that he receive more training before he began the job, explaining: "If I'm going to come back to a full-time job, I would really like to broaden my background more. The difference between my experience with Dr. Salmon, and my experience in the Air Force, and then my experience here in St. Louis has made me realize there's a diversity of opportunities, even though you are focusing in one field."[9]

Blattner agreed, ultimately arranging for Daeschner to continue his training at Harvard Medical School and the Harvard-affiliated Children's Hospital Boston. Scheduled to stay for two years, Daeschner arrived full of expectations. "Soon after I got there, I found that I had more experience than some of the others, so they made me acting chief resident for about two months, while the chief resident was in Europe," he recalled. "And then, after that, they made me an instructor and chief resident in the outpatient department, where I worked for Dr. Sydney Gellis."

While at Harvard, Daeschner worked closely with Dr. Charles A. Janeway, the chairman of the department of pediatrics who was physician-in-chief at Children's Hospital Boston. The two became close friends. "I was tremendously influenced by his teaching skills," Daeschner said. "He's one of these real plainspoken New Englanders who doesn't beat around the bush, and his concern for total accuracy and honesty is just contagious. He can make any patient's history and physical a fascinating story. He was another person who really made me think I wanted to stay on teaching, and he offered me a full-time position to stay there and teach at Children's Hospital Boston."

It was an offer that Daeschner seriously considered. If he were to accept, he did not envision staying in the new field of immunology with Janeway. Instead, he was interested in continuing his work with Dr. James L. Gamble, who specialized in the area of salt and water disorders. "He was a very quiet, shy man, but when you got to know him, he was another one of these remarkable humans whom you wanted to be like," Daeschner said. "Having analyzed the composition of body fluids, he developed a methodology for intravenous feeding in 1922. Every person that gets an IV, adult or child, owes a debt of gratitude to the pioneering work of Dr. Gamble."

Impressed with these and the many other accomplishments of physicians at Harvard, Daeschner was tempted to accept Janeway's offer to remain there. But he realized that he owed his allegiance to Blattner. At the end of his first year in Boston, that allegiance was tested when a letter from Blattner arrived, asking: "Could you possibly come sooner, we are really desperate for help." Daeschner cut short his residency and immediately returned to Houston.

Back at Baylor, Daeschner became a consultant to the then-developing Southwestern Poliomyelitis Respiratory Center adjoining Jefferson Davis Hospital. Supervising all of the laboratory work for that unit, he also had a laboratory of his own. "When I first came there, there was nobody, except

Dr. Blattner, who had any background in diabetes and kidney diseases and in endocrine and metabolic disorders," said Daeschner. "My main area of focus during my residency had been in the metabolic disorders, diabetes being the principal one, and kidney diseases. And that was because those were the principal interests of Dr. Hartmann and, subsequently, Dr. Gamble. Because my knowledge and interests in those areas was greater, I sort of, by default, began working in those areas with Blattner's support."

Named head of the pediatric renal-metabolic section at Baylor College of Medicine and chief of the pediatric program at Jefferson Davis Hospital in 1951, Daeschner began conducting clinics for diabetes, kidney diseases, and other metabolic and endocrine disorders. When pediatric endocrinologist Dr. George W. Clayton arrived at Baylor College of Medicine in 1954, Daeschner happily relinquished endocrine disorders to him. "He was well-trained," explained Daeschner. "I had only superficial knowledge in endocrinology."

However, the responsibility for one particular endocrine disease remained with Daeschner. This occurred when Clayton readily accepted Daeschner's offer to continue his efforts in the treatment and management of juvenile-onset diabetes. This arrangement was not unexpected. Like most other pediatric endocrinologists who had trained at Johns Hopkins under Dr. Lawson Wilkins, the first recognized pediatric endocrinologist in the world, Clayton had limited interest in diabetes.

Clayton and Daeschner joined forces in the renal-metabolic clinic at the newly opened Texas Children's Hospital in 1954. Held every Saturday morning in the Junior League Diagnostic Clinic of the outpatient department, the renal-metabolic clinic served children with kidney disease, diabetes, and other metabolic disorders. "George Clayton joined us and we started at 8:30 a.m. in the morning," recalled Daeschner. "We would see patients with the students and then we would go into the Greer study and have a conference. George was the main organizer and leader of that conference, and I learned a tremendous amount from George Clayton during those years."

Daeschner's appreciation of colleagues who shared their knowledge was a direct reflection of his love of teaching. Inspired by his mentors, he quickly garnered a reputation for being a brilliant teacher.

He was also well-known for instilling his interest in diabetes into his students. Championing a unique approach to patient education, Daeschner felt that children with diabetes should lead a normal life to whatever extent possible, and that education was the way to achieve that goal. He encouraged his residents to publish educational material for patients and their families. A strong believer in the psychological aspect of treatment, he emphasized that over-treating patients might cause them to become psychologically and emotionally dependent.

Many of those inspired by Daeschner at Baylor College of Medicine maintained a strong interest in diabetes throughout their careers. A former resident, Dr. Luther Travis, published one of the first instructional books for children with diabetes mellitus. An immediate bestseller, the 82-page book and its subsequent 11 editions sold more than one million copies.[10]

"I think most of the ideas Luther and I had about diabetes came from Bill Daeschner," said Dr. L. Leighton Hill, his chief resident in 1956–57 and the first renal-metabolic fellow in 1957–58. "And how much of what he taught came from Alexis Hartmann I don't know, because I did not personally know Dr. Hartmann, but Daeschner talked about him a lot."[11]

For Hill, listening to whatever Daeschner had to say proved beneficial to his career. "I was fortunate to spend two years with him," Hill said. "I learned a lot about attention to detail, and what it really takes to take care of patients. I think I learned many teaching techniques from him—and, of course, a great deal about integrity. I suppose he has more integrity than anybody that I've ever come across in medicine. He was a brilliant teacher and a very good investigator, too. He was a very powerful influence on a lot of lives."[12]

One of those lives was Hill's. After completing his fellowship with Daeschner in 1958, Hill wished to continue his research training in water and electrolyte metabolism, kidney diseases, and diabetes. When offered a position by one of Gamble's former associates, Dr. Bill Wallace, a Daeschner mentor who had gone to Western Reserve School of Medicine, Hill accepted. "He ran Dr. Gamble's lab at Children's Hospital Boston and then became chairman of the department of pediatrics at Western Reserve in Cleveland," Hill said. "He was of the same caliber as Drs. Hartmann, Salmon, Gamble, Janeway, and Daeschner."[13]

Returning to Baylor as a permanent member of Daeschner's renal-metabolic section, Hill planned to assist Daeschner, teach, do clinical work, and also start a lab and begin research projects. To his surprise, this was not Daeschner's plan.

Within two months of Hill's arrival in October 1959, Daeschner announced that he was leaving Baylor for a position at the University of Texas Medical Branch in Galveston. When offered Daeschner's job at Texas Children's Hospital and Baylor College of Medicine, Hill was hesitant. He eventually accepted the position. In 1960, he assumed leadership of the renal-metabolic service, the nephrology training program, and the diabetes program at Texas Children's Hospital.

Under Hill's leadership, the renal-metabolic service grew steadily over the following decades. A major focus of its efforts at Texas Children's Hospital continued to be in the management of children with diabetes mellitus. As well as overseeing the management of children who came to the Saturday morning clinic, Hill's service provided consultations to other physicians who cared for children with diabetes. "By the late 1950s it was well known that childhood diabetes had to be treated with insulin and that the majority of adults had a non-insulin dependent type of diabetes," Hill said. "Radioimmunassay measurements of insulin in the late 1970s and early 1980s reconfirmed this clinical distinction."[14]

In order to provide quality clinical care for children with diabetes mellitus at Texas Children's Hospital, Hill assembled a team consisting of faculty members, renal fellows, pediatric residents, renal-metabolic nurses, and two diabetes educators, who were brought in during the late 1970s. When Houston pediatricians and other Texas physicians referred patients whose symptoms indicated a strong possibility of diabetes, Hill and his team followed a strict procedure. "When a diagnosis was made, or strongly suspected, the child was admitted to Texas Children's Hospital for other tests," Hill explained. "Then the day-to-day regulation of the diabetes began, along with an intensive teaching program."[15]

By 1979, the educational program originated by Daeschner more than two decades earlier had grown beyond recognition. It now included such topics as a general explanation of diabetes, principles of nutrition and nutritional aims, urine testing for sugar and acetone, types of insulin, techniques of insulin administration by injection, goals of therapy, the importance of regular exercise, the management of emergencies, and home blood sugar testing. "We began to use home blood sugar testing in the late 1970s, when glucometers became very reliable and required only tiny amounts of blood," Hill said. "Prior to that time, urine testing was the chief measure of control."[16]

With continuing advances in equipment and techniques, updating pertinent information for diabetes patients and their families at Texas Children's Hospital was an ongoing effort. "Many hours were spent by the entire team on the educational process," Hill said. "They were joined in the care and education of these patients by dedicated social workers, psychologists, dietitians, physical therapists, and psychiatrists. After a patient was diagnosed or discharged from the hospital, faculty members talked daily to each family in the early mornings for the next one to three weeks."[17]

Always anxious to ensure the normal psychological, emotional, and social development of each child with diabetes, Hill and his team stressed goal setting not only for patients, but also for their families. "We attempt to engender a feeling by the youngster and the family that he/she is not so different from others," Hill said. "We want them to have confidence that whatever major objectives in life that are decided upon are still possible, despite the diabetes."[18]

Also stressed was the importance of self-discipline in the control of diabetes. To effectively manage diabetes at home, patients had to perform urine tests to measure sugar and acetone concentrations and record the results; administer their own injections of insulin; maintain a well-balanced diet using an exchange system to ensure constancy of calorie, carbohydrate, and protein intake from day to day with regular timing of meals; follow a rigorous exercise program; and, beginning in the 1970s, perform blood sugar testing. To prevent future hospitalization, patients were aware that the avoidance of severe insulin reactions and ketoacidosis were constant goals. The achievement of normal physical and emotional growth and development was of paramount importance, as was the avoidance, to the extent possible, of diabetic complications that adversely affected the eyes, kidneys, and nervous and cardiovascular systems.

Encouraging patients and their families to call Texas Children's Hospital with any of their questions or if their control of diabetes deteriorated, Hill established a 24-hour page call number by which they could reach someone in the renal-metabolic service at any time.

To further support children with diabetes and their families at Texas Children's Hospital, Hill formed a diabetes patient education task force in 1982 to develop teaching materials and a resource guide. Although the diabetes book by Travis contained comprehensive information, Hill felt that it did not completely meet the needs of the diabetes educational program at Texas Children's Hospital. Headed by Hill, Kay Bartholomew of the health education department at Texas Children's Hospital, renal-metabolic diabetes nurse-educator Andrea Forbes, and psychologist Danita Czyzewski, the education task force consisted of the entire renal-metabolic team. Incorporating many of Hill's ideas from his early days with Daeschner, along with multiple contributions from individual team members, the task force produced a series of detailed booklets concerning the medical, emotional, and psychological aspects of diabetes in children and adolescents. Printed in two sets, one for patients and one for parents, the booklets titled *Learning to Manage Your Child's Diabetes* debuted in 1984. Soon after, orders for copies came in from all across the country. It was an accomplishment that evoked this modest description from Hill: "We were trying to teach patients and the families how to take care of children."[19]

As Hill's diabetes program at Texas Children's Hospital continued to expand its services, the number of diabetes patients began to increase. Actively involved with the management of more than 400 children with diabetes mellitus, the renal-metabolic team began using new modes of therapy. Starting in 1979 and continuing through 1985, approximately 30 children with growth-onset diabetes mellitus received treatment through an open loop system of continuous insulin therapy via programmable insulin pumps. The constant subcutaneous infusion of insulin obviated the necessity for multiple insulin injections, allowing more latitude in the timing and size of patients' meals. This breakthrough mechanical device was the precursor to the smaller and more portable insulin pumps made available in the 1980s.

Other advances in diabetes treatment underwent investigations in the renal-metabolic service at Texas Children's Hospital during the 1960s, 70s, and early 80s. "We were very interested in the treatment of ketoacidosis and I think, personally, that we were way ahead of the country on this because, as nephrologists, our area of expertise lay in renal physiology and water and salt metabolism," Hill explained. "In diabetic ketoacidosis, which unchecked can progress to diabetic coma and death, there are very high blood sugar levels causing the patient to spill huge amounts of sugar in the urine. This glucose drags out a large quantity of water and electrolytes with it, producing profound dehydration. Also, ketoacids accumulate, causing a severe acidosis. Altogether, diabetic ketoacidosis produces one of the classic water and electrolyte, acid-base disturbances."[20]

The effectiveness of low-dose continuous intravenous insulin infusions in children with ketoacidosis by Hill, Dr. George Edwards, and Dr. Ed Kohaut at Texas Children's Hospital resulted in the first paper published on this breakthrough treatment in 1977. Other accomplishments of this renal-metabolic team in the late 1970s and early 1980s included the early use of glycosylated hemoglobin levels to assess the long-range control of diabetes. Because the required lab test was not initially available in the laboratories at Texas Children's Hospital, for several years the determinations took place in the renal-metabolic research laboratories at Jefferson Davis Hospital.

During the 1970s, the pediatric renal-metabolic service at Texas Children's Hospital introduced a noteworthy advance in the treatment of children with diabetes—blood pressure control. "I think we recognized before many the benefit of blood pressure control in the child, adolescent, and young adult with diabetes mellitus and we had the expertise to manage this serious complication of diabetes," Hill said, noting how pediatric nephrologists in the renal-metabolic service had particular insights because they were the subspecialists who cared for children with hypertension.[21]

The introduction of blood pressure control in the treatment and care of children with diabetes was among an array of accomplishments credited to the 31-year Daeschner-Hill era of diabetes care and management at Texas Children's Hospital. When Clayton stepped down as chief of pediatric endocrinology in 1985, a new era began with the arrival of Dr. Kenneth H. Gabbay, named head of the pediatric endocrine and metabolism section at Baylor College of Medicine and chief of the diabetes service at Texas Children's Hospital. An internationally renowned diabetologist, Gabbay was respected both for his clinical expertise and for research advances in the field. Therefore, after 26 years of treating children with diabetes mellitus as chief of the renal-metabolic service at Texas Children's Hospital, Hill relinquished his diabetes responsibilities to the new chief.

Gabbay, the former chief of the diabetes unit at Children's Hospital Boston, immediately embarked on a major program to develop a children's diabetes center at Texas Children's Hospital. Announcing the August 1986 opening of the new clinical and laboratory center at 8080 North Stadium Drive, Gabbay wrote in a *WATCH Magazine* article: "The newly expanded and reorganized endocrinology and metabolism section provides an integrated program in pediatric endocrine and metabolic diseases, with juvenile diabetes mellitus and growth disorders as two of its main interests."[22]

Of major interest to Gabbay was the basic science research program at the children's diabetes center. Heavily oriented towards the development of laboratory discoveries with eventual clinical relevance, the program included the genetic foundation of susceptibility to diabetes and its complications; the mechanisms of beta cell destruction in the young diabetic; and the mechanisms of long-term complications. Fascinated by this aspect of diabetology, in 1987 Gabbay decided to step down as chief of the endocrinology and metabolism service to devote himself full-time to diabetes research.

"Dr. Gabbay had a career that was very much involved with the molecular aspects of diabetes and I think he wanted to be more involved in the molecular work," recalled Dr. John L. Kirkland III, named acting chief of the endocrinology and metabolism service at Texas Children's Hospital in 1987.[23] Also chief of the endocrine clinic, Kirkland assumed Gabbay's former responsibilities at the children's diabetes center.

During Kirkland's tenure as chief of the children's diabetes center, noticeable changes occurred in the nationally accepted nomenclature for the disease. When researchers utilized radioimmunassay technology to measure insulin in the blood, they discovered that some people with diabetes still made their own insulin. They identified that group as "non-insulin-dependent" diabetes mellitus (NIDDM), or Type II diabetes. The other group became known as "insulin-dependent" diabetes mellitus (IDDM), or Type I diabetes.[24]

"Type I is much more common in children, is more life-threatening in children, and requires imminent treatment," said Texas Children's Hospital pediatric endocrinologist Dr. Lori Sherman in a *Developments* magazine article published in 1992. Estimating that there were between 400 and 500 children with Type I diabetes in the Texas Children's Hospital program at the time, Sherman stated: "There are less than 30 Type II diabetes patients who are being treated and monitored at Texas Children's."[25]

The treatment program for all patients at the children's diabetes center also was to undergo a change, one inspired by the 1993 release of the Diabetes Control and Complications Trial (DCCT) documentation. A clinical study conducted from 1983 to 1993 by the National Institute of Diabetes and Digestive and Kidney Diseases (NIDDK), this was the largest and most comprehensive diabetes study ever conducted. Having compared intensive treatment with standard treatment, the DCCT conclusively proved that blood sugar control with intensive treatment can prevent or substantially delay the onset of microvascular complications in people with Type I diabetes.[26]

"They had very close contact, weekly telephone contact, with patients," Kirkland said. "Those patients in the intensive group used either multiple daily injections or an insulin pump. They also tested their blood sugars four times a day, and kept their blood sugars under control by changing their insulin doses as often as needed with the help of their diabetes educator and doctors. They had weekly contacts and counseling with their diabetes educator, dietitian, and social worker, and there was a significant reduction in complications. It was one of the most important studies, ever."[27]

To incorporate the recommendations of the DCCT into the diabetes program at Texas Children's Hospital, physician-in-chief Dr. Ralph D. Feigin named Dr. Kenneth L. Copeland as director of the newly named Diabetes Care Center in 1993. "Dr. Copeland was the one who named the center," recalled Kirkland, who was named chief of the endocrine and metabolism service the same year. "He played a big role in its development."[28]

Instituting a number of changes in the management of children with diabetes, Copeland introduced a comprehensive diabetes education program. Patients and their parents received an initial ten to 15 hours of education focused on self-management of the disease to prevent hospitalization. Taught to check their own blood sugar levels at least four times a day and encouraged to purchase a glucose meter, patients and their parents began learning one of the basics of self-management.

"Our primary focus at Texas Children's is to empower the patient," Copeland explained in 1994. "The best way to manage disease is for the patient to become independent with the hospital's team providing education, psychological, and social support and expertise when patients get medically sick. My vision of a Diabetes Care Center is to teach patients to become their own best doctor and to give patients confidence and control over their disease."[29]

To accomplish his vision, Copeland staffed the Diabetes Care Center at Texas Children's Hospital with eight endocrinologists, two nurse educators, a diabetes nutritionist, a psychologist, and a social worker. After further enhancing the 24-hour telephone support system that had been instigated more than a decade earlier by Hill, Copeland credited this as being a critical part of his program's success.

Succeed was what the program measurably did. Within two years of Copeland's arrival, the Diabetes Care Center at Texas Children's Hospital had grown to become one of the largest diabetes treatment centers in the United States. In 1995, more than 180 new patients entered the diabetes self-management program, bringing the total number of patients in the center to approximately 800.

National recognition of Copeland's successful efforts to set noteworthy standards in self-management education came in 1995. After embarking on a lengthy and labor-intensive application process, the Diabetes Care Center at Texas Children's Hospital received credentialing from the American Diabetes Association (ADA). In so doing, the center became one of the very few pediatric diabetes care centers in the United States to be awarded recognition by the ADA in accordance with the National Standards for Diabetes Self-Management Education Programs. This accomplishment gained Texas Children's Hospital the right to include the American Diabetes Association's Education Recognition logo on all printed material concerning the Diabetes Care Center.

"The American Diabetes Association only recommends programs that are recognized," explained Barb Schreiner, RN, MN, CDE, who served as an outside consultant during the application process in 1994 and 1995. "Being a recognized program puts Texas Children's Hospital in an elite group, especially with the insurance companies. The patients benefit because the education is reimbursed by the insurance companies."[30]

Hired as associate director of the Diabetes Care Center at Texas Children's Hospital in 1996, Schreiner assumed responsibility for coordinating the education program. "Dr. Copeland wanted someone who would actually do program planning and development," she said. "I just took what already was here and extended it in a couple of different directions and added more staff."

Schreiner coordinated the curriculum, the educational material, and the audio visual materials created in-house. She also guided the staff not just in teaching approaches and motivational approaches, but also in a model called "case management." Schreiner explained: "Each nurse has a group of patients, about 200 to 300 children, whom they follow. They help remind them about visits, follow their laboratory tests, and provide additional education if they need it."

For each patient in the program, Schreiner's staff prepared and distributed a loose-leaf binder filled with basic information about Type I diabetes. Written for patients, parents, other caregivers, and siblings, the "book" stressed that these were the most important members of the diabetes care team. "There was a tremendous commitment from Dr. Copeland and Dr. Kirkland to get the recognition that we had a beautiful program," Schreiner said. "As soon as we began collecting data and demonstrating that, patients started to come. The other thing that happened was Texas Children's Hospital got really good at garnering a lot of managed care. When they said, 'Thou shalt go to Texas Children's Hospital,' we were ready for them."

Schreiner ensured that the program gave individual attention to each patient. With the patient population growing, she also coordinated group classes for patients. "We keep evolving new classes, depending on what comes our way," she explained. "For instance, the new explosion of children with Type II diabetes. I designed a program that is now being run by one of our research nurses and our dietitian, our social worker, and an exercise therapist. We have had some really good outcomes from that."

Over the next few years, the need for Type II diabetes education programs did not diminish. Rather, demand increased threefold. By 1999, there were more than 84 children with Type II diabetes treated in the Diabetes Care Center at Texas Children's Hospital—nearly three times the number treated in 1992. "An epidemic of 'extra-large' kids has caused an alarming rise in the number developing Type II diabetes," Dr. Morey H. Haymond stated in a 1999 report. A diabetes researcher at the USDA/ARS Children's Nutrition Research Center and professor of pediatrics at Baylor College of Medicine since 1996, Haymond included the following statement: "Fifteen years ago, less than 5 percent of children diagnosed with diabetes had the Type II form. Today, the number being diagnosed with the Type II form is over 20 percent."[31]

With this increase in the number of Type II diabetes patients and the steadily growing influx of children with Type I diabetes, the Diabetes Care Center at Texas Children's Hospital experienced more than 3,000 visits from approximately 1,160 patients in 1999. The year saw another milestone as well—the stepping down of Copeland as director of the Diabetes Care Center to accept a position elsewhere.

"Dr. Copeland made some major changes here," said Haymond, named director of the Diabetes Care Center in October 1999. "What he started with the patients, I have continued, but more radically. There are three questions I expect the kids to know the answers to: 'Why are you doing this?' 'To stay healthy.' 'How do you do that?' 'Keep my blood sugars near normal.' 'Who is your diabetes doctor?' 'I, the patient, am.' I tell them that I'm not the doctor, because 'you make the decisions of what you eat in the morning, what you eat at lunch, when you take your insulin, whether you checked your blood sugars, what you adjust, and all your responsibilities.' I tell them my job is to be a consultant, to give advice and bail them out of trouble when needed."[32]

It was to be a philosophy that Haymond and his diabetes team would instill in more than 1,500 children with diabetes during 4,000 patient visits to the Diabetes Care Center at Texas Children's Hospital in 2001.

During the following three years, the record-breaking number of patient visits and patients continued to increase. And, with its fiftieth anniversary in 2004, what began as a small Saturday-morning clinic in 1954 had become the second-largest clinic at Texas Children's Hospital.

"Before Claire's diagnosis, what I knew about juvenile diabetes you could put in a thimble, and most of it would have been wrong," Liz Conroy said four and a half years later. "Now, I feel like I could almost write a textbook about it."[33]

The learning process began with Claire's diabetes diagnosis at Texas Children's Hospital. Within hours, the team from the Diabetes Care Center met with the family and emphasized the medical care and diabetes education necessary for Claire's well-being. After teaching the new skills needed to safely manage diabetes at home, the team presented an outline for the management training essential for proper diabetes care.

From the Texas Children's Hospital team, Claire and the Conroys first learned how to test blood glucose using a meter, how to test urine ketones, how to record information about diabetes, how to prepare and give insulin injections, and what food to eat. From a three-day diabetes self management training course, they learned about management plans, insulin adjustment, nutrition, exercise, and possible medical complications and their treatment.

"They can only give you so much information at a time," Liz said, recalling their crash course in Type I diabetes. "We have a big binder from Texas Children's Hospital with lots of information in it. They always said that you will get to the point where you will know more about your own situation than others do."

But, in the beginning, Liz did not have that reassuring confidence. She readily accepted the team's offer to be of service at any time of the day or night. "I have to tell you, when you needed them, they were there," she recalled. "We were calling them once and twice a day because we were not comfortable adjusting Claire's insulin. We were simply reporting back to them the results, and they would make the corrections. There was never any sense of feeling like we were bothering them. They were always positive and supportive, and very much brought us up to the comfort level to where we thought we could handle it for the most part."

Already handling the realities of her disease was Claire, who began giving herself the insulin injections within two weeks of leaving Texas Children's Hospital. Always hungry in the beginning weeks as she adjusted to the insulin injections, Claire began eating three times more than usual yet continued to lose weight. To address her hunger at school, she began taking an ice chest filled with food and snacks instead of a lunch box. "I was eating a lot," Claire remembered. "Like, right after breakfast, I would say, 'When's lunch?'"

"It was her body trying to play catch-up," Liz explained. "As soon as her numbers came down and the insulin began to be effective, her body was able to gain a little bit of weight. As her diabetic issues came under control, her appetite dropped off. So, she only was carrying her ice chest for about a month."

Once again, just as she had reacted to all the other unexpected changes in her routine behavior, Claire easily adapted to her diabetes needs. Her ability to do so was, her mother believed, attributable not only to her "you got to do what you got to do" spirit, but also to her age at the time of the diagnosis. "She was old enough to have some understanding of what the issue was, but she was not old enough to really have a stigma associated with it," Liz said.

Claire was a quick learner. Within two years, she had mastered the art of testing her blood glucose levels and adjusting her insulin when needed. An active participant in sports, she continued her gymnastics year-round, played soccer and basketball in the winter, and went swimming in the summer. Because exercise affected the rate with which her body absorbed insulin, Claire always had to factor her activities into her daily diabetes management. To keep from giving herself insulin shots all day long, she would mix a "cocktail" of short-acting, long-acting, and ultra-long-acting insulins. Consequently, she would then have to eat, hungry or not, at predetermined times in response to the amount of insulin she had given herself earlier.

Because Claire had a very good understanding of managing her diabetes by the time she was nine years old, the diabetes care team at Texas Children's Hospital recommended that she wear an insulin pump to control her diabetes. A small, computer-programmed device, the pump was designed to deliver insulin 24 hours a day via a thin plastic tube called an infusion set that is inserted beneath the skin. Containing a small reservoir of insulin, a small battery-powered pump, and a computer that controls its operation, the insulin pump offered Claire the ability to manage her diabetes more effectively.[34]

"One of the Texas Children's Hospital diagnosticians trained us on the pump," Liz said. "It took us several months to get the basal rate fine-tuned. Since the pump gives her a programmed basal rate dose of insulin 24 hours a day, the process of managing Claire's diabetes is, on its most basic level, a carbohydrate counting exercise. She needs to determine how many carbohydrates she is eating, and then give herself that amount of insulin with the pump to match it. And that's what keeps her blood sugar levels in the appropriate range. She still has to do the finger pricks to get a glucose reading, but she no longer has to give herself insulin shots."

For Claire, the insulin pump introduced a new flexibility to her formerly rigid daily regimen. To her delight, instead of having to eat meals at predetermined times, she could eat not only when she wanted to, but also what and how much she wanted. "I can eat more if I want to, and not eat if I don't want to," she happily reported.

The pump also facilitated Claire's participation in school and extracurricular activities. She attended Camp Rainbow, the American Diabetes Association's day camp for diabetes patients and their siblings, with her sister Kate and brother Clint. She also attended the weeklong Lion's Camp in the Texas Hill Country.

A straight A student with an outgoing personality and lots of friends, Claire never used her disease as a crutch or an excuse. Competent in her diabetes management skills from the beginning, by the time she was 11 years old Claire had accepted her fate with undeniable maturity. "At first, I was kind of wondering if diabetes was going to cramp my lifestyle," she said. "I thought I was not going to be able to do what I did before, but now it's just another aspect of my life. It does not affect most of my activities, and it really is not that bad."

Such optimism and self-confidence did not surprise her proud parents. "Claire's a pretty remarkable little girl in terms in how she handles life in general," Liz said. "So this really did not set her back at all. I would like to think that we as parents and Kate and Clint as siblings offered her a good support group."

"We also had the incredible support of Texas Children's Hospital and the diabetes and endocrinology clinic," said Liz. "They were just an amazing help. The technical, medical, and emotional support that we got was just priceless."

13

🖐 DIAGNOSTIC IMAGING 🖐

I̲T̲ ̲W̲A̲S̲ ̲T̲H̲E̲ ̲O̲F̲F̲I̲C̲I̲A̲L̲ ̲B̲E̲G̲I̲N̲N̲I̲N̲G̲ of his professional career, and it was not what he had expected.

"I had a desk there with nothing to do," recalled the first physician on the staff at Texas Children's Hospital, Dr. Edward B. Singleton.[1]

Having recently completed his residency at the University of Michigan, Singleton was a graduate of the University of Texas Medical Branch in Galveston. He arrived at Texas Children's Hospital in February 1953 to assume the role of chief radiologist at both Texas Children's Hospital and St. Luke's Episcopal Hospital. It was to be his first job.

Although he had been accepted for the position in 1952 and told that the hospitals were opening in the spring of 1953, Singleton discovered that this was not to be the case. Neither facility was available for occupancy because of construction delays. Consequently, he found himself not in the Texas Medical Center hospitals, as promised, but miles away in temporary offices located in the Gulf Building in downtown Houston.

While sharing this space with the administrator of the hospitals, Lee C. Gammill, Singleton became restless. Thinking back to his first few months there, he later said, "I'm not sure what I did then; I don't guess I did anything except listen to Mr. Gammill."[2]

Anxious to do more, Singleton pored over the construction plans with Gammill and helped order the initial X-ray equipment for the designated space reserved for the radiology department, located in the connecting link between the two hospitals. To the trained radiologist, the unfinished facilities already appeared to be inadequate. That each hospital had only a single X-ray room was not a practical way to do radiology, he thought. However, since plans were unalterable during construction, he vowed to remedy the situation at the first opportunity.[3]

Singleton also deemed it impractical to be sitting idly in an office while waiting for the hospitals to be completed. To occupy his time more effectively, he devised an immediate solution: "I went off to Children's Hospital Boston to get a little more education."

After studying briefly in Boston with renowned pediatric radiologist Dr. Edward B. D. Neuhauser, Singleton returned to continued construction delays. He worked for a short time in the radiology department at M. D. Anderson Hospital. Finally, in the summer of 1953, Singleton began the job that he had been hired to do, albeit in makeshift quarters. Carved out of space in the recently completed lobby area of Texas Children's Hospital—a space that later became the cardiac catheterization lab—Singleton's long-awaited X-ray department consisted of himself; a technician, Dean Frizzell; and one X-ray examination room. Even though the hospital did not open until February 1954, the services of this new department were available beforehand to children referred there as outpatients.

To Singleton's dismay, the first patient was neither a child, nor had he been referred there by a physician. It was Texas Children's Hospital's 80-year-old gardener, Joseph Kostrewski. Along with his wife, Josephine, Kostrewski had been involved in an altercation with a worker who apparently had dared to walk on the lovingly manicured lawn in front of the hospital. "Old Joseph was very protective of the new grass he was growing, and he got after him and the worker hit Joseph and knocked him down," Singleton said. "Then Josephine, who was older than her husband, jumped out of the truck and got after the worker with a hoe and the worker, I think, knocked her down, too. Well, they brought both of them in and it was a chance for us to test out our new X-ray equipment, and I'm happy to say no one was seriously hurt."

Also not referred by an outside physician was the first child to undergo an elective X-ray examination at Texas Children's Hospital. The grandchild of the housekeeper at the hospital, Clara Roberts, came at the request of Singleton. "Mrs. Roberts described how her grandchild was constipated all the time, and I thought this would be a chance for our first pediatric X-ray examination," he remembers. "So, she brought her grandson in, we gave him a barium enema and, surprisingly enough, he had legitimate causes for constipation. He had a condition called Hirschsprung's disease, which is a relatively rare condition. It was interesting that the first examination and diagnosis happened to be a somewhat unusual case. I think it was prophetic of the years to come and our ability to handle the unusual as well as the usual."[4]

The fact that these first two patients were from the inner circle of employees at Texas Children's Hospital also was out of the ordinary, considering the size of the staff. When all the hospital's employees signed an X-ray consultation form for Singleton's thirty-third birthday card on October 22, 1953, the total numbered less than 20, each of whom he knew well. Not only that, the names were not to be forgotten.

With that treasured memento in hand more than four decades later, Singleton pointed to each signature and recited: "There is the housekeeper Roberts and X-ray technician Dean Frizzell; hospital administrator Gammill and his daughter, who worked as the personnel director; telephone operator Maxine Moody; purchasing agent Barney Walker; maintenance engineers Weathers and Williams; bookkeeper Jane Long; nurses Betty Weinert and Bonnie Shoemate; janitors Andrew and Cleveland; future outpatient clinic director Winifred Spencer; and secretaries Pat Smith and Marguerite Garner, who was my secretary and a lovely, lovely lady."

For that secretary, who observed the limited number of patients during the X-ray department's first six months of operation at Texas Children's Hospital, listening to her boss' predictions about the future was a necessary part of her job. "Someday we'll have 50 patients a day," she remembered Singleton's saying in 1953. Such an increase seemed impossible, "His figure seemed exaggerated at the time," Garner recalled.[5]

Nonetheless, Singleton remained stubbornly optimistic about the potential growth of his newly established X-ray department. It was an optimism he was to maintain indefinitely, regardless of the unexpected challenges that came his way.

After all, he already knew from his experiences at Texas Children's Hospital how to adapt successfully to change.

The field of pediatric radiology was an emerging specialty when Texas Children's Hospital opened in 1954.

Although pediatric problems were diagnosed within the specialty of radiology in the 1940s, interest in both diagnostic and therapeutic approaches began to increase with the growing awareness of specialized problems with young patients.

Becoming one of the pioneers in this blossoming medical field was not the original goal of Dr. Edward B. Singleton. Instead, his career path was one altered by circumstance. Fittingly, it was a routine chest X-ray in 1947 that served as the impetus.

"I had a history of tuberculosis and it reactivated, as evidenced by the chest X-ray, when I was a surgical intern at the University of Michigan," Singleton said. "They put me to bed 'the Michigan Way,' which meant you would be completely flat in bed for three months to a year. You weren't even allowed to sit up to read. And then, when your X-ray picture was stable, you sat on the edge of the bed for five minutes and let your feet dangle. Then, the next week you could do that for ten minutes. When you could do that for 30 minutes, the big day came and you sat in a chair by the side of the bed for five minutes."

During his lengthy hospitalization, Singleton realized that his childhood dream of becoming a surgeon like his father, Dr. Albert Olin Singleton, was unattainable. Knowing that he should avoid the extra efforts and activities of a surgeon, he was ambivalent about entering an alternate area of medicine. After receiving devastating news from home, he made the decision that dramatically influenced not only his own future but also, ultimately, that of Texas Children's Hospital.

"I was wheeled on a stretcher to the phone in the hall and my mother and brother told me on the phone that Dad had died," he recalled. "All I could do was just mourn for him. My desire to work with him some day was obviously impossible, so I decided I had to do something. I was advised by Jack Holt, who was interested in pediatric radiology and on the faculty of the University of Michigan, to go into radiology. He, along with the chief of radiology, Fred Hodges, had just written a book called *Radiology for Medical Students,* and he gave it to me."[6]

While still hospitalized, Singleton began reading the book. It was an enlightening experience. He learned that the field of radiology concerned more than just skeletal fractures, foreign bodies, and chest examinations of a primitive type, as he had previously thought. Radiologic diagnosis now included an established reliability in gastroenterology, urology, chest diagnosis, and neurosurgery, as well as numerous other specialties.

Rapid developments in the field were to be expected, given its short history, Singleton learned. First observed in 1895 by German physicist Conrad Roentgen, who named it "X-ray" because of its mysterious properties, the discovery of the hitherto unknown ray's ability to penetrate objects and subjects completely opaque to sunlight was revolutionary. The 1896 publication of Roentgen's first "radiograph"—a photograph taken of his wife's hand with X-ray instead of sunlight—and his description of the ability to see through the body startled the scientific world.

Since the apparatus utilized for Roentgen's discovery was readily available, scientists and inventors around the world immediately began to experiment with replicating the new X-ray. Within one year, inventor Thomas Alva Edison had created an innovative apparatus called a Vitascope. Later known as a fluoroscope, the device consisted of a tapered box with a calcium tungstate screen and a viewing port. First marketed for commercial sale in 1896 by General Electric, it was to become the standard tool for the viewing of X-ray images by physicians and those in the rapidly developing field of radiology.

Roentgen was awarded the first Nobel Prize in physics in 1901. He and his discovery also received unprecedented public recognition. In newspapers around the world, the potential usefulness of the X-ray was debated. Cartoons demonstrated the comical side of X-ray vision and see-through clothes, inspiring the sale of lead underwear for the timid. Unaware of the possible radiation effects, entrepreneurs set up crude equipment in X-ray portrait studios and began offering people the opportunity to purchase their own ghostly images on film.[7]

The danger of exposure to massive doses of radiation soon became evident to scientists and inventors. Having experienced severe burns from his daily work with X-rays, Clarence Daily, Edison's assistant, died in 1904. Awareness of the possible cause of Daily's death prompted the use of lead barriers to shield the operators of X-ray equipment. It also inspired the rapid invention of equipment that abbreviated exposure times, along with the recommendation that only trained technologists operate the equipment.[8]

Four decades later, in the early 1940s, X-ray technology was universally accepted as one of the most important inventions of the nineteenth century. Yet the technology was still in its infancy. As an instrument-based medical specialty, radiology benefited greatly from the accelerated advances made in X-ray equipment to meet the needs of the military during World War I and World War II. Contemporaneously with the 1947 publication of *Radiology for Medical Students* by Holt and Hodges, this newly improved X-ray apparatus was apparent in most major hospitals, as was the growing importance of radiologic diagnosis.

As for the future of radiology, Singleton believed it would be like its past—both unpredictable and limitless. Supporting this view was a prescient prediction in the book: "The brilliance of today's accomplishments in medical radiology will become the commonplaces of tomorrow; it has been so since the beginnings of the specialty. Medicine must not hesitate to abandon individual applications the moment a better method becomes available and the limitations of intellect alone will determine when progressive change will cease to occur."[9]

Enticed by such possibilities, Singleton made his decision to abandon his surgical career to become a radiologist. While still hospitalized, his exact thoughts at the time were decisive, if somewhat reluctant. "Well, I have to do something, I might as well try this radiology," he recalls thinking.[10]

Accepted into Hodges' radiology program at the University of Michigan, Singleton soon found himself especially interested in pediatric radiology. Fueling his fascination with the field were his encounters with its recognized leader, Dr. John Caffey, author of the definitive 1945 textbook *Pediatric X-Ray Diagnosis*. A close friend of Hodges' and a frequent visitor to the University of Michigan, Caffey lectured to Singleton and the other residents on several occasions.

"I got to know him then," Singleton recalls. "He knew about my interest in pediatric radiology. Later, when he organized the John Caffey Society, I was one of the hand-picked people asked to join."[11]

After completing his radiology internship and residency at the University of Michigan in 1952, Singleton became aware of the plans to build St. Luke's Episcopal Hospital and Texas Children's Hospital in Houston. Born on Galveston Island, where his mother and brother still lived, and married to a Houstonian, Singleton longed to return to his native state. Although he enthusiastically applied for a job at the new hospitals, he honestly did not expect to be hired. He soon was.

"I was very fortunate to jump from just finishing my residency to being chief of a radiology service of two hospitals," he recalls. "I thought I was pretty hot stuff to get this job, but in retrospect, I think one reason was no one was interested in pediatric radiology back then. I think there may have been some other applicants, but I don't think they were overrun with applications."[12]

What there was an apparent abundance of, Singleton discovered upon his arrival, were fluoroscopy areas. Construction plans called for one to be placed on each floor of Texas Children's Hospital. "Back then it was common practice, I guess, for the pediatrician to fluoroscope all his patients," he said. "We were beginning to recognize that this radiation was not the best thing for a child and that it should be done by people who were trained in its use, so that it won't be overdone. During construction, I was able to get those areas out of the plans and get all fluoroscopy moved down to the radiology department."

This did not mean that there would be an array of equipment when the radiology department opened. Quite to the contrary, at first there was just one item. Placed in the department's temporary location, a small area off the lobby of Texas Children's Hospital, the X-ray machine was the newest apparatus available at the time.

To perform the initial X-ray examinations, Singleton and his technologist worked in complete darkness in order to see the fluoroscopic images. Both wore specially designed red goggles, enabling their vision to adjust to the absence of light. Patients, however, were not so fortunate. Frightened by the dark, they immediately became apprehensive and unruly. For the radiologist and technologist, "it was not a pleasant thing to hold a struggling child down in the dark."[13]

This discomforting situation was soon remedied by a technological development of the 1950s, the image intensifier. A new type of fluoroscope, the device increased the brightness of the image and allowed much more accurate studies in a lighted room. How this new apparatus became a part of the radiology department was memorable. "Mrs. Leopold Meyer was in St. Luke's Hospital, and we had done some X-ray work on her," Singleton recalled. "Mr. Meyer was in the room when I pointed out that if we had an image intensifier we could do the study much quicker, and with a great deal more accuracy than we were doing with the antiquated equipment we were made to use. I had not been able to get the hospital administration to buy one. The next day, the administrator told me that we had an image intensifier in the budget after all and it would soon be received."[14]

Also remedied quickly in 1954 was a logistical problem in the newly opened radiology department. Located in the connecting link between Texas Children's Hospital and St. Luke's Episcopal Hospital, the department originally consisted of two rooms, one for children and one for adults. After its first month of operation, in which there were more than 200 radiographic procedures performed on children, the department had to expand. One month later, two new radiographic rooms were available for pediatric patients. Usurped from planned storage space in the basement of Texas Children's Hospital, the rooms boasted colorful paintings executed by Singleton's sister-in-law, artist Joan Singleton.

Immediately utilized by a growing pediatric patient population, this ancillary area solved one problem and created another. For the radiology department's one and only radiologist and his technologist, attempting to correlate the work done in two areas became a frustrating experience. Nonetheless, Singleton said, "We did the best possible job under difficult conditions."[15]

Another radiologist was hired in 1955—not to assist Singleton, but to replace him for two years. "I was drafted into the Air Force," he explained. "Before leaving I needed help, obviously, and Dr. E. W. 'Wiley' Biles was working at Memorial Hospital, and I asked him to join us. While I was in the Air Force, he carried this department, even though he was not a pediatric radiologist. He brought in additional part-time people to do the work. A little later on, Dr. C. T. Teng, a Baylor radiologist, joined the team."[16]

It was unfathomable to Singleton that he had been drafted and assigned to Alaska one year after the opening of Texas Children's Hospital. At the time, he thought "my career had suddenly started and then ended." Years later, however, he deemed the experience "the best thing, professionally, that ever happened to me, because it gave me the time to write a book on pediatric radiology at a time when there were few books published on the subject."[17]

It was while writing his *X-Ray Diagnosis of the Alimentary Tract in Infants and Children* that Singleton began to harbor concerns about his future. Convinced that his lengthy absence from the department of radiology at Texas Children's Hospital and St. Luke's Episcopal Hospital was detrimental to his academic goals, he felt dejected and alone in 1956. On a rainy day in Alaska, his sinking spirits were immediately buoyed by a drenched copy of the *American Journal of Roentgenology*.

"I still get emotional thinking about this," he said. "I opened it up and the lead article was about the history of pediatric radiology and was written by Dr. John Caffey. In this article, he listed those whom he thought to have been the most productive, or promising, I forget his exact words. And here my name was on this list of about 12 pediatric radiologists. It was quite a moving experience."[18]

Caffey had identified Singleton as one of "the enthusiastic, well-trained, young clinical scientists who man pediatric roentgenology in the several major clinics and children's hospitals in the United States." These, Caffey declared, "are men of great promise and we can expect a splendid yield from their endeavors." Singleton was ebullient and also further inspired to complete his first book.[19]

Returning to his job in 1957, Singleton found that the radiology department was continuing its rapid growth. With more than 1,000 X-ray examinations performed each month on pediatric patients, pediatric radiology at Texas Children's Hospital was no longer a novelty but an established entity. Already well known in the local medical community for its diagnostic capabilities, particularly in difficult cases, its reputation was about to flourish both nationally and internationally.

With a wealth of interesting and unusual pediatric illnesses seen at

Texas Children's Hospital in the 1950s, the pediatric radiology department had participated in nine national medical meetings since the hospital's opening. Also instrumental in establishing its national standing was the presentation made by Singleton at the inaugural gathering of the Society for Pediatric Radiologists in 1957.

"This was a group of pediatric radiologists who got together to organize their own society," Singleton said of that newly formed organization, one that he later served as president. "Practically everybody presented papers. There weren't that many members, maybe 20 or 25 of us."[20]

Regardless of its size, the membership roster of the Society for Pediatric Radiology boasted the top names in the field at the time. Through Singleton's prominent association with that organization, as well as the John Caffey Society and countless other radiological organizations, events, and publications, Texas Children's Hospital gained worldwide recognition.

Also garnering attention in the late 1950s and early 1960s were technological advances in radiology. Although individual radiographs—the standard still photos taken with X-ray—still required development by hand, "electronic type" fluoroscopic studies came into use. Enabled by the quality results produced by image intensifiers, technologists began to record radiological examinations—first on movie film and eventually on videotape.

Radiologists Singleton, Biles, and Teng incorporated this electronic advance into the department in 1965. With a television camera permanently mounted to the X-ray machine, they could record each pediatric examination at Texas Children's Hospital. With these additional studies performed on an ever increasing number of patients, the staff grew to include 12 technologists. Yet for the next six years, the burgeoning pediatric radiology department remained in its original makeshift setting, spread among multiple locations.[21]

Despite these cramped conditions, efforts to deliver excellent patient care never wavered and academic pursuits continued unimpeded. Dr. Milton Wagner and later Dr. Robert Dutton, two dedicated pediatric radiologists, joined the service. Praising his colleagues, Singleton said: "I look back over those difficult years and take considerable pride. Even working under those frustrating conditions, the radiologists of this department have written two textbooks on pediatrics radiology, contributed 15 chapters to other texts of pediatrics and radiology, and written 100 individual publications for scientific journals."[22]

At long last, the radiology department moved into spacious new quarters in 1971. Located on the ground level of the new 26-story tower at St. Luke's

Episcopal Hospital, the 20,000-square-foot area provided adequate space for the comfort of patients as well as staff. In addition to the pediatric radiologists, there was one radiology fellow, numerous residents from Baylor College of Medicine and M. D. Anderson Hospital, 22 X-ray technologists, and 12 aides.

Designed with patients and their families in mind, the two separate waiting areas—one for adults and one for children—afforded much-needed privacy to each group. Each of the five X-ray rooms designated for pediatric patients had its own dark room and processing area. Equipped with the most modern form of electronic fluoroscopic equipment and monitoring available, Singleton's "magnificent structural department" was a welcomed change. That it was to become just as cramped and inadequate as before was unthinkable at the time.

In retrospect, such an outcome was a certainty. For one thing, there was an increase in the patient population almost immediately. Following the 1972 expansion of Texas Children's Hospital from 106 to 267 beds and the enlargement of the Junior League Outpatient Department, pediatric X-ray examinations totaled more than 2,000 each month.

Also dramatically affecting the future of the department was the advent of technological advances that revolutionized the ability and accuracy of diagnostic studies in pediatric patients. The first of these innovations was in ultrasound studies, the non-invasive use of high-frequency sound waves inside the body to produce echo images on a video screen. Originally developed as an ultrasonic underwater detection system after the sinking of the *Titanic* in 1912, it eventually became known as SONAR during World War II. Utilized by the military to determine the location of German submarines at sea, the technology proved to be invaluable.

"Diagnostic ultrasound resulted from the minification and refinement of SONAR in the 1960s," said Singleton, remembering its introduction at Texas Children's Hospital. "It improved remarkably and became a very vital part of obstetrics. It is especially important for pediatric use because it utilizes sound waves rather than ionizing radiation. It is extremely valuable in determining if a child with a tumor has a solid mass or whether it's a cystic structure, and this is of great help to the surgeon in evaluating preoperatively the malignant lesion from a benign lesion, for example."[23]

The next technological advance, introduced in the 1970s, was Computed Axial Tomography, known as CT or CAT scan. Combining diagnostic X-ray studies with a computer to form a computerized, three-dimensional, cross-sectional image, CT enabled the evaluation of intracranial abnormalities and other diseases of the brain.

"One main advantage is that not only does it provide a different view, but it is also noninvasive, in that the insertion of catheters and the injection of contrast media into the arterial system of the body frequently are unnecessary," Singleton said. "Computed tomography can be justifiably considered the greatest advance in diagnostic radiology since Wilhelm Roentgen first discovered the X-ray in 1895."[24]

Invented in 1971 by British engineer Godfrey Hounsfield of EMI Laboratories, the original CT scanned only the head. Total body CT scanners first became available in 1976. The first of its kind in Texas was installed in the department of radiology of Texas Children's Hospital and St. Luke's Episcopal Hospital on April 20, 1976. Two years later came the installation of the department's second CT scan, reported to be 75 times faster than the original.

By 1979, the previously unimaginable need to enlarge the radiology department was clearly evident. Already expanded to seven radiographic rooms, pediatric radiology shared its diagnostic equipment with adult radiology out of necessity. In addition to its original X-ray machines, there were two CT scanners, an ultrasound suite, a neuroradiology section, and portable radiographic equipment for intensive care patients and newborns. Crowded but not cramped as before, the department had little or no unused space. And, although unbeknown in the late 1970s, another technological advance was on the horizon.[25]

Introduced in the 1980s was nuclear magnetic resonance, or NMR. Using magnetic fields, rather than ionizing radiation like the CT, NMR imaging produced computerized anatomic images or cross sections known as "slices." Initially used in research laboratories to analyze the composition of compounds, NMR scanning involved the use of a giant magnet to scan the magnetic nuclei found in hydrogen, carbon, fluoride, sodium, and phosphorus.[26]

Discovering that the nuclei of hydrogen atoms in the cells of a patient aligned themselves to the powerful magnetic field generated by the NMR scanner, scientists introduced its revolutionary capabilities to the medical profession. Wary of using the word "nuclear" because of its perceived negative connotation, hospitals and companies dubbed it "magnetic resonance imaging," or MR imaging. Over time, it became known as MRI.

Initially utilized at Texas Children's Hospital and St. Luke's Episcopal Hospital only for scanning the head for research purposes, the radiology department's first MR imaging equipment arrived in 1985. Though at first skeptical of the full potential of MR imaging, Singleton soon became a convert.

"It has the unique ability of determining the chemistry of the area under study, detecting types of tumors and potentially differentiating cancerous from noncancerous tissue," Singleton explained. "In simple language, it means that the science of anatomic image of the body and detecting abnormal areas whether they be the result of trauma, tumors, infections, congenital defects, or arteriosclerosis has reached a degree of sophistication and accuracy which has surpassed anyone's previous expectations."[27]

What also was to surpass Singleton's expectations were the approved plans for the new pediatric radiology department. Instead of being jointly operated with St. Luke's Episcopal Hospital, as in the past, the new department was to be an entity in itself. Announced after the 1987 separation of the two hospitals' jointly operated and managed services, the pediatric radiology department was to be located in the newly built West Tower of Texas Children's Hospital.

In a salute to the diverse technological advances that dramatically influenced its past, shaped its present, and guided its future, Singleton named the new department "diagnostic imaging services."

Opened in 1991, diagnostic imaging services contained state-of-the-art diagnostic equipment and had the capability to perform 75,000 diagnostic examinations a year. At its helm were the original three pediatric radiologists—Singleton, Dutton, and Wagner—and a rapidly expanding staff of technologists, clerical workers, and aides.

Singleton's unique career path, stretching from a one-room X-ray department in 1953 to one of the largest pediatric radiology departments in the United States, came to its official end in 1995. Before retiring as the first and only chief of the pediatric radiology department at Texas Children's Hospital, Singleton handpicked his replacement. His choice was Dr. Bruce R. Parker, a pediatric radiologist at Stanford University School of Medicine and coauthor of the textbook *Pediatric Oncology Radiology.*

"I came in 1994," Parker recalled. "I had known Ed Singleton for many years. Sometime in 1993, he called me and asked me if I would be interested in taking the position, since he was retiring. I told him I really was not interested, and he said, 'Well, look, why don't you come down and take a look. It will be a nice weekend for you and your wife, and we'll have a good time together, and if you don't like it, you don't like it.' So, how could I refuse an offer like that?"[28]

After several visits to Texas Children's Hospital, Parker changed his mind and accepted Singleton's offer. "I was very honored that he wanted to turn over his department to me after 42 years," Parker said. "I also had known Drs. Dutton and Wagner, the other two pediatric radiologists, for many years and I liked the situation here."

Perceiving his job to require bringing the department to the forefront technologically, Parker immediately embarked on an ambitious project. Turning a futuristic concept into a reality, he shepherded the implementation of computed radiography (CR) and picture archiving and communication systems (PACS) at Texas Children's Hospital.

Beginning in 1995 and continuing through 1997, Parker found that CR demanded changes in practice by the technologist, radiologist, and referring physician. Accustomed to viewing radiographic images on films, each had to adjust to viewing these images on a computer screen instead. For those unfamiliar with computers and entrenched in the ways of the past, adapting to this revolutionary change usually took three months.

Although it was a steep learning curve, Parker reported that the clinicians soon came to appreciate the excellent image quality, the immediate availability of images, and the juxtaposition of images and reports available electronically.[29]

"As with all technical innovation, an initial period of confusion, trial-and-error testing, and exasperation was followed by a rush to acquire systems as they prove themselves in active clinical settings," Parker said. "But what we developed is what is called a 'filmless' department. It's a very expensive project, one that I was very fortunate Texas Children's Hospital was able to support."[30]

Known nationally as the first full-service children's hospital to be "filmless," Texas Children's Hospital played host to countless medical professionals from all over the country. Curious to see how PACS worked in a clinical setting, the visitors wished to determine whether or not to invest in a system of their own. Inevitably, each left with a favorable impression.

"It's quite professional," Parker explained. "It's all done on computers. If a patient goes somewhere else and we have to give him some film, we just print it out from the computer. As for access to the PACS archives, with the correct computer equipment, I can look at images from Europe or Hong Kong or anywhere."

Six years after its initial implementation and two years after its completion, a major system upgrade required that CR and PACS be shut down for 12 hours during one weekend in 2001. "It was awful," Parker recalled. "Going back to reading films after two years of not looking at one was just amazing. I'm so spoiled by this, I could never go back."

This was a sentiment shared by all the pediatric radiologists in the department. With the successful implementation of PACS, the ability to review a patient's images within two minutes of an examination was an invaluable tool—and a necessary one, given the more than 300 examinations performed each day. "When I came in 1994, this department already was a little small," Parker recalled in 2001. "It had been built to do about 75,000 examinations a year and, by the time I got here, it was already over 80,000. We're up to more than 125,000 now."[31]

Just as it had in the one-room X-ray department that Singleton established in 1953, and in all the subsequent reincarnations throughout its existence, the diagnostic imaging service at Texas Children's Hospital experienced a demand that exceeded the supply of space. To position this rapidly expanding service for continued growth in the future, Parker designed multiple facilities.

When Parker's redesign was completed in 2002, instead of just one central area for diagnostic imaging there were three separate locations. The general radiographic procedures and ultrasound occupied the eighth floor of the new Clinical Care Center; nuclear medicine was located on level B1 of the West Tower; and MRI, CT, ultrasound, radiographic fluoroscopy, and general radiographic and interventional procedures were performed on level 1 of the West Tower.

No matter how spacious and up-to-date the new diagnostic imaging center appeared in 2002, it was certain to be enlarged again in the near future. "One of my goals is to position this department so that it will be considered one of the top five departments in the country," Parker said. "My prime goal is outstanding patient care and education goes along with it."[32]

In 2004, with more than 125,000 radiographic examinations a year, the diagnostic imaging service at Texas Children's Hospital was one of the three busiest services in the country. To ensure that it was also one of the best, Parker had recruited new members to his team continuously ever since his arrival.

"When I came to Texas Children's as chief in 1994, I was the sixth radiologist," he said. "We now have 16. The most important thing for any chief to do is hire good people; if you don't hire good people, you don't have anything. I brought in some really superb pediatric radiologists, all with an academic background. Every one is subspecialty trained in pediatric radiology, pediatric Ultrasound, pediatric CT, and pediatric MR. Each is certified by the American Board of Radiology in Pediatric Radiology, as well as general."[33]

This accomplishment, along with Parker's other major contributions to the diagnostic imaging service at Texas Children's Hospital, took place at an accelerated pace in the ten years following his 1994 arrival. Aware from the beginning that his tenure as chief of diagnostic imaging would not span decades, he explained his motivation, "I was older when I got here so I am not going to be around for 40 years like Dr. Singleton. I look at my job as trying to create the infrastructure so that the next person who comes in after me can really move it into a very high level."[34]

Satisfied that he had achieved his mission, Parker stepped down in July 2004. Named as his successor was Dr. Taylor Chung, who had been a member of the service for the previous five years. "It's an honor to succeed Dr. Parker," Chung said as he assumed his new role. "He has built a world-class department that very few children's hospitals around the country can match."[35]

Chung was only the third chief of diagnostic imaging in the 50-year history of Texas Children's Hospital. He accepted the challenge of his new job by making a promise for the future that also paid tribute to the past. "We take pride in offering the latest technological imaging advances, maintaining the highest standards of patient care, and providing responsive diagnostic consultations," he said. "The top priority for diagnostic imaging is, and always will be, the delivery of excellent care and service to our patients and referring physicians."[36]

Chung's commitment to the established pattern of always offering the latest technological imaging advances in the diagnostic imaging service at Texas Children's Hospital also echoed a passage in *Radiology for Medical Students,* the 1947 textbook that had inspired Singleton 50 years earlier.

As accurate in 2004 as it had been in 1947 was this prescient statement in that book: "The brilliance of today's accomplishments in medical radiology will become the commonplaces of tomorrow; it has been so since the beginnings of the specialty. Medicine must not hesitate to abandon individual applications the moment a better method becomes available and the limitations of intellect alone will determine when progressive change will cease to occur."[37]

As always, the diagnostic imaging service at Texas Children's Hospital eagerly anticipated the progressive changes that lay in its future.

As the official ending of his professional career in 1995, it was not what he had expected.

Forty-two years after becoming the first physician on the staff at Texas

Children's Hospital, Dr. Edward B. Singleton found himself to be in another singular position. Incredibly, his first job remained his only job. At the time of his 1995 retirement, he was the hospital's sole remaining original employee—a distinction held since 1973.

Recognized nationally and internationally by his peers, Singleton garnered countless tributes for building an outstanding pediatric radiology department at Texas Children's Hospital. Under his direction, what had begun as a one-room X-ray department in 1953 grew to become one of the five largest pediatric diagnostic services in the United States.

Characteristically modest about his myriad accomplishments, Singleton preferred to extol the achievements of his medical specialty, pediatric radiology. "I am more amazed by the development of technology that happened during those years," he said.

With his vivid memory of each new technological advance and its dramatic impact on patient care at Texas Children's Hospital, Singleton easily recalled amusing anecdotes associated with every one. The memories ranged from early days, when he wore the red goggles necessary to operate the fluoroscope and told the nurses and secretaries that those glasses gave him the power of X-ray vision, to later times, when "some of the paramedical people are trying to teach some of us old guys which buttons to push on this computer. If you don't know how to type now, you are lost. It's amazing how these younger people are so good at it. I just hunt and peck."[38]

The subject of typing skills and the advent of computers reminded Singleton of how his first secretary, Marguerite Garner, had laboriously transcribed every word he dictated into a recording device called a Dictaphone. Utilizing that now-antiquated procedure, she typed countless papers and publications for Singleton, as well as the manuscript for his first book, *X-ray Diagnosis of the Alimentary Tract in Infants and Children,* in 1959. Every correction or addition made by Singleton required her to retype the entire chapter or page. It was an extraordinary effort by Garner, one that Singleton continued to praise.

From the 1970s, he recalled an occasion when a physicist from Rice University came to inspect the newly arrived ultrasound equipment. "Charlie Squire, a friend of mine, read about our new ultrasound in the local papers," he said. "He came by and was so excited to see the application of ultrasound to diagnosing diseases. In World War II, he had been on a submarine chaser, one of those big SONAR things. Soon afterward, when he was a physicist at the Massachusetts Institute of Technology, they brought one of those huge, two-story SONAR things back to study its possible future applications. He told me they decided there was no way to minify to use in a practical way for medical purposes. So, he was very excited to see our ultrasound. It was very refreshing to see."

Although each technological advance was awe inspiring in itself, what Singleton appreciated most was its application to patient care at Texas Children's Hospital. He was convinced that the best patient care resulted from exploiting the latest technology and its advanced diagnostic capabilities. Singleton championed that cause from the beginning of his career to the end.

He believed passionately that pediatric radiologists had to seize every opportunity to deliver better patient care, a philosophy that he practiced for more than four decades. "Our philosophy has been that we always talk to the parents and explain what we have found," Singleton said. "Relating to the parents is something a lot of radiologists don't do, and I think it's important they know our role in their child's care."[39]

With endless recollections about countless patients and their families, Singleton fondly recalled the innumerable physicians, nurses, technicians, volunteers, and other individuals with whom he worked. "I don't really recall the business part," he explained. "I remember the people."

This was not selective memory on his part, but confirmation of something he had learned from his father. "He was a very wise doctor who believed it's not the bricks and the mortar that make a hospital; it's the qualifications and the dedication of the people who are doing the work," Singleton said.

For further confirmation of that sentiment, Singleton needed to look no further than his retirement dinner on October 22, 1995, the evening of his seventy-fifth birthday. Surrounded by colleagues and friends from the past and present, he received their heartfelt expressions of adulation and respect. At such a celebration, this type of attention was to be anticipated by even a modest pediatric radiologist. What came next, however, was not.

It was an announcement. In honor of Singleton's unparalleled accomplishments and contributions, the pediatric radiology center at Texas Children's Hospital was to be named the Edward B. Singleton Diagnostic Imaging Services. Completely surprised by this tribute from Texas Children's Hospital, Singleton returned the favor. Instead of retiring permanently, as planned, he soon came back to work part-time in his namesake area.

Back at work, Singleton became familiar with yet another technological advance—PACS. "We don't have X-ray film any more," he explained. "We don't have all those films to fuddle with, pull out, put back into the envelope. We just archive it all on a computer. It's just been wonderful."[40]

Not at all intimidated by the new technology, Singleton was, rather, charmed. "I can brighten the image, magnify it, enhance the detail, and sharpen it," he said. "I would give anything to be able to look into the future to see what other advances may be on the horizon."[41]

As he expertly observed digital images of a patient's X-ray examination on a computer screen, Singleton exemplified one of the trademark aspects of his legendary career at Texas Children's Hospital.

Once again adapting to an unexpected change, Dr. Edward B. Singleton embraced it wholeheartedly.

14

❦ EMERGENCY CENTER ❧

Suddenly, their twenty-two-month-old daughter could not breathe and was desperately gasping for air.

In a matter of moments, the child had expended so much energy that her tiny body became as limp as a rag doll. Terrified as they watched helplessly, not knowing exactly what they could do to help, the child's mother and father scooped her up, jumped in the car, and rushed to the emergency center at Texas Children's Hospital.

With the child cradled in their arms, they arrived at the emergency center and "the nurse just eyeballed her and knew she was in severe distress," her mother recalled. "Immediately, they put a pulse oximeter on to measure the amount of oxygen in her blood, and that's when they knew what to do. They started her on oxygen, started an IV, and started her on medication."[1]

When told that their daughter was having an asthmatic attack, the parents were stunned. Although she had previously suffered a similar, although less acute, breathing problem and her pediatrician had diagnosed it as either bronchitis or asthma, they nonetheless "were shell-shocked. We didn't have a family history of asthma," the mother said. "We did not know what we were dealing with when we first started. And then we learned. We learned a great deal."

This in-depth educational process about asthma continued in earnest for the following three days. After being observed for several hours in the emergency center, the child was admitted to Texas Children's Hospital. Her parents knew that they would not leave her there alone. They decided that one of them would stay overnight, while the other went home to care for their older child before returning the next morning. Unknowingly, they established a routine that would be followed again and again in the future.

"My husband would come back in the morning, after he had had his shower and breakfast, and I would come home, shower, sleep for four or five hours, and then I would go back and relieve him," the wife said. "And then he would swing by in the evening, bring our son, say 'Hey,' and then we'd do the same thing all over again. It was exhausting. It's like having a newborn because you don't get any sleep. And I think what makes it worse is that anytime you're so fatigued, your emotional state is just that much more fragile."

Trying to recall the precise details of that initial visit to the emergency center at Texas Children's Hospital, the mother admitted that her memory was "all a little fuzzy about that first time." But she clearly remembered the lessons learned at Texas Children's Hospital about the best way to treat her child's asthma. Staying with her daughter each night, she watched and worried as the child reacted poorly to theophylline, her pediatrician's newly prescribed, caffeine-based medication. Concerned that her normally active infant was exhausted, motionless, and wide-eyed while on that medication, she called the pediatrician from the hospital.

While the mother was telling the doctor that the medication was not delivering its desired effects, a nurse in the room interrupted her and said, "I don't mean to eavesdrop, but I couldn't help but overhear and I'm about ready to give that medication to your child." In response, the appreciative mother quickly handed the phone to the nurse so that the pediatrician could discuss an alternative medication. "The staff at Texas Children's are so good," said the mother, thinking not only of that moment, but also of how they patiently taught parents how to administer the medications to their children and how to operate the equipment.

After closely observing the respiratory therapist as she gave breathing treatments to their child four times a day in the hospital, both parents learned how to work with a nebulizer, a little machine that creates a mist, and how to put the machine's mask on the child so that they could do breathing treatments at home. "Before you are released, they show you how all of this works," the mother said. "And then you basically have to repeat it back to them to show them you know how to do it."

Satisfied that they had successfully completed their crash course in asthma treatments, the family happily checked out of the hospital after three days. They took their recovered daughter back home, never dreaming that they would have to return to the emergency center at Texas Children's Hospital anytime soon. What they did not expect to happen did happen—and more than once.

Six times the following year, the child had to be rushed to the emergency center at Texas Children's Hospital. Typically, there was an established pattern. The onset would begin and she would get very ill very quickly, and one of her parents would immediately take her to the emergency center. "Once she got treatment at the hospital, she would bounce back pretty quickly," her mother said. "After several visits to the emergency center, our initiative was always to get her home where she would be more comfortable."

The child usually responded rapidly to the treatment she received in the emergency center at Texas Children's Hospital. Her parents often had to explain this to the attending physician. On one memorable occasion, their explanation was unnecessary. A respiratory therapist recognized the frequent patient and said, "Hey, Peanut, what are you doing back here?" Then the therapist turned to the doctor and said, "You watch this one. She's going to surprise you."[2]

Although always anxious to take their daughter home immediately after these treatments, her parents often did not. Three of the visits resulted in the child being admitted as a patient at Texas Children's Hospital. On each occasion, her parents simply fell into their established routine of the mother's spending the nights and the father's covering the day shifts.

Also becoming second nature to the parents were the physical surroundings of Texas Children's Hospital. "It got to the point in the emergency center that I knew where the crushed ice machine was and I would just go help myself," the mother said, laughing at the memory. "I remember one time when I did that, I thought, 'I am way too comfortable with this emergency center.' I really know my way around this place."

The mother also found herself to be extremely familiar with the medical jargon used in emergencies with asthmatic patients. "The doctor would come in and I would say, 'The onset was at this time; the respiratory rate is this; her pulse rate is this; and I gave her an albuterol mist or whatever.' And once I did that, the doctors would snap to and realize what they were dealing with," she said, reflecting on her newfound knowledge. "When they are dealing with asthma on the TV show ER, I know exactly what they're talking about. Like, someone says, 'OK, we're going to push two CCs of albuterol,' and I know what they're doing."

Her husband became expert at the art of navigating the hallways of the different buildings at Texas Children's Hospital. During one Thanksgiving visit, with the IV pole in one hand and pulling his daughter in her little red wagon with the other, they explored every corner of Texas Children's Hospital without getting lost.

During their exploratory tours of Texas Children's Hospital, both parents became aware of the critically ill children who were not as fortunate as their daughter. Always hopeful that the future would bring a healing change to the child's fragile health, her mother said, "Everything is relative. I don't like this. I wish she didn't have it. But you know what? I can deal with it."

W hen Texas Children's Hospital opened its front doors in February 1954, it also opened a set of gray double doors marked "Emergency" in the rear of the building.

"The emergency room, back in those ancient days, was a little room right across from the red elevators on the first floor," recalled Dr. Allen H. Kline, the chief resident at Texas Children's in 1959.[3]

Accessible by ringing a bell and staffed with one registered nurse, the emergency room did not have a physician on staff, but was the responsibility of the chief resident, who could muster the hospital's medical personnel into action 24 hours a day, if required. "But it was not like today," Kline said. "People were sent there by their doctors because they had some acute, serious problem that should be seen in a hospital."[4]

One particular acute, serious problem that occurred in the first few months of the center's opening in 1954 was unique, according to nurse Helen A. Dunn, who worked the night shift on the fourth floor and in the emergency room at Texas Children's Hospital. Whenever a patient who required emergency services arrived at night, the nurse followed a specific procedure. "They would ring the bell and I would go down and take care of the emergency," she said. "Then I would come back up to the fourth floor."[5]

After hearing the bell ring at 5 a.m., Dunn rushed downstairs to see what the problem was. Standing in the room was a family with a child who had been bitten by a snake. Dunn asked what kind of snake it was. To her surprise, a family member replied, "This kind," and handed her the snake. "Luckily, they brought that snake in," Dunn says. "From that particular snake, the laboratory made an anti-venom which worked extremely well."[6]

Other emergencies were handled just as effectively. For each specific need, the chief resident had the ability to call in, at a moment's notice, the necessary interns, doctors, laboratory technicians, X-ray technicians, and nurses. However, such instantaneous response was required only on rare occasions. "I would not see a patient in there every day," Kline recalled, echoing published reports of the emergency room becoming a "beehive of activity" when two patients were there at the same time.[7]

Ten years later, the pace in the emergency room at Texas Children's Hospital had become accelerated and a record number of 433 cases were treated during August 1964. The permanent staff of the emergency room at Texas Children's Hospital consisted of a registered nurse-in-charge, who was aided by a nursing supervisor. Responsible for "a steady steam of traffic through the gray doors," that two-person emergency room staff, and the large number of physicians on the premises called in to assist, expertly handled myriad emergencies, ranging from children with bruises and cut fingers to those who were critically ill.[8]

As the number of patients steadily increased year by year, the little room behind the double gray doors soon was at maximum capacity and often overflowing. A solution to this problem of unbridled growth was found when construction began in June 1967 on the expansion of Texas Children's Hospital, St. Luke's Episcopal Hospital, and the Texas Heart Institute. Abandoning its original space, the emergency room at Texas Children's merged with the existing emergency room at St. Luke's Episcopal Hospital, located on the first level of the south side. This joint operating arrangement was to continue until 1991.

To accommodate the needs of both adult and pediatric patient populations, the facility at St. Luke's Episcopal Hospital was expanded to include a spacious reception and waiting area, seven examining and treatment rooms, ten observation beds, a trauma treatment room for seriously ill or injured patients, an isolation room, and storage and office space for medical personnel.[9] Named the "emergency center" and opened on May 1, 1972, the newly combined facilities at St. Luke's Episcopal Hospital treated more than 1,000 patients in the first month of operation.[10]

Throughout the next six years, the chief resident of Texas Children's Hospital continued his responsibilities as the physician-on-call for pediatric patients in the emergency center. With the number of pediatric emergencies steadily increasing, this arrangement was no longer optimal.

A much-needed change occurred on July 1, 1978, when the Texas Children's Hospital emergency center was included in the training rotation for pediatric residents at Baylor College of Medicine. With the implementation of this program, at least one resident and one intern were on duty throughout the day in the Texas Children's Hospital emergency center. During the night hours, one resident remained in the center and the other residents and interns were available on call.[11]

One of those interns in 1981 was Dr. Joan E. Shook, who in 1987 became director of the Texas Children's Hospital emergency center. Memories of the early days of Shook's career at Texas Children's Hospital remained vivid decades later. "As an intern, you worked every third night from 6 in the evening until the following morning," Shook recalled. "You were there with a second-year or third-year resident and it was the two of you seeing the children. There was never a senior person there, never. There was a general emergency physician there on the St. Luke's side, but we really never talked to one another."[12]

When the number of pediatric patients escalated to more than 16,000 in 1987, questions about which patient population took precedence in the combined emergency center became a source of tension. "We were rapidly increasing much more than on the adult side, which made St. Luke's pretty unhappy with us, not surprisingly," Shook said. "I can't blame St. Luke's and I'm not indicting them here; it was a very difficult situation. Our patients really were kind of crowding out the St. Luke's patients and the St. Luke's patients probably were not getting the services that they deserved."

With communications at a minimum, the sharing of a defined area of space was often a contentious ordeal for those from St. Luke's Episcopal Hospital and Texas Children's Hospital assigned to duties in the emergency center. Attempting to manage this combined effort was a committee consisting of the director of nursing, the chief operating officer, and the medical director of St. Luke's Episcopal Hospital and Texas Children's Hospital. Organized to handle the various issues that arose in the emergency center, the committee met on a weekly basis with the single nurse manager.

Each weekly committee meeting lasted for hours, an experience Shook remembered in exacting detail. "Fortunately, I was young and inexperienced then and I didn't know that that was abnormal," she said. "I thought people always sit down and fight for three hours on Thursday. And we did. We fought over every last thing. Whether we should draw lines on the floor, whether we should change the colors of the nurses' smocks, depending on where they are working that day. Should adults get precedence over children? It was just wild and crazy stuff."

It was a dilemma that intensified during the next two years. When the number of pediatric visits escalated to more than 20,000 in 1988, Shook began to improvise, introducing ways to stretch the space and alleviate the overcrowding. "We did several things in that era to try and mediate those problems," she said. "One was, we opened upstairs, in the old Junior League clinic space, a rapid-turn-around area for about five hours every evening, just to have another place to see children and try to get them out of the emergency department downstairs. We also brought child life in at that time to keep the kids entertained and focused in this very tight space so that they would be somewhat less disruptive to the adult side."

Child life specialists were able to alleviate the common anxieties experienced by children and parents alike in the Texas Children's Hospital emergency center. Since each specialist was appropriately trained and educated to provide professional assistance to children and their families, the impact of their services was immeasurable. Able to explain various procedures and tests in simple, everyday, and easy-to-understand language, child life specialists brought calm to the often-chaotic emergency center.

The innovative child life program, which provided therapeutic play activities and emotional support to hospitalized children and their families, was already in place at Texas Children's Hospital. "We just brought them downstairs," Shook said. "We kind of toyed with a number of possibilities. Did we want child life? Did we want patient advocates? Did we want other things? And it was my hope that having a child life specialist there would change the nurse assistant's activities. With the ability to concentrate more on the patients, nurses would begin to understand how you can handle a child in a different way from an adult and make the world work a little bit better in a pediatric facility."

As Shook continued to implement strategies for improved delivery of emergency services, a solution to the ever-increasing need for additional space came in 1988 with the announcement of the $149 million expansion plan for Texas Children's Hospital. Since an emergency center exclusively for Texas Children's patients was to be on the first floor of the newly constructed critical care and surgical building, Shook enthusiastically took part in its initial planning.

In 1988, faced with what she thought was an overabundance of space for the delivery of emergency care to pediatric patients, Shook looked over the plans and decided to include individual office spaces in the unused back alcove of the proposed new emergency center. But, with the 12 to 14 percent growth in pediatric emergency cases continuing over the next five years, she began worrying that her plans for the new emergency center were becoming outdated. Indeed, by 1991, the center was treating more than 26,000 pediatric cases each year. Shook decided to redesign the space completely, even though construction had been completed.[13] "Before the emergency department opened, the individual offices in the back alcove were gutted and redone into patient care space," Shook said. "We didn't even get to the point of opening it because I was so concerned about this mushrooming growth."[14]

The projected increase in patients affected not only the physical surroundings in the new emergency center, but also the staffing requirements, which underwent significant changes. To accommodate the clerical needs of the growing staff and since office spaces no longer existed in the emergency center, Shook created new offices in space carved out of the lobby.

Having worked to create an ideal facility for pediatric emergency care, Shook set out to perfect the delivery. "The first thing we did was train our nurses differently," she recalled. "I was able to bring in a staff of physicians. We had 24-hour pediatric medicine coverage in the emergency department, which was the first one in the state. We brought in a computer system. We really expanded our scope and our quality of service. I think we really raised our level of care to a new height."

When the Texas Children's Hospital emergency center opened on October 1, 1991, there was a newly trained team of nurses, an expanded staff of physicians, and great expectations of providing loving care to the children in need. Named the Meyer and Ida Gordon Emergency Center in honor of the late Houston philanthropists, the center was prepared to provide extensive lifesaving procedures and to treat children with fevers, earaches, and sore throats, as well as asthmatic patients who required many different types of medications and, possibly, intubation and advanced life support.

Also established in the newly opened Meyer and Ida Gordon Emergency Center at Texas Children's Hospital was a pediatric emergency medicine fellowship. It was only the second pediatric emergency medicine fellowship in Texas and one of the first in the United States. At the time, pediatric emergency medicine was a relatively new field. The discipline was not recognized as a subspecialty until the mid-1980s and was not sub-boarded until 1992.

The three-year pediatric emergency medicine fellowship program at Texas Children's Hospital was designed around the skills required to be a competent pediatric emergency physician. Included in the training schedule was a rotation in orthopedics, anesthesia, critical care (ICU), surgery, otolaryngology (ENT), ophthalmology, and a variety of other departments. With hands-on experience available 24 hours a day in the emergency center, fellows observed the myriad activities and problems that arise in a rapidly growing and ever-changing pediatric emergency care center. It was an invaluable teaching tool. "The spectrum of illnesses in children is very different," Shook said. "And the way they respond to various illnesses is different. That is why it is essential to have people who have had wide-ranging experience with children to make the decisions about the best direction to take in their treatment."

The need for such specialized care continued to escalate at the newly opened Texas Children's Hospital emergency center. Within the first 18 months of operation, the remarkable increase in pediatric emergency cases necessitated expansion of the facilities. How to accomplish that mission required some improvisation from Shook, who had already utilized every inch of patient-care space available. She found the answer in one of her previous alterations, the last-minute offices created in the lobby in 1991. Gutting those, she created the acute treatment area in 1993.

"It's what we call ATA, the minor medicine area," Shook explained. "And it was there we brought in our first group of mid-level practitioners, they were physician's assistants, to help us staff that area. Because a different level of expertise is required there, it is also staffed by general pediatricians instead of sub-boarded physicians."

Shook considered minor emergencies to be illnesses or injuries that were not life threatening. With five of its 11 beds equipped with heart monitors, the ATA was expected to treat 20 percent of the daily volume in the Texas Children's Hospital emergency center. It was a goal quickly reached. While treating those 20 to 50 patients a day, the physicians working with mid-level practitioners in the ATA enabled the emergency center medical staff to devote full attention to those patients who required urgent care.[15]

This improvised solution proved successful and the next three years brought exponential growth in emergency care cases at Texas Children's Hospital. Once again, Shook had to expand the capacity of the emergency center. "In 1996 we looked at our whole operation and in that five-year interval we had grown from 26,000 visits to 52,000 visits," Shook said. "We realized we had really outgrown our space. So we did a design change and ripped out any administrative or support space we had and turned it into patient-care space."[16]

The design changes implemented aspects learned from past experience and research. Realizing that patients' complaints could be categorized into distinct areas of patient care, Shook incorporated those areas into the new design of the Texas Children's Hospital emergency center. "We organized the emergency center around three different zones or bays, based on people's chief complaints. We have a respiratory zone, a medical zone, and a surgical zone," Shook explained. "All that really means is that we concentrate supplies and expertise in that area so that if a patient comes in with what looks like a fracture, we make sure he goes back to the surgery area because that's where I know the splinting materials are and that's where the appropriate equipment is to handle those kinds of complaints."

This division of the emergency center into bays also necessitated changes in the day-to-day activities in the center. "Nurses rotate among all the areas, but if they are on surgery that night, they know that they will be expected to assist with laceration repair, surgical repair, and so on," Shook said. "It also helps the community doctors who come in or some specialists, because if the patient is a surgical patient, they're always in the surgical area. So, rather than having these guys wandering all over the department looking lost, they just walk right back to surgery and say, 'Where's the patient?' So it's helped from many points of view and has allowed some streamlining of our process."

Also fine-tuned was the method in which patients from the emergency center were admitted to Texas Children's Hospital. Since 60 percent of all the patients of the hospital were admitted through the emergency center, Shook emphasized the importance of the pediatric emergency physicians "eyeballing" each child downstairs "before we let them upstairs."

There were several reasons for such scrutiny. "The most significant is that children can look pretty good to somebody in the emergency center, and by the time they get to the hospital, look pretty bad," Shook said. "The delay of receiving care upstairs is usually not too bad, but it can be long enough that it can be significant. There's also the issue that a child can look pretty bad in the outside practitioner's office, but by the time he has gone home, had a soda, and then come into the emergency center, he can look pretty good and may not require hospitalization. So we intervene on both sides of that."

Another impetus for knowledgeable scrutiny of the needs of patients in the emergency room was the near-capacity census of the hospital for a large percentage of the year. "I don't want to promise somebody a bed and then make them wait in the lobby for seven hours pending that bed," Shook explained. "It's better that they receive their care as soon as we can deliver it to them. So that's a piece of it. But it really speaks to the acuity of the patients that we see in our department. There's no question that our kids are getting sicker. We're intubating more kids and sending more to ICU."

The escalating illnesses of children seen in the emergency center were puzzling to Shook, who thought the reasons were varied. The fact was that some ill patients were waiting longer than usual to come into the emergency center. Whether this was because they indulged in self-care a little longer, or because they felt constrained by their health plans or by their physicians, Shook knew only that they chose to delay seeking help. The result was sicker children in the emergency center at Texas Children's Hospital.

On the other hand, there were some families with sick children who always sought help immediately and often. Some were in the emergency center at Texas Children's Hospital so frequently that the hospital became their second home. "I don't know how they do it," Shook said, shaking her head. "The majority of them take it with equanimity, I'm not quite sure how. But they walk in the emergency center and say, 'Oh, hi, Dr. Shook. We're back.' And I think, 'Why aren't you screaming at me?' I would be screaming."

The habitual return of families with chronically ill children was not an occurrence singular to Texas Children's Hospital. Nor was the escalating number of new patients seen annually in its emergency center, a national trend projected to continue. National statistics in the 1990s indicated that although children's hospitals were treating 25 percent of the total population of pediatric children in need of emergency care, most young patients continued to seek treatment in an adult emergency center. Once its reputation for excellence in the treatment of pediatric emergencies became established, Texas Children's Hospital experienced a steady increase of referrals from adult hospitals to its emergency center.

This influx of referred patients brought a new dimension to the spectrum of illnesses seen at the emergency center at Texas Children's Hospital. In addition to the traditional group of children who were sick with earaches, asthma, and colds, there was now a group of patients who were more ill and had been referred there for treatment. To better serve all the patients and provide a timely response to each need, Shook instituted a color-coded triage system in the emergency center.

The moment a patient arrived in the emergency center, the triage nurse assessed his or her needs and assigned one of three color-coded stickers to the necessary paperwork. Designating Code Red for a crisis, Code Yellow for urgent, and Code Blue for non-urgent, the triage nurses prioritized and stacked each code's papers. Even when most stickers were Code Blue, there was an established priority order of needs, superceded only when a Code Red or Code Yellow arrived in the emergency center.

Among these patients in the emergency center at Texas Children's Hospital was a growing number of sexually abused and assaulted children, as well as physically abused children—an alarming trend throughout Houston hospitals.[17] After a physician evaluated each child who was either physically or sexually abused, there was a consultation with a social worker. "Physically abused children are typically brought to the emergency room by their own parents," said Dorothy Black, the director of the Texas Children's social services department. "Parents usually want to stop abusing their children and are indirectly asking for help when they bring their abused children to the hospital."[18]

Depending on what the issues were, abused patients and their families were referred either to other agencies for follow-up, or to the Texas Children's Hospital protective health services. "All of those children, if the perpetrator is in the household, are also referred to the Children's Protective Services (CPS) and all those families get a CPS evaluation," Shook explained. "Occasionally, the perpetrator is in the school or the daycare or somewhere, and in those cases other agencies are invoked."[19]

Created to respond to the needs of abuse victims in 1976, Texas Children's Hospital protective health services was under the direction of a committee that consisted of a pediatrician, registered nurse, social worker, psychiatrist, child life specialist, occupational therapist, and chaplain.[20] Its stated purpose was to provide medical, social, and psychological assessment and treatment, acute crisis intervention, counseling, and patient advocacy. From its inception, that multidisciplinary team supervised the care and treatment of children and adolescents evaluated as child abuse victims at Texas Children's Hospital emergency center and throughout the hospital.

Although the number of abuse cases seen at Texas Children's Hospital was not expected to grow in the 1980s, it did. After the United States Department of Health and Human Services predicted in 1980 that there would be a 25 percent reduction in the number of children who were being injured and killed by their abusing parents, the late 1980s proved this to be only wishful thinking. At Texas Children's Hospital alone, the number of abuse cases rose from six in 1983 to more than 600 in 1989, mirroring a national trend that showed no signs of slowing down in the near future.[21]

Acutely aware of this alarming trend was Dr. F. James Boland, the founding chairman of the Texas Children's Hospital protective services team in 1976. "It was my gut feeling we had to stop these kids from falling through the cracks in the system," he explained.[22] By 1986, Boland and his team had seen more than 1,000 child abuse cases over a ten-year period at Texas Children's Hospital. As the number of cases seen by the team steadily climbed in the late 1980s, Boland declared: "The increase in child abuse seen at Texas Children's Hospital is due to the increase of awareness, prevention, and reporting of child abuse."[23]

By 2004, there were more than 1,000 children evaluated annually for child abuse in the emergency center at Texas Children's Hospital. Nationally, three children died each day from abuse and neglect at home, with children under the age of five the most frequent victims. At Texas Children's Hospital in 2003, there were 26 deaths directly attributed to child abuse, a fact that deeply disturbed Shook. "It's especially tragic that the very individuals responsible for a child's care and supervision are often the abusers," Shook said. "Today's parents and caregivers are under enormous stress. When that pressure is not productively released, built-up tensions can trigger a dangerous situation. Unfortunately, whether the abuse is verbal or physical, an innocent child may be the recipient."[24]

As the number of those recipients of abuse continued to grow among the patient population of the emergency center of Texas Children's Hospital, so did another type of victim. Classified as pediatric trauma, this grouping included children who suffered from an intentional or unintentional injury. Although not formally recognized through the American College of Surgeons as a qualified "trauma center," the emergency center at Texas Children's Hospital nonetheless treated a variety of accident-traumatized patients. However, not treated to any extent were children with penetrating injuries, such as gunshot injuries or stab wounds, and complex multisystem trauma, such as devastating life-threatening injuries resulting from car accidents. Those patients tended to be transported to the established trauma centers at either Hermann Hospital or Ben Taub Hospital.

Along with its vast variety of acute illnesses, abuse victims, accident-traumatized children, and unique pediatric cases, the emergency center at Texas Children's Hospital counted children with high fever among its predominant groups of patients. Another major area of treatment was asthmatic attacks and seasonal ailments such as the flu, making respiratory disorder the most common diagnosis.

Although these statistics reflect the average patient population on an annual basis, the needs of patients changed constantly on an hourly, daily, and weekly basis. The ability to respond effectively to such unpredictable needs was an integral aspect of pediatric emergency medicine. "It is somewhat different than other specialties," Shook explained. "Rather than knowing everything there is to know about one thing, we have to know something about everything."[25]

One area of knowledge into which Shook delved was pain management. Her goal was to provide the least painful methods of treatment to patients in the emergency center at Texas Children's Hospital. After spending countless hours researching the available options, Shook repeatedly introduced measures to ensure that children experience as little pain as possible at Texas Children's Hospital. "Rather than remembering us as causing pain, we wanted them to remember us as relieving it," Shook said. "We really have changed our philosophy considerably, backed up by the research that we've done."

Other research projects undertaken in the emergency center at Texas Children's Hospital included a study of blood lead levels in children, an analysis of pediatric emergency room visits by parents of children with minor illnesses, the use of helium-oxygen in pediatric patients with reactive airway disease, and the neurobehavioral outcome of head injury in children. With such diverse areas of interest, Shook found that the constantly evolving needs addressed by pediatric emergency medicine created a limitless realm of study opportunities.

Always eager to learn more about her profession, Shook constantly kept track of research activities performed at other institutions, as well as published reports of incremental advances made in the field. "The way we practice emergency medicine now is really very different than it was ten years ago," she said. "My whole staff is always pushing me to keep up, so I know I have to keep reading all the time. It's rapidly changing."[26]

One such change came to the emergency center at Texas Children's Hospital during the 1990s, in response to the needs of patients and their families. It was the emergency center pharmacy, a service that was open 24 hours a day, seven days a week. "It is not the cheapest pharmacy, by any means, but it is very convenient if you're in need of a certain medication for your sick child and you're walking out of the emergency center at 2 in the morning," Shook said.

Although many new services were introduced at the emergency center throughout the years, the center's unique and colorful decor remained unchanged. Believing that the display of children's artwork could change a child's perception of the hospital, art consultant Pamela Marquis introduced an imaginative project, The Art of Texas Children's Hospital, in the mid-1990s. After enlisting the participation of numerous school and community groups, Marquis installed the donated artworks throughout the hospital's hallways.

Designated for one of the emergency center's corridors and donated by students at the Presbyterian School was a bright blue mural of the sea, swimming with handmade tissue-paper creatures. With its vibrant colors and amusing content, the mural represented the vitality that Marquis wished to impart through art. "The atmosphere is based on stress reduction for patients as well as staff," Marquis said, pointing out that this was one of the major goals of her art project. "Texas Children's sends a message to children and their parents that healing works through the mind as well as the body."[27]

To further achieve this goal, Marquis placed individually framed artwork from elementary schoolchildren throughout the emergency center. Each artwork was a handwritten and illustrated reply to the question, "When I'm sick, what makes me feel better?" These colorful and heartfelt documents received appreciative praise not only from patients and their families, but also from emergency center staff members. "Pam said it would make the kids feel safer, and she was right," Shook said. "It must tell them that children have been here before and they have been safe. It's really cute to watch the families as they wander around and read all these. If you have a five-year-old child, it makes perfect sense to him."

To illustrate that point, Shook recalled the emergency center patient who related to the illustration and sentiment expressed in the artwork known as "Number 20." After this little girl read the message, "When I'm sick, I want my puppy to make me feel better," she was inspired. Days after receiving treatment, she returned with a puppy to give to Shook and the nurses in the Texas Children's Hospital emergency center.

While the artwork offered immeasurable comfort to patients, their parents found reassurance in one the fundamental policies of the emergency center at Texas Children's Hospital. Unlike most other emergency centers, Texas Children's Hospital allowed parents to accompany their child into the examining rooms.[28] "The only time we don't is when the child is very ill and we are doing a particularly unpleasant procedure," Shook explained. "If the child is intubated, or the child has a fairly invasive procedure or something going on, we may ask the families to step out. If it's a family with a lot of experience with a child who has been chronically ill, and they want to stay in while he is being intubated, then I go ahead and let them."

In another policy instituted on behalf of parents, Shook arranged for an additional staff member to be present whenever a physician was performing a resuscitation. It also benefited the emergency center physician, who did not have time to stop and answer questions from parents during complicated procedures. "It's by necessity," Shook explained. "When we're doing a procedure we're very businesslike and I think it's sometimes hard for the family to see us be that dispassionate. So the staff person narrates and says, 'Now Dr. Shook is doing this, and then she's going to do that, and this is why she's doing it.' And some families handle it very well, and I think it relieves some of their anxiety."

Shook knew that anxious moments, and sometimes hours, were the norm for all parents and caregivers of children who awaited treatment in the emergency center at Texas Children's Hospital. With the efficient color-coded triage system of treating patients in order of need, some of the less ill often were forced to wait indeterminately for their consultation with a physician. Fully aware of this problem, one that also existed in emergency centers throughout the country, Shook was always in search of a solution. "There is not anybody in the world who wants, who truly wants, to wait for four hours to hear their child is not critically ill," she said. "It's not that I am not pleased to see patients with minor complaints, but it's not an effective use of the family's time to come to the emergency center at Texas Children's Hospital and wait four hours to hear me say, 'Yes, your child sure does have a cold.' It would be better for them to seek another source of care. For a child who is not critically ill, there are a lot of other resources available for comprehensive treatment."[29]

Although there were practical alternatives, these were not easily achieved. Most families who came to the emergency center with children who were not critically ill were either unaware of other resources available, or were unable to take advantage of these options for various financial or personal reasons. A definitive solution to the problem was elusive. "Even if they do have a primary doctor who is only open from 9 a.m. to 5 p.m., and both parents work from nine to five, then they really do have few alternatives," Shook said. "In the future, I am hopeful that we will do some better matching of family and patient needs with service suppliers."

One way to achieve this goal was to educate families more effectively on how to use the services of the emergency center at Texas Children's Hospital more effectively, if at all. In the case of accident trauma, Shook stressed to parents that prevention was the preferred way to guarantee the best outcome. Unintentional injuries caused more deaths annually than any other childhood disease and remained the leading killer of children under the age of 15.[30] "We see at least one drowning a week during the summer," she said. "Drownings are 100 percent preventable, so one a week is too many. Bicycle and playground injuries are similar in that they also are preventable. I think there must be a lot more emphasis on just trying to prevent things from happening."[31]

Despite these and other such worthwhile efforts to prevent the need for children's emergency medical treatment, more than 63,000 children were seen in the emergency center at Texas Children's Hospital during 1999. The cases treated ranged from colic to meningitis to bad car accidents, with more emergencies resulting from illness than accidents.[32] Over the following five years, the number of emergency cases steadily increased to an annual average of 80,000, with more than 14,000 admitted to Texas Children's Hospital for further treatment. By 2004, the Meyer and Ida Gordon Emergency Center at Texas Children's Hospital was the largest pediatric emergency center in south-central Texas.

Since its opening in 1991, more than 650,000 patients had been treated for a variety of pediatric medical emergencies. Open 24 hours a day, seven days a week, and staffed by full-time sub-boarded pediatric emergency physicians and nurses, the emergency center at Texas Children's Hospital had grown to 48 emergency beds and 19 observation beds by 2004. With state-of-the-art equipment, computerized bedside registration, timesaving lab-testing procedures, and a centralized communications center, it was "a very different operation" than the one Shook had first joined in 1981.

"To watch this evolution unfold in front of my eyes in the last 23 years has really been a professional gift that I couldn't have asked for," Shook said. "When we moved in 1991, I was it, the only full-time person there. There were two other people who were part-time ambulatory, part-time emergency medicine, but I was the only person full-time."

As the center evolved into one of the largest pediatric emergency centers in the nation, Shook saw its staff grow proportionately. "Today, we have more than 95 on the nursing side, and approximately 25 physicians, including my pediatric emergency physicians in training and general practitioners," Shook said. "So we've come a long way and developed a quality of service that really is unparalleled. You can't do better than what we deliver anywhere."

Although the phenomenal growth of the Meyer and Ida Gordon Emergency Center at Texas Children's Hospital mirrored that of emergency medicine across the country, Shook believed that "Ours was a story unto itself."

After repeated visits to the emergency center at Texas Children's Hospital throughout 1992, the three-year-old asthma patient was not showing any signs of improvement. Her parents grew increasingly concerned.

A glimmer of hope about the future treatment of their daughter's chronic illness came in December 1993, when the parents heard about the recent opening of a new asthma center at Texas Children's Hospital. At that moment, they realized that "we are a blessed family," the child's mother recalled.

"I heard about it, not from the hospital, but as most moms do, from the mother of another child who had trouble with asthma," she recalled. "And another father of one of my son's friends is a pediatric pulmonologist at Texas Children's, who had told her, 'You ought to check into the asthma center.' Since you had to have a referral from your physician, I asked my doctor and he said, 'Absolutely, you should go over there,' and I beat a path to their door."

Opened in October 1993, the Texas Children's Asthma Center was established to develop and maintain appropriate systems of primary care for the 55,000 children in the Houston area with asthma. Specifically designed to enhance asthma care for children by functioning as a resource center for referring physicians in the areas of treatment, care, prevention, and research, the center's primary goal was to serve as a consultant and to implement an evaluation and treatment plan.[33]

"The frustrating thing about asthma is they don't know what causes it," the mother said. "There are a number of triggers that they have identified. Some people have asthma that is triggered by physical exertion; others have asthma that's triggered by allergens. We just weren't sure what was causing our daughter's. But at the asthma center, they began this incredible history of trying to track down what was the trigger."

To achieve this goal, the mother was asked to complete a detailed history not only of each family member's individual personal medical background, but also of specifics about the home—such as whether the furnishings were upholstered or wooden; whether the floors were covered in tile, wood, or carpet; and whether there were dogs or cats.

"They asked me all the medications she was on and then they asked me this wonderful question: 'Well, does it work? In your opinion, is it working?' I felt some were and some weren't," she recalled. "Their whole philosophy is that the parent is an integral part of the treatment team. It was so refreshing. So radically different from when I was a child in the hospital in Oklahoma and my mother used to fight the nurses to stay overnight with me."

Given a brand new treatment protocol at the Texas Children's Asthma Center, the daughter also was given a red, green, and yellow flow meter, especially designed for children, and a little bag in which to carry it. As her mother observed and listened, the child was told by a therapist to "blow into your flow meter and if you are at the green level, you can go anywhere, do anything. If you blow into the yellow level, it's caution, slow down, watch your medication. If you get into the red level, all bets are off. Now you're on your full treatment protocol."

The positive results from this first visit to the Texas Children's Asthma Center were measurable, a fact the child's mother attributed to the therapist's helpful color-coded instructions about the flow meter. "It was a wonderful concept because even a three-year-old understands red, yellow, and green from stop lights," the mother said.

As hoped, her daughter easily adapted to the flow meter and to the new protocol treatment. In addition, she loved going to the Texas Children's Asthma Center, especially because of the wonderful playroom.

Also charmed were her parents, who found the answer to their prayers at the Texas Children's Asthma Center. During their first visit, they met with pulmonologist Dr. Marianna Sockrider, who explained what she hoped to accomplish in terms of home environment, medication, and treatment at the asthma center. She advised that the center was created not just to rescue children in the emergency center, but also to eliminate the need to go there in the first place. "Instead of having their child's asthma develop to the point where you are in the emergency center and she is barely able to breathe, what we do is manage the condition to keep you from getting to that point," she told the appreciative mother.[34]

To the family's delight, this stated mission was a success. "In our case, the asthma center did exactly what it was supposed to do," the mother reported. "We have never been back to the emergency center at Texas Children's Hospital with an asthmatic attack."

What did prompt a return visit was an accidental injury that the child suffered while coming home from school on the bus. After tripping over somebody's foot, she fell down and split her lip. When her big brother ran into the house for help, everybody on the bus, including the bus driver, followed him. Crying breathlessly, he called his mother at work and said, "She busted her lip and she's bleeding," and then handed the phone to the housekeeper, who confirmed his assessment.

The distraught mother hung up the phone and raced home. "By the time I got there, they had put ice on it and it wasn't that bad," she recalled. "But I thought, 'This is her face. This is her lip. Let's go have her checked out.' So I took her to the emergency center at Texas Children's Hospital and it was my very best visit there."

Arriving at the emergency center with her child, the mother showed the injury to a nurse. After examining the lip, the nurse indicated that she saw no need to suture the wound, but would verify her opinion with one of the physicians. Minutes later, the physician came out to see the child and agreed that no suture was necessary and that she could go home. "I was out of there in 30 minutes," the mother said. "The nurse gave the children popsicles and the policeman gave them stickers. We didn't fill out a single form. It was wonderful, but it was like, 'Oh, this is too easy.' It was fabulous."

Although that visit turned out to be an enjoyable experience, the mother hoped never to repeat it. But should there be another traumatic event or medical emergency in her children's future, there was no doubt where she immediately would take them for help.

"The emergency center at Texas Children's Hospital is just this beacon in the night," she said. "You arrive there and you know you're going to be taken care of, especially with such a scary thing like what our daughter had in the beginning. With a broken bone or a cut lip, you figure it's painful and it's awful and you hope that it didn't happen. But when you've got a really sick baby, it's nice to know they're there."[35]

Because of Texas Children's Hospital, everyone in her family could breathe easier.

15

🖐 GASTROENTEROLOGY, 🖐 HEPATOLOGY AND NUTRITION

FOURTEEN-YEAR-OLD SOCCER AND FOOTBALL PLAYER Benjamin Sellers thought he had shin splints, the common cause of leg pain in athletes.

To the contrary, the cause of his pain was decidedly uncommon. It was polyarteritis nodosa (PAN), an autoimmune disease that affects arteries. Since occurrence of the disease in children is rare, Ben's diagnosis was not immediate. In fact, it took weeks.

"It all started around the end of February in 2001, when I had high fever for five weeks and I had no feeling in my left leg," recalled Ben. "I had been diagnosed with tendonitis and neuritis in both of my ankles, but I was in so much pain. That's when the doctors told me to rush to the emergency room at Texas Children's Hospital."[1]

After being admitted as a patient, Ben began five weeks of extensive medical testing, all of which produced no definitive diagnosis. All the while, the pain in his legs continued to escalate. "They did not know what was wrong with him," said his mother, Roberta Sellers. "The pain in his legs kept getting worse and worse. The doctors referred him to a cardiovascular surgeon, Dr. George Reul, at St. Luke's Episcopal Hospital. They ran a dye through his legs and found out both his legs had total blockage."[2]

To alleviate the blockage, Reul immediately performed bypass surgery on both legs. Ben's operation began at 8 a.m. one morning and lasted until 1 a.m. the next day. Immediately after the surgery, the doctor told Ben's family that he had been able to save both legs. But, four hours later, the arteries in both legs were blocked again and Ben was rushed back into surgery. "They saved the right leg," Roberta said. "When they came out of surgery, the doctor said he lost the left leg and that they would make the call in 24 hours about whether they would amputate or not. The next day was April

1, April Fool's Day."

Recalling the moment when the doctors advised him of their decision to amputate, Ben said with a laugh, "Thank God I did not know what day it was."

Ben's left leg was amputated above the knee on April 2 at St. Luke's Episcopal Hospital. After spending one week in that hospital's ICU, Ben was transferred back to Texas Children's Hospital, where he stayed for two months. While there, the effervescent Ben charmed his nurses. "I have the home email addresses of two of them, they are my friends," he said. "And one of them wanted to adopt me."[3]

With this increasing crowd of admirers, Ben continued to recuperate. He also underwent testing to determine the extent of the inflammation of arteries caused by PAN. Because vessels in any of Ben's organs or organ systems were susceptible areas, as characterized in PAN patients between the ages of 40 and 50, the testing was extensive.

"The disease is so very, very rare, and you don't see it in children often," Roberta said. "Ben was one of the rare ones. He's the most severe pediatric case they had ever had so all his tests were done at St. Luke's. He had blockage in both arms and his legs, so it hit him in the extremities instead of his internal organs. They did an angiogram in his brain and everything was fine in his brain."[4]

The next step was to begin treatment to decrease the inflammation of arteries by suppressing the immune system. Ben was prescribed high-dose intravenous and oral cortisone medications. "He had to be put on several different steroids," his mother recalled. "When we were in Texas Children's Hospital, every three days they gave him a heavy dose of those steroids. We watched his body just balloon, which is a side effect of the prednisone. When we got home, we were on 40 milligrams of prednisone every day, plus once a week a nurse would come out to the house and give an IV treatment through the summer."

By the time fall came, although he did not have a prosthesis, Ben felt strong enough to go back to school in his wheelchair. Unfortunately, after two weeks of class, the ninth-grader contracted a staph infection and was rushed back to Texas Children's Hospital. "Dr. Reul had to open up the right leg at St. Luke's," his mother said. "Cysts had formed there and they had to drain it and see if the bypass grafts were all OK. Those were fine, but we stayed another week in Texas Children's Hospital. It was a major setback for Ben."

Afraid that another staph infection might impede his recovery, Ben's mother decided that home schooling was preferable. "Because of his being autoimmune, he can pick up anything from anybody," she explained. "So I opted to have the teacher come to him and do the whole ninth grade at home. He still went to school functions, football games, and soccer games."

Ben also consumed copious amounts of food. Always hungry, he continuously ate and seemingly was never full. In addition to the ballooning side effects of the steroids, his insatiable appetite resulted in an accumulation of more than 80 pounds of extra weight. Aware that Ben was overeating, his mother did not have the heart to tell him to stop. "He was such a large child to begin with," she said. "But after the second surgery, he didn't have his prosthesis yet, so he just sat there in his wheelchair, wondering what he was going to do. All he did was eat, eat, eat. When he would say, 'Mom, I'm hungry,' what was I going to do? What can you do with a 14-year-old at that time? Tell him, 'No, you can't have'?"

That Ben's weight was becoming a health threat became evident in October. In a visit to the physical therapist at Texas Children's Hospital, he displayed no energy and shortness of breath during therapy. Alarmed at his condition, therapist Adrienne Tilbor picked up the phone and called Ben's rheumatologist, Dr. Maria D. Perez, and said, "Something must be done."

Although unsure of exactly what was said to whom, Ben was aware of the chain of events: "Dr. Tilbor called Dr. Perez. Dr. Perez called Dr. Klish, the chief of gastroenterology and nutrition, and Dr. Klish got us into the Weigh of Life program."

Simultaneously in October, another impetus for a lifestyle change happened. It was an incident that Ben later credited with inspiring him to lose weight. "It was meeting David Baty, the prosthetic guy from Dynamic Orthotics who casted me for my leg and makes all the adjustments for my leg," he said. "He came to see us at Texas Children's Hospital. If it wasn't for him, I wouldn't have a new leg and be learning how to walk again."

Baty, a certified prosthetist/orthetist, not only measured Ben for his prosthesis, but also explained its many benefits. "I told Ben that with his new prosthesis, he was only limited by his mind," Baty recalled. "I also told him he could choose the material to cover the socket and he chose purple camouflage."[5]

When fitting and adjusting Ben's purple "camo" prosthesis at two-week intervals thereafter, Baty showed concern for his client's escalating weight. Noting that the extra pounds Ben was carrying made the prosthesis hard to manage, Baty advised him that losing weight would enhance his agility.

Motivated by Baty's insight and his own desires, Ben entered Texas Children's Hospital's Weigh of Life program in December with a set goal. The determined former soccer and football player had a game plan, one in which losing meant winning.

The gastroenterology and nutrition service at Texas Children's Hospital began to address the increasing need for research and treatment of children's eating disorders in 1984.

Established and directed by Dr. William J. Klish, chief of the gastroenterology and nutrition service at Texas Children's Hospital, the eating disorders clinic concentrated primarily on overweight children and adolescents. Offering this opportunity to help patients identify the eating behavior that caused weight gain, Klish stressed behavior modification, dietary management, and exercise.

"I brought that program with me when I came back in 1983," Klish explained. "It's gone through three revisions since and it has developed into its present form, Weigh of Life. It has been a very successful 13-week program for those who complete it, but there is a huge drop-out rate, as one would expect in weight control. Only one out of five actually make it through the program. But of the 20 percent who make it through, all are successful."[6]

Research into the reasons for its successes and failures enabled the eating disorders clinic to provide healthcare professionals with up-to-date information on helping overweight children lose weight and maintain the loss. In fact, before the clinic's 1984 opening, children's nutrition had been an integral area of research at Texas Children's Hospital for 20 years.

Although officially established in 1970, the gastroenterology and nutrition service at Texas Children's Hospital actually started in 1964, with the arrival of physiologist Dr. Buford L. Nichols, Jr., as the associate director of the newly established Clinical Research Center (CRC) at Texas Children's Hospital.

Funded under a grant from the National Institutes of Health (NIH) on June 1, 1964, the CRC at Texas Children's Hospital was one of 12 such centers in the United States. Established and financially supported by a 1959 federal mandate, the General Clinical Research Centers Program (GCRC) evolved to supply the demand for highly specialized facilities and personnel to meet the needs for conducting controlled studies in a laboratory specifically designed for research.

The designation of Texas Children's Hospital as one of the sites for such a facility was the direct result of concentrated efforts spearheaded in 1962 by physician-in-chief Dr. Russell J. Blattner, endocrinologist Dr. George W. Clayton, and nephrologist Dr. L. Leighton Hill. Over a period of two years, Clayton and Hill visited existing CRC units at Johns Hopkins and

The Children's Hospital of Philadelphia, initiated the grant proposal, and eventually planned and executed the unit's physical design for a suite of rooms on the fourth floor of Texas Children's Hospital.[7]

With the CRC plans approved and its November 1964 opening scheduled, Blattner assumed the role of principal investigator of the CRC and named Clayton as program director. Outlining his responsibilities, Clayton stated: "The primary aim of the federally funded GCRC is to increase the knowledge of human physiology and pathophysiology; provide an optimal setting for controlled studies by clinical investigators; encourage disciplinary interaction and develop technological and therapeutic advances; and increase the knowledge of disease, thus leading to improved healthcare."[8]

During the planning stages, Blattner and Clayton already knew whom they wanted as associate director of the CRC. It was Nichols, the Baylor College of Medicine alum who had once worked in Clayton's endocrinology lab and clinic at Texas Children's Hospital. Subsequently, Nichols had studied at Yale and Johns Hopkins before returning to Yale as chief resident. A trained physiologist, he embraced the opportunity for creative development in nutrition, a newly emerging field in pediatrics, and planned to pursue it.[9]

Exactly where Nichols would go to achieve his goal was uncertain; there were few postdoctoral fellowship programs in nutrition in the United States at that time. When approached with an offer to return to Texas Children's Hospital to work as the associate director of the proposed CRC, Nichols was hesitant to accept. "George Clayton came to visit me at Yale during a blizzard to ask me about coming back," he recalled. "He had been at an endocrinology seminar in New York and took the train to New Haven. He told me about the grant proposal for a new Clinical Research Center at Texas Children's Hospital, and that he wanted me to become involved with it. George told me that I could come and work on nutrition as the associate director of the Clinical Research Center."[10]

Simultaneously offered a similar position at two other existing CRC units, Nichols did not immediately accept Clayton's offer. However, when he discovered that the chairmen of pediatrics at both institutions "wanted to specify very strictly a very defined plan of what I was going to do in my career," Nichols lost interest in their offers. His decision to accept Clayton's invitation came following an encounter with Blattner at an Atlantic City seminar the following spring.

"I asked Blattner what intellectual freedom I would have to develop the field of nutrition," remembered Nichols. "He said, 'Whatever you want to do.' The fact that Blattner offered me the intellectual freedom to develop my own thing here, plus the fact that George Clayton soon thereafter got the grant, brought me here. Part of the package was that I had a lab at Texas Children's Hospital and start-up funds. I got to bring a PhD, Dr. Carlton Hazlewood, with me to help me develop the research, and I had a technical staff. They had no restraints or restrictions on what I could do research on. It was a wonderful opportunity."[11]

Also receiving Blattner's promise of intellectual freedom was Clayton, who envisioned the CRC at Texas Children's Hospital as unique in its scope. While other NIH-supported research units across the country emphasized endocrine and metabolic research protocols, the CRC at Texas Children's Hospital had no such limiting parameters. Both Blattner and Clayton believed all of the hospital's specialty services were eligible for inclusion and planned the six-bed unit and professional staff accordingly. When the CRC opened on November 2, 1964, among the expected protocols were those dealing with infectious diseases, cardiology, immunology, dwarfism, genetics, and nutrition.

That there would be an emphasis on nutritional research was attributable to Nichols' persistent influence. His desire for definitive studies of children's nutrition was clearly demonstrated on the opening day of the CRC. "I had a poster made of an old-fashioned scale, one that weighed one side to the other," he recalled. "It had a baby on one and a rat on the other. The rat was smaller, but it weighed more than the baby and the message was, 'We need more human research.'"[12]

Poised to accomplish this mission in the Clinical Research Center at Texas Children's Hospital was a highly skilled team. Consisting of physicians and nurses, the unit's personnel also included a research dietitian and diet technicians, which was unique—as was the unit's metabolic kitchen for the preparation by dietitians of special diets and formulas, the execution of balance studies, and the determination of various constituents of CRC patient diets.

Recruited to oversee this area was Elaine Potts, one of the dietitians at Texas Children's Hospital. "Dr. Clayton and Dr. Nichols knew that I was very interested in nutrition and being sure that the children were fed properly, and they wanted me to take the job," she said. "When they opened the CRC, they hired someone but she didn't stay. I don't know why. When they started on me to take the job, I told them I had never been in research, and they said that they thought I would just be fine. They just would not quit, so I came here in October of 1965. The first year was terribly hard for me, getting used to learning everything."[13]

One lesson Potts quickly became aware of was the trial-and-error aspect of dietary research, particularly during Nichols' efforts to improve survival in acute and chronic diarrhea of infancy. Second only to pneumonia as a leading cause of mortality during the early years of life, chronic diarrhea resulted in more than 20 deaths each year at Texas Children's Hospital in the late 1960s.

"The residents called these children 'slick gut' syndrome," explained Nichols. "You put anything in the mouth and it would just come straight out. As we began to do biopsies, it seemed to be appropriate, because instead of having a nice velvety-like structure, the gut was just as flat as a mirror. It was just terrible, and we were desperate. At least one-fourth of all the patient days in the CRC back in the 60s were these malnourished children with chronic diarrhea."[14]

Aiming to manage these diverse cases of chronic diarrhea and to find a cure, the CRC study and treatment produced measurable results in the form of a modular formula for the management of infants with specific or complex food intolerances. In order to perfect the safe and proper use of this formula, which was designed to meet the needs of each individual infant, Potts spent countless hours preparing and feeding various combinations of the formula to more than 100 infants who had been admitted to the CRC. The result of those efforts was the first modular formula. Introduced in 1968, the breakthrough treatment was known as the Baylor Core Formula. Since the inception of this modular-formula concept, many infants have gone from a hopeless condition to full recovery—not only at Texas Children's Hospital, but also throughout the United States.[15]

For those malnourished patients with chronic diarrhea who could not tolerate the modular formula, Nichols sought another solution. He found one in 1967 when the University of Pennsylvania's Dr. Stanley Dudrick introduced Total Parenteral Nutrition (TPN), a technique that enabled nutrients to be introduced intravenously by catheter. Although the first attempt to use TPN with a desperately ill child with chronic diarrhea at Texas Children's Hospital in 1968 was ultimately unsuccessful, the concept of feeding a patient by vein remained promising.[16]

Particularly interested in TPN was Klish, a pediatrics resident at Baylor College of Medicine in 1970. Aware that sick infants and children often must go for prolonged periods without oral intake of any kind, leading to malnutrition, starvation, and death, he began concentrating his efforts on how to perfect TPN technique. "I was chief resident at Ben Taub when we introduced TPN in the pediatric unit in 1971," Klish recalled. "By taking Dudrick's ideas, I set up my only little micro-pharmacy, where I mixed my solutions; I gathered surgeons together to put in catheters for me; I created a little team to do TPN. It worked beautifully. We cut the mortality rate in that ward in half in one year's time. We then introduced it at Texas Children's Hospital."[17]

Also arriving at Texas Children's Hospital in 1970 was its first trained pediatric gastroenterologist, Dr. George D. Ferry. A Baylor College of Medicine alum and pediatric resident, Ferry returned to Houston after receiving gastroenterology training at Johns Hopkins. Encouraged by physician-in-chief Blattner, Ferry agreed to devote one-third of his time to Texas Children's Hospital and two-thirds to private practice. It was an agreement destined to last more than 17 years.

Once Ferry had accepted Blattner's proposal, the physician-in-chief immediately capitalized on the combined interests of Ferry and Nichols, whose studies of diarrheal diseases had evolved into an interest in other intestinal diseases. Recognizing the potential, Blattner created the gastroenterology and nutrition service at Texas Children's Hospital in 1970, naming Nichols as chief of the service. Headquartered in the CRC, this was one of the first such services in a children's hospital in the United States. "Although nutrition has long been a primary interest in pediatrics, gastroenterology as a subspecialty has only recently attracted the interest of pediatricians," explained Ferry. "The merger of these two fields is appropriate since childhood intestinal disorders are frequently complicated by nutritional disturbances. In fact, recovery may be more related to malnutrition than the bowel disturbance itself."[18]

As the newly established gastroenterology and nutrition service at Texas Children's Hospital began to grow, its clinical services expanded and the newly named gastroenterology and nutrition clinic in the Junior League Diagnostic Clinic of the outpatient department at Texas Children's Hospital met on a weekly basis. Originally created in 1968 as a follow-up clinic for nutrition patients seen in the CRC, its mission now included gastroenterology problems. Each Monday morning, Ferry and nutritionist Corinne Montandon, along with residents, fellows, medical students, and visiting fellows in nutrition, conducted the clinic. Concentration centered on common and rare disorders, including acute and chronic liver disease, malabsorption syndromes, ulcerative colitis, and a variety of severe nutritional disturbances.

This growing scope of the service was not limited to clinical services in the hospital. Nichols was gaining international recognition for his research studies in malnutrition and into the causes, treatment, and prevention of diarrheal diseases. After receiving approval from the Pan American Health Organization, he began a major effort to combat diarrhea and malnutrition on an international basis. To survey conditions and implement new techniques,

Nichols and a team of researchers traveled to Jamaica, Mexico City, and Guatemala in the early 1970s.

Nichols also addressed the malnourishment that existed in Houston, where an estimated ten to 15 infants died each year from starvation. Convinced that one solution was breast-feeding, he began a concentrated campaign to put "babies on the breast" instead of feeding them store-bought formula. "The greatest thing we could do is to give every infant a ready-to-serve formula for the first six months of life," he said. "If we can put a man on the moon, there's no reason we can't put healthy babies in the first grade."[19]

With its diversified areas of interest, multiple research studies, and increasing patient load, the gastroenterology and nutrition service had grown sufficiently enough in 1973 to begin a fellowship program. Accepting the offer to become one of the first fellows was Klish, whom Nichols immediately sent to Mexico for a four-month research project devoted to metabolic studies of children suffering from malnutrition. "I really hadn't thought about fellowship," recalled Klish. "I wanted to be an adventurer, go into private practice. The first four months of my fellowship in Mexico were indeed an adventure. There were good times and bad times, but that's why I ended up in the field that I'm in, because of this sense of adventure. We got an award by the president of Mexico for the research that we had done in Mexico on Kwashiorkor, protein calorie malnutrition."[20]

Upon his return, Klish joined Nichols' efforts to perfect the TPN technique at Texas Children's Hospital. Since TPN had the capability to reverse the dire effects of malnutrition, whatever the cause, the multidisciplinary effort involved an organized team of physicians, nurses, and pharmacists. With the successful implementation of TPN by many services at Texas Children's Hospital, the survival rate, particularly of infants, greatly improved.

By 1974, the impact of TPN and new formulas such as the modular Baylor Core Formula was measurable. In a 25-year period in Texas, the number of deaths from diarrhea had been reduced from 1,200 to 120. "Despite that fact and the fact that those starving have a better chance for a normal life, much remains to be done," stated Ferry in 1974. "The gastroenterology and nutrition service has an on-going program into the causes and prevention of such severe diarrhea."[21]

To find a solution to the "slick gut" problem, Nichols required additional funding from the NIH. "The experience with nutritional research, internationally and in our own work with these malnourished children as a clinical investigator, led us to an awareness that we needed to get more deeply into the mechanisms in that particular disorder," he explained. "We were submitting two or three grant proposals a year for investigations of these children and were not getting a very good response. Because the NIH was problem oriented rather than basic science oriented, we began to look around at other possibilities for funding."[22]

What Nichols found was a new nutrition research center in Grand Forks, North Dakota. Funded by the Agricultural Research Service of the United States Department of Agriculture (USDA), this was the first in a series of planned regional centers to be established. Inspired by the possibility that one center could be located in the South, Nichols embarked on what would become a years-long journey to bring that center to Texas Children's Hospital and Baylor College of Medicine. Proposing that the center study the nutritional needs of mothers and infants, Nichols first appeared with Houston Congressman Bob Casey at a public hearing before the appropriations committee of Congress in 1974.

With the enthusiastic support of Texas Children's Hospital board members, colleagues, and eventually new physician-in-chief Dr. Ralph D. Feigin, who arrived in 1977, Nichols doggedly continued his quest. After four years, following various feasibility studies, multiple trips to Washington, D.C., for hearings, and countless conferences and telephone calls to various congressmen and USDA officials, Nichols' dream finally came to fruition.

On hand to make the November 2, 1978, official announcement of the world's first center devoted solely to research on nutritional needs of children were congressional leaders, USDA administrators, and Houston medical authorities. Supported by a $1.5 million federal appropriation from the USDA Science and Education Administration, the National Children's Nutrition Center established at Texas Children's Hospital and Baylor College of Medicine was to be operated in existing laboratory and office space. The possibility of a separate facility existed, but was dependent on the allotment of future funds.

When Nichols addressed the gathered crowd, he stressed the fact that more than 150 million children around the world suffered from nutritional problems. He acknowledged that existing scientific data was "awfully weak," and that there were "literally thousands" of questions that needed answers. "Ultimately, the scientific data gathered by the researchers in the National Children's Nutrition Research Center will be translated into new standards for promoting the health of our nation's and the world's children," he said. "This is personally a joyous day for me because of what all this means—the future is only as bright as our children."[23]

In tandem with such advances in nutritional research in 1978, Klish and

Ferry experienced what became known as "one of the major diagnostic advances in pediatric gastroenterology in this decade," fiber optic endoscopy.[24] In concert with Dr. David Graham, an adult gastroenterologist at Baylor College of Medicine, Klish and Ferry published one of the first accounts of the value of flexible gastrointestinal endoscopy in infants and children.

A well-established technique in the diagnosis and management of gastrointestinal diseases in adults, endoscopic procedures previously were a rarity in the pediatric population. This was due to the lack of suitable instruments and adequately trained physicians, the three gastroenterologists stated in their publication. With the introduction of fiber optics and smaller instruments, Ferry, who received endoscopy training at Johns Hopkins, and Klish, who received that training from Graham, learned this breakthrough technique together. From 1973 to 1975, they performed fiber optic endoscopy on 52 patients between the ages of two months and 16 years.[25]

"We reported how the recent introduction of a forward-viewing fiber optic endoscope of small diameter has allowed the pediatric gastroenterologist to accomplish heretofore almost impossible tasks," Klish said. "It changed the whole flavor of pediatric gastroenterology. We were very much a metabolic specialty until that happened, and then we became a procedurally oriented specialty."[26]

These procedural advances also helped propel pediatric gastroenterology to the forefront, creating immense interest in the medical community. Hospitals and medical schools across the country became anxious to have a service similar to the one established at Texas Children's Hospital and Baylor College of Medicine. One such institution, Strong Memorial Hospital and Rochester School of Medicine in Rochester, New York, contacted Klish in 1978. "David Smith, who was the incoming chairman at the University of Rochester, called me one day and said, 'I need somebody to develop a pediatric gastroenterology unit here,'" said Klish. "My research interest was always in nutrition, and there was a very famous nutritionist there by the name of Gilbert Forbes. I decided that it looked like a good place to go, so I did. I developed a nice little unit and had been there five years when Buford Nichols and Ralph Feigin called to ask me to come back."[27]

Accepting the offer, Klish returned to Texas Children's Hospital and Baylor College of Medicine in 1983 as the newly named chief of the gastroenterology and nutrition service. Nichols, who had stepped down from that position, wished to devote more time to his directorial responsibilities and scientific research at the rapidly growing Children's Nutrition Research Center (CNRC).

Encouraged by Feigin to develop a center of international stature for the evaluation and treatment of childhood gastrointestinal and nutritional disorders at Texas Children's Hospital, Klish began to expand existing services and to introduce new ones. The first of these was an endoscopy suite. "When I came back, all the endoscopic procedures were being done in the St. Luke's emergency room that Texas Children's kind of shared," Klish explained. "It always was an adventure to go down there. You would grab a nurse and whoever else was there to assist you in doing whatever needed to be doing. To develop our own endoscopy suite in the CRC, I converted a little itty-bitty lab into two rooms so we could do two procedures at the same time. It was nothing to write home about, archaic by modern standards, but it worked and we managed to work out of that endoscopy suite for ten years."

Though small, Klish's converted lab with a big name, the gastrointestinal diagnostic procedures laboratory, was unique in Houston. In addition to endoscopic procedures, it offered the on-site ability to run tests of gastrointestinal and metabolic function in infants and children. For the physicians who treated the myriad diseases of the intestine, liver, stomach, and pancreas, the latest diagnostic aids and treatment modalities were available.

Other new services were introduced in 1984. In concert with Nichols and the CNRC, Klish created the lactation support program and the milk bank at Texas Children's Hospital. Designed to teach mothers how to maintain milk production while their infants were in the hospital, the program offered a bank in which to store the milk. This innovative program eventually served as a model for children's hospitals elsewhere.

Importing the parameters of the program that he had introduced and managed in Rochester, Klish created the eating disorders clinic at Texas Children's Hospital. Initially established to encourage weight reduction in infants and adolescents, the behavior modification clinic was expected to widen its scope. Projected for the future was the treatment of anorexia nervosa, bulimia, infant eating disorders, and problems with breast-feeding.

The next area to be fine-tuned by Klish was the program involving TPN, the intravenous and nasogastric feeding technique he had championed as a resident in the early 1970s. Known since its inception as the nutritional support program, the service now included a multidisciplinary team, under the direction of Dr. Robert Shulman, to monitor the technical feeding methods. "Texas Children's Hospital can boast of having one of the best organized Nutritional Support Programs for children in the United States," Klish stated in 1984. "I am very proud of our nurses who travel throughout the country to speak about TPN."[28]

Klish's pride in that program and in all other aspects of the gastroen-terology and nutrition service at Texas Children's Hospital was justified. In less than a year, the number of outpatients seen by the service increased fivefold. With a referral base broadened to encompass patients with gastrointestinal disorders coming on a regular basis from Mexico, South America, Louisiana, and Oklahoma, Klish foresaw further expansion possibilities. Not complacent with the status quo in 1984, he predicted another new area of service for the not-too-distant future: liver transplantation. "It was George Ferry who really took an interest in liver transplantation and helped develop that program," said Klish. "He was the leader in that and pushed it forward."[29]

Ferry had displayed an interest in liver disease since his arrival as the first pediatric gastroenterologist at Texas Children's Hospital in 1970. Over the years, when confronted with a desperately ill child with chronic liver disease who was in need of a liver transplant, Ferry had only one option. He had to refer the patient to one of the three liver transplant centers in existence, all of which were in other states. Faced with this geographical problem and its inconvenience for the patient, Ferry campaigned for what he felt was the obvious solution in the early 1980s: a liver transplant center at Texas Children's Hospital.

The probability of Ferry's proposal was enhanced greatly in 1983 with the Federal Drug Administration's approval of cyclosporine, the immuno-suppressant drug used to minimize the rejection of solid tissue transplantation. "That was the turning point," said Ferry. "It took liver transplants from less than 50 percent survival to 70 to 80 percent survival. It doubled it. That drug turned transplantation overnight from a research tool to a clinical tool."[30]

Motivated by this medical breakthrough, Ferry began organizing familiarization trips so that surgeons and nurses from Texas Children's Hospital could observe other liver transplant centers throughout the United States. Finally, after years of planning and preparation, the first pediatric liver transplant in Houston occurred in February 1986.[31] Performed by Baylor College of Medicine surgeon Dr. Hartwell Whisennand, the liver transplant surgeon at The Methodist Hospital, the transplantation represented a joint effort of the two hospitals. Even though this long-awaited event did not take place at Texas Children's Hospital, as Ferry had hoped, it marked the beginning of a program that eventually would. Estimating that there were more than 30 children at Texas Children's Hospital in need of a liver transplant at the time, Ferry hailed the first Houston liver transplant as the dawning of a new era and said, "It was really a great day."[32]

Another triumph Ferry celebrated in 1986 was the formation of the Pediatric Gastroenterology Collaborative Research Group (PGCRG) at Texas Children's Hospital. Interested in finding a new drug therapy for inflammatory bowel disease, ulcerative colitis, and Crohn's disease, Ferry designed a study to test Dipentum, a new drug for children with ulcerative colitis.

Invited by Ferry to participate in this study to evaluate the safety and effectiveness of Dipentum was a group of leading pediatric gastroenterologists from 15 medical centers throughout the United States. "Through the generosity of Mimi and Tom Dompier and the Bob and Vivian Smith Foundation, funds were given to Texas Children's Hospital to establish a permanent coordinating center for the PGCRG at Texas Children's Hospital," Ferry said. "The success of that first study led to ongoing meetings of the group and multiple studies to find new and improved treatment for children with inflammatory bowel disease."[33]

While Ferry continued to pursue treatments and cures for gastroenterological disorders, Klish supported and participated in these efforts while maintaining his own interest in nutrition. Through his direction, the nutrition support service at Texas Children's Hospital was becoming one of the most active in the country. Also achieving new heights was Nichols, whose goal of a permanent facility for the CNRC had been reached on October 7, 1988. The 11-story, 200,000-square-foot building, located adjacent to Texas Children's Hospital, was built with $49 million in funds appropriated by Congress. As one of the five human research centers established by the USDA, the service remained the only one dedicated to determining the needs of infants and children as well as pregnant and nursing women. Having completed more than 100 nutritional research studies in the CNRC since its founding at Texas Children's Hospital in 1979, Nichols continued his dedicated efforts to ensure the successful future of this joint project of the USDA, Texas Children's Hospital, and Baylor College of Medicine.

Vital to the future growth of the gastroenterology and nutrition service at Texas Children's Hospital was the symbiotic relationship of Klish and Ferry. "We complement each other very well; it's always been that way," Klish said. "We both do the same thing, gastroenterology, but our interests and goals are different. I think the thing that really brought the service together was that I recruited George Ferry out of private practice and brought him into academics in 1987. When he came full-time, not only did a bunch of patients come with him, but it created a clinical presence at Texas Children's Hospital."[34]

Named chief of the gastroenterology and nutrition clinic in 1987, Ferry was also made head of the new hepatology unit at Texas Children's Hospital. Charged by Klish to develop a liver transplant program, he succeeded in doing so. By 1992, more than 15 children had received liver transplants at Texas Children's Hospital. In the years that followed, the number each year fluctuated between a high of 20 and a low of only one. After the arrival of Dr. John C. Goss as director of pediatric liver transplantation at Texas Children's Hospital in 1998, the program again began to excel.

Goss also served as surgical director of the new liver disease center at Texas Children's Hospital. Established by Ferry and Klish in 2000, the new center provided multidisciplinary medical assessment and treatment for pediatric patients with a wide variety of acute and chronic liver disease. For those patients who required surgical treatment, Goss performed liver resections, bile-duct resections, and liver transplantation. Serving as director of the new center was Dr. Saul Karpen, a former faculty member at Yale University School of Medicine. "Texas Children's has assembled an eminent team of liver-disease experts offering a unique blend of services, not only to patients in Houston but to the southwestern United States," Klish said. "The center will be dedicated to developing new and innovative treatments for all forms of pediatric liver disease."[35]

One of the newest procedural advances in liver transplantation had been implemented at Texas Children's Hospital in 1999. This was the introduction of a surgical procedure to divide a cadaver's liver while it was still in the donor's body, thereby doubling the number of recipients who could receive transplants from a single liver. Known as in-situ splitting of the liver and performed by Goss and Dr. Philip Seu, director of the liver transplant program at Baylor College of Medicine, this type of transplant was the first of its kind in Houston.

Also implemented in the liver transplantation program at Texas Children's Hospital were living-related-donor transplants, also the first of their kind in Houston. Utilizing a portion of an adult relative's liver, this technique virtually eliminated the need for a child to wait for a cadaver donor program. With more than 800 children placed on the national waiting list for liver transplants each year, fine-tuning the medical and surgical treatment options was a priority to Goss. "I think the future will see the recipient list continue to grow, and the split-liver and living-donor transplants will continue to grow as well," he said. "New trials will test immunosuppressive agents and create preservative solutions for liver storage. In coming years, we also expect to see positive results from gene therapy and immunotherapy."[36]

Positive results were immediate at the new inflammatory bowel disease center, another first for the gastroenterology, hepatology and nutrition service at Texas Children's Hospital. Established in 2000, the center was unique in the Southwest and offered a comprehensive multidisciplinary approach to the diagnosis and treatment of inflammatory bowel disease (IBD) in pediatric patients. Under the direction of Ferry, the center became one of the six founding members of the National IBD Consortium and was able to offer its patients access to the latest advances in therapies and clinical trials.

This enhanced ability to provide support for patients and families who were dealing with the difficult issues related to IBD and its symptoms fulfilled one of Ferry's missions at Texas Children's Hospital. "I am actually seeing some of my dreams come true; I have wanted an IBD Center here for a long time," Ferry said, pointing with pride to the other achievements of the gastroenterology, hepatology and nutrition service at Texas Children's Hospital. "There are things happening here that are just fulfilling. We have a true liver center with true liver specialists who have been trained in liver disease. We have an incredible liver transplant program. We are unlocking a lot of keys to all these different diseases we take care of. We're finding incredibly better medications. These are all things that I have wanted to see happen for a long time and they are happening."[37]

The gastroenterology, hepatology and nutrition service at Texas Children's Hospital also continued to gain recognition for breaking new ground in the area of gastrointestinal procedures. "We are learning how to do new things through our endoscopes," Klish explained. "Pentax Corporation, who makes endoscopes, designed our procedures laboratory and we are a demonstration laboratory now for all the new equipment that is being developed by that industry."[38]

No longer confined to the tiny makeshift lab Klish had cobbled together in the CRC in 1983, he and other Texas Children's Hospital physicians discovered they were not the only ones to revel in this spacious new state-of-the-art laboratory. "When I bring friends from other medical centers here and show them around, they just start drooling when they go into our endoscopy suite," Klish said. "It is the best in the country. The way it is set up, it is beautiful."

Klish also took great pride in the steady growth of the fellowship program in pediatric gastroenterology, hepatology and nutrition at Texas Children's Hospital. Having been Nichols' first fellow in 1972, Klish was followed during the next three decades by more than 49 others—36 of whom he had trained after becoming chief of the gastroenterology and nutrition service at Texas Children's Hospital in 1983. Beginning with the 1989 addition of Dr. Susan Henning as director of research and the subsequent recruitment of additional mentors in the basic sciences, Klish emphasized research training, with opportunities ranging from clinical research to the forefront of molecular medicine.

By 2004, what had begun as Nichols' one-person gastroenterology and nutrition service at Texas Children's Hospital in 1970 had become one of the largest pediatric gastroenterology, hepatology and nutrition services in the United States, with more than 16 faculty members, seven fellows, and a 50-member support staff. With one of the busiest clinical programs in pediatric gastroenterology, hepatology and nutrition in the United States, the service at Texas Children's Hospital saw more than 10,000 patients each year in its outpatient clinics and averaged more than 1,000 inpatient consultations each year.

Although justifiably proud of the phenomenal progress made in the pediatric gastroenterology, hepatology and nutrition service since its beginnings at Texas Children's Hospital, Klish expected further expansion to be rapid in the not-too-distant future. "Gastroenterology is coming into its own in a lot of different ways," he said. "There has been an explosion in technology that will allow us to get into areas that we have never been in the past."[39]

As for the future of nutrition services at Texas Children's Hospital, Klish referred to the past and the mission he had first embraced in 1983. "Obesity is the most important medical problem in America today," he said. "If we are going to control the epidemic of obesity, we have to start the only way we can start, and that is with children. Prevention has to happen in youth."

After entering Texas Children's Hospital's Weigh of Life program, 16-year-old Benjamin Sellers became one of its stars when he quickly lost 24 pounds.

"I think he is a superstar," said psychologist Vernisha Shepard, clinical coordinator of the program. "He is just an amazing young man. He has done the program better than others who are not amputees."[40]

Shepard, who counseled Ben throughout the three-and-one-half-month program, attributed his success to personal motivation, his own need for change. "Very seldom do we have a child who goes through the program and loses 24 pounds in three months, and that's what Ben did," she said. "He is in follow-up now. I want him to feel comfortable and confident to make the program his own, so that he will apply these principals the rest of his life."

Also credited for contributing to Ben's accomplishments was his mother. An enthusiastic supporter of his efforts, she further inspired Ben by embracing his behavior modification program as her own. "It has been marvelous," Roberta Sellers said. "I mean, absolutely marvelous. It has made us rethink our whole life."[41]

For both mother and son, the lifestyle metamorphosis began when they applied to enter Weigh of Life. Arriving at the eating disorders clinic at Texas Children's Hospital for the first time, they each were asked to fill out extensive questionnaires about their individual eating attitudes, their attitudes towards dieting, and their nutritional knowledge. Questions about parental activity level, family history of weight problems, eating patterns, and Ben's motivation to lose weight also were included, as were many others about their relationships with food and diet.

After completing the questionnaires, Ben and his mother met for several hours with psychologist Carmen Mikhail, director of Weigh of Life and the eating disorders clinic at Texas Children's Hospital. Following Mikhail's comprehensive psychological screening, Ben was accepted into the program. When to begin was not a question. "It was late December, and there was just one week left in the year," Ben's mother recalled. "I said to Ben, 'Let's just get going.' So, that's what we did. We started moving fast, and we've been here ever since."

Seven months into the program, motivation remained the key to Ben's continuing enthusiasm. "My goal is to get back to my normal weight," he said. "I want to lose about 60 more pounds."[42]

To accomplish this and to maintain his desired weight after reaching his goal, Ben realized that he had to continue living his new Weigh of Life. Although he successfully completed the program's 14 projects and was not required to return to the clinic for more projects, he planned to continue his follow-up sessions and counseling. "I like to see my kids for at least a year," Shepard explained. "Weight was not gained all at once, and it's not going to be lost all at once. If a patient takes the time to learn how to manage behavior, he is going to acquire the skills needed for lasting weight control. But sometimes there are relapses. Sometimes you take one step back to take two steps forward. Sometimes it's difficult, but it is very doable."[43]

Rather than being apprehensive about missteps, Ben's mother worried about the effect that medications might have on Ben in the future. Although still fighting PAN, he had been taken off steroids for the time being, but might possibly have to take them again. However, knowing what the side effects might be, she was confident that they now had the tools to control them.

That was because both Ben and his mother embraced the program's lifestyle changes. Their newly formed eating habits became an integral part of their daily lives. "The program makes you plan," explained Ben's mother. "I get up in the morning and I think, 'What are we going to cook today, or what are we going to fix today that is within the right program?' It's not a diet; it's a change of life. It makes you question your actions. 'Do I really want this cookie? No, I don't really want to eat that cookie. I would rather have a fat-free yoghurt or a fat-free pudding or something because look at the fat content of this cookie. Even though this cookie looks good, I can have more yoghurt or more pudding versus that one cookie.' We have learned to rethink. I have been on every type of program you can name, but this one has really made a major impact."[44]

One major result, particularly rewarding to the mother who had once been unable to say no to her hungry son, was Ben's unwavering commitment to the program. Instead of constantly nibbling on something at odd hours throughout the day, he religiously consumed only an allotted amount of food at a specified time.

When not at home, Ben and his mother continued to follow a plan. On their weekly visits to Texas Children's Hospital for appointments with Ben's various physicians and therapists, they planned what they were going to eat and where.

Often at the hospital three times a week, and sometimes more, they found that practically living in the familiar surroundings had become second nature to them. "We call it our 'home away from home' now," she said. "We know someone everywhere we go. I remember when we first came to Texas Children's Hospital with Ben over a year ago. I noticed a family in the waiting room who seemed to know everybody there. I thought, 'Boy, I bet their child is really sick, since they know everybody and everybody knows them. I hope that doesn't happen to us.' And it did, but in a good way. Without this hospital, my child would not be alive today. We are very comfortable here."

Ben and his mother also adapted to social situations away from home and the hospital. When traveling to other homes, like that of Ben's grandmother in Louisiana, they knew what food to expect and planned the rest of their day accordingly. When entertaining Ben's friends at home, his mother prepared recipes from the Weigh of Life cookbook, authored by senior clinical dietitian Laura Laine at Texas Children's Hospital. "My mom is a great cook," says Ben. "She was before the program, and she is now with that cookbook."[45]

Ben's mother took no credit for the accomplishment. "The whole program is in that book," she said. "We haven't found a recipe in there that we don't like. Chicken enchiladas are a family favorite and I prepare it once a week. It's simple and only takes 30 minutes. It's geared towards kids and they love it. One of Ben's friends had some the other day, and he said to me, 'Can you teach my mom how to make these? It's so good.'"[46]

Her son heartily concurred. "They really, really like it," says Ben. "And the prosthesis guy loves it, too."[47] That was David Baty, who had happened to mention during one of Ben's prosthesis fittings that his own doctor wanted him to lower his cholesterol. "They brought me the Weigh of Life cookbook the next time they came for a visit," he said, genuinely pleased by the gesture. "I was so proud of Ben's losing all that weight, and he wanted me to learn how he did it."[48]

Ben also gave Weigh of Life cookbooks to his home-school teacher, numerous friends, several mere acquaintances, and anyone else he and his mother thought "lived in the fast lane" lifestyle. Always scouting for other potential converts, the head cheerleader and the superstar of the Texas Children's Hospital Weigh of Life team had also become two of its most enthusiastic recruiters.

For former soccer and football player Benjamin Sellers, Weigh of Life had become a new kind of sport, one in which his success as a loser represented a gain for him, as well as for the many fans he converted.

16

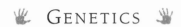

SOMETHING WAS WRONG with Gina Guerrero, and her parents knew it.

Although the one-year-old appeared to be a normal, happy baby, she could not walk or even crawl. Nor could Gina pick up anything with her hands, or sit up on her own without assistance.

When parents Eugene and Vi Guerrero took her to their pediatrician, they feared the worst. Referred to a neurologist, they grew more anxious. But the parents were relieved to hear the specialist say that Gina's problem was "just slow growth" and that "we'll send you to physical therapy at Texas Children's Hospital."[1]

Their relief was to be short-lived. After seven months of physical therapy at Texas Children's Hospital, Gina had not shown much progress. "One of her therapists told us something else was wrong, but they didn't know what it was," recalled Eugene. "They referred Gina to the Meyer Center for Developmental Pediatrics at Texas Children's Hospital in November 1993."[2]

To the Guerreros' surprise, after months of unanswered questions about their daughter's condition, it took less than 15 minutes at the Meyer Center for them to receive an unexpected answer. After observing and playing with Gina, Dr. Robert G. Voigt told her parents that he suspected she might have Angelman syndrome. He explained that the syndrome was a rare genetic condition first identified in 1965 by British pediatrician Dr. Harry Angelman.

Voigt explained that the symptoms of Angelman syndrome included a happy demeanor, developmental delay, a nearly total lack of speech, and unique behaviors such as inappropriate bursts of laughter and hyperactivity. When Angelman treated three patients with these symptoms, who also displayed jerky movements he likened to characteristics of a puppet, he grouped his findings and published a paper titled "Puppet Children" in 1965.[3] This condition eventually became known as the "happy puppet syndrome," a term with which the parents of similarly afflicted children were not pleased. The name was changed to Angelman syndrome in the early 1980s.[4]

The Guerreros learned that Angelman syndrome was often misdiagnosed as cerebral palsy or autism. For an accurate diagnosis, Voigt advised that Gina required genetic testing. He referred the family to the Kleberg Genetics Clinic at Baylor College of Medicine. There, the Guerreros met with a geneticist and answered questions about their family histories, while blood was drawn from Gina for fluorescence in situ hybridization (FISH), the standard for genetic diagnosis of Angelman syndrome. Utilized to detect abnormalities in chromosome number or microscopically visible duplications or deletions of chromosomal material, FISH analysis required several months to produce a diagnosis.[5]

While waiting to hear the results of Gina's genetic testing, her parents were anxious to learn more about Angelman syndrome. They soon discovered that little or nothing had been published about the genetic condition. They tried to look it up in medical books, but found nothing. They asked friends who were in the medical profession, "Have you heard about this?" only to find, "No one had a clue."[6]

Frustrated by this factual void, in November 1993 the Guerreros came to the only conclusion available to them. Eugene explained, "Since Dr. Voigt said Angelman syndrome used to be called 'happy puppet syndrome' because they flapped their arms and were always happy, just like a puppet, and the fact that the word 'Angel' was part of its name, we decided it can't be all bad."

Their optimism waned on Christmas Eve, when Gina became ill with a high fever and sinus infection. When she began to have grand mal seizures, her father was the only one home with her. Eugene "didn't know what the heck was going on, so I just called the ambulance," he said. "The ambulance driver wanted to take us to another hospital, I forget which one was closer, and I told them, 'No, we have to go to Texas Children's Hospital because all of her records and all of her doctors are there.' I argued with the driver about it for some time, and finally said, 'If you can't take me there, I'll go by myself,' and he finally took us there."[7]

Upon arriving at Texas Children's Hospital, Gina began to suffer more seizures. The doctors in the emergency center searched for a cause. "They checked her for everything," Vi said. "They did a CT scan and they did a spinal tap because they thought she had meningitis. After it was all said and done, the neurologist came out and said she was low on salt, and that's why she was having seizures. He said they would keep her overnight and pump her up with salt and everyone would be happy."[8]

Although Gina recovered the following day, the most probable explanation for her seizures was not known until two months later. The answer came when the FISH results from the Kleberg Genetics Clinic confirmed the diagnosis of Angelman syndrome. Although relieved to know exactly what was wrong with their daughter, the Guerreros found their consultation with the geneticist to be unsettling. "We went in and they said this is what you have, and this is what your child is going to be, and it was the worst scenario they can give you," remembered Eugene. "That's when we learned about the possibility of seizures and abnormal EEG tracings."[9]

In addition to the possibility of seizures, the Guerreros were told of the other consistent features of Angelman syndrome. Traditionally, these include developmental delay, functionally severe; speech impairment, none or minimal use of words; movement or balance disorders; and behavioral uniqueness, including frequent laughter, a happy demeanor, an easily excitable personality, a short attention span, and hand-flapping movements.

They also learned that the ability to diagnose Angelman syndrome definitively had only become available in 1987, when geneticists recognized a small deletion of the long arm of chromosome 15 to be the cause. Although the known incidence of Angelman syndrome was rare—estimated to be between one in 15,000 and one in 30,000—the geneticist at the Kleberg Genetics Clinic told the Guerreros that Gina's FISH results conclusively confirmed that there was a deletion in her maternal chromosome 15 and that she had the condition.

After leaving the clinic, the Guerreros were given a small pamphlet about Angelman syndrome. Although limited in scope, the brochure was the first printed information they had seen on the subject. At that point, what little they already knew about Angelman syndrome had traumatized both of them, particularly Vi. "When they said that this actually was my gene, maternal chromosome 15, that wasn't fully developed, I felt really bad about it," she explained. "I thought, 'What did I do during my pregnancy?' But I soon learned that it occurs during conception, not during pregnancy."

Although comforted to know that she was not to blame, Vi remained depressed about the situation for some time. "I don't remember how long it was," she said. "I do know my adrenaline just started pumping, and I became determined not to institutionalize Gina. I said, 'I am going to make this child as independent as possible. She's going to have a life that is as normal as possible. One day she is going to live in a group home or she is going to live with me until I am no longer here. Her world is going to revolve around me, I'm not going to revolve around her world.'"[10]

Accomplishing this goal was to become the Guerrero family's shared mission.

W hen Texas Children's Hospital opened in 1954, the medical subspecialty of genetics was in its early infancy.

The birth of genetics was attributed to a major scientific breakthrough, the identification of the double helix structure of the deoxyribonucleic acid (DNA) molecule by James Watson and Francis Crick. Published in 1953, the news instigated a revolution in the world of medicine. The specific impact that this medical milestone would have on Texas Children's Hospital was unknown at the time, but five decades later it was measurable.

"I distinctly remember reading that paper in junior high school," said Dr. Arthur L. Beaudet, chief of the genetics service at Texas Children's Hospital and chairman of the department of molecular and human genetics at Baylor College of Medicine, in 2003. "I decided then that I wished to pursue research in what we would now call molecular genetics."[11]

Beaudet pursued his interest in this new field at Holy Cross, graduating magna cum laude with a bachelor of science degree in biology in 1963, and at Yale University School of Medicine, graduating cum laude with a medical degree in pediatrics in 1967. As he began his internship on the Harriet Lane Pediatric Service at Johns Hopkins Hospital in Baltimore, Maryland, in 1967, his chosen field of pediatric genetics was beginning to grow throughout the country.

One cause for the growth of pediatric genetics was a national campaign spearheaded by the March of Dimes National Foundation. Having achieved success in the early 1950s with its original mission to cure polio, in 1959 that organization redirected its efforts to preventing birth defects. Among the first 90 recipients of the foundation's financial support for congenital birth defects and genetics research was Texas Children's Hospital.

Made possible by a $49,296 grant from the Harris County March of Dimes, the birth defects center at Texas Children's Hospital opened on July 1, 1967. Named as director was Dr. James J. Nora, a pediatric cardiologist and geneticist interested in the causation of congenital heart disease. The emphasis on cardiology was due to the growing reputation of the pediatric cardiology service and the existing "large numbers of cardiac cases," explained physician-in-chief Dr. Russell J. Blattner.[12]

Referrals to the new center came from other disciplines as well. "Following the rubella pandemic of 1964–65, the most common manifestation of the rubella syndrome was congenital cardiovascular disease," said Nora. "Furthermore, there was an appreciable risk of mental retardation, visual problems, and deafness following maternal infection in the second trimester."[13]

To address the needs of patients, the birth defects center at Texas Children's Hospital consolidated the hospital's existing programs involving birth defects. Although most programs concerned congenital heart defects, Down syndrome, muscular dystrophy, and spina bifida, the center also offered programs that had previously been developed for inborn errors of metabolism, cystic fibrosis, hypothyroidism, sickle cell anemia, phenylketonuria (PKU), and Tay-Sachs disease.

The clearly defined purpose of the birth defects center at Texas Children's Hospital was outlined in its first brochure: to conduct clinical research to explore the causes of birth defects; to develop improved techniques in prevention and treatment; to provide diagnosis and genetic counseling for patients and their families; and to educate other health professionals in the treatment, rehabilitation, and community relationships vital to the well-being of patients with birth defects. "Each child brought to the birth defects center will be examined by a clinical geneticist who then mobilizes, as needed, the services of other specialists," Nora stated in that brochure. "Together they evaluate the child's problems and plan treatment in a coordinated way."[14]

In addition to the services of the multidisciplinary medical team, the center offered genetic counseling to help parents evaluate the risk of birth defects in other children they might have in the future. A social worker was also available to help families solve the multiple problems associated with birth defects.

In correlation with the clinical activities was a laboratory research program instigated by Nora in 1967. With research assistant and scientist Anil K. Sinha, Nora explored the relationship between hereditary and environmental factors in the development of birth defects. Their work included studies on chromosomes, genetic mapping of human autosomes, and miscellaneous patient data collected in the clinic.[15]

"Monday was clinic day, held in the Junior League Outpatient Department at Texas Children's Hospital," recalled Nan O'Keeffe, the center's first executive secretary. "I worked closely with Dr. Nora and kept the birth defects registry indexes and cross-indexes by patient and diagnosis.

Because Dr. Nora also was on the heart transplant team at St. Luke's, I kept track of all those transplant patient records, too. From 1968 to 1970, there were more than 21 operations performed by the transplant team, so Dr. Nora was really busy with that."[16]

Unquestionably, Nora had a hectic schedule, given his diverse areas of responsibility. In fact, he once rushed from the St. Luke's Episcopal Hospital operating room to a March of Dimes dinner in his honor. Still dressed in his green scrub suit, Nora arrived late. After sitting at the head table for 20 minutes, he accepted a $9,985 check for the birth defects center at Texas Children's Hospital and promptly excused himself to return to his heart patient. Because of his association with the newsworthy transplant team, the incident was chronicled in the local newspapers.[17]

"On top of all that, he also was writing a book, *Medical Genetics: Principles and Practice,* with Dr. F. Clarke Fraser," O'Keeffe said. "I helped type the manuscript for it, but it wasn't published until 1974, which was several years after Dr. Nora had left to go to Colorado in 1971. That's when Dr. Dan McNamara, chief of the pediatric cardiology service, took his place for a few years."

Named to replace McNamara as director of the birth defects center in 1973 was Beaudet, who had just completed his two-year postdoctoral fellowship in the genetics section of the department of medicine at Baylor College of Medicine. "C. Thomas Caskey and I came here together in July 1971," said Beaudet. "Tom, who had his training in adult genetics, was about three or four years senior to me and he was recruited to start a section of genetics at Baylor. I was trained in pediatrics, and I was interested in the clinical aspects of genetics in pediatrics."[18]

Before coming to Houston, the two doctors had performed research together in the laboratory of Dr. Marshall W. Nirenberg at the National Institutes of Health (NIH) in Bethesda, Maryland. "The experience at the NIH was very exciting and it reaffirmed my plan to pursue a career in molecular genetics," Beaudet said. "The deciphering of the genetic code was being wrapped up and Dr. Nirenberg later shared the Nobel Prize for this effort. The understanding of the genetic code was completed in the 1960s, although reading during my college years had suggested that this task would extend into the next century."[19]

Surprised by the rapidity of that and other scientific breakthroughs in genetics, Beaudet instinctively knew that many more advances in the field were forthcoming. Unlike his expectations concerning the genetic code, he believed that most would occur before the end of the century. The optimism of Beaudet and others in his field was confirmed when a Harvard Medical School team isolated the first gene in 1969 and University of Wisconsin researchers synthesized a gene in 1970.[20]

Although the impact of such findings was to be long-term, other medical advances had an immediate effect on the birth defects center at Texas Children's Hospital. Chromosomal analysis through amniocentesis testing for prenatal screening was one such breakthrough in the 1970s. "I distinctly remember the first time a mother came into the birth defects center for screening," said executive secretary O'Keeffe. "Amniocentesis was such an exciting concept to all of us."[21]

The introduction of amniocentesis, along with countless other such technological advances, enabled a dramatic change in the emerging medical subspecialty of genetics. With more than 2,000 genetic diseases identified by 1972, geneticists possessed the means to diagnose and not just observe, as before. Utilizing prenatal screening, chromosomal studies, amino acid analysis, and enzyme assays, Beaudet's genetics service now offered specialized diagnosis.

"There were dozens and dozens and dozens of disorders we could diagnose by laboratory methods that we couldn't before," recalled Beaudet. "The clinical activities began to grow and we began to see more and more patients." With its change of emphasis recognized, the newly named genetics and birth defects center at Texas Children's Hospital emerged in 1973.[22]

Already given a new identity was an area in Caskey's adult genetics section at Baylor College of Medicine. Named the Robert J. Kleberg, Jr. Center for Human Genetics at Baylor College of Medicine in 1972, the center was made possible through the generosity of the Kleberg family. Its mission was to further the study of genetic disease and its diagnosis, treatment, and—where possible—prevention. In 1973, Beaudet became head of the center's pediatrics section and also head of the genetics section of the department of pediatrics at Baylor College of Medicine.[23]

Mirroring the growth of genetics as a medical subspecialty at Baylor College of Medicine, the genetics and birth defects center at Texas Children's Hospital experienced exponential growth. Its patient population had quadrupled since its 1967 inception, with more than 320 patient visits for diagnostic screening in 1973. No longer a small unit focusing mainly on cardiac malformation, the center had become a complex facility offering diagnosis, genetic counseling, biochemical studies, cytogenetic studies, and prenatal diagnosis.[24]

"Most people who come to the clinics appear because they have had one child affected with a genetic disorder, such as mongolism or cystic fibrosis, and they want to know the chances of another child having the same defect," Beaudet explained in 1975.[25] "The major province of the center is genetic counseling. An accurate diagnosis and an extensive family history provide the basics for counseling. Long hours are spent talking with families, discussing reproductive plans, and providing written summaries of the relevant information. In fact, geneticists probably talk with their patients more than most physicians, with the exception of psychiatrists."[26]

Geneticists Beaudet and Caskey also had lengthy conversations with the physicians in virtually every diagnostic facility and consultation service at Texas Children's Hospital. With the diagnostic opinion of neurologists, ophthalmologists, radiologists, pathologists, and others, the geneticists were able to distinguish between genetic and nongenetic disorders and to learn whether the disorders had varying inheritance patterns. These extensive evaluation procedures were followed because "accurate diagnosis forms the foundation for proper treatment and counseling," Beaudet explained.

The accurate recognition and diagnosis of single gene defects, such as cystic fibrosis, sickle cell anemia, and Tay Sachs disease, depended on the close examination of family patterns and chemical tests. For Tay Sachs disease and sickle cell anemia, testing to detect the carrier condition was available in the 1970s. "If such testing could be developed for cystic fibrosis, all couples would have reason to consider genetic testing before childbearing," Beaudet said in 1978, stressing the necessity for further research.[27]

"Advances in clinical genetic services have been highly dependent on laboratory research," he explained. "It is an important priority in our program. The great majority of genetics staff, both here and nationally, spends more than 50 percent of their time in a research laboratory. Patients with rare genetic diseases, in a sense, represent the experiments of nature which can teach us numerous lessons in normal body function and body chemistry."[28]

The opportunities to learn more from patients and families multiplied in 1979. In that year, the genetics service at Texas Children's Hospital served more new families in the outpatient area than did any other subspecialty service at the hospital. The 995 new families seen during that period illustrated the rapidly increasing demand for genetic services.

The reasons for that increased demand were twofold. First, there was growing community awareness of the prenatal services offered at the genetics and birth defects center at Texas Children's Hospital. Second, there were more technological breakthroughs that increased the geneticists' abilities to diagnose a number of chromosomal and biochemical disorders during pregnancy. Because a vast majority of prenatal diagnosis studies provided reassurance that the fetus was not affected with a specific condition, referrals for those services began to increase markedly.

Faced with the challenge of meeting this increasing demand, Beaudet added a major educational component to his service. Beginning in 1981, there were two postdoctoral fellows in training in genetics, Dr. Robert Nussbaum and Dr. Hans-Georg Bock, and numerous PhD scientists in training in medical genetics research. In addition, pediatric residents rotated on an elective basis in the genetics service.

Following the development of board certification in medical genetics in 1982, the number of postdoctoral fellows in Beaudet's service began to multiply—mostly because the genetics program at Baylor College of Medicine, funded by an NIH training grant, became an approved site for training. With its expanded medical staff and large patient population, by 1982 the clinical pediatric genetics program at Texas Children's Hospital and Baylor College of Medicine had become one of the largest of its kind in the United States.[29]

At the same time, technological advances in genetics were taking place globally. In 1982, genetically engineered insulin became the first recombinant DNA drug approved by the FDA. Recombinant DNA techniques, also known as gene cloning, began to offer great promise. The 1983 invention of the polymerase chain reaction (PCR) technique enabled scientists to reproduce bits of DNA rapidly, making copies of genes and gene fragments possible. The entire genome of the HIV virus was cloned and sequenced in 1984. Also that year came the development of "genetic fingerprinting," the use of DNA to identify individuals, and the first genetically engineered vaccine.[30]

"The really big development that kind of revolutionized our laboratory work, I think, was the recombinant DNA methods," Beaudet said. "These methods allowed you to take DNA work to the bedside and to start to do analyses on patients and families. We could now give very different kinds of information, very specific answers to genetic questions."[31]

These technological advances and the introduction of new techniques were "the primary reason that we can mark 1982 to 1984 as the time when the exact molecular basis for cancer began to unravel at a rapid rate," said Beaudet in 1984. "Recombinant DNA techniques are already in widespread use for diagnosis of genetic disease. We can anticipate that genes for most of the important human genetic diseases will be cloned soon. With DNA analysis, the next step will be to characterize the disease genes with the hope that this will bring with it an effective treatment."[32]

With the ability to analyze DNA from the amniotic fluid cells, safer and more accurate prenatal diagnosis became possible through the chronic villi sampling (CVS) procedure. DNA analysis also became useful for identifying the carriers of genes that bear great risk for future children. The development of more sophisticated carrier-testing procedures was expected to follow.

"Among human genetic diseases, in addition to sickle cell anemia, for which the gene is already cloned, the 'big three troublemakers' might be listed as cystic fibrosis, muscular dystrophy, and Huntington disease," explained Beaudet in 1984. "Recombinant DNA techniques are being used to identify cloned pieces of DNA near these genes, something which is already done for muscular dystrophy and Huntington disease. This will be more difficult for cystic fibrosis, but still should be accomplished soon."

As Beaudet applied recombinant DNA techniques to his ongoing research program on prenatal diagnosis and genetic treatment of cystic fibrosis, Caskey continued his own efforts directed towards muscular dystrophy and the genetic diseases that cause mental retardation. Together with other researchers in their laboratory, the two also began to conduct preliminary studies designed to investigate gene therapy, the replacement of the defective gene for a permanent and complete cure of a genetic disease. "I am predicting that a patient will be helped by gene therapy before the end of this decade," Beaudet stated in 1984. "I believe the obstacles will be overcome well enough for patients to benefit soon."

Such optimism was to be expected. Advances in genetics were occurring monthly, if not weekly or daily. Beaudet's personal experience in newsworthy laboratory research studies at Texas Children's Hospital was no exception. In the early 1980s, its laboratory research studies involved recombinant DNA technology, white blood cell function and type 1b glycogen storage disease, neurofibromatosis, and other human chromosomal disorders. These efforts resulted in significant publications in the medical literature in the areas of biochemistry, pediatrics, and infectious diseases.

With the resulting peer-group recognition and increased public awareness, the demand for genetics services at Texas Children's Hospital continued to expand significantly in the early 1980s. Clinical care now involved prenatal screening with CVS, ultrasound, and amniocentesis; the diagnosis of birth defects and genetic diseases; the treatment of biochemical genetic disorders; and the provision of genetic counseling to families with regard to both the care of an affected child and reproductive options for the future. With the rapid onset of technological developments, existing services were refined and new services were added, when possible. To describe this ongoing escalation in 1984, Beaudet simply stated: "Genetics is exploding."[33]

Aftershocks of this explosion included the 1985 establishment of the

Institute for Molecular Genetics at Baylor College of Medicine. Appointed as the institute's first director was Caskey, whose responsibilities included genetics research and the coordination and unification of all genetics-related studies at Baylor College of Medicine and Texas Children's Hospital.[34] To achieve those goals required a consolidation of efforts and restructuring. "All of us who had primary appointments in either pediatrics or internal medicine in the sections of genetics moved to the Institute for Molecular Genetics," Beaudet said. "We continued to have the genetics service at Texas Children's Hospital, but the research laboratories were at the institute."[35]

Coincidentally, the year saw another significant breakthrough in genetics—one that had a specific impact on Beaudet. It was the discovery of various genetic markers for cystic fibrosis. Simultaneously found on chromosome 7 by independent research teams in the United States, England, and Denmark, the markers enabled the development of more sophisticated prenatal screening tests for cystic fibrosis. One such test, the first in the United States, was to be initiated by Beaudet.[36]

Introduced in January 1986, the test was given to three women, each of whom had previously given birth to a child with cystic fibrosis. Knowing the location of the markers and utilizing CVS techniques, Beaudet and his team of geneticists were able to diagnose whether the fetus of each patient was destined to develop the disease. By the end of the year, more than 26 families with two or more individuals affected with cystic fibrosis had been tested. The results, published in the *American Journal of Human Genetics,* confirmed that DNA markers were useful for prenatal diagnosis within affected families.[37]

With this initial success, Beaudet and his team increased their efforts to perfect a test that would identify carriers of cystic fibrosis for parents with no family history of the disease. Because the effective treatment of cystic fibrosis depended on recombinant DNA techniques to clone the responsible gene, "that's the current focus of our research efforts," Beaudet stated in 1986.[38]

During this time, the Institute for Molecular Genetics was focusing on another genetic disease, Duchenne's muscular dystrophy. The genetic markers of the disease were also discovered in 1985, and the gene responsible for this common form of muscular dystrophy was identified. In prenatal screenings through amniocentesis and CVS, Caskey and his team of geneticists were able to use those genetic markers to diagnose the disease in a fetus.

The overwhelming response to such advances brought about specific changes in the genetics service at Texas Children's Hospital during the late 1980s. "Prenatal diagnosis has been a major aspect of genetic care over the past 20 years," Beaudet explained. "We have evolved to have a separate prenatal clinic. It functions in another building, Smith Tower, where we are dealing with couples who are currently pregnant, as distinct from Texas Children's, where everybody has had their baby. Although when we are dealing with a couple who has a child with a problem, we are routinely discussing future pregnancy questions."[39]

Despite the increased ability to diagnose genetic diseases in a fetus, geneticists remained unsure about the potential for a treatment or cure. Laboratory research at the Institute for Molecular Genetics continued to address this question. "There's every promise that the gene replacement therapy is going to work," Caskey stated in 1986. "What has been accomplished, you probably would not have predicted five years ago. But it is a goal worth tremendous effort. If successful, it alters totally your approach to the treatment of heritable disease and the way you view heritable disease. It's like finding a miraculous drug that does away with something that's lethal."[40]

Because there was widespread optimism that cystic fibrosis might be a reasonable candidate for this approach, Beaudet concentrated his efforts on further research involving that disease. While performing the chromosome analysis of a cystic fibrosis patient in 1988, he discovered something unique. "There had not been anything comparable described up to that time," he recalled. "It was a patient who had inherited two copies of her mother's chromosome, or the chromosome seven, and none of her father's. It's a patient I discovered through a sample sent to us from out of town, New York, and we spent huge amounts of research effort."[41]

What had been discovered by Beaudet and his research team was the first known case of "uniparental disomy," meaning two bodies from one parent. "Uniparental disomy in an individual with a normal chromosome analysis is a novel mechanism for the occurrence of human genetic disease," Beaudet's research team concluded in 1988.[42]

This highly regarded, laboratory-based breakthrough led to further worldwide research into the adverse outcome of uniparental disomy. The resulting phenomenon, the recognition of the differential expression of genetic traits based on inheritance from the mother or father, became known as "genomic imprinting."[43] Within a matter of months, geneticists announced that the first recognized examples of genomic imprinting were Prader-Willi syndrome (PWS) and Angelman syndrome (AS). Distinct human disorders characterized by neurobehavioral abnormalities and mental retardation, both were caused by deficiency of paternally (PWS) or maternally (AS) expressed genes on chromosome 15. Studies of genomic imprinting, concerning both the basic biology and the genetics of the process, became Beaudet's major area of interest. Specifically focused on PWS and AS, he and his laboratory team began their search for the responsible gene in 1989.

Beaudet's other laboratory research included continuing studies of cystic fibrosis. After the 1989 discovery by another team of researchers of the gene coding for the cystic fibrosis transmembrane conductance regulator protein (CFTR) on chromosome seven, the efforts of Beaudet and other geneticists to develop gene therapy for cystic fibrosis intensified. Although measurable advances had been made, there was no set date for implementation. "It's a tricky area," said Beaudet at the time. "We have to find the right balance of optimism and caution. Most people are not willing to make any absolute predictions as to what's going to happen by what date."[44]

While there was uncertainty about the future use of gene therapy in cystic fibrosis, additional opportunities to find cures and treatments for all genetic diseases came in 1988. Announced that year was the Human Genome Project, a 15-year program to locate and identify all of the estimated 100,000 genes on the 46 chromosomes. Since the identification of a gene responsible for causing a disease enabled geneticists to accurately diagnose that disease and expedite efforts to find a cure, expectations in the field of genetics were high.

In 1990, the NIH designated Baylor's Institute for Molecular Genetics as a Human Gene Research Center. Accompanied by a five-year, $10 million grant, the designation made the institute one of six such centers in the United States. Named as lead scientist for the NIH grant was Caskey. With 40 researchers assigned to the gene research center, Caskey announced that its focus would be on the X chromosome, chromosome six, and chromosome seven. "Another mission of the Houston center will be to transfer the basic science into medical applications as quickly as possible," he said. "We have the scientific backup at Baylor to meet all of our goals. We have the largest DNA diagnostic laboratory in the country."[45]

Such confidence was warranted. Within three years, Caskey's genetics team had identified more than 16 genes. With each new discovery at Baylor's Institute for Molecular Genetics, its reputation was enhanced further, both within the medical community and among the general public. Patients from around the world were referred to the institute for consultation or diagnosis and counseling. Between 70 and 80 percent of these referrals were pediatric patients.

The end result was an escalating number of families coming to the Kleberg Genetics Clinic and to the genetics service at Texas Children's Hospital in the early 1990s. With nine board-certified geneticists and the increased ability to diagnose patients through advances in laboratory testing, the genetics service had expanded. However, the original clinic had not changed.

"In reality, the Thursday morning clinic has been doing the same thing from 1971 to the present, except it has gotten a lot bigger," Beaudet explained. "Over the years, more specialized clinics were added, like neurofibromatosis, which is a common disorder and there's a lot of need for ongoing care. The cardiovascular genetics clinic is another. We also have a metabolic clinic for all the disorders we have some ability to treat with medications and drugs. Also, one of our geneticists will go and participate in a particular clinic, like spina bifida, Down syndrome, Prader-Willi syndrome, cleft-palate craniofacial, and many others."[46]

Another direct result of the worldwide advances made in the identification of genes was the 1992 establishment of the Laboratory for Genetic Therapeutics at Texas Children's Hospital. "The vast majority of gene therapy research has involved experiments in animals in attempts to develop successful methods," Beaudet stated in 1992. "Gene therapy protocols designed to treat patients are just being initiated throughout the United States. It seems certain that the number of gene therapy studies performed will increase successively during each year of this decade. It is realistic to hope that patients from around the world might come to major medical facilities such as Texas Children's Hospital for curative treatments based on gene therapy."[47]

In 1994, Beaudet's area of responsibility was vastly increased. Replacing Caskey, who resigned, Beaudet was appointed acting chairman of Baylor's new department of molecular and human genetics, formerly the Institute for Molecular Genetics. When Beaudet took charge of the department, what had begun in small quarters with two geneticists—Caskey and Beaudet—in 1971 had grown to include more than 15 primary faculty members in a space that measured more than 30,000 square feet. Under Beaudet's direction, the department was to grow even more.

One major influence on this growth was the 1996 establishment of the Human Genome Sequencing Center at Baylor College of Medicine. Designated by the National Human Genome Research Institute, the center was one of the six pilot programs for the final phase of the Human Genome Project. Funded by a $1.5 million grant and headed by Dr. Richard A. Gibbs, the center became part of Beaudet's department. After pioneering new methods for genomic mapping and sequencing, Gibbs began generating more than 40,000 sequence reads per month. Over the next three years, funding increased to a total of $12 million. In 1999, the center was selected as one of the three centers to complete the Human Genome Project and received a five-year $80 million grant. By 2001, Gibbs and his team of 220 were generating

1,400,000 DNA sequence reads per month.[48]

While progress was being made on the Human Genome Project, Beaudet continued his laboratory research studies in genomic imprinting, the phenomenon he had helped identify in 1988. After more than nine years of concentrated efforts, in 1997 he and his team of researchers announced the identification of the gene for Angelman syndrome (UBE3A), on chromosome 15. Also announced were the team's ongoing efforts to probe the biology of genomic imprinting in both Prader-Willi syndrome and Angelman syndrome. "Thirty years ago, so little was known about Angelman syndrome," Beaudet said. "Today, we are able to explain to Angelman syndrome patients the origin and mechanics of the disease and we can provide some hope that new gene therapies might be available to them one day."[49]

One area in which gene therapies were already beginning to make great strides in the late 1990s was pediatric cancer. Research studies proved that gene therapy made tumor cells more susceptible to drug treatments. In addition, there were indications that gene therapy made patients more resistant to the side effects of chemotherapy.

In 1997, an internationally recognized leader in the development of cell and gene therapy, Dr. Malcolm Brenner, joined Texas Children's Hospital. Named director of cell and gene therapy and of the cell and molecular therapy laboratory in the cancer center, Brenner began introducing effective gene therapy protocols for inherited and acquired disorders.[50] However, he also pointed out that "due to the complex nature of diseases, just knowing the particular gene that causes the problem doesn't always give us the solution."[51]

Accordingly, by the end of the twentieth century, Beaudet's prediction that gene therapy would be providing cures for some patients had not come to fruition. "We can now point to maybe one or two successes here or there, but they are very, very minimal," he said in 2001. "I thought by this time we would have seen gene therapy beginning to make a significant difference, but I remain convinced that certain disorders are perfect for treatment."[52]

As in the past, Beaudet remained optimistic about future developments in the field of genetics. His initial enthusiasm about the possibilities offered by genetics had come from the discovery in 1953 of the double-helix structure of DNA. Beaudet's continuing inspiration was derived from the technological and medical advances made in the field at Texas Children's Hospital and Baylor College of Medicine.

Throughout his three-decade career, Beaudet's ability to transform the endless possibilities of genetics into realities was evident in the genetics service at Texas Children's Hospital. Since his 1973 arrival at Texas

Children's Hospital and Baylor College of Medicine, the genetics service that had begun with the weekly birth defects clinic of the March of Dimes in 1967 had grown to become one of the largest pediatrics genetics services in the country. By 2003, the genetics service at Texas Children's Hospital included the Kleberg Genetics Clinic and various other genetics clinics and patient care centers for spina bifida, neurofibromatosis, Prader-Willi syndrome, skeletal dysplasia, cancer genetics, cardiovascular genetics, metabolic disorders, and inborn errors of metabolism.

The training programs in molecular and human genetics that Beaudet had established in 1980 continued to thrive in 2003. Of the more than 27 geneticists trained by Beaudet at Texas Children's Hospital and Baylor College of Medicine, most chose to continue their careers with him. As chief of the department of molecular and human genetics at Baylor College of Medicine, Beaudet and 30 other primary faculty members shared facilities that encompassed 70,000 square feet of space equipped with state-of-the-art instrumentation for research in molecular, cellular, and biochemical genetics.

Throughout its existence, the molecular and human genetics department at Baylor College of Medicine had received numerous competitive research grants, as well as national recognition and support from foundations and private organizations. Having helped Caskey establish the two-person department in 1971, Beaudet was justifiably proud of its three-decade evolution and the resulting accomplishments in the field of genetics. "We currently rank second in the NIH funding among genetics departments in the United States medical schools and rank first as measured by the number of NIH grants by a wide margin," he said in 2001.[53]

As to exactly what lay ahead for the genetics service at Texas Children's Hospital, given the five-decade history of the field of genetics, Beaudet was confident that his expectations would be met, if not surpassed. "Before looking forward, it is instructive to look back at some of the major advances of the last 25 years," he said. "The field of genetics has progressed way beyond whatever we could have imagined in high school. We didn't know what the genetic code was, and most people thought we would not unravel it until after the turn of the century. By the end of the 1960s, we were awarding Nobel prizes for unraveling the genetics code. No one would have had a clue about sequencing the genome, and now we have a situation in which lay people are learning about it in leaps and bounds. First of all, if not before the O. J. Simpson trial, they learned that DNA can identify people. They see billboards for paternity testing by DNA. They have heard a lot about the Human Genome Project. We have now a huge industry of biotechnology with recombinant growth hormone being administered to people. Molecular genetics and molecular biology has provided a solution to the AIDS and the hemophilia patients. So, yes, what has happened has been extraordinary."[54]

Whatever exciting discoveries and advances the future brings to the field of genetics, Beaudet planned to embrace them at Texas Children's Hospital and Baylor College of Medicine. More importantly, he expected them to occur sooner, rather than later, saying, "I'll still be here, but not for another 30 years."

E leven-year-old Gina Guerrero was included in everything the Guerrero family did in 2001.

Whether it was going to church or the grocery store, attending a baseball game, or dining out in a restaurant for dinner, Gina participated. Rather than be confined at home, she was visible to the community. "People always come up and speak to her by name, but they only know us as 'Gina's parents,'" Eugene Guerrero said, laughing at the thought. "I always introduce myself, but they never remember my name, only Gina's."[55]

Memorable to acquaintances was Gina's happy-go-lucky demeanor and her endearing affection for others, the same qualities that made coming home to her each day such a pleasure for her parents. "You are thinking, 'Boy, I sure have had a bad day,' and you walk through the door and she comes running up and gives you a big hug and you just melt," Eugene said. "This happens every day. It's like you've been on vacation for two weeks and you've just come back."

Gina's unbridled affection was also evident each and every morning. "When she wakes up, she has to hug you and love you," said Vi Guerrero. "Hugs and smiles and kisses and all kinds of stuff; we call her our fallen angel. We also think she sees angels, because she will be in her room and just looking up and laughing and moving her arms like wings. I'll say, 'Gina, are you talking to your friends again? Just tell them Daddy and I are taking care of you just fine.'"[56]

When Eugene confided to a priest that he and his wife thought Gina could see angels, the priest replied: "Who is to say she cannot? She has no concept of her limits." Embracing his philosophy as their own, the Guerreros applied it to Gina's bad days, as well as her good ones. Erratic behavior was not typical for Gina, but when it occasionally occurred her parents learned to cope with the disruption through creative and calming solutions. "It hasn't been easy," Vi said. "It's tough, but you learn to compromise."

Another difficulty was establishing effective communication between Gina and her family. Over the years, a pattern of recognizable sign language and gestures eventually evolved, but Gina remained almost completely non-verbal. Although some Angelman syndrome children never learn to speak words, Gina was able to use three words consistently—"Momma," "Po" for her father, and "Bubba" for Michael, her 14-year-old brother.

Always very protective of his little sister, "Michael has been there since day one and they are very close," explained Vi. "He was there every minute of the day when we were trying to figure out what was wrong with Gina. He's been through therapies with us. He's been to Texas Children's Hospital with us. He knows everything, because he's been there. I don't know how we decided to get him involved when we did, but it's another thing that has made us stronger."

One source of their strength came from the family's determination to ensure that Gina has as normal a life as possible. Since the day of her Angelman syndrome diagnosis at the Kleberg Genetics Clinic in 1993, the Guerreros remained focused on that goal. "We were persistent," Vi said. "Right away, we started physical therapy, extensive muscle therapy, speech therapy, occupational therapy, and anything else we could find to get her as independent as possible. She was going to Texas Children's Hospital three times a week."

As Gina continued to progress, milestones were reached. At the age of three and a half, she walked for the first time without assistance. By her fourth birthday in 1995, she had entered the half-day classes of the early childhood development program in the Pearland School District. On the three afternoons she had therapy, her grandmother, Amelia Garcia, picked her up and drove her to Texas Children's Hospital. "Thank goodness for my mother," Vi said. "Eugene and I work full-time, and I couldn't do this without her help. She does everything for Gina when I am at work. I am very fortunate because a lot of people are not that lucky."

The misfortunes of other Angelman syndrome families became apparent to Eugene and Vi. After contacting those diagnosed at the Kleberg Genetics Clinic, they soon discovered that there was a small loosely organized parent support group, one that the Guerreros found to be ineffective for their needs. "We wanted to know more," Eugene explained. "What we already had learned about Angelman syndrome ourselves was basically from being one-on-one with Gina. We knew we could learn more from other child-parent relationships and we wanted to build a strong support group to help others. It wasn't there for us to benefit from when we found out about Gina, but we hoped it would be there for somebody else. We also wanted to raise money for research."[57]

To accomplish these goals, Eugene and Vi developed a new support group, Houston Area Angelman Syndrome Association (HAASA). Beginning with just a few families in 1994, HAASA soon grew to become a vital organization. Within a few years, after hosting several golf tournaments to raise funds for genetics research, HAASA had $40,000 in its savings account. "It was a lot of money for a small group, we thought," Eugene said. "We decided to go over to Dr. Beaudet's office at the Kleberg Genetics Clinic in 1996, and said, 'Hey, we've got money. Where can we put it?' Dr. Beaudet explained, 'That's lots of money, but it only pays the salary for one year for one individual. But I'll tell you what to do.' So he led us in the right direction to where our money could do the most good. He told us how to get matching funds and how to put our money into existing research. In other words, he told us how our $40,000 could be doubled or tripled by somebody else."

Another successful HAASA effort was to increase awareness and knowledge about Angelman syndrome in the medical community. "From the beginning, we realized the doctors depended on us parents to educate them about Angelman syndrome," Vi said, remembering the information void in 1993 and the small pamphlet she had received from the Kleberg Genetics Clinic after Gina's diagnosis.

"When we started our first genetic research study at the clinic, they knew so little about the capabilities of children with Angelman syndrome," Vi said. "They were amazed, not just of Gina, but of the other kids who had the supervision of parents who were working with their kids day-in and day-out. Dr. Beaudet was amazed Gina understood us when we told her to do things like, 'Pick up the phone and call daddy,' and she would go and pick up the phone. He was just amazed she could understand my request. So our involvement has made not a small step, but a big step possible in research."[58]

Aware that previous Angelman syndrome research studies mostly involved institutionalized patients, the Guerreros seized the opportunity to effect a change in future studies. When volunteers were needed for research studies at the Kleberg Genetics Clinic, Eugene and Vi actively recruited participants from HAASA. "We were trying to get the parents involved, to come in and spend the night," Eugene said. "We would say, 'Look, we need the research. They need your kids to come in. They have got to have them in this study.' The first time we had more than 20 patients and their families come in."

Involved in Angelman syndrome conferences throughout the United States, Vi and Eugene began to network with other families outside of

Houston. After learning from a Dallas woman that her ten-year-old son had only recently been diagnosed with Angelman syndrome, the Guerreros were stunned. "Dr. Voigt at Texas Children's Hospital knew right away it was Angelman's syndrome," Eugene said. "Gina was only two and a half then, and this poor woman's son was ten years old and just barely diagnosed."[59]

Gina's parents believed that their daughter's early diagnosis had been integral to her steady progress. "That's why I am just so grateful we live here and that we have the Texas Medical Center," Vi said. "I think that is one of the reasons Gina has developed the way she has developed. I give us credit, too, but it's because right away Texas Children's Hospital started her therapy. Right away, those therapists knew what to do, how to get her independent, how to get her to walk, how to get her to sit up. Of course, we had to take her there three times a week."[60]

What Vi and Eugene were equally proud of was the amount of printed information and emotional support that had become available to members of HAASA. Such accomplishments reflected not only the astounding genetic advances of the last decade, but also the passionate pursuit of those goals by the Guerreros and other dedicated Angelman syndrome families.

The impact of those efforts was noticeable, if not measurable. "You see hope in the eyes of these new parents," Eugene said. "They come and see our kids. They see Gina running, or they see another kid's gesturing, and it gives them hope. They see you have to work with these kids on a daily basis, not shove them away. If you get involved, you are going to have results similar to what we have with Gina."[61]

Something was right with Gina Guerrero, and her parents knew it.

17

HEMATOLOGY-ONCOLOGY

Iᴛ ᴡᴀꜱ ᴊᴜꜱᴛ ᴀ ꜱᴛᴏᴍᴀᴄʜᴀᴄʜᴇ, a slight one at that. But his head felt hot, too, he thought.

So, when ten-year-old Laurence Bosworth Neuhaus, Jr., affectionately known to family and friends as "Bo," came home after school that December day in 1982, he told his mother and she took his temperature.

Bo had only a low-grade fever of 100 degrees, but his mother did not wait for more symptoms to appear as she had done in the past. Instead, she immediately put Bo in the car and headed for the pediatrician's office. "Don't ask me why," Lindy Wyatt-Brown Neuhaus said. "I don't know why I did it."[1]

At the pediatrician's office, the doctor examined Bo and called in a colleague for a second opinion. "Of course, I was thinking it must be appendicitis," Lindy recalled. "And my first reaction was, 'I can't handle an appendicitis. This is right before Christmas. I can't do this. This is horrible.'"

Little did Lindy know how horrendous it really was. The doctor administered numerous tests and ordered a blood test, advising Lindy that he would call her soon with the results. That the doctor had felt an unidentifiable mass in Bo's abdomen was not mentioned until the next day, when he also told Lindy to take Bo to Texas Children's Hospital for an ultrasound. "And from that point on, Texas Children's took over," Lindy said. "The first week, with all the tests and surgery, I was pretty much in a fog."[2]

It would take three days of extensive testing—including ultrasound, X-rays, and an arteriogram—at Texas Children's Hospital to learn that the cause of Bo's slight stomachache and low-grade fever was a life-threatening tumor on his liver, one that had to be removed immediately. "Our surgeon was Jim Harberg, who was absolutely the most compassionate man I've ever known," Lindy said. "He was the dearest, sweetest man and he just wept with us. He was so dear, because he knew it was bad by just looking at the ultrasound. It didn't look good."

More bad news came immediately after Bo's surgery. The pediatric oncologist told the Neuhauses that the tumor they had removed from Bo was an undifferentiated mesenchymal hepatic sarcoma, a rare and deadly type of cancer. "It was so rare that the doctors were only able to come up with 60 cases and only two survivors," Lindy said. "And those two survivors were still classified as high risk as the recurrence is almost inevitable. Because it was such a rare type, there was also very little literature on it and drug therapy was strictly experimental—a guessing game, we were warned."

When Harberg told them he hoped that Bo's "surgery will stave it off for a while, but you need to get ready to deal with this child's not being here in about three or four months," Lindy and Larry were devastated. "We resented every doctor who entered Bo's room because each one seemed to only want to tell us more bad news."

For Bo's parents, there was no denying the bleak picture painted by the surgeon and the oncologist, who told them that with aggressive experimental chemotherapy treatments, Bo had three months to live. He would probably have one good month and then go down from there, one doctor said. Lindy and Larry were stunned. How had all of this happened so suddenly to their perfectly healthy little boy? "He had appendicitis, or what we thought to be appendicitis, on Wednesday, and a tumor that was deadly on Friday," Larry said.[3]

Remembering how devastated they were at that precise moment, Lindy later said: "I have to say, in retrospect, that those doctors were amazing. They were able to relate to us this impending nightmare, and yet did not jerk every bit of hope from us. I suppose at the time they were quite sure that Bo's case was hopeless, but they were still able to give us a glimmer of hope."[4]

When the realization of Bo's predicament finally sunk in, the next step was an obvious one—not just for Bo, but also for the entire family. "I think when they said 'three months' to us, we had to do some fast peddling," Lindy said. "Whereas, if they had said this is a low-grade tumor and it may be five years and who knows if there will be a cure, then I don't know what we would have done then. But we had to peddle fast for the other kids as well."

Deciding exactly what to tell Bo's brother and sisters—seven-year-old Charlie, 12-year-old Mary Kessler, and three-year-old Alexandra—was difficult. The children really were too young to comprehend the dire consequences of Bo's recently diagnosed illness, their parents thought. And, although Bo certainly looked weak after the surgery, he did not look seriously ill. "We simply told them that we had a hard battle ahead of us and that there were going to be some bad times ahead for Bo, but that there would also be some good times, too," Lindy remembered. "They seemed very receptive, but I don't think they were really able to grasp what we were telling them."

As to when Bo became completely aware of his fragile condition, Lindy and Larry remembered a conversation they had with him in the hospital after the first surgery. It was when they had learned that he was going to have chemotherapy. "We said, 'They got the bad tumor out but they're afraid they might have left the cancer cells in there.' We didn't want to say, 'You have cancer.' And he said, 'Cancer cells? Oh, my gosh. If they left cancer cells, I could have caught cancer from it.' So, at the beginning, Bo did not know. He gradually learned. Lindy pretty much told him that there was a good chance he was not going to be here very long."[5]

"But we also said God was the only one that knows when any of us will die; any day anyone of us could be run over by a truck," Lindy said. "So, he was aware of it, in a gentle way, and somehow he understood. Bo had a remarkable Christian foundation." Enrolled at River Oaks Baptist Church School, he had been studying the Bible since the first grade and knew a lot more than Lindy did, she said. "I really do think he was spiritually touched. He had some sort of inner peace that it was going to be okay. I think, for some reason, a lot of these kids, when they're sick, learn to find out what's important in life."[6]

When Bo first mentioned that he was scared by the thought of dying, his mother told him that there was no reason for him to be afraid, because dying is like going to spend the night with your best friend. "She asked me who did I like to spend the night with the most and I said Hunter, my cousin who lives in Austin," Bo said. "So my mom said heaven would be like going to stay with Hunter, only even better. I did not feel as afraid of dying as I did before."[7]

That Bo not only understood his fate, but also decided to fight it was something at which his parents marveled. "Children who are very sick really mature quickly, because they've seen something that adults don't even know how to deal with," Larry said. "They understand their situation."[8]

Since Bo had decided to "beat this thing, either in this life or the next," he began chemotherapy treatments in the hematology-oncology clinic at Texas Children's Hospital the week after Christmas 1982. It was the beginning of a courageous battle.

A pproximately 9,000 children under the age of 15 were diagnosed with cancer in the United States in 2002.

Fortunately, with the development of effective treatments for childhood malignancies throughout the previous five decades, a diagnosis of cancer was no longer the universal death sentence it had once been for children. One out of every 900 adults in the United States in 2002 was a survivor of childhood cancer, and it was estimated that by 2010 one out of every 250 adults under age 55 would have survived childhood cancer.

Unfortunately, childhood cancer still was the leading cause of non-accidental death in children in the United States. "Although cancer remains a serious threat to the health of children, great strides have been made in treatment," said Dr. David G. Poplack, director of the Texas Children's Cancer Center and Hematology Service at Texas Children's Hospital since 1993. "Prior to 1960, maybe 5 to 10 percent of children with cancer were being cured, primarily when they had surgical removal of their tumors, but most would not survive. And now we're curing over 70 percent of all children with cancer."[9]

The achievement of such dramatic results in the field of pediatric hematology-oncology represented a milestone in the history of medicine in the twentieth century. This success was attributed not just to one particular individual, discovery, event, or cure, but to thousands of physicians and scientists who diligently researched, experimented, and produced the necessary anti-cancer drugs and treatment protocols. And, with the goal of completely eradicating childhood cancer, the tireless research and intensive clinical trials continued in pediatric hematology-oncology research laboratories, clinics, and cancer centers throughout the world.

At Texas Children's Hospital, these Herculean efforts began in 1957, when the survival rate of childhood cancer was less than 10 percent. The desire to eradicate childhood cancer resulted in the establishment of a hematology-oncology service in a basement laboratory at Texas Children's Hospital. In less than five decades, what had begun as a one-person lab grew to become one of the largest and most prominent pediatric cancer and hematology services in the United States.

More than 22,000 pediatric cancer patients from 35 states and 26 countries were seen at the Texas Children's Cancer Center and Hematology Service at Texas Children's Hospital in 2002. With between 375 and 400 new pediatric cancer patients and more than 850 new patients with hematological disorders referred each year, Texas Children's Cancer Center and Hematology Service utilized a team approach to facilitate the delivery of optimal care to each child. Each diagnosis-specific healthcare team comprised physicians, nurse practitioners, nurses, and social workers, with a senior physician as the primary doctor. Having the same team of caregivers on an ongoing basis, along with access to a full range of social services, the patients and their families benefited from continuity, familiarity, and trust.

With an expert medical staff of 75 faculty members and 500 employees, the Texas Children's Cancer Center and Hematology Service had a 22,000-square-foot clinical care unit with 11 examination rooms, procedure rooms, an infusion room, an on-site pharmacy, and multiple conference rooms. In addition, there was a 36-bed inpatient clinical care unit and a 15-bed bone marrow transplantation unit. A nationally recognized site for new drug development and research into innovative therapies for childhood cancer and blood diseases, the service included 21 different research laboratories dedicated to the cure of these diseases.

"Texas Children's Cancer Center and Hematology Service offers innovative therapies for all forms of childhood cancer and blood disorders," Poplack said in 2002. "The Cancer Center is working to improve the outcome for all patients afflicted with these diseases and to develop and perfect new treatment approaches that are born from the most extraordinary scientific insights. The staff at the Texas Children's Cancer Center and Hematology Service is committed to a future free from the threat of childhood cancer and blood diseases."[10]

Such sophisticated services, progressive expansion, and national prominence were not even imaginable to Dr. Donald J. Fernbach during the humble beginnings of the hematology-oncology service in the basement of Texas Children's Hospital. "I started the hematology unit from scratch," he said. "I was right out of fellowship training at Children's Hospital Boston. The word 'oncology' was not a word even most doctors were familiar with then, so we didn't even use it. Because I was interested in platelet research at the time, I called it the research hematology laboratory."[11]

Three years before the creation of the research hematology laboratory, Fernbach had begun his career at Texas Children's Hospital as one of its initial first-year pediatric residents in 1954. He was impressed with a senior resident, Dr. John Griffin, who "was sharper than everybody else." Fernbach learned that Griffin had spent a year in pathology at Children's Hospital Boston with Dr. Sidney Farber, known as the founder of pediatric pathology in the United States. "So I talked to Dr. Blattner, who was the physician-in-chief at Texas Children's Hospital and head of the department of pediatrics at Baylor, about that and said, 'I would like very much to go to

Boston and spend a year in pathology,' and he said he would help me out," Fernbach recalled.[12]

While studying in Boston, Fernbach discovered that he didn't want to spend all of his time in the pathology lab. Although he liked working with microscopes, he also wanted to work with patients. Because hematologists did a little of both, he became interested in pediatric hematology, a service that was being pioneered at Children's Hospital Boston by Dr. Louis Diamond, the founder of pediatric hematology. "So, I decided I'd like to go back and do that," Fernbach said. "It was a unique opportunity to have been able to work under these two giants in their fields."

With this plan in mind, Fernbach completed his fellowship in pathology and returned to Texas Children's Hospital, becoming its chief resident in pediatrics. At the end of his senior year of residency in 1956, he was accepted into Diamond's program and returned with a Jesse H. Jones fellowship to Children's Hospital Boston to study hematology. Although Fernbach hoped to come back to Texas Children's Hospital after his training, he knew that there was no job for him at the time. His own fate was uncertain, but he believed that Texas Children's Hospital would have a remarkable future.

After completing his year with Diamond, Fernbach spent a few more months in the clinic service where Farber, who had introduced the use of chemotherapy as a treatment for childhood leukemia in 1947, was continuing his history-making advances in the treatment of that disease. "Dr. Farber said, 'Before you go back, you have to see cancer patients,'" Fernbach remembered. "He wouldn't let me go home. I was one of the few people who worked with Dr. Farber and Dr. Diamond after they had feuded, but both of them knew what I was going to be doing and they both wanted to be sure I was well trained. So, when I came back, I was one of the few people who had experience in both cancer and hematology."[13]

In September 1957, Fernbach was back in Houston and hoping for a position at Texas Children's Hospital. He was at first rejected by Blattner, who lacked funding for another faculty member. "There wasn't any place for me to do anything, and I don't think Dr. Blattner actually had funds for me at that time. But he soon found funds, which basically were for a technician's salary, from Dr. Harvey Rosenberg, head of the pathology department," said Fernbach. "So I came in, technically, as a technician, at least on the books, and an instructor in pediatrics at Baylor. I also became the director of the new blood bank at Texas Children's Hospital."[14]

Fernbach and Rosenberg were good friends, having met in the service during World War II. While at Children's Hospital Boston, Fernbach had been so impressed with the hospital's blood component therapy blood banking program for pediatric patients that he wrote to Rosenberg about it, promising to bring him the technique needed to establish the program at Texas Children's Hospital.

What Fernbach had seen was the first use of plastic containers for blood collection, a concept introduced in 1950 by Boston surgeon and innovator Dr. Carl W. Walter. It was the heart of a flexible blood-processing system that made all subsequent advances in blood processing possible.[15] Fernbach wasn't the only one who was impressed by this breakthrough. Decades later, the replacement of breakable glass bottles with durable plastic bags was recognized as one of the single most influential technical developments in blood banking, according to the American Association of Blood Banks.[16]

"When I came back from Boston, with the help of Dr. Rosenberg, we installed the new system and became the first hospital in the southern part of the United States to use blood component therapy in plastic equipment," Fernbach said. "We were the first hospital in Houston to give platelet transfusions, years before any other hospital here even went into plastic blood banking and even before the National Cancer Institute began to use platelet transfusions."

Immediately appointed as director of the hematology and transfusion services in the diagnostic laboratories of Texas Children's Hospital in January 1958, Fernbach began administering the highly specialized service. With capabilities of dividing the original adult-size pint of blood (500 milliliters) to a smaller pediatric unit (50 milliliters) for transfusions, and efficiently separating whole blood into its own various components, the newly introduced blood banking system offered distinct technical advantages in providing special blood products for special needs in children. Also, because blood survival is slightly better in plastic containers, platelets lasted long enough to be useful in the treatment of certain bleeding disorders.[17] "It worked very well after we taught people how to use it," Fernbach said. "I was very proud that we were one of the first hospitals in the country to have, from day one, a working blood bank with plastic equipment that provided all of the different components that were available at the time."[18]

What was not available at the time, however, was adequate workspace for Fernbach. While developing and administering the blood bank, Fernbach and Rosenberg decided to take matters into their own hands—literally. "We decided I needed a place to work," Fernbach recalled. "So one night, the two of us stayed late and we put on scrub suits from surgery. We went down to the basement and the two of us moved all of this furniture and equipment out of an area in the basement where it was in storage. We collared a couple of men in the maintenance section and said, 'We need to put up a wall over here.' These fellows were good friends of ours and, before anybody knew it, we had created a partition there and that became the hematology lab."[19]

With an office consisting of a desk and chair and with laboratory benches outside, the small hematology lab backed up to Rosenberg's office on the other side of the plywood. It was an informal arrangement, they agreed. In fact, it was so informal that Fernbach and Rosenberg would communicate with each other by banging on the wall and talking over the top. This method of communication was finally deemed unsuitable when Rosenberg was talking to some of the hospital's board members in his office while Fernbach was yelling at him from his. "Like a one-room schoolhouse, this area served as an office, a laboratory, a treatment room, and an examining room," Fernbach recalled. "There also was a desk out there for a secretary that I didn't have at that time."

The addition of a secretary, Ann Robinson, came in 1958. Her arrival coincided with the official launching of the hematology-oncology service at Texas Children's Hospital, which occurred after Blattner and a number of other departmental chairmen from other Southern medical schools helped organize the Southwest Cancer Chemotherapy Study Group (SWCCSG). In order to participate in that group, Blattner designated Fernbach chief of the hematology-oncology service at Texas Children's Hospital and assistant professor of pediatrics at Baylor College of Medicine.

"Through the Southwest Cancer Chemotherapy Group, we received our first grant from the National Cancer Institute," said Fernbach. "With which we were able to buy equipment for our little lab set-up and could go to work. Mary Nagai became the first technician there. Everybody in those days knew Mary Nagai; she was sort of the dean of medical technologists in Houston. She'd been at the old Jeff Davis Hospital, taught a lot of the technologists there. She was an absolute perfectionist, which is what I needed because we were mixing up some of the potent experimental chemotherapy in our lab. They would send it to us from the National Cancer Institute in powder form, and we had to prepare it. We had to filter it and sterilize it so we could give it to patients."[20]

That first grant was the beginning of an ongoing relationship between the National Cancer Institute (NCI) and Texas Children's Hospital. Fernbach reported in 1999 that financial support from the NCI had continued uninterrupted every year since 1958.[21]

Also firmly established was Texas Children's affiliation with the SWCCSG.

Fernbach, as one of approximately 20 doctors in the country at that time who had had training in pediatric hematology-oncology, became one of the lead investigators with that primarily pediatric organization.

Thus, in 1958, when the number of drugs available to treat childhood cancer was still at a minimum and government funding was becoming available for cancer research programs, the SWCCSG began developing a cooperative study program that ultimately became a model for the development of cooperative cancer clinical trial groups. In subsequent years, SWCCSG evolved and renamed itself the Southwest Oncology Group (SWOG) and then the Pediatric Oncology Group (POG). After the POG merged with all of the other childhood cancer cooperatives in the United States in 2000, the collective group became the Children's Oncology Group (COG).

"It was, and is, one of the older cooperative groups and was one of the most productive pediatric groups in the world until the others caught up," said Fernbach. "Texas Children's Hospital continues to be one of the largest single contributors to the studies in the group. So what Dr. Blattner did in helping to found this group and becoming one of its charter members was to be in on the beginning of the era in which all the dramatic changes in the survival of children with cancer occurred."[22]

One such advance was made at Texas Children's Hospital in 1959. It was the study Fernbach conducted on a new anti-cancer agent, cyclophosphamide, a drug designed to maintain complete remission in children with acute leukemia. Previously deemed ineffective by the National Cancer Institute, Memorial Sloan-Kettering, and the Children's Cancer Foundation in Boston, the drug was administered to a child at Texas Children's Hospital who was in the terminal stage of leukemia. The child went into remission and survived for an additional 15 months. Fernbach was the lead author of a manuscript titled "Clinical Evaluation of Cyclophosphamide: A New Agent for Treatment of Children with Acute Leukemia," the SWCCSG report published in the *Journal of the American Medical Association* in 1962.

"It was one of the milestones in chemotherapy," Fernbach said. "Since then, cyclophosphamide has become widely used not only in just childhood malignancies, but also in adult malignancies as well. It has been used not only in cancer treatments, but also as an immunosuppressant agent. It was a major contribution."[23] This development subsequently laid the groundwork for the first report on the comparison of cyclophosphamide with other drugs in "Chemotherapy of Acute Leukemia in Childhood," an article by Fernbach that appeared three years later as the lead article in the prestigious *New England Journal of Medicine* on September 1, 1966.

Also during the early 1960s, another collaborative venture to study the possible role of viruses in childhood cancer was begun by the research hematology laboratory and the department of virology and epidemiology at Baylor College of Medicine, spearheaded by Dr. Joseph Melnick and Dr. Matilda Benyesh-Melnick. Awarded a major $300,000 resource grant from the National Cancer Institute, the hematology-oncology portion of the project included the monitoring of newborn baboons delivered by cesarean section and caged individually in a carefully controlled, locked, and air-conditioned environment.

"They were locked up mainly to keep people out of there because they wanted to play with them," Fernbach said. "Simon, the first one we had, I brought home and my wife raised him for three weeks. All the kids in the neighborhood thought it was great, and I became the pediatrician for the baboon. The baboon began talking to us, and my wife and kids could translate it. Simon would make certain sounds when he was hungry, and when he wanted to get out and exercise, and when he was bored. He was a funny little animal."

Simon was the first of more than 600 baby baboons that were used over a period of years to investigate whether humans could transmit leukemia. None ever showed the faintest glimmer of a blood disease. Although a tremendous amount of research was conducted and an enormous amount of information was gained about baboons and baboon hematology, the project was eventually terminated and the baboons were donated to zoos and animal parks. To Fernbach's dismay, the *Houston Chronicle* summarized the experiment with this headline: "Million Dollar Project Failure."

However, something good did come out of that ill-fated project—and it happened before the project had even begun. When representatives from the NCI came to Texas Children's Hospital to discuss the possibility of the grant, one mentioned to Fernbach that money could be allocated for the expansion of his laboratory. Told that the NCI could not subsidize the building of anything new, but could fund renovations, Fernbach had an inspiration. He suggested that the laboratory could be accommodated in the residents' building in the hospital parking lot. Built in the late 1950s to house the hospital's residents and nurses, the two-story building was more than adequate for a "renovated" laboratory. "We received the money to renovate one end of the downstairs part of the building and physically moved out of the basement of the hospital and above ground, with windows and all, in April 1964," Fernbach said. "And that became the research hematology laboratory and the outpatient building."[24]

The NCI grant also made possible the addition of new personnel, including an assistant hematologist, Dr. A. Thomas Adkins, the first hematology fellow. With the arrival of Dr. Kenneth A. Starling and several technicians, the staff was able to conduct extensive research on childhood cancer, with an emphasis on leukemia.

In the newly renovated eight-room research hematology laboratory at Texas Children's Hospital, Fernbach and his five-member staff entered the era of childhood-cancer chemotherapy research in the 1960s. Their goal was to find a drug or a combination of drugs that specifically destroy or damage malignant cells. In an independent study, they demonstrated the dramatic impact of the introduction of chemotherapy on the treatment of childhood cancer. In a 1965 paper presented by Fernbach, the group reported a 95 percent survival rate with the use of Actinomycin-D in the treatment of Wilms' tumor, a rare kidney tumor in children. These results were the first of their type to be presented. It was almost ten years before the results were later duplicated and confirmed by the National Wilms' Tumor Committee.[25]

In the hematology clinic, which was under the direction of Fernbach and met every Tuesday in the Junior League Outpatient Department at Texas Children's Hospital, there was a growing patient population. "Pediatricians all over the state of Texas and Mexico referred patients to us," Fernbach remembered. "I was in the Texas Pediatric Society and had been introduced to the membership as a pediatric hematologist, the first in the state. So, if someone would ask a pediatrician, 'Where do I send this kid?' they would reply, 'There's a pediatric specialist at Texas Children's Hospital in Houston.' And that's how we got them. That's how the service grew from the very start."

As the hematology-oncology service at Texas Children's Hospital evolved throughout the 1960s and 70s, it became responsible for the diagnosis and management of children with red blood cell, white blood cell, platelet, and bone marrow disorders, as well as those with disorders of blood coagulation and malignant and non-malignant tumors. Fernbach's stated purpose for the hematology-oncology service at Texas Children's Hospital was to contribute knowledge of the cause of the disease where the cause remained obscure, to develop improved methods of diagnosis, and to strive continuously to develop improved methods of therapy.

Among the patients referred to the hematology service at Texas Children's Hospital in 1959 was a three-year-old boy who had bone marrow failure, aplastic anemia, a disease that had a mortality rate of over 75 percent and no known cure. "Interestingly, this boy had an identical twin brother who appeared to be well at the time," Fernbach recalled. "I had been working with the late Dr. John Trentin, in the department of experimental biology at Baylor, who was studying bone marrow transplantation in mice. He irradiated mice to destroy their bone marrow making them aplastic, and then administered normal marrow from healthy mice. The transplanted marrow would grow in the damaged marrow and spleens of the irradiated mice. It seemed reasonable to us to assume that marrow from the healthy twin might similarly help the sick twin to recover."[26]

After discussing this idea with the parents of the twins, Fernbach and Trentin confirmed the identity of the twins by blood tests and by swapping small full-thickness skin grafts. They were convinced that this was a unique opportunity to provide a lifesaving human tissue transplant, as the downside risk was small because the tissues were identical. "The boys were placed side-by-side in an operating room and marrow was aspirated from the healthy boy and injected intravenously into the sick twin," Fernbach explained. "A series of three transplants was performed over the next three months, during which time gradual improvement was noted. No transfusions were required for the next five months. Although bone marrow transplants are now done for a large number of malignant diseases, commonly for children who have leukemia, this transplant was years ahead of its time."

Decades later, Dr. Don Thomas, who was awarded the 1990 Nobel Prize for his phenomenal work with bone marrow transplantations, recognized Fernbach and Trentin's 1959 bone marrow transplantation as the first of its kind anywhere in the world. "He teased me by saying he thought there was one that had been done before ours, but that he could not find it," Fernbach said.[27]

Another first for Fernbach was the publication in 1973 of the only multidisciplinary book on childhood cancer in existence, *Clinical Pediatric Oncology*. Published with fellow editors Dr. W. W. Sutow from M. D. Anderson Hospital and the Tumor Institute in Houston and Dr. Theresa J. Vietti from Washington University in St. Louis, *Clinical Pediatric Oncology* became the acknowledged text in the new subspecialty of pediatric hematology-oncology, which was formally recognized in 1974.

Targeted to the clinicians responsible for the diagnosis and management of children with cancer, the book included information, in practical terms, about topics designed to enhance clinical knowledge and performance. The book also provided medically detailed therapies for the specific disease entities. Immensely popular, it was updated and republished in four editions over the following 17 years.

By the time the book was published, milestone advances had been made in the treatment of childhood cancer. "During the 1970s we saw incredible progress in extending the survival rate of patients with leukemia, the most common of the childhood cancers. This was in large part due to chemotherapy," said Fernbach. "At the same time we began to use these drug treatments as a supplement to surgery and radiotherapy in all types of cancer in children. This adjuvant therapy was designed to destroy microscopic spread of the tumor after the primary tumor was removed."[28]

As improved treatments were introduced and Fernbach's reputation as one of the recognized specialists in the new field of pediatric hematology-oncology continued to grow throughout the 1970s and 80s, the number of cancer patients at Texas Children's Hospital also increased. With more than 500 new patients annually, the independent and cooperative-group research projects quickly multiplied. By the late 1980s, the medical staff at the hematology-oncology service at Texas Children's Hospital had more than doubled in size. With ten full-time staff positions and more than 30 other employees, workspace was at a premium—even after expanding to encompass both floors of the former residents' building in the parking lot, now referred to as the hematology-oncology building. Because the number of children with hematological disorders outnumbered those with childhood cancer, an established pattern since the service was founded in 1957, the patient population mushroomed. Finding his service to be woefully overcrowded in the late 1980s, Fernbach eventually moved the hematology-oncology service at Texas Children's Hospital off campus and across the street to the Medical Towers Building, where it occupied the entire fifth floor.

Also affecting the growth of the service was the hemoglobinopathy laboratory, established in 1973 at Texas Children's Hospital to screen blood specimens from the City and County Health Clinics and Health Department. By 1983, more than 40,000 specimens derived from all newborn umbilical cord blood of infants born in the Harris County Hospital District had been screened for hemoglobin abnormalities. The purpose of the screenings, which totaled more than 60,000 specimens and was conducted in conjunction with the medical genetics section at Baylor College of Medicine, was to identify babies at risk from severe anemias during the first two to three years of life.

When serious hemoglobin abnormalities were identified in this laboratory, the hematology-oncology service at Texas Children's Hospital provided counseling to the families. The parents of infants and children with serious hemoglobin abnormalities, including sickle cell disease, thalassemia, and hemoglobin E, became an integral part of the ever-increasing traffic flow and crowded facilities in the Medical Towers Building.

The limitations of physical space and its effect on patients deeply concerned Fernbach. Stressing the need for additional funds for renovation and expansion, he wrote in 1987: "Many patients and their parents are required to spend long hours in less-than-ideal circumstances while the patient undergoes long chemotherapy infusions or blood transfusions. The waiting areas, where a great many sick children will spend a great portion of their young lives, are limited and often crowded and lack the comforts that would make outpatient visits a more pleasant experience."[29]

Wishing also to enhance the experiences of critically ill patients who were admitted to Texas Children's Hospital for treatment, as well as those children who had to return to the clinic repeatedly, Fernbach learned of a revolutionary concept that had come to fruition for cancer patients and their families in Philadelphia in 1974. It was the home-away-from-home Ronald McDonald House, underwritten by McDonald's restaurants and community donations. A place where a family could stay while a child was undergoing treatment, it was the only facility of its kind. Fernbach envisioned another one for Houston. "Everyone can identify with the value of a low-cost lodging," he said. "And most people can appreciate how much better this might be for emotionally distraught parents who would otherwise have to retreat to a strange and lonely hotel or motel room."

When a second Ronald McDonald House was announced for Chicago, Fernbach immediately contacted the advertising offices of the McDonald's restaurant cooperative in Houston. He was referred to a pediatric oncologist in Chicago, Dr. Ed Baum, a recently appointed member of the newly formed National Advisory Committee for McDonald's. Told by Baum that there had been a rapid increase in the number of cities seeking to have a house, Fernbach realized the urgent need to elicit strong local support for his idea to build one in Houston.

Where to begin this quest was not a problem. Fernbach started with the families of present and former patients—many of whom he had known before the early 1970s, when most children diagnosed with cancer were given a virtual death sentence. Back then, the parents appreciated anything that Fernbach could do for them. Aware of his research involvement with the National Cancer Institute and fully cognizant of the physical and financial limitations of the hematology-oncology service at Texas Children's Hospital, these parents always wanted, and offered, to help in some way. "When his son Troy was sick with lymphoma, Don Mullins had made it clear that someday he wanted to 'help' however he could," Fernbach remembered. "After listening to my description of the two existing houses, he said, 'Let's go look,' and so we invited ourselves to Chicago. The beautifully renovated old mansion had a friendly look from top to bottom, including the living rooms, bedrooms, play areas, kitchen, laundry room, and a host of other amenities. That look was all it took and the Houston house was on its way."

Joining Mullins in the effort first was Liz Kelley, whose son Sean had leukemia. An energetic dynamo, she spearheaded the fund-raising efforts. Next came many other parents, most of whom had lost children to cancer. Then there were attorneys, builders, designers, publicists, and a host of volunteers.

In the beginning, Mullins, Kelley, or Fernbach addressed any organized group in Houston that would let them present a proposal for funds. Astonishingly, no group refused, Fernbach recalled. One, in particular, jumped at the chance to be associated with the project. Because the Ronald McDonald House had been supported in Philadelphia by the Philadelphia Eagles and in Chicago by the Chicago Bears, the plan for a house in Houston was presented to Bud Adams, owner of the Houston Oilers professional football team. Adams not only enthusiastically endorsed the project as the official charity of the Oilers, he also became a member of the organizing committee.

The next step was to find an appropriate house. After an extensive and futile exploration of the homes available to renovate in the Texas Medical Center area, the organizing committee decided to build the house from scratch. Mullins, who had used the raised funds to form the non-profit organization Oncology Services of Texas, Inc., became its president and assumed responsibility for the building project. With most of the services and materials donated or provided at cost, a 21,000-square-foot building accommodating 21 families was built. The Houston Ronald McDonald House opened in May 1981. "When so many people spend so much of their time to do so many things for so many other people, it is difficult to believe that things can be so bad in this old world," Fernbach said. "When the house opened it had no mortgage, it had a pure heart, and it had as much love built into it as the law and God allow."

That "house that love built," as it became known, was located less than two miles from the Texas Medical Center and provided a warm, caring atmosphere to more than 750 families a year. After outgrowing its facilities in September 1997, the haven moved to the newly built Ronald McDonald House, a 65,000-square-foot building accommodating 50 families.

Still owned and operated today by Oncology Services of Texas, Inc., the Houston Ronald McDonald House is maintained by a network of volunteers who help through donations, as well as contributions of time and effort. In appreciation to Fernbach for his guidance and inspiration, the surplus funds raised by the non-profit organization are earmarked, in perpetuity, for the research hematology laboratory at Texas Children's Hospital. It is a generous stipulation written into the charter of the organization and one that uniquely differentiates the Houston house from the more than 200 Ronald McDonald Houses that are now scattered throughout the world.

Also providing substantial support to the ongoing efforts of the hematology-oncology service at Texas Children's Hospital in 1989 were the trustees of the John S. Dunn Research Foundation, which established the Elise C. Young Chair of Pediatric Oncology at the Baylor College of Medicine. The Foundation provided $500,000 for the chair and a committee of Baylor College of Medicine and Texas Children's Hospital trustees raised matching funds.

Named in honor of Elise C. Young, Dunn's executive assistant for more than 30 years, the chair had been established at Baylor because Young selected Texas Children's Hospital as the recipient. She stated: "My heart told me this is where I can help. Most of us have had a full life, but these children need us desperately. I'd like to give them a chance for life on earth. I appreciate the Trustees of the Foundation giving me the opportunity to choose where to establish the Chair."[30]

"The first occupant of the Elise C. Young Chair of Pediatric Oncology is Donald J. Fernbach, M.D., chief of the hematology-oncology service at Texas Children's Hospital," physician-in-chief Dr. Ralph D. Feigin announced in 1989. In a salute to Fernbach's many accomplishments at Texas Children's Hospital since founding the hematology-oncology service in 1957, Feigin praised him as "the physician–scientist whose research has increased the life expectancy of children with cancer."[31]

The establishment of the Elise C. Young Chair stabilized the financial resources of the hematology-oncology service and also permitted the appointment of two new staff members. Joining the faculty at Baylor College of Medicine and Fernbach's team at Texas Children's Hospital were Dr. ZoAnn Rightmire Dreyer and Dr. Angela Kent Ogden. With its newly enlarged medical staff, the hematology-oncology service at Texas Children's Hospital was poised to move to a new and bigger location in 1991, the tenth floor of the newly constructed Clinical Care Center, later known as the Feigin Center at Texas Children's Hospital.

It was not the only big change to occur that year. After almost four decades at Texas Children's Hospital, Fernbach decided that it was time to retire. In 1991, more than 50 percent of children who developed cancer were expected to be cured and to live normal, happy lives—a situation to which Fernbach had significantly contributed. Yet he lamented the fact that there was still much left to be done. "Cancer is a battle that is being won; the fight has been long and hard, and at times emotionally exhausting for the participants, but the rewards have been worth all the labor," he said. "In 30 years the hematology-oncology service at Texas Children's Hospital is one of the top ten pediatric cancer centers in the country and its staff members are among the most widely known, frequently published, and highly respected medical professionals in the world."[32]

Fernbach's career had been long and fulfilling. In addition to his lengthy affiliation with Texas Children's Hospital and Baylor College of Medicine—and his extraordinary contributions to the field of pediatric hematology-oncology—Fernbach had also excelled in his extracurricular activities. These included serving as vice president and president of the medical staff at Texas Children's Hospital and serving on virtually every other committee of the medical staff. He had also served as president of the American Cancer Society's Texas Division in 1981–82. Fernbach was awarded an American Cancer Society professorship in clinical oncology for six years, the first such honor ever awarded to a pediatric hematologist/oncologist. An active participant in numerous professional organizations, he had also volunteered his services to various community organizations— including the building of the Houston Ronald McDonald House, which remained one of his proudest accomplishments.

"It's time for somebody else to take the hematology-oncology service to its next level," Fernbach told Feigin in 1991. While waiting for the search committee appointed by Feigin to complete its nationwide search for his successor—a task that took two years—Feigin appointed Dr. C. Philip Steuber as acting chief of the hematology-oncology service at Texas Children's Hospital. A former fellow during the 1970s and an assistant professor of pediatrics at Baylor College of Medicine, Steuber had worked with Fernbach over the years, successfully treating the increasing numbers of childhood malignancies seen at Texas Children's Hospital.

Along with their successes in treating childhood cancer came unanswered questions about the long-term effects of toxic cancer therapy in the children who survived. With a grant from the Ronald McDonald House, Fernbach and Dreyer established the long-term survivor program in the hematology-oncology service at Texas Children's Hospital. "The important thing is that now we have survivors to study," Fernbach noted.[33]

The need for a central place where this ever-growing number of survivors could go for follow-up appointments with the specialists who treat cancer survivors was evident to pediatric oncologist Dreyer in the late 1980s. "As our survivor rates started going up, we started noticing more side effects from cancer and treatments that a survivor's regular internist or pediatrician might not notice or know how to treat," Dreyer said.[34]

Opened in 1989 and headed by Dreyer and a team of individuals dedicated specifically to the care and support of childhood cancer survivors, the long-term survivor program at Texas Children's Hospital began tracking the long-term effects of cancer therapy in childhood cancer survivors. The program was established to track survivors treated at Texas Children's Hospital and those referred from a variety of other hospitals throughout the United States. Within ten years, more than 600 childhood cancer survivors were participating in the program, one of the largest of its kind in the world.

Dryer attributed the growing number of childhood cancer survivors throughout the world to the research-based treatment protocols used in childhood cancer. "Less than 20 percent of adults are treated with research-based protocols because there are so many adult cancers," she explained. "The children's population and types of cancers are much smaller. Fully 85 percent of the treatments we do at Texas Children's Hospital are research-based treatment protocols, which are proven to be much more effective. We also intensify the treatment and we diagnose and begin treatment much quicker."[35]

As the survival rate of childhood cancer continued to climb, serious complications from some research-based therapies began to develop, sometimes not until decades after treatment. The late effects of some such toxic treatments became evident in studies performed in the long-term survivor program at Texas Children's Hospital. Within two years of the program's inception, Fernbach already had begun to eliminate several toxic therapies deemed no longer adequate by the study.[36]

Also obsolesced in 1991 was Fernbach's role as one of the editors of *Clinical Pediatric Oncology*, which had remained the leading pediatric hematology-oncology textbook since its first publication in 1974. "When we were preparing the fourth edition in 1991, the book by the National Cancer Institute's Dr. Philip A. Pizzo and Dr. David G. Poplack, *Principles and Practice of Pediatric Oncology*, came along. Their book was much more comprehensive than ours. It's really a very good book," said Fernbach. "I agreed that we would finish the fourth edition of our book, because it was a popular book and serves more of a use for pediatricians as well as oncologists, but we wouldn't go any further. There wasn't any point in it. Pizzo and Poplack had really covered it very well."[37]

At the time, Poplack was already known as one of the premier investigators in the field of pediatric leukemia and cancer pharmacology. He previously had been credited with rapidly advancing the understanding of the central nervous system pharmacology of anti-cancer agents, particularly those administered intrathetically or into the cerebrospinal fluid. An internationally known clinician, researcher, teacher, and author, Poplack was also recognized by his peers as an "enthusiastic leader capable of motivating students, fellows, and faculty to perform at their best level."[38]

When Feigin approached Poplack in 1992 with an invitation to come take a look at the position of chief of the hematology-oncology service at Texas Children's Hospital, Poplack was hesitant. Admittedly, he was curious, but not overly enthusiastic about the prospect of making a move. "I had been at the National Institutes of Health for 20 years and was quite happy with my position," he said. "I headed a large and very productive research laboratory program, was responsible for the National Cancer Institute's intramural pediatric leukemia program, and was deputy director of the pediatric branch of the National Cancer Institute."

Aware of Texas Children's Hospital and the Texas Medical Center primarily through his knowledge of Fernbach's textbook, Poplack also knew Feigin. They had both been honored as distinguished alumni of the Boston University School of Medicine many years earlier. "I remember saying at that time to my wife, 'Gee, isn't it interesting, he went all the way from BU to Texas,' and, of course, I knew about him through his reputation," said Poplack. "So, when Dr. Feigin called, I said, 'Well, it doesn't hurt to look.' I came down and I was really blown away by what I saw. And, needless to say, Dr. Feigin can be very persuasive."

What persuaded Poplack was the stated desire of Feigin and Mark A. Wallace, president and chief executive officer of Texas Children's Hospital, to bring the already outstanding hematology-oncology service to another level, developing it into a nationally and internationally recognized center of excellence. "Their vision to make it the premier pediatric cancer hematology service in the country was music to my ears," Poplack recalled. "It was exactly what I wanted to hear. And, even though I previously had no aspirations to run a service, I felt that I had the experience. And, if I was going to do it, I'd only do it if I had the opportunity to build the best pediatric cancer and hematology program in the country. And Dr. Feigin and Mark Wallace were very, very supportive of that vision and concept."[39]

Although never dreaming of suddenly becoming a Texan himself, three factors convinced Poplack to accept the position: First, he was impressed with Texas Children's Hospital, a "first rate clinical facility on its way up" with "excellent leadership." Second, he was very impressed with Feigin and Wallace's enthusiasm and their shared common vision, with which he heartily concurred. Third, he was drawn there by both the Texas Medical Center, "because in cancer research it is very important to have a large critical mass of investigators and researchers," and Baylor College of Medicine's "strengths in genetics, cell biology, and molecular medicine, the very disciplines that are required to perform first-rate cancer research."[40]

Poplack also was impressed by the strength of the faculty at Texas Children's Hospital, particularly in the hematology-oncology service. "Phil Steuber and Don Mahoney were accomplished and experienced, and both were nationally known in the field, and Ken McClain and ZoAnn Dreyer had also established themselves as outstanding clinicians," he said.

The complexities of childhood cancer required that the pediatric oncologist work as a member of a multidisciplinary team. Poplack found that an outstanding team of nurses, social workers, psychologists, nutritionists, child life specialists, pharmacists, rehabilitation therapists, and specialists in pain management and supportive care was already in place at Texas Children's Hospital. "The key to taking care of children with these diseases is having close interaction between the hematology-oncology service and the other subspecialties, including pathology, diagnostic imaging, surgery and neuro-surgery, radiation therapy, infectious diseases, intensive care, neurology, cardiology, and intensive care," he said. "At Texas Children's Hospital, the sub-specialists are the very tops in their field."[41]

Knowing in 1993 that all of the necessary ingredients to achieve his vision existed at Texas Children's Hospital, Poplack enthusiastically accepted Feigin's offer. He became professor of pediatrics as the occupant of the Elise C. Young Chair of Pediatric Oncology in the department of pediatrics at Baylor College of Medicine and chief of the hematology-oncology service at Texas Children's Hospital.

Poplack arrived in Houston in January 1993 with aggressive plans for expanding the hematology-oncology service. He immediately instituted a five-year plan, with priorities to hire additional clinical faculty, to optimize psychosocial support for the hematology-oncology patient population, and to build a more robust clinical and laboratory research program. Poplack was particularly interested in developing significant laboratory programs in molecular oncology/cancer genomics and genetics, clinical pharmacology and developmental therapeutics, neuro-oncology, tumor cell biology, and tumor immunology.

To increase the clinical support service so vital to ensuring excellent patient care, Poplack recruited some of the finest pediatric hematologist-oncologists in the nation, including Dr. Marc Horowitz, nationally recognized for his expertise in solid tumors. Poplack also developed a strong nurse practitioner program, which later became one of the finest in the country. "We also have been committed to providing strong psychosocial supports for our patients and families," he explained. "First and foremost, one must provide superb clinical care. In dealing with the devastating diseases we treat, it is critical to provide comprehensive family-centered care that is focused on making certain that the patients and their families are supported through their illness. We added social workers, psychologists, and a vast array of patient and family-oriented services to achieve that goal."[42]

Poplack's development of a clinical infrastructure to support clinical research quickly followed. Specific clinical teams were established for leukemia/lymphoma, solid tumors, neuro-oncology, bone marrow transplantation, hematology, long-term survivors, cancer genetics, and pharmacology and investigative therapies. "Each team is comprised of physicians, nurse practitioners, nurses, social workers, and research nurses with unique experience, expertise, and knowledge in its specific area," Poplack said. "This helps insure that every patient receives state-of-the-art treatment."[43]

Another area that Poplack was committed to expanding was the bone marrow transplant program initially created by Fernbach. After designing the new bone marrow transplant unit at Texas Children's Hospital with a unique patient-friendly environment, Poplack introduced innovative treatment methods to increase its capabilities. "The field of transplantation has changed dramatically," he said. "With the new approaches available, such as cellular therapy and gene therapy, we were committed to having the best program anywhere."

To accomplish that goal, Poplack recruited noted scientist Dr. Malcolm K. Brenner and his research group from St. Jude Research Hospital to establish a cell and gene therapy program at Texas Children's Hospital, The Methodist Hospital, and Baylor College of Medicine in 1998. With the inauguration of what soon would become the most innovative and advanced cell and gene therapy program in the world, Brenner predicted, "Centers like this will be at the forefront of a coming shift in the way disease is treated. Not tomorrow, not five years from now, but 20 years from now medicine won't be something you take from a bottle. It will be like surgery was going to be 50 years ago."[44]

Aware of this progressive change—as well as all of the immediate ones—

occurring in the treatment of childhood cancer, Poplack accelerated his original five-year plan. To the surprise of no one who knew him, or his reputation, he achieved these initial goals in less than three years. Poplack attributed this rapid advance both to the fact that he, Feigin, and Wallace shared a common vision and to the extraordinary support he received from the department of pediatrics at Baylor College of Medicine and from Texas Children's Hospital. "We've undergone dramatic growth in the past six years," he stated in 1999. "When I came here in 1993, there were seven faculty members and 42 employees. In 1999, there are 55 faculty members and 430 employees. And the growth has been in all areas—clinical, research, and education."

As for the new facilities built in 1991 for the hematology-oncology service in the recently named Feigin Center, almost two-thirds of the tenth floor quickly underwent changes to accommodate Poplack's vision. "Initially, we had about 4,000 square feet of laboratory space," he explained. "Since then, we've grown almost sixfold. We will be getting additional laboratory space in the future as our research efforts expand."

Although Poplack's long-range plan was an ambitious one, he was confident it could be achieved. "Being a center of excellence, we want to be the place that develops the innovative new therapies that then get transferred into use on a more global basis," he said. "That's our focus. I think we have been extremely successful in recruiting the best young pediatric cancer and hematology researchers in the country to this center. I think we have been very, very effective in that. We have a wonderful group of young researchers now. We are steadily becoming more successful and productive in the research arena. We are highly motivated to find new therapies and to make cure a reality for all children with cancer and blood disease."

With an ever-expanding hematology-oncology service, the need for more clinical space became evident after the 1995 redesign at the Feigin Center. Reconfigured to accommodate an anticipated increase in the patient population over the next decade and renamed the Texas Children's Cancer Center and Hematology Service, the new space was outdated in less than four years. With a 25 percent increase in patients over a two-year period—from 10,400 outpatient visits in 1997 to more than 15,500 in 1999—the space had to be extended along the hallways, reminiscent of Fernbach's overcrowded conditions in the hematology-oncology building in the parking lot during the 1970s and 80s.

The reasons for the overcrowding were multiple. Because there had been only a slight statistical increase in childhood cancer each year, the phenomenal growth that the Texas Children's Cancer Center and Hematology

Service had experienced was attributed to several other important factors. "I think the increase in patients reflected a number of things," Poplack said. "I think it had to do with the increasing visibility and presence of Texas Children's Hospital in the community and the development of Texas Children's Hospital Pediatric Associates. Also, the fact that we're doing our job well and have become noted as a center of excellence, getting referrals not only locally and regionally, but also nationally and internationally."[45]

This increase in the number of referrals to the Texas Children's Cancer Center and Hematology Service at Texas Children's Hospital was largely due to its pioneering development of a variety of important new treatment approaches for childhood cancer during the 1990s. Included among these achievements was the treatment of Hodgkin's disease with cell therapy; gene therapy for retinoblastoma and other tumors of the eye; new intrathecal therapies for central nervous system tumors; a novel chemotherapeutic approach for infants with leukemia; innovative new agent treatments for refractory childhood cancers; and the successful use of matched unrelated donors in stem cell transplants.

There were many other noteworthy accomplishments during the 1990s in the Texas Children's Cancer Center and Hematology Service. More than 20 new research laboratories were established to improve the diagnosis and treatment of children with cancer. Recruited for those laboratories were more than 60 of the finest cancer researchers in the field. Gaining financial support for the increased research activities through federal and scientific granting agencies, researchers at Texas Children's Cancer Center saw funding grow to more than $10 million annually in 2002.

With this substantial increase in research funding, the Texas Children's Cancer Center and Hematology Service became one of the nation's most comprehensive clinical research programs in childhood cancer. New research efforts introduced to the service in the 1990s included a unique cancer genomics program, a clinical pharmacology and developmental therapeutics program, and a comprehensive brain tumor treatment and research program.

Also established was a childhood cancer epidemiology and prevention center, a joint effort of Texas Children's Hospital, Baylor College of Medicine, and the University of Texas M. D. Anderson Cancer Center. The mission of this new center was to identify the causes of childhood cancer through research studies focused on molecular epidemiology, prevention, long-term survivorship, quality of life, and treatment outcomes.[46] "Our real goal is to prevent these diseases," Poplack said. "This is the most exciting time in the history of cancer research, and I truly believe that in the next few years we will be using new genomic-based technologies to identify molecularly defined therapeutic targets for which we will then be able to develop specific therapies."[47]

Poplack predicted that the ability to treat these diseases in a more advanced and comprehensive way would revolutionize the future treatment of cancer in children as well as adults. "It's worth noting that pediatric cancer research is important not only in its own right, but also because of its impact on the entire field of cancer research," he said. "Most people are not aware of the fact that 75 to 80 percent of the anti-cancer drugs currently in use for adult cancers actually were first used to treat childhood cancer. The concept of combination chemotherapy, administering together multiple drugs that have different mechanisms of action but non-overlapping toxicities, is a concept that evolved out of the treatment of childhood leukemia."[48]

Also learned from the treatment of childhood cancer and blood disorders in the past were ways to address the psychosocial requirements of patients and their families. Since repeated clinical and hospital visits over prolonged periods of time are often required for children on cancer treatment, Poplack developed an arts in medicine (AIM) program to provide enjoyable, educational, and meaningful arts opportunities for patients and their families. An annual *Making a Mark* exhibition of more than 200 art, writing, sculpture, crafts, and photography contributions from patients and siblings touched by cancer attracted worldwide participation in the 1990s. Each year, the juried exhibition of artwork submitted from patients at Texas Children's Hospital and all over the world debuted at Texas Children's Hospital and then traveled to museums and hospitals throughout the country. "This exhibit provides an opportunity to gain a unique insight into the experiences faced by childhood cancer patients and survivors," Poplack said. "The artwork is a window into the spirit and strength of these children."[49]

Immediately embraced by cancer patients and survivors throughout the nation, this innovative program garnered enthusiastic participation and support, particularly from Houston individuals and organizations. Such community interaction was not uncommon for the Texas Children's Cancer Center and Hematology Service. In fact, it was routine, with Poplack attributing much of the service's rapid growth to its community partners. "They have been supporting us, our patients, and families over the years and have been phenomenal," he said. "We have lots of them and they are wonderful. And they include the Cancer League, the Thetas, Houston Junior Women's Club, the Parents Against Cancer, Mothers Against Cancer, Candlelighters, Cancer Counseling, the Leukemia and Lymphoma Society, and the Houston Ronald McDonald House, which has been a truly wonderful partner, providing services to our families and supporting research. It's just a great relationship."[50]

Impressed with the generosity not just of the community partners, but also of Houstonians in general, Poplack said: "If you ask me what single thing has made this experience unique, it has been Houston. I came here from Washington, D.C., the national center of cynicism, to a place where optimism reigns. People in Houston have a 'How can we help others?' type of mentality. I think that's what makes this city absolutely unique."

With the optimism of the entire Houston community as his inspiration, Poplack had limitless expectations for the Texas Children's Cancer Center and Hematology Service. Expecting to devote more attention to the further development of research programs in the area of hematology, he planned "to execute the same, excellent research approach that we established in cancer. There is a whole population of patients who we are treating for whom we can improve their lot through increased research efforts," he said. "We eventually want to become as well known for our excellence in hematology as we are now known for our excellence in cancer."

One area in which Poplack already had excelled was education, particularly in the area of a fellowship program for pediatric hematology-oncology. Believing that fellows needed at least three years of training in the lab as a starting point, Poplack established a four-year training program at Texas Children's Hospital. "Previously, maybe one or two fellows per year would be training here and only in clinical pediatric hematology-oncology, not in research," he said. "We have developed a fellowship training program that is one of the most sought after pediatric hematology-oncology fellowship programs in the country. It's very difficult to be accepted into the program. Last year we had more than 100 inquiries for five positions. And each year the number of applicants continues to grow."

Reflecting the phenomenal growth of the entire service during Poplack's ten-year tenure was the new 22,000 square-foot outpatient clinic in the recently constructed Clinical Care Center at Texas Children's Hospital, opened in 2001. Located on the fourteenth floor, this child-friendly, state-of-the-art Texas Children's Cancer Center and Hematology Service clinic included multiple waiting and play areas, as well as the Johnny Klevenhagen Family Education Room and Joan and Stanford Alexander Learning Center. Activities such as arts and crafts, videos and computer games also were available to an ever-increasing number of patients and families. By 2004, there would be more than 25,000 outpatient visits annually at the clinic, with patients' coming from 35 states and 26 countries.

Another expansion in the service took place following the 2003 completion of the West Tower at Texas Children's Hospital. On the ninth floor of that new building, the Texas Children's Cancer Center and Hematology Service inaugurated a 36-bed unit for inpatients. Also in the West Tower and located on the eighth floor was a new 15-bed bone marrow transplant facility, the largest of its kind in the Southwest. Because this unit featured a specialized HEPA air-filtration system, bone marrow transplant patients were able to freely roam around the unit and interact in the unit's playroom and exercise facilities with limited risk of infection. In addition, visitors did not have to wear masks or gowns, making the bone marrow transplant child feel less isolated.

These and all the other attentive details incorporated to assure the delivery of loving care to patients and families reflected Poplack's vision for the Texas Children's Cancer Center and Hematology Service at Texas Children's Hospital.

By 2004, the inevitable steady growth of the service had continued unabated, reflecting both the past and the future at the Texas Children's Cancer Center and Hematology Service. From its 1957 inception in the basement to becoming one of the top-ranked in its field, the hematology-oncology service at Texas Children's Hospital no doubt would ascend to even greater heights in the coming decades.

The courageous battle that Bo Neuhaus waged against cancer was to include more than two years of chemotherapy and three surgeries at Texas Children's Hospital.

Bo had defied his three-month prognosis of certain death. Hoping to help other children who were coping with cancer, 12-year-old Bo decided to write a book. Lindy Neuhaus said that her son hoped that through his day-to-day observations, he could bring his readers "closer to God, to know the power and love of God as he knew it."[51]

He was also able to document his experiences as only a child could. Remembering every detail about his very first visit to the hematology-oncology clinic at Texas Children's Hospital, Bo wrote: "The children did not look very well, they looked strange. They did not have much hair. The nurse fussed at my mom for being five minutes late. That day I got sick late in the afternoon. I didn't think I would get sick. We talked about how I might and probably would lose my hair. We made jokes about my possibly being bald. My mom said she thought it was great that I could laugh about it and that she hoped I'd be a good sport about it when it really did fall out. I said I didn't want to go to school, but my mom said it would be okay. And when it did start falling out it was okay. It itched a lot, but it was okay."[52]

To Lindy, that first visit was "one of the worst days that I can recall. I felt this avalanche of fear coming down on me. It must have shown on my face, because one of the mothers signaled me to come sit by her. She seemed so in control of her situation, and I was awed by her composure. She didn't even seem concerned that her six-year-old daughter didn't have a hair on her head."[53]

The young mother introduced herself and told Lindy that her daughter had undergone chemotherapy for two years and was doing fine. "Having her daughter diagnosed with cancer and told she would not survive more than two months, the mother had decided that she was not going to give up fighting this disease, and that it was this attitude that had gotten her this far," Lindy remembered her saying. "She told me the first trip to the clinic was always the worst and that someday I would feel very comfortable there."

Upon hearing this unsolicited advice and "realizing she, too, could handle the situation and not give up," Lindy also "vowed to myself that I would, someday, do the same for some poor mother bringing her child into the clinic for the first time." The opportunity to assure others presented itself on countless occasions. Bo went to chemotherapy every three or four weeks as an outpatient and spent several days at a time as an inpatient receiving the cancer-fighting chemicals intravenously. "It was an unpleasant fact, but it was bearable," Lindy said.

It also afforded her the opportunity to spend many "almost enjoyable hours" with Bo—mostly because, even in the most uncomfortable circumstances, he remarkably retained his sense of humor. To break the tension during his treatments and even later, when his health was declining, Bo raised his head from the bed, smiled at his mother, and said something funny, such as, "Next time they give you an option of going through this experience, let's turn it down, okay?" Everyone always cracked up, Lindy fondly recalled.

"Humor was vital to our sanity," she said. "As important as it is to laugh during one's good times, it is even more important to be able to laugh during the bad times. Humor kept us from expending our energies worrying about what tomorrow would bring." On the days when Bo was feeling better, the family used to joke about how the hospital must have mixed up the records and given them misinformation about his health. Some other little boy with a similar name was probably the one who was so sick, not Bo, they said. Such joyful jesting amused them often, Lindy and Larry agreed, recalling how the family learned to find something funny in each situation encountered. From irate nurses at the hospital to an insensitive child at Bo's school who made fun of the hat he wore to cover his bald head, every incident provided fodder for mirth.

Comfort and support for Lindy and Larry also came from the other parents and families of children with cancer, as well as the doctors and nurses at Texas Children's Hospital. "When you have inpatient treatment, you really do walk up and down the halls and compare notes with the other families," Lindy said. "One interesting thing, we were meeting with some parents one night, just informally. We all realized that not one of us would trade illnesses or diseases or anything with one of the other parents. Even though this child over here had leukemia with an 80 percent chance of being cured, I wouldn't dare take a chance and trade ours, who had zero chance, with that parent, or vice versa. Every parent agreed."

Another opportunity afforded by Bo's intermittent inpatient visits to Texas Children's Hospital was that of getting to know all of the hospital's staff, whom Lindy and Larry admired and appreciated. "The nurses on the inpatient floor were divine; they were wonderful," she said. Larry agreed, saying, "I thought they were incredibly dedicated. They are what I call 'real doctors and nurses' who are really in it to help you."

One of those "real doctors" during Bo's courageous battle with cancer was Dr. Donald J. Fernbach, the director of the hematology-oncology clinic and director of the research hematology lab at Texas Children's Hospital. "Dr. Fernbach told me, 'You were a pretty spoiled guy until you ran into this.' And I said, 'You're right. I was,'" Larry recalled. "He became my father, sort of. I have incredible respect for Dr. Fernbach; he started that clinic with nothing."

In conversations with Fernbach, Larry often discussed the overcrowded and understaffed condition of the hematology-oncology clinic at Texas Children's Hospital. Once, when Bo had to receive his chemotherapy treatment while on a gurney in the hallway because there were no rooms available, his father found the conditions incredulous. "Here Bo is taking life-threatening drugs, it's 12 degrees outside, and the doctors are coming in and out, opening the doors to the outside right by Bo's gurney in the hall," Larry remembered. "It was just craziness. They didn't have any place to put him. And I thought, 'There's something wrong here.' Nonetheless, they took great care of him, that was the amazing thing."

Bo was aware of his father's concerns about the conditions in the clinic and wrote about them. In his description of the time he was freezing on that gurney in the hallway, he said: "Mom and Dad decided that they were going to accomplish two things: they were going to fix me and they were going to fix the clinic."[54]

What ultimately could not be fixed was Bo. After a valiant two-and-a-half year battle, Bo died in the arms of his mother and father in the parking lot of Texas Children's Hospital on April 1, 1985. Minutes before, too weak to enter the clinic for a scheduled appointment, he mumbled something that Lindy and Larry could not hear. They asked him to repeat what he had said. "He very belligerently answered, 'I'm talking to Jesus!' It was as though he was telling us that he didn't need his earthly parents anymore, that he had found something even better," Lindy said. "It gave Larry and me such security as Christian parents, knowing that Bo went from our adoring arms into those of our Savior, Jesus Christ. There was no fear, no worry, and no agony for him. What more could a parent ask?"

Although Bo had accepted that he would soon to die, his father did not fully comprehend that fact himself. "I don't know that I realized it," he said in retrospect. "I couldn't get it in my head that he was going to be dying that fast. We knew the day he died, but we didn't know before then. You look back and wonder how he lived that long; he was so sick." .

Remembering her son's courageous battle with cancer, Lindy said: "Bo truly believed that God's plan is a perfect plan and there was no reason to question it. With God's help, Bo took a wretched situation and turned it into a beautiful and special two years with a glorious ending. He taught many people, his family included, how to live life and realize what is really important on this earth."

Bo's lessons in living and dying were documented. In 1986, one year after his death, his inspirational book *It's Okay, God, We Can Take It,* which included comments written by Lindy, was published. All proceeds from the book were designated to the research hematology lab at Texas Children's Hospital. Although Lindy and Larry could not fix Bo, they could do something to fix the clinic, as promised. And donating the proceeds from the book was only the beginning of their tireless efforts to achieve that goal.

Since Bo's death, the Neuhauses have devoted their energies to helping other families that have suffered a devastating loss. They offer constructive criticism and advice to doctors about patient care and bedside manner, contribute their time and efforts to the Houston Ronald McDonald House, and raise funds for the Texas Children's Cancer Center and Hematology Service at Texas Children's Hospital. The Neuhauses also established Bo's Place, where children who have lost siblings and other family members can gather and talk.

Their contributions are a living and loving tribute to Bo's short life and to the people at Texas Children's Hospital who prolonged it. "These guys, 'the real doctors,' are the ones in there pitching to do something for you," Larry said. "That's why you stick around and work for them. Even though you lose your child, you know that they did all they possibly could to help you through a terrible problem."[55]

As for the future, Lindy and Larry Neuhaus planned to continue their efforts on their son's behalf for the benefit of other patients at Texas Children's Hospital. "People used to say to me when Bo was sick, 'What will you do when your life is back to normal?' And I thought: 'This is normal.' The hospital, especially with an illness like cancer, becomes your family," Lindy said almost two decades after Bo's death. "So, I think it's a therapy for the parents to continue working with the hospital. It's part of their lives. It really is a part of their lives."[56]

The fact that the courageous spirit of Bo Neuhaus lived on and became a part of so many lives had not been unexpected by the little boy who had never lost his hope or his faith. "I don't know what is ahead for me," he wrote on the last page of his book in 1985. "But I have a feeling that it is going to be great, whatever God has planned for me—whether it's on this earth or in the next life."[57]

18

 INFECTIOUS DISEASES

FOURTEEN-YEAR-OLD MATTHEW "THE BEAST" YKEMA had earned his nickname in junior high.

Fearless on the wrestling mat, where he displayed his pin-to-win determination, and on the football field, where he played the role of hard-hitting linebacker with dedicated zeal, the Beast lived up to his billing admirably. The confident yet easygoing athlete was also known for his dry sense of humor and for his gentleness with children, making him the favorite babysitter on his block.

Very muscular, with broad shoulders and tree-trunk legs, Matt had grown more than six inches in height during the summer before he entered Klein Oak High School as a freshman in 2003. Suiting up for the first football practice on the Saturday before school began, he was enthusiastic about the opportunity to demonstrate his prowess for the coaches and his teammates.

Although playing football in the sweltering heat of August had been exhausting, Matt felt fine both during and after the practice session. Following a brief nap at home that afternoon, he began feeling pain in his knee. Matt was not overly concerned; nor were his parents, Kathy and Rick "Ike" Ykema, who assumed that their son's after-practice aches would eventually disappear.

"When I looked at his knee Saturday night, it was not swollen," Kathy said. "The next day, although he said it still hurt, it was still not swollen and he went to church and to the mall. On Monday morning, he went to school, his first day in high school, planning to see the trainer after classes."[1]

Matt was convinced that he was not badly injured, and the trainer agreed with him. They discussed the possibility of a hyperextended knee, but nothing else, and addressed the pain by treating it with ice. That night, the pain got worse instead of better. "I got some crutches we had at the house," Matt recalled. "The next morning, my knee was puffy, but not swollen, and Mom went to see the trainer before school, who still thought it was just a hyperextended knee."[2]

Aided by crutches, Matt could navigate from class to class fairly well. He soon found that he had another problem. Although usually energetic, he was exhausted and could barely keep his eyes open in class. The only thing that kept him awake was the rapidly escalating pain in his knee. By the time he got home on Tuesday afternoon, the pain was excruciating and all Matt wanted to do was go to sleep.

When his mother awakened him early in the evening, he felt warm to her touch. She decided to take his temperature. "I didn't have a clue at this point that I had a fever," he recalled. "It was 104! Mom asked if anything else was bothering me and I realized my chest hurt as well. At this point, my knee was swollen and blotchy and there was a blotchy ring around my neck as well. Mom called the doctor and he suggested we head to the hospital, just to be on the safe side."

When he arrived at the emergency room of Houston Northwest Medical Center with his parents, Matt was given a Motrin and told to take a seat until a doctor could see him. After waiting for three and a half hours, the entire Ykema family became increasingly frustrated. They discussed whether they should stay any longer. "Mom almost took me home because we really didn't know there was anything seriously wrong with me," Matt said. "When the doctor finally took a look at my knee, he kind of freaked out and sent us right to ultrasound."

Then, in rapid succession, Matt had blood drawn and a CAT scan. He recalled that "when I got back to my little cubicle, the doctor came in and told me and Mom that they knew I had a blood clot behind my knee, a septic emboli in my lungs, and an enlarged heart." There was more bad news. "The doctor also said that I was in septic shock and that it was possibly due to an infection that apparently had gone straight to my bloodstream. At this point, they told me they were going to transfer me to Texas Children's Hospital and an ambulance from there was coming to get me."

When told that Matt would be transferred by Texas Children's Hospital's intensive care transport service—the Kangaroo Crew—his parents knew that he was critically ill, but they did not fully grasp the severity of his condition. "Here we had gone to the emergency room thinking, oh, he'll come home with a brace," Kathy said. "We just didn't understand that he was dying right before our eyes."[3]

The full realization that Matt was the victim of a "new kind of silent killer," Kathy said, was when the Kangaroo Crew arrived in the emergency room. After the intensive care doctor on the Texas Children's Hospital team stabilized Matt for transport, she looked at the Ykemas and said, "If this is what we think it is, by the time he gets to Texas Children's Hospital he might go downhill so fast he will be on a ventilator, so if you want to tell him you love him, you better tell him now."

Both parents were stunned. With great anxiety, the Ykemas watched as Matt was placed in the state-of-the-art vehicle equipped as a portable intensive care unit. Matt's father joined the doctor, nurse, and respiratory therapist on board for the 25-mile trip to Texas Children's Hospital, while his mother followed "inches behind" in her car.

Matt would not remember the journey, or his immediate admission to the pediatric intensive care unit (PICU) after arriving at Texas Children's Hospital. He was aware of being "surrounded by teams of doctors coming in to check on me during the first few hours," but otherwise recalled little except the fact that he was never afraid.

At the time, Matt did not know that he had a severe community-acquired methicillin resistant *Staphylococcus aureus* (CA-MRSA) infection. The aggressive bacterial "superbug" was resistant to the most commonly used antibiotics and could lead to a fatal outcome.

Matt also was unaware that he was not expected to live through the night.

When Texas Children's Hospital opened in 1954, the most common reason for an infant or child requiring hospitalization was an infectious disease.

This was not a peculiarity, but an established pattern evident since the first century.

Documented initially by Hippocrates and continuously thereafter, infectious diseases historically comprised the major cause of sickness and death in children.[4] The first half of the twentieth century saw substantial progress in the care and treatment of children with infectious diseases, but the evolution of the subspecialty of pediatric infectious diseases was still in its infancy in 1954. The phenomenal growth of this dynamic new discipline in the second half of the century closely mirrored that of Texas Children's Hospital, where many of the pioneering efforts took place.

In the 1930s, 20 years before the opening of Texas Children's Hospital, the highly specialized field of pediatric infectious diseases was only beginning to emerge. Areas of concentrated interest were contagious childhood diseases, those transmitted from person to person, such as measles, mumps, chicken pox, influenza, and tuberculosis; disease processes caused by microorganisms, such as bacteria, viruses, fungi, and parasites; and wound and burn infections.

This broad spectrum of infectious diseases had exacted a deadly toll in the United States at the beginning of the twentieth century. The leading cause of child mortality in 1900 was diarrheal diseases, diphtheria, measles, pneumonia and influenza, scarlet fever, typhoid and paratyphoid fevers, tuberculosis and whooping cough. Since the concept of prevention was virtually unknown, only a handful of physicians were in the emerging specialty of pediatrics, and their time was devoted to caring for sick children, rather than those who were well.[5]

The introduction of the compulsory smallpox vaccination in public schools in 1911 marked the beginning of preventive medicine for children in Texas. Internationally, the establishment of medical standards to understand and treat infectious diseases in children began to evolve after landmark microbiologic advances achieved in the twentieth century.[6] The first of these occurred in 1910, when scientists perfected the ability to identify chemical compounds that act selectively to target specific bacterial diseases. This landmark achievement enabled the advent of "miracle drugs" known as antibiotics and a new era of medicine called chemotherapy.

What marked the beginning of the antimicrobial era was the introduction of sulfonamide antibiotics to treat bacterial infections, such as meningococcal meningitis, in the early 1930s. It was the first of the so-called miracle drugs to control bacterial infections. A decade later came the introduction of penicillin, the bacteria-destroying compound first discovered by Alexander Fleming in 1939, and streptomycin, the first antibiotic to treat tuberculosis, a common and serious problem of childhood.

In addition to these new antibiotics to treat infectious diseases, there was newfound scientific knowledge of how the body's immune system protects itself from infections. These discoveries made in the early twentieth century resulted in new tests for diagnosing bacterial infectious diseases and new vaccines to prevent them. In the 1930s, scientists began to grow viruses in laboratories and that newfound ability led to vaccines against viral diseases such as yellow fever and the first effective influenza vaccine, introduced in the early1940s.

Also impacting the morbidity and mortality rates of children in the

United States during the early 1900s was the introduction of specific vaccines invented for epidemic diseases. In 1914, the first such vaccine to be licensed for universal use among children was for pertussis, also known as whooping cough, which was followed 15 years later by one for diphtheria. In 1937, the third, a vaccine for tetanus, was licensed, followed by the fourth, a combined diphtheria-tetanus vaccine in 1938. A decade later, a critical innovation in immunization, a combination vaccine for diphtheria, pertussis, and tetanus, was introduced and its use in American infants became widespread.

With only these few antibiotics, modern vaccines, and medications available for childhood infectious diseases in the United States, the fate of children afflicted continued to remain uncertain during the first few decades of the twentieth century.[7]

After the formation of the American Academy of Pediatrics to promote the welfare of children in 1930, a specific committee was appointed to address prevention procedures for communicable diseases, followed by one for immunization procedures in 1936. Another organization emerged in 1931 with a specific mission to foster research in pediatrics. Named the Society for Pediatric Research, the organization boasted many members with a particular interest in infectious diseases in childhood.[8]

Although the field of pediatric infectious diseases was beginning to emerge in the 1930s, the science of microbiology—the study of bacteria, viruses, and fungi—was also relatively new at the time. Progress was slow but steady, and incremental advances in biomedical research in the United States during the late 1930s and early 1940s were achieved in privately funded laboratories in medical schools and universities.

One such triumph occurred in 1941 at the Washington University School of Medicine in St. Louis, Missouri, where the research efforts of Dr. Russell J. Blattner focused on encephalitis and its cause and diagnosis. Blattner—who six years later would become chairman of the department of pediatrics at Baylor College of Medicine and subsequently the first physician-in-chief at Texas Children's Hospital—and Dr. Florence M. Heys demonstrated that an arachnid, a dog tick, could be infected with the virus and that it could transmit that virus to susceptible animals by bite. The published results of their efforts demonstrated for the first time how a virus persists in an arachnid.[9] Blattner and Heys subsequently showed that the mite could be a vector that permitted the St. Louis encephalitis virus to persist in a community for many months or years. Their continued investigations also concluded that infected mosquitoes could transmit the virus to humans and to other animals.[10]

While other such pioneering biomedical research continued throughout the world in the early 1940s, each proved to be a costly and time-consuming effort. Although several private foundations supported research in specific infectious diseases, only limited federal support was available at the time. Biomedical research in the United States therefore lagged far behind its well-established and generously government-funded European counterparts. But by the end of the 1940s, this no longer was the case.

The impetus for this dramatic change in fortune for biomedical research in the United States was World War II. Even though the health of children became secondary to the war effort, this era marked the advent of unprecedented advances in the field of infectious diseases. During the war, large numbers of medical researchers in the private sector were mobilized by the United States armed forces to join in the government-funded effort to help advance military medicine. Other federally funded wartime efforts, including the Manhattan Project to research and develop the atomic bomb, also recruited countless scientists and researchers from the private sector. The resulting scientific achievements of these collaborative efforts inspired the United States Congress to pass legislation that transformed the relationship between the scientific community and the federal government. Enacted in 1944, the Public Health Services Act became the legislative basis for a major federal commitment to support biomedical research through the newly renamed National Institutes of Health (NIH) and defined the shape of medical research in the postwar world.

Financially supported by the newly empowered NIH, the field of biomedical research in the United States began to grow exponentially in the late 1940s and early 1950s. Having begun with a budget of just over $4 million in 1947, the NIH grants program was to grow to more than $100 million in 1957 and expand annually by more than 40 percent to more than $1 billion in 1974.[11] This funding made possible a growing number of grants to private academic institutions and enabled greater federal assistance in both the construction of research facilities and the establishment of fellowship and training programs.[12] The direct impact of this legislation was measurable, particularly in the field of pediatric infectious diseases.

For pediatricians, the results of the enhanced ability to perform more sophisticated biomedical research were to become increasingly apparent in the postwar years. Immediately recognized in the late 1940s and early 1950s was the beneficial effect of antibiotics in the care of children with infectious diseases.

One of the antibiotics not available to civilians during the war years was penicillin. Even though large quantities of that drug were issued for military use, only a scarce amount was accessible to the public. When Houston pediatrician Dr. Edward O. Fitch learned that this miracle drug had cured soldiers with lobar pneumonia in two days—when the condition otherwise took weeks to overcome, if it could be overcome at all—he knew he had to obtain the drug to care for a Houston child who had been diagnosed with lobar pneumonia. Unable to secure a supply from Brooke Army Medical Center in San Antonio because of government regulations, Fitch was undaunted. Through mutual acquaintances, he was able to secure the required amount of penicillin from Johns Hopkins University School of Medicine in Baltimore. "That child made a quick, and to us, a marvelous recovery," Fitch recalled, noting that it was the first Houston use of the wonder drug that soon would revolutionize the control of bacterial infections in children.[13]

Along with the euphoria that Houston pediatricians experienced after the increased availability of antibiotics in the postwar years came a new-found fear associated with the outbreak of an infectious disease that had no cure or effective treatment. When the first seven cases of poliomyelitis, or polio, were reported during a two-week period in 1948, local pediatricians feared that it was the beginning of an epidemic. Following a conference with the new chairman of the department of pediatrics at Baylor College of Medicine in Houston, Blattner, who had arrived from St. Louis the previous year, the pediatricians concurred that it was not a polio epidemic after all, but rather an unusual occurrence of the disease.

What this group of pediatricians did not agree on was the source or means of the disease. Many believed that it was transmitted by flies and mosquitoes, while others attributed transmission to personal contact. Without the benefit of scientific knowledge as to the exact cause of this crippling disease or how it was transmitted, health officials in Houston sided with the experts, who believed that insects were the culprit. The city began to spray DDT in ditches and public areas and urged residents to clean up and spray their own premises.[14]

In Houston, as in many other major metropolitan cities, aggressive precautions previously instituted to stop the spread of influenza and the plague were also recommended by health officials. Mindful parents dutifully followed instructions to keep their children well bathed, well rested, well fed, and away from crowds.[15] Aware that most polio cases during earlier epidemics were known to occur during the summer months, parents forbade their children to swim in public pools, attend summer camps, or go to a movie in an enclosed theater.

What caused such public paranoia was the memory of the polio epidemics in the southeastern United States in the early 1900s and in the northeast in 1916. Primarily affecting children during the summer months, the epidemics peaked in 1916 with more than 27,000 people disabled and 6,000 dead. Another epidemic in the summer of 1921 illustrated that adults also were susceptible to the debilitating disease, which struck a future president of the United States, 39-year-old Franklin Delano Roosevelt, while he vacationed in Canada with his five children.

Seventeen years later, after extensive therapy that included learning how to stand and how to walk on crutches, President Roosevelt helped found the National Foundation for Infantile Paralysis (NFIP) to "lead, direct, and unify the fight of every phase of this sickness." To raise funds for the biomedical research necessary to help Roosevelt's foundation find a cure for polio, Broadway comic Eddie Cantor suggested during a 1938 national radiobroadcast that listeners send their dimes directly to the president in the White House, an idea that he called the "March of Dimes."[16]

Within three days of Cantor's radio appeal, the White House had received more than 30,000 letters filled with contributions and encouraging messages of hope to eradicate polio. At the end of five months, NFIP representatives announced that the amount of money received at the White House totaled $1.8 million—including 2,680,000 dimes. These funds, as well as subsequent fundraising campaigns, financed the concentrated efforts of the NFIP to achieve its mission to conquer polio through medical research.

One goal of the NFIP-funded nationwide research program was to develop a safe vaccine for polio and to find other possible preventative measures. Because of the pioneering work that Blattner and Heys had previously performed on St. Louis encephalitis, the NFIP provided a grant in 1949 to help fund research to determine where the newly identified poliovirus harbored during off-epidemic periods.[17] Once again working with Heys, who joined him at Baylor College of Medicine in 1947, Blattner and a team of researchers began a concentrated effort in search of answers that proved to be elusive.

When the research grant from NFIP was renewed in 1950, the team expanded to include research fellow Dr. Martha Dukes Yow, a pediatrician in training who had previously served as a teaching assistant in microbiology at Baylor College of Medicine. Both she and her husband, Dr. Ellard Yow, the newly recruited assistant professor in the department of medicine at Baylor, had developed a mutual interest in infectious diseases during the war years while working together at North Carolina Baptist Hospital and Bowman Gray School of Medicine in Winston Salem, North Carolina.

The genesis of their shared field of interest was based on differing needs and circumstances. "Ellard did diagnostic work on patients with infections and began to do special procedures not yet performed routinely in the hospital laboratory, such as testing the sensitivity of bacteria to penicillin," Martha Yow said. Although her lifelong fascination with infectious diseases began in childhood, she initially began working in the lab with Ellard "because such a large percentage of the patients admitted to the pediatric service had infectious diseases. The rapid need for diagnoses in all these seriously ill children led me to begin taking specimens to the lab to study them myself, frequently with Ellard's help."[18]

When offered the two-year research fellowship on Blattner's research team in 1950, Yow enthusiastically embraced the opportunity. The experience marked her introduction to the study of viruses and viral diseases—especially the group to which the poliovirus belongs, the enteroviruses. The myriad diseases resulting from enteroviruses were just beginning to be discovered at mid-century and although Yow "never thought that I would use any of the experience I gained working with the poliovirus again," she eventually devoted most of her career to working with various other infectious diseases resulting from enteroviruses.[19]

Yow and the other members of the 1950 poliovirus research team were involved in a very tedious and laborious effort. Because sophisticated methods of tissue culture were yet to be perfected, the poliovirus had to be grown in a colony of monkeys in the laboratory at Baylor. Dressed in protective clothing and apparatus resembling welding masks, the team worked with the polioviruses, investigating whether flies and mites were the reservoir for poliomyelitis. The results of this dangerous and exhaustive research were to the contrary.

What their work, as well as that of other researchers at the time, did indicate was that humans were the only reservoir for the poliovirus. "I spent two years finding out something that was negative," Yow said. "Just at the end of that time was when tissue culture became available, and that meant you could study polio rapidly and in much more depth."[20]

The landmark development of a method of growing poliovirus in nonnervous tissue took place in 1949 at Harvard. A seminal achievement that garnered John Enders, Frederick Robbins, and Thomas Weller the 1954 Nobel Prize, this breakthrough led to the development of a safe and effective polio vaccine and revolutionized vaccinology. As scientists in the laboratories continued their quest for a polio vaccine in the late 1940s, Blattner and the department of pediatrics at Baylor, which at the time comprised four full-time faculty members, tackled the responsibility of providing care not only for the children, but also for the adults in Houston who were already afflicted with the paralyzing disease. Although space was provided at Jefferson Davis Hospital (JD), the Baylor teaching hospital, for those in "iron lungs," the arrangements became woefully inadequate when a national outbreak of polio reached epidemic proportions in 1949.

A possible solution to the overcrowding at JD came with Blattner's receipt of another generous grant from the NFIP. These funds, earmarked for the establishment of 15 regional respiratory and rehabilitation centers throughout the United States, enabled the construction of an annex to JD for the Southwestern Poliomyelitis Respiratory Center, which opened in 1952. Supervising the long-term patients who required ventilation devices and rehabilitation there was Dr. William A. Spencer, a Johns Hopkins University School of Medicine graduate whom Blattner had recruited from Brooke Army Medical Center in San Antonio.

As the vacant hospital wing at JD was being reconfigured to accommodate the new center in 1950, there was no end in sight for the epidemic. During the next three years, there were more than 57,628 cases nationally, with 3,900 cases in Texas alone. By 1953, the number in Houston had peaked at 783, and JD was the only hospital in five states that accepted "polios."[21] A resident at the Southwestern Poliomyelitis Respiratory Center in 1953 recalled seeing a succession of 42 patients, both children and adults, in 42 days who required iron lungs.[22]

This experience was not unique. The number of patients afflicted with polio began to escalate in Houston and throughout the region. "They came from everywhere," said Mary Owen Greenwood, a volunteer who worked with polio victims at JD from 1953 to 1955. "All up and down the halls we had patients in iron lungs lined up; there was never enough room. The worst part was not knowing what caused it; it was just something lurking out there—an unknown."[23]

This fear was universal among Houstonians in 1954, particularly for the parents of young children. Strangers, friends, and family members shunned anyone diagnosed with polio, or suspected of carrying the poliovirus. Although JD was the city's designated hospital for the care of polio victims, anxious parents who suspected that their child had contracted the dread disease often went to the newly opened Texas Children's Hospital instead.

Five decades after his own childhood experience, one Houstonian recalled how fearful everyone was of contracting the disease and how he had to be secretly admitted for diagnostic tests at Texas Children's Hospital in the dark of night. The necessity of such clandestine efforts underscored the rampant paranoia that existed in Houston at the time, as Yow distinctly recalled at the end of her career. "Of all the diseases I was to observe during my 50 years of medical practice, paralytic polio was the one that created the most terror," she said. "It struck the rich and poor alike, without warning, leaving patients paralyzed for life or dead within a few days."[24]

This reign of terror was nearing its end two months after the opening of Texas Children's Hospital. Heralding its conclusion was the national field test in April 1954 of a vaccine developed by Dr. Jonas Salk at the University of Pittsburgh and spearheaded by the March of Dimes, the new name of the former NFIP. Documented as the largest medical test ever attempted, this mammoth undertaking involved 217 communities in 40 states, including Houston. Involved in the national effort were 200,000 lay volunteers, 20,000 physicians, 50,000 teachers, 40,000 nurses, and nearly two million schoolchildren.[25] Known as "Polio Pioneers," all of the children were inoculated, but only 650,000 of them received the vaccine. The others were given a placebo.

One year later, the resulting success of this unique field test made medical history. On April 12, 1955, officials from the March of Dimes, which had financed the research leading to the development of the Salk vaccine, announced that virologists had declared the vaccine to be "safe, effective, and potent."[26] Shortly thereafter, the first U.S. secretary of health, education, and welfare, Houstonian Oveta Culp Hobby, affixed her signature to the licensing agreement for the manufacturing of enough vaccine for more than three million children. Hobby told the gathered dignitaries and press, "It's a wonderful day for the whole world."[27]

Once licensed, the Salk vaccine rapidly was incorporated into the childhood immunization schedule. Over the following decade, Salk's vaccine, which was given by injection, and a subsequent vaccine developed by Dr. Albert Sabin, which was given orally, had an enormous impact. The incidence of paralytic polio plummeted from 20,000 to less than 1,000 cases a year. By 1988, polio had virtually been eradicated in the United States, with less than ten cases per year.[28]

This triumph, along with the other milestones in the prevention and treatment of infectious diseases, marked the beginning of what became known as "the era of modern infectious diseases."[29] For pediatricians with special interests in infectious diseases in 1955, such as Yow, the scientific advances made in the postwar boom promised a future filled with exciting possibilities for the care and treatment of children with infectious diseases. In what would later become known as the subspecialty of pediatric infectious diseases, the 1950s spawned an onslaught of pioneering efforts.

Soon to be recognized as one of the pioneers in the field, Yow joined the department of pediatrics at Baylor College of Medicine as an instructor in 1955, after a year of pediatric residency at Baylor-affiliated hospitals. When she joined the department, Yow filled the only opening available at the time, that of assistant to Dr. Charles William Daeschner, Jr., at Jefferson Davis, where she "would help run the general in-patient service, but was expected to concentrate on infectious diseases."[30]

Yow's responsibilities for children with infectious diseases at JD included not only outpatients and those admitted to the pediatric floor, but also those placed in the isolation area on a separate floor of the hospital. In addition, she provided consultations to Dr. Murdina M. Desmond in the newborn area and established a small laboratory for clinical research in the cramped space known as her office. Over the following two years, Yow "gained vast experience working with large numbers of children whose disease processes were frequently far advanced."[31]

After becoming board certified in pediatrics in 1957, Yow was promoted to assistant professor at Baylor and named head of the pediatric infectious diseases section, in which she was the only faculty member. Retaining her office at JD, she experienced an epidemic of antibiotic-resistant staphylococcal infections that occurred worldwide in the late 1950s. The infections at JD grew to be rampant in the nursery, as well as other areas of the hospital, in 1957, with more than 324 individuals diagnosed with staphylococcal disease, including 123 newborns and 201 older children and adults. "As head of infectious diseases at Baylor, my husband Ellard coordinated the efforts to control the epidemic," Yow said, noting how the outbreak at JD was probably the worst of the entire nationwide epidemic. "The first thing he did was to establish a hospital infections control committee, one of the first in the nation. This was a stroke of genius. He realized that to solve such a massive problem, the cooperation of many services was essential."[32]

Also spearheaded by Yow's husband was an urgent request for help issued to city and state health departments and to the national Centers for Disease Control (CDC) in Atlanta. The response to this plea was immediate, resulting in a larger laboratory for his study of antistaphylococcal antibiotics and a new research lab for Martha Yow. To staff her newly enlarged area of responsibility, "the state provided money for a technician in my lab and the CDC supplied me with two epidemiology nurses and a secretarial salary."[33]

Joining her husband in the study of antistaphylococcal antibiotics, Yow began her first in-depth study of an antibiotic. It was a new antibiotic, kanamycin, one studied in adults by her husband and in children by Yow. After extensive use and careful assessment of its side effects, the husband-and-wife team determined that kanamycin was highly effective against a number of bacteria other than staph and was responsible for saving many lives. They were soon jointly invited to present papers describing their experiences at the New York Academy of Sciences and the American Medical Society. Individually, Yow presented their experiences in treating children with kanamycin at the International Pediatric Conference in Montreal.

Another result of Yow's successful efforts was measurable in terms of her future career path. "The staphylococcal epidemic not only thrust me onto the national scene, but it also launched me locally," Yow said, recalling how she first began to consult at Texas Children's Hospital and other Houston hospitals in 1958. "I also was asked to consult at a number of Texas hospitals that were having nursery outbreaks of staphylococcal disease and I think it was at this time I began to be viewed as an expert in infectious diseases and antibiotic management."[34]

With this acknowledged expertise, Yow began to obtain small grants supported by pharmaceutical companies to study new antibiotics in her lab at JD Hospital. Her desire to study infantile diarrhea, a major cause of serious illness and death at JD, led Yow to apply for a large research grant from the NIH. After receiving this generous grant in the early 1960s, she and her research team moved to a new laboratory at Baylor, where she established one of the first pediatric infectious diseases research laboratories in the nation.

While most of Yow's pediatric infectious diseases research studies took place at the Baylor laboratory, she continued her collaborative work with her husband at JD until his untimely death in 1965. Also continuing were the consultation rounds that she made at the other Baylor-affiliated hospitals in the mornings and at Texas Children's Hospital in the afternoons. "The pediatric infectious diseases consultation service at Texas Children's Hospital was very small in comparison to the other services there," she said. "Dr. Blattner was a remarkably imaginative person and he decided that the best way to develop pediatrics in Houston was to not duplicate efforts within hospitals, so the faculty member who was head of a section took care of that type of problem in all the different hospitals all over the city."[35]

In addition to these consultations, Yow's efforts in the early 1960s involved diseases such as cytomegalovirus, a congenital virus first isolated in 1957. To care for the afflicted children and to learn more about this little-known illness, she required patient beds in a special area not available at JD. When the Clinical Research Center (CRC), a federally funded self-contained unit designated for research in patients, was established at Texas Children's Hospital in 1964, Yow seized the opportunity to submit a protocol for the study of congenital virus diseases there.

Yow's immediate plans to study cytomegalovirus were circumvented by the 1964 outbreak of congenital rubella, an intrauterine infection of the infant resulting from the mother's contracting German measles or three-day measles during pregnancy. Nationally, the congenital rubella epidemic resulted in 11,000 fetal deaths and more than 20,000 infants born with defects. When the number of rubella-infected infants began to escalate rapidly at JD in the fall of 1964, Yow and Desmond quickly became aware of the need for long-term care of these infants with multiple problems. Many required corrective surgery in the first few months of life to address birth defects of the heart, spleen, and liver. Cataracts blinded many and others displayed early signs of deafness. It also became clear that the rubella virus remained in infants after birth, causing other afflictions and the need for isolation in special wards at JD. "These children encountered one problem after another," Yow said. "It rapidly became clear that we had to make some special arrangements for these very sick infants."[36]

Because most of the terribly ill children were born to young mothers and fathers who could not afford the medical expenses they incurred, Yow and Desmond created an alternative approach for the constant care that these children required. With permission to use grant moneys that had previously been allocated to other protocols and to use a certain number of beds in the CRC at Texas Children's Hospital, Yow and Desmond embarked on a monumental project. Since congenital rubella affected so many parts of an infant's body, they began to recruit a team of experts to care for these infants. Named the Baylor Collaborative Study Group, the team eventually expanded to include more than 18 members.

The coordinated efforts of this group were the responsibility of Yow and Desmond, assisted by virologist Dr. Joe Melnick at Baylor. The multidisciplinary team comprised neonatologists, cardiologists, ophthalmologists, neurologists, radiologists, otolaryngologists, pathologists, virologists, and any other specialists needed by a patient born with rubella. Because the same team of experts saw every patient, "we were able to really see the picture of rubella," Yow said. "By three months into the epidemic, we had worked with 25 rubella babies and were now familiar with what Dr. Blattner termed 'the expanded rubella syndrome' and were able to publish our early findings."[37]

Published in the *Journal of the American Medical Association* in March 1965, this was the first paper on the expanded rubella syndrome and the study represented a major contribution to solving the rubella problem. Because of Yow's involvement in this landmark effort, she became one of the key participants in the national workshops where rubella vaccine developments and control measures were discussed.

Often a topic of conversation at those rubella workshops was the work of the Baylor Collaborative Study Group created by Yow and Desmond. "One of my colleagues in New York University said, 'Well, we've got the biggest rubella study in New York, but you have the best,'" Yow recalled.[38] "Our rubella study was so controlled and the CRC at Texas Children's Hospital allowed us to do such magnificent work. We were in a position to give all these children optimal care, rich and poor alike. And we, with other investigators around the country, were able to define the rubella problem clearly so that within five years a vaccine was available to prevent this terrible illness."[39]

This rewarding experience of working with rubella had a noticeable impact on Yow's future clinical investigations in the CRC at Texas Children's Hospital. When the rubella epidemic subsided, Yow continued to work with infectious diseases in children of all ages, but her research became focused on perinatal infections, those affecting the infant while in uterus, during the process of birth or in the first few weeks after birth. Yow was acutely aware of the possibilities of providing state-of-the-art care for patients and adding new knowledge to the field of pediatric infectious diseases. In 1966, she approached Blattner with a proposal.

Yow—who remained the only faculty member in the section—shared with Blattner her vision of the pediatric infectious diseases section at Baylor and the pediatric infectious diseases service at Texas Children's Hospital. She wanted to establish a service composed of numerous faculty members, each with a special area of expertise in infectious diseases, bacterial infections, viral infections, and immunologic problems. Her plan was to emulate Blattner's technique for building the department of pediatrics. However, rather than send promising residents away for subspecialty training as Blattner had done, Yow proposed the recruitment of outstanding residents to spend fellowship training with her. She would encourage these fellows to acquire additional skills, either at other schools or in the basic science departments at Baylor, and would try to provide faculty positions for them after they completed their training. Endorsing this proposal for the establishment of a fellowship program in pediatric infectious diseases—one of the first in the country in 1967—Blattner also allowed Yow to recruit her first two faculty members, Dr. Mary Ann South and Dr. John Montgomery.

With the arrival of South and Montgomery in 1966, Yow was able to expand the clinical research efforts in pediatric infectious diseases. After turning over the coordination of the rubella program follow-up clinic at Texas Children's Hospital to Montgomery in 1967, she began a survey of children diagnosed with bacterial meningitis at JD to determine the importance of group B streptococcus. When this intense survey grew to include 122 cases over a period of seven years, Yow recalled how "my life was taken over by a new bacterium that shifted my direction on my research."[40]

That new direction was the quest for effective methods to prevent the transmission of disease from pregnant mothers to their newborns. Although group B streptococcus was an organism that rarely caused diseases in adults, it could be passed from pregnant women to their babies, who were at great risk for serious illness such as meningitis and pneumonia. Yow's research efforts also included other agents, such as rubella, cytomegalovirus, herpes virus, and toxoplasma, that were responsible for serious intrauterine diseases that may cause heart defects, mental retardation, deafness, and blindness. Because children could fall prey to these infectious diseases before birth, Yow frequently consulted with obstetricians and neonatologists and became actively involved in the diagnosis and, when possible, the prevention of congenitally acquired diseases.

These consultations in Houston-area hospitals were in addition to the rounds in pediatric infectious diseases that Yow, South, and Montgomery made to Baylor-affiliated hospitals in the morning and to Texas Children's Hospital in the afternoon. As Yow's areas of responsibility continued to expand in 1969, the need for pediatric infectious diseases consultation services at Texas Children's Hospital continued to grow, demanding more and more of her time. "We had moved from Jeff Davis to Ben Taub, and my office was at Baylor, but as head of pediatric infectious diseases at Texas Children's Hospital, I really felt I needed to be based there," she said. "The only way I could get an office at Texas Children's Hospital was to assume some more responsibility there, so I asked Dr. Blattner to let me be medical director of the Junior League Outpatient Department. After one year there, I realized I wasn't accomplishing what I needed to because I was too diverted by the administrative work of the clinic, and I stepped down. I needed to be with the children who were in the CRC, and I needed to be running the lab, so I decided that somebody else who wanted to do that kind of work ought to be doing it, and not I."[41]

Relinquishing her position in the Junior League clinic in 1970, Yow was able to concentrate more of her efforts on clinical research in the pediatric infectious diseases lab at Baylor. As she and her faculty members continued their seemingly nomadic consultations in Houston-area hospitals, they eventually found that most of their time was devoted to patient consultations at Texas Children's Hospital. One such case, the placement of a newborn with suspected severe combined immune deficiency (SCID) in a protective bubble in the CRC at Texas Children's Hospital, garnered worldwide attention. "Dr. Mary Ann South, who was in infectious diseases and immunology, conceived the idea and she has not gotten the credit she should have for that, because eventually he became Dr. Shearer's patient," said Yow. "She and I spent lots of time talking about the fact that she was going to try this before he was born. She thought, of course, that we could try to reconstitute his immunity, something that had never been done before in humans. She was deeply involved, but I kept myself discreet from it. I thought it was important for her to run it."[42]

Both South and Montgomery were among the members of the medical team that delivered the baby straight from the womb into a germ-free environment in 1971. "When David was conceived, we knew he was at risk for SCID and we delivered him by cesarean section into an isolator," South recalled decades later. "David quickly became known as the 'boy in the bubble,' a designation invented by the press. David proved to have SCID and lived in the protective bubble for 12 years before his death. There was a made-for-television movie, The Boy in the Plastic Bubble, starring John Travolta, in 1976, and I was really surprised how that movie oriented people. They remember that, although they don't remember the extensive press coverage of the real David in newspapers, magazines, and medical journals."[43]

With South's and Montgomery's concentrated involvement with David in the CRC at Texas Children's Hospital, Yow became even more determined to establish a permanent physical presence for the pediatric infectious diseases service at the hospital. Her goal was eventually accomplished with the assistance of South and Montgomery and two additional faculty members, Dr. Larry Taber and Dr. Fred Barrett. "All four helped obtain financial support to establish an infectious diseases laboratory at Texas Children's Hospital in 1972," she said. "A sixth faculty member, Dr. Ed Mason, a microbiologist, was recruited to supervise the lab."[44]

Located in close proximity to the CRC in Texas Children's Hospital, the Charles Thomas Parker Memorial Laboratory, named in memory of the late Houston philanthropist by members of his family, was established on February 15, 1972, and opened in 1974. Funded with contributions from Parker's family, friends, and business associates, the laboratory was designed to facilitate the diagnosis of infectious diseases, to study antibiotics for use in bacterial diseases, and to study the prevention, diagnosis, and treatment of virus diseases. By its existence, the new laboratory enabled Yow and her growing number of faculty to apply for foundation and federal grants to pursue special studies at Texas Children's Hospital.

One of the first NIH grants for the new Parker Memorial Laboratory of Texas Children's Hospital came in September 1972. Awarded to Montgomery, it was a grant of $118,000 for the study of cytomegalovirus, one of Yow's major research interests since the early 1960s. Affecting one in every 1,000 infants born in the United States, cytomegalovirus disease could be devastating. First isolated in the late 1950s, the cytomegalovirus disease was congenitally acquired and could lead to heart defects, mental retardation, deafness, and blindness. Not limited to the newborn, cytomegalovirus could cause serious illness throughout life. The diagnosis, prevention, and treatment of cytomegalovirus infection were to become one of the major research efforts of the pediatric infectious diseases service at Texas Children's Hospital.

Another continuing research effort was group B streptococcus. In the 1960s, Yow began seven years of research into group B streptococcus transmission; in the 1970s, she continued to investigate methods of prevention by treating the infected mother with antibiotics at the onset of labor and during the birth. Twelve years after her initial efforts began, Yow completed a longitudinal study of 52 mother-infant pairs at The Woman's Hospital of Texas and the successful results were published in 1979. "This small, intense study led to the funding of a large study in Chicago that proved our method to be effective in preventing group B streptococcal disease in the first week of life," Yow said. "This method is now the standard of care advised by the American Academy of Pediatrics and the American College of Obstetrics and Gynecology."[45]

Justifiably proud of this accomplishment, Yow insisted decades later that one of her fellows deserved the most praise for her life's work with group B streptococcus. "Dr. Carol J. Baker became one of the world's leading authorities on group B strep," Yow said.[46] "I started it, but Dr. Baker hung with it all these years and has the most recognition for it, and she deserves it. I did different things from what she was doing. I was working on the prevention of transmission from mother to baby, and she was working on the immunology of group B streptococcus and whether or not a vaccine could be made."[47]

Baker began her group B streptococcus research as one of Yow's fellows in the 1970s. She continued it as one of the new faculty members in the pediatric infectious diseases service at Texas Children's Hospital. Also joining

Yow's team in 1977 was Dr. Ralph D. Feigin, a nationally recognized pediatric infectious diseases expert and the newly named physician-in-chief at Texas Children's Hospital and chairman of the department of pediatrics at Baylor. Formerly director of the division of pediatric infectious diseases at Washington University School of Medicine in St. Louis, Missouri, Feigin recruited one of his fellows, Dr. Sheldon L. Kaplan, to join the pediatric infectious diseases service at Texas Children's Hospital in 1977. Having previously worked together in St. Louis on an NIH-funded grant for laboratory and clinical studies of bacterial meningitis, Feigin and Kaplan planned to continue their collaborative efforts on this grant at Texas Children's Hospital.

Yow enthusiastically welcomed Feigin's protégé, who was equally pleased to have the opportunity to work with one of the renowned authorities in the field of infectious diseases. By 1977, Yow had served as chairman of the American Academy of Pediatrics committee on infectious diseases and as chairman of the board of scientific counselors of the National Institute of Allergy and Infectious Diseases. She served as the 1974 editor of the *Red Book* and was on the editorial board of the *Journal of Infectious Diseases*. Yow was also a charter member of the Infectious Diseases Society of America and a member of the American Pediatric Society. In recognition of her work with group B streptococcal disease, she received the Jefferson Award from the American Institute for Public Service in 1977. "She was one of the senior established pediatric infectious disease people in the country who was internationally known," Kaplan recalled. "She was a very outgoing, funny, friendly person, who certainly looked out for me, and we always got along well."[48]

Yow also bonded well with Feigin, to the surprise of their peers in the field of pediatric infectious diseases who had predicted the opposite. Mutual respect for the other's expertise was the key to the relationship, evidenced by Feigin's recognition of Yow's previous accomplishments. "Children with serious infectious disease problems traditionally have been well served at Texas Children's Hospital," he stated upon his arrival. "We share a sense of pride in knowing that this institution remains a resource for these patients and is in the forefront of research efforts designed to further our understanding of infectious disease problems so that better methods of diagnosis, treatment, and prevention can be devised and implemented."[49]

The necessity of such future advances in the field of pediatric infectious diseases was not evident to the lay public in the late 1970s. The twentieth-century development of vaccines that were generally effective in preventing tetanus, diphtheria, poliomyelitis, smallpox, measles, mumps, and rubella had dramatically reduced the prevalence of these infectious diseases in the

United States. Together with the reduction in morbidity and mortality attributed to antibiotics developed to treat diseases caused by bacterial microorganisms, these accomplishments were responsible for the widespread feeling among the lay public that infectious diseases were conquered. To the contrary, as Feigin stated in 1978: "Infectious diseases remain the most common reason that children are brought to a physician for medical care. Human lives remain caught in a precarious equilibrium with the microparasites that cause human disease. Infectious diseases remain an ever-present threat."[50]

Rather than eradicating that threat, as presumed by the public, the scientific developments of the previous five decades had instead created new challenges. Many problems remained, and "new disease problems have emerged," Yow explained in 1979. "We might say old problems are presenting new faces and at least three factors contribute to the changing faces of infectious diseases—1) the ability of microorganisms to adapt and change in response to unfavorable circumstances (such as antibiotic treatment), 2) the ability of modern medicine to save the lives of individuals who formerly would have succumbed to noninfectious diseases, 3) and the development of diagnostic tools which permit doctors to diagnose 'new infectious diseases' which may in realty have been with us for centuries. At Texas Children's Hospital, the pediatric infectious disease service is deeply involved with dealing with each of these faces."[51]

Reflecting the growing need for solutions to ever-changing problems, by 1979 Yow's service had expanded to include ten faculty members and four postdoctoral fellows. In addition to Yow, Feigin, and Kaplan, the faculty members included mainstays Taber and Mason, along with newcomers Baker, Dr. Morven Edwards, Dr. Paul Glezen, Dr. Arthur Frank, and Dr. Donald Anderson, named director of the newly established infection control department at Texas Children's Hospital. "All communities and hospitals must be constantly alert to changes in the types of antibiotic susceptibilities of organisms present in their individual environments," Yow said. "The rapidly changing population of Houston and the large number of patients cared for at Texas Children's Hospital from all parts of the world necessitate constant and unusual vigilance. In this way, appropriate antibiotics can be utilized for individual patients and to prevent hospital outbreaks of disease."[52]

Although every faculty member in the pediatric infectious diseases service at Texas Children's Hospital had his or her own special area of interest and expertise, just as Yow first had envisioned when she proposed the new service to Blattner decades earlier, they collectively shared a unified mission. "One of the greatest things about our section is that we all shared the same idealism about dealing with patients and their families," Yow said. "As section head, it was wonderful for me to know that no matter who was on call, the patients would not only have expert medical care, but they and their families would also be treated compassionately."[53]

Each of these specialists in infectious diseases interacted with physicians from the growing number of subspecialties at Texas Children's Hospital. Accurate diagnosis and optimal management were achieved through in-depth consultations and conferencing involving other specialists. "The expertise of a number of individuals from a variety of disciplines, pediatrics, obstetrics, surgery, pathology, radiology, virology, microbiology, and immunology can be brought to bear on a single patient's problem," Yow said. "The changing aspects of infectious disease problems present an unending challenge. The agents capable of infecting humans range in size from ultra microscopic viruses to bacteria of microscopic size to parasites visible to the naked eye."[54]

In addition to the growing number of patient consultations and conferences with other subspecialties, all faculty members of the pediatric infectious diseases service were involved in the detection of new types of infection, the investigation of new antibiotics, and the development of new approaches to treatment and prevention. One of the major problems addressed at Texas Children's Hospital and throughout the world in the late 1970s was the emergence of organisms resistant to commonly employed antibiotics. First experienced during the pandemic of antibiotic-resistant staphylococcal infections during the late 1950s, that unexpected fallibility of one of the miracle drugs introduced in the 1930s foreshadowed an alarming trend. "Antibiotic resistance became increasingly evident in Haemophilus influenzae, an organism which can cause meningitis and bloodstream infections in children, meningococcus, and many other bacteria," Yow said in 1979. "Most startling of all is the emergence of pneumococci resistant to penicillin and many other antibiotics."[55]

Immediately addressing these unforeseen developments were Mason and Kaplan, who performed ongoing testing of alternative antibiotics for particular organisms in the Parker Memorial Laboratory at Texas Children's Hospital. "Pneumococci, the most common cause of ear infections and sinus infections, as well as the most common bacteria found in the blood of children under two years old with fevers, was known to be the common cause of bacterial pneumonia and the second most common cause for meningitis in children," Kaplan said. "The most common organism responsible for bacterial meningitis in children is type b and many strains have become resistant to ampicillin, the antibiotic which is most frequently utilized for this infection."[56]

Other laboratory and clinical studies by the pediatric infectious diseases service at Texas Children's Hospital included the investigation of solutions to new problems encountered among an emerging patient population, one that was distinctly different from any seen in the past. Because an increasing number of children with non-infectious diseases were being cured, or their illnesses were being modified by drugs or surgical treatments, these lifesaving procedures could render the child more vulnerable to both common and unusual organisms. In order to maintain the health of these children with a special risk of infection, the pediatric infectious diseases service at Texas Children's Hospital developed sophisticated laboratory procedures and unusual drugs and drug combinations for their treatment.

Also requiring immediate attention, and partially attributed to the advances made in medical technology, was the emergence of new and unusual bacterial and viral diseases. To facilitate the rapid diagnosis and treatment of these diseases in children, the pediatric infectious diseases service developed specific techniques in the bacteriology and virology laboratories in the Texas Medical Center and the research laboratories at Texas Children's Hospital. Through the ongoing collaboration of Yow and Taber, tools that had been developed in the laboratories were placed into service at the bedside of the patient.

Yow credited advances in the diagnosis and treatment of infectious diseases to these refined laboratory techniques, as well as the introduction of sophisticated radiologic techniques. "Nuclear scanning and ultrasonography have made diagnoses more specific and rapid than could have been imagined a decade ago," she said in 1979. "All of these methods are available at Texas Children's Hospital."[57]

In 1980, little was lacking to advance the treatment of pediatric infectious diseases throughout the Texas Medical Center—except, in Yow's opinion, a comprehensive investigation of congenital cytomegalovirus (CMV), which had remained one of her major interests since the early 1960s. Having only "done a few simple studies of this complex problem,"[58] Yow yearned to participate in a large-scale investigation. That opportunity came in 1980, when she received the Senior Investigator Award from the National Institute of Child Health and Human Development, along with the funding for a one-year sabbatical in the laboratory of CMV specialist Dr. Charles Alford at the University of Alabama School of Medicine.[59] "Few people had ever heard of cytomegalovirus and most doctors did not understand it, but it was the leading infectious cause of mental retardation and deafness," Yow said. "I was thrilled about studying cytomegalovirus infections in mothers and their infants and about learning how to conduct some worthwhile cytomegalovirus research when I returned."[60]

After completing her sabbatical in 1981, Yow hoped to establish a virus diagnostic laboratory at Texas Children's Hospital. But, due to a lack of available space, this was not feasible. Determined to achieve her goal, Yow devised an alternative solution. She accepted a joint appointment as professor of microbiology and immunology and became director of the virus diagnostic laboratory at The Methodist Hospital, established a decade earlier to service all Baylor-affiliated hospitals. After turning over her pediatric infectious diseases laboratory at Baylor to Baker for her continuing studies of group B streptococcus, Yow began applying for grants to pay a fellow and a technician for the study of CMV.

Arranging for a diverse group of physicians from varying disciplines to serve as consultants to the laboratory, Yow predicted great progress in the rapid diagnosis, prevention, and treatment of virus diseases. With the addition of Dr. Gail Demmler, an infectious diseases fellow who later became a faculty member, Yow began to build the strong CMV unit she had envisioned. "Our goal was to join other scientists in adding knowledge that would lead to prevention of cytomegalovirus infection in mothers and their newborn infants," Yow said. "There were many questions that had to be answered."[61]

To achieve this goal, Yow decided to devote the rest of her career to full-time research of CMV. In 1982, after more than 25 years as the first and only head of the section of pediatric infectious diseases at Baylor and chief of pediatric diseases at Texas Children's Hospital, she asked to be relieved of her infectious diseases administrative responsibilities, planning to remain as a member of the pediatric infectious diseases section at Baylor and of the service at Texas Children's Hospital until her retirement. Once again, a disease had determined her future efforts. "My whole career was never planned," she said in retrospect. "It always just was what disease demanded my attention. It was whatever disease said, 'I'm here; you've got to deal with me.' It was one disease after another, and it was never dull. Somebody asked my daughter one time, 'Your mother's a pediatrician, she must love children,' and she said, 'No, she loves germs.'"[62]

Named to assume Yow's former leadership positions were faculty members Baker, who became head of the section of pediatric infectious diseases at Baylor, and Kaplan, who became chief of the pediatric infectious diseases service at Texas Children's Hospital. As Yow and Demmler embarked on in-depth research projects with CMV, Baker continued her studies of the diagnosis, treatment, and prevention of group B streptococcal infections, including bacterial meningitis in infants, and Kaplan maintained his specialized research in *Haemophilus influenzae* bacterial meningitis at Texas Children's Hospital.

Since his arrival in 1977, most of Kaplan's research projects had involved *Haemophilus influenzae* type b, the organism known to cause not only meningitis, but also septicemia, septic arthritis, pneumonia, epiglottitis, ear infections, and skin infections in children six years or younger. Working with specialists Anderson, Mason, and Feigin, Kaplan evaluated new antibiotics for the treatment of all life-threatening *Haemophilus influenzae* infections, particularly the ampicillin-resistant strain first identified in 1979. "We are pursuing studies designed to further our understanding of this infection so that an effective vaccine may be developed that can prevent this disease," Feigin said in 1981. "The crude death rate from *Haemophilus influenzae* infection today exceeds the death rate that was noted for tetanus, whooping cough, or poliomyelitis in the years before immunizations were available to prevent these life threatening diseases."[63]

Considered one of the world's leading experts in pediatric infectious diseases, Feigin was the coeditor of the *Textbook of Pediatric Infectious Diseases,* the first reference text to address infectious diseases in children comprehensively. Published by the W. B. Saunders Company in 1981 and coedited with Dr. James D. Cherry, chief of the division of infectious diseases at the University of California at Los Angeles School of Medicine, the 1858-page, two-volume manual was to become the definitive and authoritative resource in the field of pediatric infectious diseases for decades, with the fifth edition published in 2004.

As this textbook emphasized, the prevention of all infectious diseases through vaccinations and immunizations remained a top priority in the field of pediatric infectious diseases in the early 1980s, but few advances had been made since the 1970s. "If you gave a lecture on vaccines in 1985, it was probably the same one you gave in 1975 about polio, DTP, measles, mumps, and rubella," Kaplan said. "There wasn't much going on until the mid-1980s, and the development of the *Haemophilus* vaccine, followed by the hepatitis B vaccine, and then the introduction of combined vaccines for *Haemophilus.* This had a major impact on patients at Texas Children's Hospital and throughout the United States. It was one of the most impressive changes that occurred in the healthcare of kids because, literally, within months, this disease essentially disappeared."[64]

Between 1960 and 1990, before the introduction of these new immunizations, more than 200 children each year had been admitted to Texas

Children's Hospital with *Haemophilus influenzae* type b infections. "In 1993, we saw no patients with this disease," Feigin reported in 1994. "The number of cases reported in the United States, which was more than 30,000 in 1991, declined to less than 100 cases per year in 1994."[65]

At approximately the same time that *Haemophilus influenzae* type b infections began to disappear in the early 1990s, there was increasing alarm in the field of pediatric infectious diseases about antibiotic resistance, particularly penicillin, in pneumococcus, the next-most-common cause of bacterial meningitis. After organizing a network of eight children's hospitals around the country to survey pneumococcal susceptibilities and outcome information of treatment of meningitis, pneumonia, and bacteremia, the pediatric infectious diseases laboratory at Texas Children's Hospital became highly regarded around the country as a reference lab for penicillin-resistant pneumococcus. "By the late 1990s, about 25 to 30 percent of pneumococcal isolates that come from kids with pneumonia, bacteremia, or meningitis are not susceptible to penicillin like they used to be," Kaplan explained in 1996. "A smaller percentage, maybe 10 percent, are not susceptible to some of the stronger antibiotics, agents we used today on a routine basis to treat meningitis. This changed our whole approach, not just here, but around the country."[66]

Even with the virtual eradication of *Haemophilus influenzae* type b infections and the advances made in the treatment of other infections, most admissions to Texas Children's Hospital in the 1990s continued to be those related to an infectious disease. Referred by general pediatricians, pediatric subspecialists, and surgeons, inpatients included those with serious bone and joint infections, bacterial and viral pneumonia, tuberculosis, meningitis, encephalitis, skin and soft tissue infections, and septic shock. Others suffered from post-operative infections, swollen lymph nodes, and fevers of unknown origins. There were also those with heart-related Kawasaki disease, endocarditis, and travel-related illnesses such as typhoid fever and malaria.

There was another group of inpatients with infectious diseases at Texas Children's Hospital in the early 1990s, one that represented an emerging population of immunocompromised children. Generated by improved treatment modalities in hematology, as well as technological advances in neonatolgy, critical care, and organ transplantation, these compromised children were susceptible to an increasing number of opportunistic viral, fungal, and bacterial infections and required expert management. "We are seeing children in the neonatal intensive care unit who did not survive years ago," Kaplan said. "A large number of patients in hematology-oncology survive now who did not survive in the past, and in the intensive care unit they are keeping children alive who would not have survived several years ago."[67]

In these infected, immune-compromised patients, the specialists in the pediatric infectious diseases service at Texas Children's Hospital concentrated on controlling the disease. "In our case, we can get rid of the infection almost always." Kaplan said. "We are talking about serious infections that we all see when we are on service here at Texas Children's Hospital. Bad bone infections, bad meningitis, encephalitis, bone marrow transplant patients, and other organ transplant patients who get an infection, those are the kind of things we are seeing primarily, as well as lots of infections in the nursery."[68]

A transformation also was taking place in the pediatric infectious diseases outpatient clinic in the late 1990s. In comparison to the diverse and ever-increasing inpatient population, outpatients seen by the pediatric infectious diseases service at Texas Children's Hospital traditionally had been relatively limited in number. "A lot of that has to do with the fact that there's not a large number of infectious disease patients that require long-term follow up," Kaplan explained. "If we're doing our job, we can fix patients who have infectious diseases. It's not like diabetes or renal disease, where you have a chronic problem. There are some infections that are chronic like a bone infection, but even then, you might follow the patient for just six months or a year, not for the rest of their life, essentially, so the need for an outpatient clinic wasn't that great when I became the chief of service in 1982."[69]

When the demand for outpatient consultations for infectious diseases began to escalate during the 1980s, it was directly attributed to Kaplan's efforts. Since his office at Texas Children's Hospital was located on the floor directly above the Junior League clinic, and not at Baylor with the other infectious diseases specialists, he could conveniently just drop down and see outpatients whenever needed. Also available to take calls from community physicians with questions about infectious diseases, Kaplan effectively established himself as an easily accessible resource. "So, for many years I did that," he said. "The outpatient business sort of grew when people knew that there was someone you could call and actually make appointments, and you could get into the clinic."[70]

By the late 1990s, the pediatric infectious diseases outpatient clinic at Texas Children's Hospital had grown appreciably, seeing between 20 and 30 patients per month—including some who required immediate consultations and hospitalization for further treatment. Staffed by one full-time faculty member with monthly outpatient responsibilities, "our clinic primarily focuses on fevers that people are working up and they can't figure out, or funny rashes, or swollen lymph nodes, pneumonias, or outpatient follow-ups of bone infections that we see in the hospital," Kaplan said. "Once a patient with a bone infection is discharged, generally, they are going to be on intravenous antibiotics at home for some time, and we will follow them and see them back in the clinic. We see lots of laboratory reports to help monitor their antibiotic treatments, but that's generally for a finite period of time that could be six to eight weeks, but for a chronic infection, it could be two years."[71]

In tandem with the dramatic changes in patient population at Texas Children's Hospital in the 1990s came an enhanced ability to prevent infections with vaccinations and immunizations. Soon after the introduction of the combined vaccines for *Haemophilus influenzae* type b came acellular pertussis vaccines for whooping cough and the development of the varicella vaccine, the chicken pox vaccine. Conducting clinical trials for this vaccine at Texas Children's Hospital was Demmler, the recently named director of the Texas Children's Hospital diagnostic virology laboratory. "Each advance opens the door to new possibilities," she reported in 1995. "Because the tiny world of viruses has been slow to yield its secrets, viruses often appear to be a fact of modern life. However, as great breakthroughs against bacterial diseases characterized 20th century medicine, vaccines against many types of viruses may well prove to be a high point of medicine in the coming century."[72]

One particular virus slow to yield its secrets was CMV. In 1991, Demmler and Yow, along with Taber, completed a ten-year longitudinal study of 5,000 women and their infants infected with CMV. The research determined that a vaccine would be valuable in preventing severe congenital CMV infection. While waiting for a safe and effective vaccine, Demmler developed rapid diagnostic laboratory techniques and began investigating other methods of protecting nonimmune women of childbearing age from the virus.

When CMV infection and disease emerged as a major pathogen in immune-compromised adults following the advent of AIDS, organ transplantation, cancer chemotherapy, and the use of other immunosuppressive agents, Yow published a landmark editorial in the 1989 *Journal of Infectious Diseases*. "Perhaps the voices of the internists and surgeons added to those of the pediatricians may reach the necessary volume to stress the urgent need for a vaccine," she wrote. "CMV is a NOW problem. We have described it long enough. Now it is time for us to monitor the problem, to educate doctors and young parents regarding prevention, to develop a safe and effective vaccine, to detect infected newborns, and to devise methods of treating this crippling disease."[73]

Following Yow's 1988 retirement, Demmler continued their shared advocacy for the urgent need of a vaccine program for congenital CMV disease. To provide the groundwork for future intervention programs and collaborative research, she helped establish the National Congenital CMV Disease Registry. Sponsored by the Centers for Disease Control and Prevention (CDC) and the Infectious Diseases Society of America and based at Baylor College of Medicine, the registry began collecting information on infants with symptomatic congenital CMV disease born since 1990. "More than 42 infectious disease specialists in 32 cities in the United States and Canada agreed to notify the registry of new patients," Demmler announced. "The registry is a confidential data base of symptomatic congenital disease cases. Data collected by the registry are then shared with the CDC."[74]

Although a CMV vaccine remained elusive, other vaccines were under development in the late 1990s—including those that might prevent pneumococcal infections, as well as a new rotavirus vaccine. "Literally every few months there is an introduction of a new vaccine or a new combination of vaccines that have major impact on patients," Kaplan explained in 1998. "As a matter of fact, one of our concerns and one of the problems is how can you deliver all of these vaccines to a baby, because right now they may come into an office and get three separate shots. That's why the combined vaccines are so important. It's changing at a really incredible rapid pace when you compare to what's going on maybe ten years ago, when it didn't change at all."[75]

Actively participating in the development of other new vaccines were faculty members of the pediatric infectious diseases service at Texas Children's Hospital. "Dr. Carol Baker and Dr. Morven Edwards have been in the forefront of developing a vaccine against group B streptococcus," Kaplan reported. "One of our other younger members, Dr. Flor Munoz, is involved with pertussis vaccine studies. A couple of the people are involved in influenza vaccines, and one of our members is interested in RSV, respiratory syncytial virus. The infectious diseases service also is heavily involved in what is called 'infection control.' Dr. Jeff Starke, whose area of expertise is tuberculosis, is the infection control officer at Texas Children's Hospital and preventing hospital infections is his job."[76]

One such hospital infection became a major area of interest for all members of the pediatric infectious diseases service at Texas Children's Hospital in the late 1990s. "It is methicillin-resistant *Staphylococcus aureus*, MRSA," Kaplan explained. "This particular staphylococcal infection is something that has been the real focus of our research and is sort of an interesting issue among us in infectious diseases. Many of us had our initial careers based on *H. influenzae* type b organism, and that went away. Then pneumococcus became a major thrust, related to antibiotic resistance, and again a vaccine was developed that has impacted this disease pretty extensively as well—not to the same degree as *H. influenzae,* but clearly the numbers of invasive pneumococcal infections are declining. The pneumococcal conjugate vaccine was licensed in 2000. A couple of years before that, we started seeing an increasing number of staphylococcal infections, and now methicillin-resistant *Staphylococcus aureus,* MRSA, and community-acquired MRSA has exploded in Houston and Texas and all across the country."[77]

At Texas Children's Hospital, more than 5,000 children with skin or soft-tissue infections caused by MRSA were seen during the late 1990s and early 2000s—including more than 200 children with life-threatening invasive infections. To investigate such infections resistant to common antibiotics, Kaplan and the infectious diseases section at Baylor and the infectious diseases service at Texas Children's Hospital participated in a nationwide multicenter study designed to demonstrate the safety and tolerance of a new antibiotic, linezolid.

Led by the Baylor and Texas Children's Hospital team of investigators, the study included 52 sites around the United States and enlisted 316 children from birth to age 11, including 63 neonates. "The incidence of these infections is increasing at an alarming rate in children in the community without typical risk factors such as recent hospitalization," Kaplan said, noting that MRSA was responsible for 60 percent of all skin and soft-tissue infections treated in the nation's emergency rooms. "This underscores the need for new treatments for children with hard-to-treat, resistant, grampositive infections. Oral linezolid may become one of the most important options for treating community-acquired MRSA in the future."[78]

By 2004, MRSA infections were the most common cause of bone infections, complicated pneumonias, and muscle infections at Texas Children's Hospital. "Most of the MRSA infections we see in children now come from the community, and it's becoming increasingly difficult to manage," Kaplan said. "This is a real mystery and people are trying to understand that. We are working carefully with a number of groups here in the Medical Center to try and understand that."[79]

What other mysteries lay ahead for the pediatric infectious diseases service at Texas Children's Hospital were unknown, but in 2004 its past accomplishments were a matter of record. From its beginnings almost five decades earlier in 1957, with Yow as its only faculty member, the service had grown to include 17 board-certified infectious disease specialists. It had become one of the premier pediatric infectious diseases services in the country. Since the inception of its fellowship program in 1967, more than 50 physicians had been trained in pediatric infectious diseases. Of these, 28 were in academic positions at 18 different medical schools throughout the world and one was a pediatric department chairman.

Throughout its existence, faculty members in the pediatric infectious diseases service at Texas Children's Hospital served in leadership positions in national and international pediatric and infectious diseases professional societies. Serving as president of the Infectious Diseases Society in 2002 was Baker. The following year, Kaplan served as president of the Pediatric Infectious Diseases Society, a group that promotes excellence in the diagnosis, management, and prevention of infectious diseases. In 2005, Demmler served as president of the Society for Pediatric Research, an international group of scientists dedicated to performing and promoting basic and clinical research that benefits children, a position Feigin had held in 1983. Feigin also served as president of the American Pediatric Society and the Society for Pediatric Research, the senior pediatric research group in the United States, in 1996.

Making major contributions to the field of infectious diseases during the past five decades, faculty members collectively published more than 700 peer-reviewed original research papers. Kaplan, who served on the editorial board of the *Pediatric Infectious Diseases Journal* from 1986 to 1989, was the author of more than 162 original publications and more than 100 review articles or book chapters. He also served as editor of the textbook *Current Therapy in Pediatric Infectious Diseases,* published in 1993, and served as coeditor with Feigin of the fifth edition of the *Textbook of Pediatric Infectious Diseases,* published in 2004.

In addition to coediting that textbook with Kaplan, Feigin published more than 500 journal articles and book chapters. He was the coauthor and coeditor of such textbooks as *Nutrition and the Developing Nervous System* and *Oski's Pediatrics: Principles and Practice.* An internationally renowned expert in pediatric infectious diseases, Feigin continued to serve as editor-in-chief of *Seminars in Pediatric Infectious Diseases;* associate editor of *Pediatrics,* the official journal of the American Academy of Pediatrics; editor of the pediatric division of *UpToDate;* and an ad hoc reviewer for numerous other journals. Often asked to share his expertise in pediatric infectious diseases, Feigin has been a visiting professor at many medical schools throughout the United States.

The beneficiaries of this collective experience were the individual children who received consultations and treatment from the pediatric infectious diseases specialists at Texas Children's Hospital. In 2004—as had been envisioned by Yow four decades earlier—the infectious diseases service at Texas Children's Hospital was comprised of a team of specialists, each with a particular area of expertise in infectious diseases, bacterial infections, viral infections, and immunologic problems. "From a patient standpoint, it's important to know that the infectious diseases doctors at Texas Children's Hospital have experience in taking care of patients with complicated infections because we are experts in many, many areas," Kaplan said. "Not every area, but, we call on each other. I would not hesitate to pick up the phone and call, for instance, Jeff Starke, whose area of special interest is tuberculosis, or I might pick up the phone to call Carol Baker, who is a world-famous authority on group B streptococcus. Or Gail Demmler, a recognized authority in congenital CMV infections, may call me about particular issues."[80]

Inspired by both the past and future pioneering efforts of the pediatric infectious diseases specialists at Texas Children's Hospital, Feigin believed that the twenty-first century held promises of new technologies, refined research techniques, and vast improvements in child health—particularly in the rapid diagnosis and treatment of both old and emerging infectious diseases. "Infectious agents remain large in number, mutate constantly, and effectively develop resistance to therapeutic agents," he said. "The emergence of severe acute respiratory syndrome, avian influenza, and other disorders constitutes extraordinary potential threat to children and adults worldwide."[81]

When Texas Children's Hospital celebrated its fiftieth anniversary in 2004, the most common reason for an infant or child to require hospitalization was an infectious disease.

This was not a peculiarity, but an established pattern evident since the first century.

A lthough critically ill with a life-threatening infection, Matt Ykema survived his first night in the pediatric intensive care unit (PICU) at Texas Children's Hospital.

The 14-year-old athlete was diagnosed with a severe CA-MRSA infection. Not evident externally, the bacteria of unknown origin had infected his blood, causing dozens of blood clots in his leg and lungs and weakening his bone marrow. From the moment he arrived in the PICU, Matt found himself surrounded by teams of doctors from infectious diseases, hematology, orthopedics, and cardiology who administered aggressive treatment.

To fight the severe CA-MRSA bacterial infection itself, there was a regimen of intravenous antibiotics. For the excruciating pain that Matt continued to feel in his leg, there were painkillers. For the blood clots in his leg and lungs, there were blood-thinning medications and a procedure to implant a filter in his inferior vena cava (IVC) to prevent further infected clots from reaching his lungs. Throughout it all, Matt retained his sense of humor.

When Dr. Sheldon L. Kaplan, the chief of pediatric infectious diseases at Texas Children's Hospital, first examined him and asked whether he was experiencing pain in areas other than his leg, Matt groaned and said, "Yes, in my stomach," and Kaplan grew concerned. "What kind of pain is it, sharp, achy, exactly what?" Kaplan asked. When Matt replied, "No, not that kind, I am just hungry and they do not allow me to eat," everyone laughed.

Many such unexpectedly light-hearted moments occurred during the harrowing two weeks that Matt spent in PICU, but he could recall only a few afterwards. However, he did not forget "a lot of stuff that happened, like I didn't like all that prodding, but I was on heavy-duty pain meds so I don't remember it all," he explained. "I remember a lot of the procedures they had to do on me, like the arterial lines and the catheter PICC lines, and when they drained fluid from my knee. But what I remember most are the PICU nurses, they were the best."

Among his fondest memories was how one PICU nurse solved a recurring problem. "Lorien Martinez made me a wonderful new invention," Matt said. "The bedpan I had to use the first few days was hard and cold, so Lorien took those gel pads that are used under pressure points for a patient in bed and taped them to the bedpan. She and my mom nicknamed it 'the cushie tushie.'"[82]

Another cobbled-together invention by one of the nurses enabled Matt to venture outside the PICU for a brief period of time. "I was really, really sick and had been in the hospital only a few days when some of my friends came to see me," he said. "My wonderful nurse Deborah Ybarra commandeered a pair of scrubs and cut them off so they would work for me. It was very difficult to get me out of bed into a wheelchair because I was hooked up to all of those machines, but Deborah was determined I would get to see my friends that day and that's exactly what I did."

This above-and-beyond care was greatly appreciated by Matt's family. "Two weeks is a long time in PICU," said Kathy Ykema. "The nurses there were wonderful and attentive to Matt and to me and my family. We were always informed of Matt's prognosis and progress and I loved the way they called me 'Mom.' It was something that was so very simple, but when your child is dying right before your eyes, it was a precious reminder of the most prized position, that of being a mom."[83]

Also making a lasting impression on Kathy was the entire care-giving team at Texas Children's Hospital. "The doctors treated Matt like he was their only patient," she said. "While discussing some of the serious decisions we had to make, many of which could have serious complications, Dr. Kennedy, who was heading up all the disciplines in the PICU, was so genuinely concerned that he sat and cried with us. Tears ran down his cheeks as we agreed on the best route to take. What an incredible sign of real compassion!"

The Ykemas found that such compassionate care continued after Matt was moved out of PICU and into a patient room at Texas Children's Hospital. During the following four weeks, Matt underwent numerous surgeries and procedures on his knee and continued to receive treatment for the bacterial infection in his blood and bones. He instantly made friends with all the doctors and nurses and "wasn't overly anxious to get home," he recalled. "Mom says I have a content character and I guess I just dealt with the hospital the best I could. Everyone was really nice to me, and my friends came to visit all the time. It also gave me a lot of time to think about how valuable life is and how much time you need to spend with your family."[84]

During his six-week stay at Texas Children's Hospital, Matt had to accept the fact that he could never participate in contact sports again. "My hematologist, Dr. Donald H. Mahoney, is very protective of my health," he explained. "The major reasons I can't participate are the IVC filter and the blood thinners. I have more of a problem not being able to wrestle than football. I love to wrestle, but I can participate in non-contact sports and I am starting to take scuba-diving lessons."

When Matt was finally released from Texas Children's Hospital, he "made the transition with much grace and dignity," Kathy said. "Not a day goes by where we're not just tickled silly to know Matthew is just a walking miracle.[85] It would have been great to do without this entire experience, but, given the circumstances, we could not have orchestrated it better or handpicked a better team. Great docs, great nurses, great hospital, and a great God that placed them all in our path for such a time as this."[86]

Having survived such a life-threatening ordeal, Matt advised others who might find themselves in a similar situation to "have a good sense of humor and a great faith in God," and to "pray a lot" as he and his family had.

Several years later, Matt had fully recovered from the effects caused by the severe CA-MRSA infection and was in perfect health. Nonetheless, he continued to see Mahoney, his hematologist, at Texas Children's Hospital for periodic checkups. After returning to school and becoming manager of the wrestling team at Klein Oak High School, the healthy 17-year-old was awarded a letterman jacket with his nickname embroidered on the back.

But instead of "the Beast," the moniker he had earned from friends in junior high, Matt's jacket boasted a name he bestowed on himself after coming home from Texas Children's Hospital: "Miracle Man."

"Nobody calls me that," Matt said with a twinkle in his eye. "I just want them to know that's what I am."

19

 JUNIOR LEAGUE OF HOUSTON

WHEN VIRGINIA HOLT MCFARLAND received a social invitation in 1955, she never expected it to have lifelong consequences.

But McFarland's decision to accept that invitation and become a member of the Junior League of Houston, Inc., had exactly that effect. The socially prominent women's organization was committed to promoting voluntarism, developing the potential of women, and improving the community. Upon joining the Junior League, the young housewife and mother embraced its altruistic mission as her own. Even though the long-term effects of this conversion were not foreseeable at first, they were to have a significant impact on the future of Texas Children's Hospital.

As a new member—known as a "provisional"—of the Junior League, McFarland was required to complete the extensive training course; work for four months in the Junior League tea room, the league's fund-raising restaurant operation; and volunteer for four months in one of the organization's numerous community projects. "We were given a choice of community projects," McFarland recalled. "I heard representatives from the entire community speak, and when Frances Heyck spoke about the Junior League Diagnostic Clinic of the outpatient department at Texas Children's Hospital, I knew that's where I wanted to be. I didn't want to be anywhere else. There never was a question about it. I went there like a homing pigeon."[1]

It was, in fact, a return to one of McFarland's previous roosts. She and husband Russell had become intimately familiar with Texas Children's Hospital when their late son Scott was a patient there in 1954, the year the hospital opened. "In the late 1940s, when Scott first became ill, he was a patient of Dr. Lane Mitchell, who soon realized it was something of a particular nature that he did not have the expertise to deal with. He said, 'Dr. Russell Blattner is here and I would like him to see Scott.' Dr. Blattner came to our apartment, climbed up the stairs, talked to us for a few minutes, looked at Scott, and he told me, 'I think this child has nephrosis or a form of metabolic disease. I cannot do with it what should be done. But very fortunately, there is a wonderful young man who has just come here from Children's Hospital Boston, Bill Daeschner.' Bill had studied with Charles Janeway at Boston, the foremost authority at that time of metabolic illness in children, particularly nephritis and nephrosis," McFarland remembered. "And so we did go to see him at Baylor, over in the old red-tiled-roof building, the only one there at the time. And Scott was given an experimental drug therapy at Baylor and was Bill's patient from then on."[2]

It also was the beginning of a lifelong friendship between the McFarlands and Daeschner. "I owe Bill Daeschner and Dr. Mitchell a vote of gratitude for the rest of my life," McFarland said. "They realized that it would help me and help everybody if I could be involved in Scott's care more intelligently, more on an active level. So they got a blood pressure manometer for me and a stethoscope and taught me how to measure Scott's blood pressure."

Daeschner, in turn, was full of praise for McFarland: "Ginny is one of those extremely remarkable people that there just aren't any others like her. She can retain her objectivity in the face of all sorts of emotional stress and pressures. Their son had a nephrotic type of chronic glomerulonephritis. At that time, and I doubt even today that we would have been able to interrupt the course. He probably would have become a candidate for a transplant today."

While making two rounds a day to see Scott at the hospital, Daeschner recalled, McFarland always had a list of questions for him. "They were not foolish questions at all. They always went right to the heart of the matter. You wonder how she knew enough about the disease to ask such intelligent questions," he said. "And so it just came naturally to teach her all that we could. She learned, and she tested his urine, and she kept records, and, as I say, she's one of these quick-learn people. You know, had she gone to medical school, she would have been an outstanding physician, because of her ability to learn, and the speed with which she learned is just short of phenomenal. I never had a nephrotic parent who knew the ins and outs of the condition and everything like Ginny did. Yet, she always had time to be helpful to all the other patients around and was just a very special person."[3]

It was that innate desire to be helpful to other patients and their families, together with her interest in medical care, her ability to learn quickly, and her respect for the medical profession that beckoned McFarland back to Texas Children's Hospital—not only while a provisional member of the

Junior League of Houston, but also ever since. "I never have deviated from the time I was a provisional," she said in 2000.

This is not to say that McFarland limited her focus. Instead, she continually expanded it. From her first moments at the Junior League Diagnostic Clinic of the outpatient department at Texas Children's Hospital, McFarland endeavored to learn all there was to know. Quickly bored with the routine duties of weighing patients, taking temperatures, and assisting with other assigned chores in the clinic, she soon was volunteering to help the physicians with more complicated medical procedures. "Luckily, I worked on Saturday morning with George Clayton and Bill Daeschner," she said. "They seemed to know that I could do a little bit and they trusted me to do a few things and they taught me to do a few things, all very rudimentary things because I had no medical skills at all. But they knew they could depend on me to do what I said I'd do. So, I would take the urine samples and I would do the tests to see if there was diabetes or if there was sugar. I was taught to do things about BUN, which was the blood urine nitrogen level in the urine. Very simple things like that. And then they gradually moved me up to entering things in the chart, which I was allowed to do when they told me exactly what to put in."

McFarland also studied and absorbed the intricate details of running the Junior League Diagnostic Clinic of the outpatient department at Texas Children's Hospital. She observed and learned how Frances Heyck skillfully interviewed the hundreds of medically indigent patients, ascertaining the clinic's sliding-scale fees for each. Once again McFarland proved to be a quick study, an accomplishment she attributed to those who taught her. "Frances was an incredible teacher and mentor; she clued me in on so many things," McFarland said. "I would sit in her office and she would interview patients to be taken in as partial pay, full pay, or whatever. And she would work with them with such sensitivity and such kindness, yet with a good grasp of business as well. She counseled them, worked with them, and did a variety of things in helping a patient come into the hospital to receive service. I learned a lot from her."

With this newfound knowledge and an obvious grasp of the intricacies of the clinic's inner workings, McFarland was asked to become chairman of the Junior League Diagnostic Clinic of the outpatient department at Texas Children's Hospital in 1958. It was a role that she expertly performed for two years, serving as a consultant for several years afterwards. "That was back in the dark ages," she said, laughing. "There was a dim light bulb in the basement where I had to go down and pick up charts. It also was when I would come home and take off my pink uniform in the garage and drop it into the washing machine, because I was afraid I might bring some infection into the house. They don't worry about that kind of transmission of disease anymore."

Such a change in thinking served as an example of the many revisions in medical care McFarland was to experience firsthand. Committed to finding new ways to serve the children in the community who needed help, she pursued her quest relentlessly. Always anxious to learn the newest course of action, she was never reticent to discard obsolete methods.

McFarland's admirable ability to adapt easily to change—a virtue that she shared with the Junior League of Houston—was one that did not go untested at Texas Children's Hospital.

F ounded by 12 Houston women in 1925, the Junior League of Houston was the first organization to provide healthcare services for underprivileged children in the Houston community.

Opening in 1927 and located in the basement of the First National Bank Building in downtown Houston, the Junior League Children's Health Clinic was the organization's first charitable project. This vital community effort was inspired by the charter league members, many of whom were young mothers, who recognized the lack of health services available for disadvantaged children in Houston.

Initially a free well-baby clinic, the Junior League Children's Health Clinic emphasized prenatal care and the prevention of illness. The center was staffed with one full-time physician and a full-time secretary, supplemented by a Junior League volunteer who assisted each morning from 10 a.m. until noon.

After offering aid to those families who could not afford medical treatment during the Depression, the center had expanded its parameters and services in 1931 to include care for medically indigent children who were ill. It provided free tonsil and adenoid operations and treatment for non-contagious diseases in children under the age of ten. "There were a lot of people in Houston who were able to pay all their bills, except those for emergency medical needs," recalled Junior League member Adele Peden, a former clinic secretary. "I think you might say this is where the idea of being 'medically indigent' versus just plain 'indigent' came into being."[4]

The services offered by the Junior League Children's Health Clinic were unique and much needed, serving 60 new patients each month. Yet members of the league realized that the clinic was isolated from and ignored by other social agencies in the city. To remedy the situation, in 1932 the Junior League established a working relationship with the newly opened Hermann Hospital, an endowed institution that provided free medical care for the eligible sick in Houston and Harris County.

Hermann Hospital agreed not only to pay for the clinic's rent, gas, light, and heat bills, but also to provide free hospitalization and laboratory work and discounted X-rays. On November 1, 1932, the Junior League Children's Health Clinic moved into the Junior League's new headquarters on Stuart Street. As part of the agreement, the clinic began furnishing a public health nurse to do follow-up work on all of the hospital's obstetrical cases. In addition, the clinic began an educational program instructing new mothers in the care of infants and in first aid.

The Junior League Children's Health Clinic on Stuart Street also increased its free services to medically indigent children. With the volunteer help of five pediatricians and nurses from the staff of Hermann Hospital, a full-time physician no longer was required. The clinic's staff now comprised a full-time secretary and two Junior League volunteers on duty daily—one to handle medical records and the other to assist the doctors and nurses during clinic hours. Open from 9 a.m. until 3 p.m. each day for appointments and two hours each day for treatments, the clinic attracted 109 patients in one of its first months of operation. "Our experiences have proved that our hope of enlarging our sphere has been more than justified," wrote a Junior League volunteer in a 1933 status report. "The welfare agencies are co-operating with us and the principals of the public schools in the poorer districts have begun sending us patients. Our preventative work is at last becoming a reality. We feel that we are on a sound basis, with expansion insured, and we feel that we are establishing the future for hundreds of children in Houston."[5]

With a steady increase in patient flow, the new clinic concentrated on children's preventative care by offering light treatments, whooping cough vaccine, tuberculin tests, small-pox vaccinations, Schick tests, tetanus anti-toxin, thymus treatments, metabolism tests, and countless other treatments.

Continuing to enhance its services over the next decade, the Junior League Health Center on Stuart Street began offering the services of attending specialists. The Junior League paid these professionals $5 per day for their services. Neurologists, allergists, dentists, laboratory technicians, and eye, ear, nose, and throat specialists were among those available.

Although patients were not charged a fee for services, there were some who could not afford to pay for prescriptions or special care. This was a problem that Junior League volunteers at the clinic were anxious to solve. Consequently, the Junior League Memorial Fund was officially established when one of those volunteers, Nellie Black, decided to make a financial contribution for that purpose on March 4, 1942. Black began encouraging others to do the same. Once established, the Junior League Memorial Fund immediately enabled the clinic secretary to give needy children the money necessary to buy medical services and supplies, including medicines, special tests, equipment, and transportation.

During the war years, Junior League provisionals were required to work in the clinic as part of their training. Provisionals also participated in the newly launched weekly story hour created for hospitalized children. Although settled into a restricted, though busy, routine by 1943, the volunteers soon discovered that the Junior League Children's Health Clinic was about to undergo another change. This occurred when Dr. George W. Salmon, the acting head of the pediatrics department at Houston's new Baylor College of Medicine, began supervising pediatric services at Hermann Hospital and the Junior League Children's Health Clinic on Stuart Street.

Because there were fewer physicians available during the war years, Salmon sought to improve the efficiency and quality of healthcare provided at the Junior League Children's Health Clinic. His idea was to move the clinic into the outpatient department of Hermann Hospital, a suggestion that was accepted unanimously by the Junior League membership. On December 1, 1944, the Junior League Health Center changed its name and its location and became the Junior League Children's Health Clinic of Hermann Hospital Outpatient Department.[6]

After combining efforts with the pediatric clinic at the hospital, the Junior League Children's Clinic began providing both well-baby and sick-baby services on a sliding-fee scale to medically indigent children. Offering free and part-pay care, the combined clinics became teaching areas for senior medical students at Baylor College of Medicine and also served as the principal diagnostic outpatient clinic in the Texas Medical Center for the treatment of children's diseases.

As the first volunteer organization to work in Hermann Hospital, the Junior League soon capitalized on new opportunities to be of service to both patients and the health community. Concerned about those medically indigent children who had to be separated from their parents and admitted as patients in the hospital, the Junior League created a special ward program. A retired teacher was hired to come in every day to engage Junior League volunteers in bedside play activities with the children in the multi-bed wards, helping allay the children's anxiety and fear of being alone. A distant forerunner of the 1970s program known as child life, it was a revolutionary concept in 1945 and marked the beginning of the Junior League volunteers' one-on-one involvement with inpatients.

Junior League volunteers also became more involved in the rapidly growing clinic, where their services always were in demand. As an integral part of the teaching and research departments of Baylor College of Medicine, the clinic expanded its services to six days a week, 12 months a year, and changed its emphasis from preventative healthcare to developing new methods of diagnosing and treating children's diseases, often with dramatic results.[7] "The very first heart operation in Houston was on a Junior League Children's Clinic child at Hermann Hospital in February 1944," said Frances Heyck, that clinic's secretary at the time. "And the Junior League Memorial Fund helped finance the surgery by providing three weeks of around-the-clock special nursing for the child afterward. Because, in those days, that's the way you took care of patients after hospital surgery, there was no recovery room then."[8]

Decades later, Heyck still had vivid memories of the child who underwent Houston's first heart operation. "She was about nine years old and she was so crippled, so blue," she said. "Her fingernails were all clubbed. She was totally incapacitated. She was very crippled and, because of the lack of oxygen, mentally retarded. So Dr. Salmon operated on her."

The procedure was performed by Dr. Howard Barkley, a Houston chest surgeon; Dr. Don Chapman, Houston's first adult cardiologist; and Salmon. This history-making surgery took place within months of the first successful one, the 1944 Blalock-Taussig "blue baby" operation at Johns Hopkins Hospital. Salmon, who had asked Barkley and Chapman to study the intricacies of the new procedure, recruited those doctors to perform the surgery. "Dr. Salmon was one of the pioneers in bringing good pediatric care to Houston," Heyck said. "And this little girl lived to be 21 years old, we followed-up on her every year. She was able to get out of bed. She was able to attend a special school. She was able to lead a fairly normal life. So, we did indeed not only extend her life, but give her a certain semblance of normality within her limitations."[9]

For Heyck, a member of the Junior League who had first volunteered in the Stuart Street clinic in 1943 and later became its part-time professional secretary, there were many vivid memories of the first few years at Hermann Hospital. Of particular interest were the many healthcare innovations introduced at the Junior League Children's Clinic. "It was fascinating because this was when all the newest antibiotics were introduced," she said. "And so, guess whose patients got the first antibiotics? It was our clinic patients. And when they discovered the first antibiotic, streptomycin, to help influenzal meningitis, Dr. Salmon would say, 'Okay, Frances, you do the fever grafts for me, do the charts.' It was fascinating. They'd start these kids on streptomycin. The fever would be way up there, and it would just come down. And I did all those charts for him. I learned real quick how wonderful it was being a part of a teaching and research service."

Intrigued with the advances in medical care that she was witnessing, Heyck was soon also working part-time in the nursing department of the Red Cross and in the record room at Hermann Hospital. In addition to her clinic duties, she served as Salmon's secretary on a voluntary basis at Baylor College of Medicine—a job she parlayed into becoming the paid part-time secretary to the department of pediatrics in 1947. "I just sort of eased in," she said, remembering her enthusiastic and progressive entrenchment in the medical milieu.[10]

Heyck's enthusiasm and interest never wavered or waned, but rather increased. As secretary to both Dr. Russell J. Blattner, the newly arrived head of the department of pediatrics at Baylor, and the Junior League Children's Clinic, she found herself to be not only an eyewitness to the planning stages of Texas Children's Hospital, but also an active participant.

As a Junior League member, Heyck was aware that Dr. David Greer had asked the organization to support the building of a children's hospital, an idea conceived by Greer and the Houston Pediatric Society. She was also familiar with the Junior League's efforts to promote the Pin Oak Charity Horse Show in 1947, and its successful selling of tickets and program advertising. Heyck was proud of the fact that the funds raised by those efforts were donated to the Texas Children's Foundation and subsequently underwrote the extensive and lengthy tour of children's hospitals in North America taken by Blattner, her boss at Baylor College of Medicine.

In her position as secretary to Blattner, Heyck was involved in the preliminary planning of Texas Children's Hospital. "When plans for the building began to take shape around 1949–1950, provisions were made for a large outpatient department in one wing of the new hospital," she recalled. "It was planned that its primary function as a referral clinic would be to develop various specialized clinics to help medically indigent parents provide care for the more complicated types of children's diseases. At the same time, the outpatient department would serve as a coordinating center for the teaching and research program to be carried on at the hospital."[11]

It was necessary to determine who would be responsible for the charity outpatient program at Texas Children's Hospital. According to Heyck, Blattner proposed that the board of trustees of Texas Children's Hospital request the Junior League of Houston to move its existing pediatric program from Hermann Hospital. This would avoid any duplication of efforts.

When the Texas Children's Hospital board formally invited the Junior League of Houston to join forces with the new hospital, president Lida Edmundson accepted "with great pride" in June 1953. Not only did the Junior League agree to serve as volunteers in the Junior League Diagnostic Clinic of the outpatient department at Texas Children's Hospital, it also offered $8,000 as a financial gift to the hospital for the first year. In addition, the organization would contribute to the salaries of the pediatrician in charge, as well as the secretary for the clinic. Thus, the Junior League made a financial promise to the new hospital, as well as its commitment of time.[12]

While continuing to provide a well-baby clinic at Hermann Hospital, the Junior League of Houston made a focused effort at Texas Children's Hospital "to provide medically indigent parents with special diagnostic care for their sick children and to provide special clinical material for teaching and research purposes." In this way, pediatricians in the Baylor College of Medicine program had an opportunity to see a wide variety of patients needing medical attention, thus learning while simultaneously providing treatment.[13]

Once the Junior League clinic's move was approved, a redirection of efforts was in order for Heyck. Relinquishing her part-time secretarial position at Baylor College of Medicine, she became full-time executive secretary of the newly relocated and renamed Junior League Diagnostic Clinic of the outpatient department of Texas Children's Hospital in 1954—a position she would hold for 20 years.

Financial support for the new clinic came not only from the board of Texas Children's Hospital and from the Junior League, but also from the patients themselves. Heyck assumed the responsibility of screening patients to determine their needs and their ability to pay. In 1954, clinic patients paid somewhere between 50 cents and $1 to see a physician. Charges for diagnostic tests were more. Based on a sliding-fee scale, some patients were part-pay, some were full pay, and some were free, but all received medical care and attention.

Many patients and their families in the Junior League Diagnostic Clinic of the outpatient department at Texas Children's Hospital received financial support from the Junior League Memorial Fund, managed and directed by Heyck. Continuing the mission with which it was established in 1942, the fund helped pay for patients' medicines, eyeglasses, special nursing care, transportation, and whatever else was deemed necessary.

In addition to providing 43 trained volunteers to work in the clinic, the Junior League made an annual monetary contribution to the board of Texas Children's Hospital for overall maintenance and also contributed towards the salaries of Heyck and Dr. Fred M. Taylor, the medical director of the outpatient department.

Under Taylor's direction, referred outpatients first were seen in the Junior League Diagnostic Clinic, a general pediatric medical clinic for outpatient consultation, examination, and laboratory study. When the patient's medical problem was satisfactorily solved, he or she was sent back to the referring source. If further diagnostic study and treatment was required, the patient was then sent to one of the specialty clinics, which offered highly specialized care for the solution of obscure problems. Although there were no restrictions regarding race, creed, color, or length of residence in Houston, all of the clinics limited patients to those 14 years of age and younger—and all had to be referred.

"In contrast to other major facilities in the city which cope with the large volume of routine health problems in the overall pediatric program, the Junior League Diagnostic Clinic reserves its facilities for the medically indigent patient and provides an unusual opportunity for giving consultation and special care to the referred child," Taylor explained in 1957. "By restricting the patient load to special consultations and to referral cases, the clinic personnel are able to provide sufficient time and adequate attention to each and every patient."[14]

Even though it was an innovative approach to the complex diagnostic and treatment problems of children, the Junior League Diagnostic Clinic of the outpatient department opened in 1954 with 11 highly specialized clinics, staffed by volunteer specialists in pediatrics and other medical sciences and the full-time faculty of Baylor College of Medicine and assisted by trained Junior League volunteers.

"The individual clinics were dental; eye; heart; metabolic and endocrine; urology; ear, nose, and throat; allergy; surgery; hematology; neurosurgery; and celiac, the fibrocystic disease of the pancreas," Heyck recalled. "Each volunteer was obligated to take a training course in the various clinics in order that her work be more efficient and helpful to the professional workers she assisted. We felt the clinic program to be a good example of the many different ways an organized volunteer group can assist in a community endeavor."[15]

Within three years, there were more than 600 patient visits each month at the Junior League Diagnostic Clinic of the outpatient department of Texas Children's Hospital. Heyck felt that the growing number of patients reflected the fact that the service being offered to the community was a living testament to the work of many minds, and—most of all—many hearts.

Reflecting on those early accomplishments, Taylor believed that it was a unique adventure in a modern pediatric organization. "The total mission of the Junior League clinic is to improve the health of children, to carry out projects in clinical investigation, and to teach sound fundamentals of medicine," he said. "An ambitious program, it is undertaken earnestly. Its force lies in the unbounded enthusiasm and clear insight of the lay boards, the administrative personnel, and the professional staff. All of whom see in pediatrics the abundant opportunities to give comprehensive individualized professional service and to advance scientific knowledge for the benefit of infants and children."[16]

Seizing one of those opportunities, Taylor included the clinics in the rotation schedule for the Baylor College of Medicine residency training program. Under his expert tutelage, many physicians received further training in one or more of the clinics' many pediatric subspecialties. But it was his utmost concern for the well-being of patients that became Taylor's legacy. "Some of those students who began their work with Fred Taylor speak of him with such reverence and such appreciation and respect. All the medical students loved him," Junior League member Virginia McFarland recalled. "He was a prince of a man, a wonderful man, a gentle man, and very soft-spoken and kind. You never saw such a kind person with patients."[17]

McFarland added to her praise: "He was Dr. Blattner's right-hand man at Texas Children's Hospital, and Blattner could not have accomplished all he did without Fred Taylor. But Fred was not a man who waved flags around about what he had done or was involved in. He was very quiet, very self-effacing. But, he was rock solid."[18]

These were attributes that Taylor displayed throughout his decade-long tenure as medical director of the clinics. During this period, the Junior League clinic once again underwent a change in nomenclature. Renamed the Junior League Outpatient Department in 1963, the clinic expanded its services to include 24 specialty clinics visited by an average of 2,000 patients each month and a voluntary staff of more than 100 Junior League volunteers. Under Taylor's direction, the clinic and its service had more than doubled in size.

Departing Texas Children's Hospital in 1969, Taylor moved to San Antonio. He was replaced as medical director by Baylor College of Medicine physician and infectious disease specialist Dr. Martha Dukes Yow. When Yow decided that she wanted to return to the research arena, neonatologist Dr. Arnold J. Rudolph became medical director in 1970. It was Rudolph who oversaw the 1971 expansion of the outpatient department to more than four times its original space. Rudolph, who went on to create the neonatology service at Texas Children's Hospital, was followed by Dr. Michael S. Ward, named medical director of the Junior League Outpatient Department in 1976.

In 1974, during Rudolph's leadership, Heyck relinquished her duties as executive secretary of the outpatient department and Junior League clinic to become director of community affairs for Texas Children's Hospital. Praising the capabilities of the woman who had become known as "Miss Pediatrics" in the burgeoning Texas Medical Center, Texas Children's Hospital executive director Newell E. France said: "Her contribution over the years to providing renewed health for children will be magnified many fold in this new capacity."[19]

More changes came to the Junior League Outpatient Department in 1977, when Blattner retired and Dr. Ralph D. Feigin became the new physician-in-chief of Texas Children's Hospital. When Feigin arrived, the Junior League Outpatient Department had grown beyond recognition in size and scope. Coexisting in its physical space were both the original diagnostic and specialized clinics for the medically indigent and the clinics and examining rooms for private outpatients of Baylor College of Medicine faculty members, an entity known as Pediatric Consultants. Although both services shared the space, they did not share duties and responsibilities. This was deemed to be a duplication of efforts and an inefficient use of space, as well as being confusing to patients. Feigin foresaw the need for sophisticated ambulatory services, predicting that this would become "the lifeblood of the future." He implemented a consolidation plan in 1978 that combined all aspects of the outpatient department into a more egalitarian approach to medical care.[20]

At approximately the same time, the Junior League of Houston was undergoing a change in the demographics of its membership. With more and more professional women as members, the Junior League found that the placement of volunteers in the daily clinics had become difficult, if not impossible. Many members could only work at night and others were interested in getting more involved in hospital areas other than the clinics. Consequently, with Feigin's restructuring of ambulatory services and the Junior League Outpatient Department, there also was a change in the duties of Junior League volunteers. League members soon began working in the emergency center, in recreational therapy, and in the playrooms on the patient floors of Texas Children's Hospital.

The repercussions of the physical changes made for ambulatory services at Texas Children's Hospital became evident in 1979, when the total number of outpatients—excluding those in the emergency center—exceeded 15,000. Appointed medical director of the Junior League Outpatient Department that year was Dr. Margaret E. Gutgesell, who began her efforts to streamline the department by concentrating on keeping accurate records, providing efficient services, and delivering excellent patient care.

By 1984, the total number of outpatients at Texas Children's Hospital exploded to more than 113,000. Such a large jump in numbers was mind-boggling, but not entirely unexpected. It was a national trend, one that Feigin had begun preaching about when medical care throughout the United States rapidly started to change in the late 1970s. Since the cost of medical care had risen rapidly, by the mid-1980s the federal government and private insurers had heavily promoted a shift from inpatient to outpatient care, applying every possible measure to shorten the duration of hospital stays.[21]

Interestingly, the astounding increase in outpatient numbers occurred before the advent of the new federal insurance programs and before the change in attitude of private insurance carriers and various corporate programs. And, without any outward attempts to market the ambulatory care program at Texas Children's Hospital, the numbers reflected an increase in private patients and a decrease in charity cases. Whatever the reasons, the Junior League Outpatient Department already had outgrown its expanded facilities by 1986.

"We got so big, we couldn't accommodate all the patients," said Mary Kana, assistant director of ambulatory services. "Several clinics moved over to the 8080 North Stadium Drive building in 1986 and left the Junior League's and some of the other clinics here. We were in something like 23 locations. We had some in the Abercrombie Building's upper floors, some over in Smith Tower and Scurlock Tower, and some down the street on Holcombe."[22]

Given the job of overseeing this growing geographic nightmare in 1984 was Dr. Rebecca Kirkland, the newly appointed medical director of ambulatory services and the Junior League Outpatient Department at Texas Children's Hospital. "By 1988, the number of outpatients had grown to 142,541," Kirkland said. "Although the outpatient department may generate only 20 percent of the overall revenue for the hospital, the 142,000 outpatients contrast with annual inpatient census of 12,000. It is a major shift from 1977 because the majority of care is now outpatient."[23]

Since most outpatients were not medically indigent, as they were during the early years of the Junior League Outpatient Department at Texas

Children's Hospital, there also was a major shift in the Junior League's role in the program. "In the early days, the medically indigent patients were subsidized in large part by the Junior League, but these expenses were somewhat more manageable," Kirkland said. "Now, the majority of patients have some resource. But the cost of the new technology can be overwhelming for parents and it is difficult for any one person or any single organization to pay for children's complex illnesses without external help or resources."

To meet these financial needs, Texas Children's Hospital instituted a pre-planned charity program, the Texas Children's Hospital's Financial Assistance Program, but the Junior League continued to give Texas Children's Hospital a considerable donation for the charity care of indigent patients. "It helps us by monetarily supporting some of our programs and indeed we are one of the major recipients of the Junior League's budget per year," Kirkland said. "It also still utilizes its Junior League Memorial Fund for patients' special needs."[24]

Renamed the Texas Children's Hospital Memorial Fund, the former Junior League Memorial Fund established in 1942 to meet the prescription, equipment, and transportation needs of medically indigent patients and their families. Through the years its purpose had expanded. "Few people realize that the Memorial Fund also finances other needs for the families, such as rent or utility bills for a month," explained Elizabeth Orsini Bunk, fund chairman. "Many times the parents of a critically ill child are unable to work while their child is in the hospital and the fund allows us to step in and provide financial support to get that family through this crisis period. It's a less obvious use of the fund, but it is just as important."[25]

Becoming more obvious throughout Texas Children's Hospital in the late 1980s were Junior League volunteers. Rather than being strictly involved with just one area, as they had been in the beginning, Junior League volunteers now worked not only in the outpatient clinics in various locations, but also in inpatient areas within the hospital. More than 150 Junior League volunteers were involved with child life, the health resources group, the emergency center, the cancer center, the safe sitter program, the wellness camp, the Pi Beta Phi Patient/Family Library, and various other programs and activities. "In the past, the Junior League volunteers were involved in menial tasks such as records and record management," Kirkland said. "In the future, they will be much more patient-oriented. It's very important to make the hospital a warm and friendly environment and it is the Junior League volunteers will help us do that. In so doing, they will enhance the level of service we can provide."

Because more than half of the Junior League volunteers were donating their time and service to Texas Children's Hospital during the evening hours and on weekends, the scope of their activities also changed. From this growing number of Junior League volunteers whose professional schedules did not permit daytime volunteering came numerous behind-the-scenes activities and services. "Today, many volunteers come in the evening hours and create arts and crafts activities for the children to do in the daytime," Kirkland said. "They prepare all the tools and materials, which is very helpful the following day."

One such behind-the-scenes activity was the muslin doll project, an effort that produced more than 1,000 stitched and stuffed muslin dolls each year. When completed, each doll was given to child life specialists for distribution to patients. Junior League member Leah Eknoyan said, "Once the doll is used as a teaching tool, the child gets to keep it and may draw on it, color it, do whatever he or she wants to do to make it his or her own."[26]

Another change for Junior League volunteers occurred in 1991, when the more than 56 ambulatory services clinics located at various locations were consolidated in the newly constructed Clinical Care Center, later named the Feigin Center. At that time, the Junior League Outpatient Department not only underwent another transformation, but also returned to its roots by being renamed the Junior League Children's Health Care Center—as it had similarly been called when the clinic was first established in 1927. With its residents' primary care and general medicine clinics, both assisted by Junior League volunteers, the new Junior League Children's Health Care Center continued its namesake's original mission to provide preventative healthcare to the medically indigent children of Houston.

As Texas Children's Hospital continued to grow in the early 1990s, so did the number of volunteers and the amount of financial support from the Junior League of Houston. In 1994, in recognition of the league's four-decade history at Texas Children's Hospital, members of the Junior League of Houston were recognized by the board of trustees for both the countless number of hours served and the more than $1 million contributed.

Five years later, when the number of Junior League of Houston volunteers at Texas Children's Hospital reached 300, Junior League president Dorothy Mathias Ables said: "I believe what has made the Junior League viable for 75 years is that our commitment to help the community has never changed while we have adapted to the changing needs of our volunteers and the community."[27]

Having begun with only 12 members in 1925, the Junior League of

Houston had grown to 5,000 members in its seventy-fifth year, making it the third-largest Junior League in the world. The organization's first community project, the Junior League Children's Health Care Center at Texas Children's Hospital, remained one of its largest in 1999, but it was only one of 32 projects to address a variety of needs in the community. Among these were projects to address healthcare, the abuse and neglect of women and children, literacy, cultural exposure for children, and issues affecting the elderly. To provide financial support throughout the community, the Junior League of Houston participated in various community collaborations and offered monetary assistance through emergency grants. The principal resource for the necessary funding of its many endeavors was the annual Junior League charity ball. Other fund-raising activities included the Junior League tea room, ballroom, and pantry, and the publication and sale of cookbooks and a children's book.

In 2000, the future for the Junior League of Houston at Texas Children's Hospital promised to be as productive as its 46-year past. Predicted to have particularly far-reaching results was the league's decision to use the hospital as the Junior League training center for each year's provisional class. Averaging 300 provisional members annually, the training consisted of a 12-week course offered three times a year and supervised by active Junior League members designated as team leaders. "A lot of other Junior League community placements have looked to our program at Texas Children's Hospital for how to train their volunteers," said Eknoyan in 2000. "It really runs like a well-oiled machine and has been credited with graduating many future Junior League leaders in the past."[28]

Many of those past leaders were on hand in 2000 to celebrate the seventy-fifth anniversary of the founding of the Junior League of Houston. As a salute to its past and to address the future health needs of children, the league celebrated its anniversary with a $1 million gift to the Houston community. This three-year commitment was to purchase and underwrite the operation of a mobile pediatric clinic and its personnel. Known as the SuperKids Mobile Pediatric Clinic, the 37-foot-long, state-of-the-art clinic on wheels was equipped with a medical staff to aid the children of one or more specially chosen Houston Independent School District (HISD) elementary schools and its surrounding area. Pointing out the historical importance of this gift, Ables said: "The first community project of the Junior League of Houston was a well-baby clinic—this is the well-baby clinic of the twenty-first century."[29]

This mobile clinic to provide acute healthcare was a collaborative effort between the Junior League of Houston, Texas Children's Hospital, Baylor College of Medicine, HISD, the Harris County Hospital District, and the City of Houston Health and Human Services Department. "We will give them inoculations, screenings for dental care, nutrition and diet guidelines, information to avoid smoking and to be sure to exercise," said Texas Children's Hospital physician-in-chief Feigin. "Ideally, we will be able to prevent illness by giving preventative care."[30]

To measure the effectiveness of taking pediatric care on the road, baseline data from each area served was kept and monitored at Texas Children's Hospital. Incidences of infectious diseases, trips to the emergency rooms, and other medical records will be studied in an effort to improve service to the community. The project also represented a possible solution to another growing problem. "We've got such a big, uninsured population that it's hard to know where to start fixing the problems, but when I see a project like this, I think, 'Here's a place to start,'" said Kirkland.[31]

Providing free introductory healthcare and preventative education to medically underserved children and their families in Houston was the stated mission of the SuperKids Mobile Pediatric Clinic. Staffed by a pediatrician and nurse practitioner from Texas Children's Hospital and assisted by volunteers from the Junior League of Houston, the fully equipped medical clinic inside a customized motor coach traveled to schools in Houston and began to provide immunizations, well-child checkups, sports physicals, miscellaneous care, and referrals for medical and social services. Focused on students who did not have insurance or access to full medical services, the mobile clinic eventually served more than 12 elementary schools in the Houston community.

With the introduction of the SuperKids Mobile Pediatric Clinic in 2000, the Junior League of Houston and Texas Children's Hospital reinvigorated their 46-year partnership. Working together since the 1954 opening of Texas Children's Hospital, they had remained true to their shared mission to provide care to medically underserved children and families in Houston.

After continuously adapting to the changing needs of the community in the past, the Junior League of Houston and Texas Children's Hospital remained positioned to do the same in the future.

Forty-five years after first becoming a Junior League volunteer at Texas Children's Hospital, Virginia Holt McFarland was still donating her time and services there.

"The real reason that I'm here is because of my love of children and their well-being," she said in 2000. "And to see the wonderful progress that's being made in medical care almost every day."[32]

When she looked back at the early years of the Junior League Diagnostic Clinic of the outpatient department at Texas Children's Hospital, McFarland was quick to acknowledge that "the Junior League saw the enormity of the need in the community and was so farsighted and truly altruistic in its wishes to do something about it at the time. It was the reason they stepped forward and gave so generously. And, years later, when the needs grew beyond the Junior League's capabilities, the generosity nonetheless continued."[33]

Just as the Junior League of Houston had played an integral part in the ever-changing history of Texas Children's Hospital, so too did McFarland. One of the first women asked to serve on the board of Texas Children's Hospital in an honorary capacity by Leopold L. Meyer in 1970, she retained her "honorary" status for two years before being granted full membership in 1972. Still serving in that capacity in 2000, McFarland said: "I guess they saw that we weren't going to sink the ship or speak up too much. But that didn't take too long for that to happen."

Although it was unusual at the time for a woman to serve as a trustee, McFarland said that she never felt ill at ease about being on the board. "I wasn't expected to run the show and I had no such aspirations," she said. "I was there because I loved medical care and I knew it was an opportunity to help children who needed it in the very best possible way. It was at the beginning, planting the seeds to watch them grow. I could do something because I loved it and I was willing to learn. I had the instincts to help children. And I still have those instincts."

An enthusiastic participant in all aspects of Texas Children's Hospital for more than four decades, McFarland finely tuned her innate instincts to help children. "She is an absolutely dedicated, not just board member, but member of the Texas Children's family," said physician-in-chief Dr. Ralph D. Feigin. "She is one of the few people who takes all the time in the world to participate basically in everything that goes on in the hospital. She makes rounds. She goes to conferences. So, I think that fundamentally she really understands what makes the hospital outstanding. And instead of just sitting in board meetings and listening to a bunch of financial reports and committee reports and other things, she fundamentally knows what it takes. Ginny is probably the most wonderful person that I have ever met."[34]

Such praise for McFarland's attributes, as well as her leadership capabilities, were not limited to just her tireless efforts at Texas Children's

Hospital. Since joining the Junior League of Houston in 1955, she had served as a member of its board of directors for two years; been president of the Sustaining Club, the organization for Junior League members over the age of 40; and become a sustaining director of the Association of Junior League International.

At Texas Children's Hospital, McFarland recognized the need for a lending library for patients. She convinced her fellow members of the Pi Beta Phi Alumnae Club of Houston to adopt the project as one of its philanthropies. To expedite planning, she personally searched for appropriate space in the already-overcrowded hospital, discovering an unused linen closet that she deemed adequate for the sorority's early efforts. Converted in 1984, the former linen closet opened as the Pi Beta Phi Patient/Family Library with 400 books on its shelves.

Less than a decade later, in 1992, the Pi Beta Phi Patient/Family Library expanded to include more than 4,000 books in English, Spanish, and French; VHS movies; cassette tapes; computer games; magazines; and paperbacks for parents. Staffed by members of the Pi Beta Phi Alumnae Club of Houston and volunteers from the Junior League and The Auxiliary to Texas Children's Hospital, the library has become one of the most popular services at Texas Children's Hospital.

In addition to her work with the Junior League, the Pi Phis, and Texas Children's Hospital, McFarland was appointed a lifetime honorary trustee of the National Association of Children's Hospitals and Related Institutions. In this role she repeatedly traveled to Washington, D.C., for more than 23 years to educate congressional members about the unique problems of children's hospitals. She also was presented with the prestigious Friend of Children award from that organization and visited all the major children's hospitals in the United States. "My eyes were opened to the quality of care that is given to seriously ill children at first-rate hospitals by both the doctors and the nurses," McFarland said. "My respect for them grew so much because of my personal experience. I've realized there is a commonality among those children with life-threatening diseases. They are so brave and wise beyond their years. Their maturity and acceptance of what they're dealing with is truly remarkable."[35]

In concert with her efforts on behalf of children's hospitals, McFarland cofounded six organizations dedicated to children's advocacy and children's health. She also served on the boards and advisory committees of more than 15 different organizations and has been recognized countless times for her tireless volunteer efforts on behalf of children. But one of the accomplishments of which she and her husband are most proud is the pediatric metabolic research laboratory, established in memory of their son Scott, who succumbed to his debilitating illness at the age of seven. "When we lost Scott, we and our friends were able to establish the laboratory. We asked that it go with Bill Daeschner, who left Baylor and Texas Children's Hospital to become the head of the children's hospital in Galveston. And that's indeed where it is and where it continues to flourish," McFarland said. "It's wonderful because children who have severe burns are moved there for treatment, as well as all the other patients who are treatable. So, it's helping a variety of children and that's a real satisfaction."[36]

Never complacent in their endless quest for knowledge, in the early 1990s McFarland and her husband enrolled in a layperson's anatomy, physiology, and medical terminology class at Baylor College of Medicine. "I was going to go and do it by myself, but the classes were at night and Russell said, 'No, you're not going to the Medical Center at night by yourself and come home by yourself at 9 p.m., so, I'll just take it with you.' And so we did. We had notebooks, and we had to study all the parts of the body, and it was fascinating. We got to work in the pathology lab a couple of nights, and it was fascinating to see the shape of a heart or a lung or a kidney. And then we took the exam, and Russell and I missed one question each—the same question. We were right proud of that," she said. "It was truly a privilege to learn."

Because of their interest in research, the McFarlands also could be found each Friday morning at grand rounds at Texas Children's Hospital. "I like to see the results," McFarland said. "Going to grand rounds, I see and hear these wonderful people who come and talk to us from other hospitals, and its absolutely electrifying to hear how excited they are about research in specific areas, and how close they are to really revolutionary findings."

To the McFarlands' dismay, although they have witnessed myriad advances in medical care and learned of innovative protocols and procedures throughout the years, the insidious disease that took their son more than 40 years ago continued to be incurable. "We have learned during grand rounds that they have better symptomatic care, but they do not have a cure to this good day," she said. "They can do kidney transplants for nephrosis and nephritis, but that still has effects which you have to deal with the rest of your life. There is no real cure because they still do not know what causes it."

But the McFarlands have not given up their hope for a cure. "At the last grand rounds Russell and I went to, there was the most wonderful presentation of the possibilities of gene therapies I've ever heard," Virginia said in early 2000. "My mouth just flies open because I am so excited about it. The potential is just thrilling. He spoke hopefully about the way it can be used in solid tumors, like brain tumors in children, which is the most terminal tumor in children. The speaker was so dynamic that I thought: 'Wow. If I were a medical student, I would sign up with you right this minute and start to work immediately!'"

Such enthusiasm had been her trademark since joining the Junior League of Houston in 1955. Personifying that organization's mission as her own, the remarkable McFarland adapted to the changing needs of the community over the years while never changing her personal commitment to help all children who are in need.

Because of her unwavering dedication to that mission at Texas Children's Hospital, untold thousands of patients and their families have benefited from the consequences of one social invitation being accepted in the 1950s by Virginia Holt McFarland.

20

He WAS A BRILLIANT CHILD, maybe even a genius, his mother thought.

By the time he was eight years old in 2001, he was never at a loss for words. Able to recite poems from memory and discuss intricate details of myriad subjects, he possessed an unusual command of verbal skills and an expansive vocabulary.

The fact that he also made lengthy statements that were pointless was dismissed by his mother, who thought that this was something he would outgrow.

Fiercely competitive at sports, but shying away from team sports like football, he excelled at individual athletic challenges such as one-on-one basketball games.

That he only played by himself and rarely interacted with children his own age was nothing unusual, his mother thought.

At times, his genius also was temperamental, displaying unpredictable mood changes. Inexplicably and without warning, the gregarious child sometimes became an introvert. Consumed with some unexpressed worry, he withdrew into himself. Seemingly unable to articulate the cause of his distress, he was unresponsive to efforts to determine its cause.

Just as puzzling to his mother was the child's inability to follow explicit instructions or grasp new concepts. Repeatedly finding his room in a mess with toys and clothes strewn in every direction, each time she patiently explained to him where to place his toys and how to fold or hang his clothes, but to no avail.

She compiled a list of written instructions for him to follow and he ignored it. Consequently, his room remained in a perpetual state of disarray.

His mother attributed this shortcoming to his fickle attention span. Easily distracted, he rarely completed any project he started. Those tasks that he did complete were his daily routines. Performed as if by rote, each task never varied from one day to the next.

Stubborn in his ways, he resisted change of any sort. When shown how to accomplish an old task in a new way, he ignored the advice. Preferring to continue in the same way he always had, no matter how time-consuming or ineffective it proved to be, he was obstinate in his refusal to compromise.

Although such peculiar behavior produced few measurable consequences at home, this was not the case at school. Instead of excelling in academics as his mother had expected, he experienced distinct difficulties. Having lovingly labeled him a genius at home, she soon found that his teachers chose an altogether different way of describing of him.

The child definitely had a "problem," they told her. Pointing to his difficulty in learning to solve mathematical problems, perform paper and pencil tasks, and pay attention to instructions, the teachers suspected he might have a learning disorder or attention deficit disorder (ADD).

To assess the presence of the behavioral signs of attention problems, the child's pediatrician administered a questionnaire to his mother. Her responses suggested that the boy did indeed experience difficulties of attention regulation. The pediatrician prescribed Ritalin to help him control his attention. The boy's mother was very hopeful that the drug would help, as she had read that the psychostimulant medication enjoyed a high success rate among children with ADD and other related symptoms. Since published reports stated that between 70 and 80 percent of children responded positively to Ritalin—often showing improvements in attention span, impulsivity, and on-task behavior—she thought that her son's problems would soon be solved.

Unfortunately, this optimism was short-lived. To her dismay, Ritalin offered no such relief to her son. Not only did the child continue to have academic difficulties, he also began to experience anxiety and sadness about his failings. Disturbed about his inability to succeed, he suffered from poor self-esteem.

Convinced that there was a viable solution to what was becoming an escalating problem, the distraught mother searched for answers. By reading newspapers and magazines, she learned that there were no specific tests for ADD. By consulting other medical professionals, she discovered that learning difficulties might cause a child to be inattentive and to appear to have ADD.

Therefore, with each new article she read, the mother questioned the accuracy of the diagnosis. Did her son indeed have ADD, or was it something else? Where and to whom should she take him? Should he see a psychiatrist or a psychologist? Should he see a neurologist or a neuropsychologist? Or, should he see them all? If so, was there a preferred sequence to the various referrals? Where should she go to accomplish this? In pursuit of the answers to these questions, she researched the diagnosis and treatment of learning disabilities and ADD at the library, surfed the Internet for further information, and talked with friends, acquaintances, and relative strangers.

It was while talking with other parents at her son's school that she learned about a program in Houston—at Texas Children's Hospital—that administered comprehensive evaluations of learning disabilities, ADD, and emotional disorders.

When told about the clinic's comprehensive screening program for learning disabilities and its extensive intervention programs for children and their parents, she instinctively knew where she and her son had to go.

The Learning Support Center at Texas Children's Hospital debuted in August 1986.

Located in the newly opened off-campus Clinical Care Center at 8080 North Stadium Drive, the Learning Support Center was established as a direct response to a voiced need in the community for the provision of individual academic assistance for children with learning disabilities, from kindergarten through college.

"Texas Children's Hospital sponsored a survey in the early 1980s to ascertain the hospital services most sought after by the Houston community," recalled Dr. Judith Z. Feigin, director of the Learning Support Center. "The patient population surveyed reported a need for a program that treated learning disabilities. The community responses suggested treatment should be offered in an outpatient setting, rather than being a part of an inpatient hospital. The opportunity to respond to the need for this service presented itself when Texas Children's Hospital opened it first outpatient building off-campus in 1986."[1]

Under the direction of Feigin, who held a master of education degree in special education with a specialization in learning disabilities, as well as a doctoral degree in educational psychology, the Learning Support Center featured a variety of teaching methods and instructional modifications used to design individualized programs for children ranging in age from kindergarten through college level.

Feigin designed the academic programs to meet the needs of students with learning disabilities or other learning difficulties that hindered their progress in the school environment. One of the first such centers to be located in a hospital setting, it was unique in concept. Yet the idea had existed decades before the Learning Support Center at Texas Children's Hospital became a reality.

"I envisioned a program that would provide a comprehensive series of services to families who had children with learning difficulties," Feigin said. "I wanted its philosophy to be child-centered, family-centered, and research-based and its interventions to be trusted. Prior to arriving in Houston in 1977, I planned to start a clinic similar to this one at the St. Louis Children's Hospital. Our family's move to Houston did not permit me to realize that plan."[2]

Although what Feigin ultimately envisioned was larger in scope, the Learning Support Center began with a smaller focus, that of teaching children with learning disabilities the academic skills required to succeed in school. At its 1986 opening, she stated: "Our purpose is to teach our students to use learning strategies to become independent learners throughout their lifetime and attain their intellectual potential and professional goals."[3]

Convinced that academic success for children was dependent on family support, Feigin encouraged the parents of students at the Learning Support Center to maintain high but realistic expectations for their child's academic achievement. To enhance each child's efforts to achieve academically and socially, Feigin commended all efforts to provide the appropriate surroundings and stressed the importance of verbal praise and encouraging hugs. So that parents could be effective advocates for their children, the Learning Support Center helped them to obtain instructional modifications for their children at school.[4]

"We wanted to provide the services children and families required to achieve success," said Feigin. "If children are to graduate from high school and college, parents and professionals must provide the necessary assistance and educational modifications to help their children achieve those goals. We wanted to help families to obtain the services required to permit their children to reach their intellectual potential."[5]

Its mission clearly stated, within its first week the Learning Support Center at Texas Children's Hospital had established what was to become a trademark pattern of operation. Always willing to add or modify services to meet the requirements of the patients referred for care, Feigin noted that many of these children had emotional, social, and attention difficulties that affected their school performance and their ability to learn. Immediately recognizing the need for additional care, Feigin expanded services from individualized instruction in reading, mathematics, and written composition to psychoeducational testing and the use of other assessment measures designed to assess difficulties of social interaction, attention focus, anxiety, and behavior. Soon after, a comprehensive social skills program for children was initiated to develop skills related to problem solving, interpersonal communication, assuming responsibility for personal actions, and developing self-control. Parents were invited to participate in a simultaneous program that taught them how to help their child practice at home the skills introduced in the social skills group setting.

"It's relevant to recognize that formal special education services were rather new in 1986," Feigin said. "The passage of Public Law 94-142, the Education for All Handicapped Children Act of 1975, mandated, for the first time in the United States, a free appropriate public education for all children with disabilities. The implementation of the law was in its infancy in the early 1980s. Although it ensured the right to due process, education in the least restrictive environment, and an individualized education program (IEP) for all children who qualified for services under the law, the application of the law to children with learning disabilities often was not immediate. The initial task for many school districts was to identify children with significant disabilities who were residing at home or in an institutional setting and to integrate them into typical school settings."[6]

The field of learning disabilities was in its infancy in the latter part of the 1970s and early 1980s. The term "learning disabilities" was itself quite new, having first appeared in a 1963 speech by educator Samuel A. Kirk to describe students who had difficulty in reading, writing, math, or other learning tasks, despite average or above-average intellectual abilities. Prior to Kirk's coining of the term, students with such difficulties were considered to have minimal brain damage or dysfunction (MBD), or to be mentally retarded, slow learners, or just plain lazy.[7] Parents welcomed the use of the learning disabilities term, as they were reluctant to label their child as having a brain dysfunction. There were few services available for children with learning disabilities in the 1960s and 70s. Parental advocacy for appropriate intervention caused learning disabilities to be included as a special education category in the public law that mandated the provision of special education services for children with "handicapping" conditions.

Public Law 94-142, the Education for All Handicapped Children Act, granted the right to special education services for children with learning disabilities. This widely accepted definition of learning disabilities first appeared in *The Federal Register* in the 1970s:

> *Specific learning disability means a disorder in one or more of the basic psychological processes involved in understanding or in using language, spoken or written, which may manifest itself in an imperfect ability to listen, think, speak, read, write, spell, or to do mathematical calculations. The term includes such conditions as perceptual handicaps, brain injury, minimal brain dysfunction, dyslexia, and developmental aphasia. The term does not include children who have learning problems which are primarily the result of visual, hearing, or motor handicaps, of mental retardation, or emotional disturbance, or of environmental, cultural, or economic disadvantage.*[8]

In the decade following the enactment of Public Law 94-142 in 1975, the number of children classified with learning disabilities more than doubled from 797,213 in 1976 to 1,811,489 in 1986.[9]

Also multiplying exponentially were public school programs for children with learning disabilities. With an increased demand that far exceeded the supply available in the late 1970s and early 1980s, there was a nationwide shortage of special education teachers. It was a side effect that clearly hampered efforts to implement the law successfully in the Houston Independent School District (HISD). In 1985, the HISD school year began with vacancies for more than 40 special education teachers.[10]

"At the time we opened the Learning Support Center, parents were concerned about the negative effects of labeling their child, such as reduced self-esteem and reduced ability to realize future goals." Feigin recalled. "We suggested parents critically evaluate the quality of special education services their child might receive within the public school prior to applying for special education services. Children with learning disabilities, by definition, have average to above-average intellectual abilities. Their academic performance is less than their intellectual potential. Parents and teachers must help these children, within the public school system or through private instruction, to acquire academic information using different instructional methods."[11]

To help children to achieve their intellectual potential and academic goals, the Learning Support Center offered instruction in academic skills six days a week, including after school on weekdays, with instructional methods and materials individualized for children from five to 18 years of age. Teaching was available to assist children to decode written information, understand written information, compose written language, and solve mathematical problems. Older children were provided with strategies to study and to develop positive social interactions.

As each new program at the Learning Support Center at Texas Children's Hospital evolved, its reputation grew and word-of-mouth referrals increased. With a growing need for services, additional staff was required. Feigin initially hired special educators and educational diagnosticians to teach the children. "Utilizing a system of continuous evaluation, intervention, and re-evaluation, the diagnostic, clinical teaching cycle was used to identify the optimal teaching methods and instructional materials required for an individual student to achieve academic success," Feigin said. "A personal education program was created for each student after a consultation with the parents, an analysis of prior assessment procedures, and an evaluation of current academic skills."[12]

Five years after it opened, with more than 260 teaching sessions per month in 1991, the Learning Support Center at Texas Children's Hospital grew to include a full-time staff of three, along with five part-time educational diagnosticians, special educators, and educational psychologists. The center had outgrown its facilities.

With its move to the seventh floor of the new Clinical Care Center—later known as the Feigin Center—on September 23, 1991, the Learning Support Center began offering expanded programs.[13] After evaluating the growth and direction of the center in the early 1990s, Feigin once again responded to the needs of its changing patient population. She instituted extensive and comprehensive neuropsychological and psychoeducational testing services by neuropsychologists with doctoral degrees in clinical psychology and an additional three or four years of training in neuropsychological testing.

The field of neuropsychology had expanded from an emphasis on identifying the nature of injuries to the adult brain, to the assessment of children using norm-referenced standardized tests. Neuropsychological assessments assisted teachers and psychologists at the Learning Support Center to intervene appropriately by accurately assessing a child's cognitive, social, emotional, and attention skills. Neuropsychologists not only analyzed test results, but could also create a profile of individual strengths and weaknesses. Feigin believed in the value of neuropsychological evaluations. Her experience working with children with learning disabilities convinced her that these assessments were necessary to evaluate the neurological development of children, as well as their social and emotional development. While pursuing her doctoral degree in educational psychology, Feigin enrolled in courses in neuropsychological evaluation and in the techniques available to assess the relationship of behavior to brain functioning.

She was convinced that it was necessary to assess the underlying abilities required for academic success.

Neuropsychological testing identified the cognitive patterns of a child and became an integral part of the assessment services for children with learning difficulties. "Our testing program helped us to identify a child's cognitive and emotional strengths and weaknesses and intervene appropriately." Feigin explained. "One cannot provide an optimal level of intervention without a comprehensive evaluation of skills and abilities."[14]

Specific areas assessed and interpreted were intellectual ability, receptive and expressive language skills, visual perception and visual motor integration, auditory perception, phonemic awareness, visual and auditory memory, executive function, and components of attention and emotional status. Identifying the individual's cognitive and emotional strengths and weaknesses, the neuropsychologist developed recommendations for intervention or provided a referral to appropriate medical personnel. "In the 1990s, many of the children referred to the Learning Support Center had 'acquired' learning disorders," Feigin said. "The neuropsychologists of the Learning Support Center were able to provide cognitive rehabilitation training for these children. Many of the instructional strategies used in exemplary special education also were used in exemplary models of cognitive rehabilitation, namely cognitive strategy instruction, environmental modifications, and the use of external aids to help track and organize information."[15]

Cognitive rehabilitation training appeared to be a natural extension of the services provided at the Learning Support Center for children with inborn learning disabilities. "Moreover, recommendations for psychosocial support for children with acquired or developmental learning disabilities suggested further expansion of our social skills training program," Feigin said.

In the early 1990s, the Learning Support Center introduced TeamMates, a comprehensive group therapy program for school-age children and their families. Mental health professionals at the masters and doctoral levels joined the staff of the Learning Support Center in recognition of the significant emotional and social difficulties experienced by many of the children referred for services. "The TeamMates program developed as an outgrowth of my research in the social skill development in children with learning disabilities," Feigin explained. "The complexity of the behavioral and emotional difficulties experienced by some of the children referred for our services ultimately suggested we move from a model that used special educators to a model that used mental health providers."

Designed to assist children to be more effective at managing themselves and their social relationships, the TeamMates program benefited from the expertise of clinical psychologists, advanced clinical practitioners, and professional counselors. Stressing increased self-awareness, perspective-taking, emotional and behavioral control, communication skills, and problem-solving skills, the program included 16 weeks of diagnosis and psychotherapy intervention services. Groups were small and tailored to meet the needs of the children and their parents. "We made a decision to hold parent and child groups simultaneously, due to the time constraints experienced by most families," Feigin said.[16]

In a separate but simultaneous program that involved specialized group therapy intervention for children and adolescents and a training program for parents, TeamMates offered assistance to children with learning disabilities, attention deficit/hyperactive disorders (AD/HD), and emotional struggles.

Differentiating students with learning disorders from those with attention or behavior disorders was to become a priority at the Learning Support Center. With more than two million students classified as learning disabled in 1990, the chances for inaccurate classifications also grew. Since evaluation procedures, disability classifications, and resulting placement decisions varied among school districts and classroom teachers, the possibilities of inaccurate diagnosis increased.[17]

One such possibility was the misidentification of AD/HD. The growing prevalence of such inaccurate assessments became evident. "Many children coming to the Learning Support Center with a diagnosis of attention deficit disorder were identified later as experiencing learning disabilities, anxiety, or depression," Feigin recalled. "We recognized we required the assistance of physicians to evaluate the children accurately and to treat them expeditiously. With the assistance of physicians in the subspecialty sections of developmental pediatrics, pediatric psychiatry, and pediatric neurology, and the neuropsychologists of the Learning Support Center, we created a multidisciplinary diagnostic clinic to evaluate attention problems."[18]

Concerned with misdiagnosis, over-diagnosis, inappropriate diagnosis, and incomplete diagnosis and treatment strategies for children with AD/HD and other attention disorders, the clinic for attention problems opened in 1994. From its inception, Feigin served as chief of the clinic. Encompassing developmental pediatrics, psychiatry, and neurology, the clinic was designed to provide both optimal care for patients and training for pediatric residents and fellows.[19]

Following an evaluation by each subspecialty and formal and informal interviews with parents, the multidisciplinary team delivered a diagnosis and proposed an intervention plan. Often included in the intervention recommendations were social skill classes for children, parenting classes, pharmacological therapy, and academic modifications. "Although we initially called it the 'AD/HD clinic' when it opened in 1994, we changed the name to the 'clinic for attention problems' in 1996, after it became apparent that less than one third of the children who were referred to the clinic had AD/HD," Feigin advised. "It was a misleading connotation that, in essence, required that you be diagnosed with AD/HD before you came to the clinic, when in fact the purpose of the clinic was to diagnose the source of your attention disorder."[20]

Many of the children diagnosed with AD/HD received assistance from the school liaison program, an existing program adopted by the Learning Support Center in 1993. Originally instigated in 1986 by Dr. Earl J. Brewer, Jr., a Texas Children's Hospital pediatric rheumatologist, the program created a partnership between families, school officials, and healthcare providers to assist chronically ill children achieve success in the educational environment. "We were happy to benefit from the skills of the school liaison professionals and assist the children referred to the Learning Support Center to gain the modifications they required at school," said Feigin. "I saw the program as a very natural addition to the Learning Support Center."[21]

Under the direction of the Learning Support Center, the school liaison program redoubled its efforts to obtain the necessary academic modifications to create an optimal learning environment for participants. As well as children with chronic illnesses such as cancer, spina bifida, juvenile rheumatoid arthritis, asthma, cerebral palsy, and AD/HD, the program began serving children suffering from the sequelae of cancer therapy, strokes, cardiac defects, diabetes, and epilepsy.

Working closely with the medical services and clinics at Texas Children's Hospital, the professionals of the school liaison program at the Learning Support Center helped healthcare providers to participate in the successful implementation of each patient's educational program. "One of the nicest things that happened to us since we moved into the Feigin Center was the opportunity for close interaction with the subspecialty physicians at the hospital," explained Feigin. "Our enhanced ability to participate in multidisciplinary clinics and to care for children with chronic illnesses permitted the expansion of our programs throughout the 1990s."[22]

In 1994, the Learning Support Center expanded the scope of its special education services once again by reaching out to the preschool population. A new program provided behavioral health services designed to increase the social abilities of these young children. "There were few community resources providing behavioral intervention for preschool children," Feigin said. "I was convinced that early intervention was the key to avoiding more problematic behavior in the school-age population."[23]

The program was developed for children between the ages of two and five who experience notable difficulties with behavior and development. It taught these children and their parents how to manage social interaction, an ability deemed crucial to learning success. A structured experiential psychotherapeutic model, the brief evaluation and intervention program (BEIP) was designed to resemble a typical preschool, complete with activity time, free play, and snack time. The setting allowed the observation of problem behaviors in a natural setting and also permitted the immediate management of socially inappropriate behaviors. As with all other programs in the Learning Support Center developed by Feigin, parents were included in the intervention. Behavioral management skills were modeled for parents to ease their ability to maintain the behavioral improvements at home and in the community.[24]

The complete BEIP program included a developmental history of the child, a home visit or school visit, 32 psychotherapeutic sessions in the clinical preschool setting, and family therapy when appropriate. "Observation of the child at home and at school assists us to gain insight into the experiences of the child and frequently explains some of his or her behavior," Feigin said. "Many times children are referred to us from daycare or preschool for severe behavioral problems, some actually having been asked to leave the school."[25]

Another new direction for the Learning Support Center came in the late 1990s with the implementation of the family therapy program. Originally developed at Baylor College of Medicine and adopted by the Learning Support Center, this was a psychotherapeutic counseling program for families coping with unanticipated life-altering events. Designed to promote adaptation to significant disruptions, such as a divorce, major physical illness or chronic illness, job loss, or unexpected death, the program provided a structured and guided approach to transitions and adjustments.

After continuously adapting to the emerging needs and wants of the community, in 2001 the Learning Support Center at Texas Children's Hospital boasted a staff of 20 mental health professionals. Consisting of four neuropsychologists, two postdoctoral fellows, and 16 psychology externs and interns, the staff also included 16 clinical psychologists, licensed professional counselors, and advanced clinical practitioners.

Stressing the necessity for a high quality of care and experience, Feigin said: "The children referred to the Learning Support Center required professionals who were trained to understand, interpret, and modify the behaviors that interfered with positive social interactions."[26]

With more than 8,000 children attending the Learning Support Center annually, the demand for neuropsychological testing and treatment for behavioral, cognitive, and attention problems was growing. "I was committed to providing the finest care for our patient population," said Feigin in 2001. "I wanted us to provide the patients of Texas Children's Hospital with the most valid, reliable, and standardized neuropsychological evaluations interpreted by the most highly trained personnel. Similarly, I wanted the intervention programs we offered to be developmentally appropriate, individualized, evidence-based, and child and parent focused. I wanted the Learning Support Center to serve the children of Texas Children's Hospital optimally. I am amazed at how the Learning Support Center has grown."[27]

To house the rapidly expanding programs, the Learning Support Center was moved to a space specifically designed to house its multiple programs. In 2001, the center's academic teaching, neuropsychological testing, family therapy, school liaison, TeamMates, and BEIP specialized interventional programs were moved from multiple locations throughout the hospital into 10,000 square feet of the newly built Clinical Care Center at Texas Children's Hospital. Divided into sections or pods for testing and for individual and group therapy, the center was furnished for preschool and school-age children. It was designed to provide the finest quality of patient care. "We are so excited about our new space and the opportunity it afforded us to work with subspecialty medical sections to integrate psychological services into the medical care of children," said Feigin shortly before the move. "With a common philosophy and common goal, we will be able to work more closely with the medical clinics and serve the needs of their patients."[28]

With its expanded facilities, growing staff, and wide constellation of services for children and their families, the Learning Support Center at Texas Children's Hospital once again demonstrated its trademark ability to adapt to the needs of the community. In 2003, with increasing scientific evidence that group programs were most appropriate for social skills deficits, Feigin once again modified the interventions offered at the Learning Support Center.

Assisted by her team of clinical child psychologists and neuropsychologists, Feigin created five new programs. In addition to the well-established neuropsychology program developed by Kevin R. Krull, PhD, ABPP/ABCN, Feigin and the psychologists of the Learning Support Center initiated an anxiety and mood disorder program, a pediatric health psychology program, an attention deficit disorder program, and an autism and attachment disorder program. Also, in an effort to provide a systematic and patient-focused process that would allow patients to access testing and intervention services in a timely manner, a diagnostic interview program was initiated. This program permitted observation of the child's behavior in an unstructured setting and allowed children and parents to be interviewed to identify the salient aspects of the child's problems. Families were then guided to the most appropriate and timely services, either at the Learning Support Center or within the pediatric subspecialty clinics of Texas Children's Hospital.

In 2003, the Learning Support Center initiated a therapeutic preschool program for children with autism. "We noted an increase in the number of children diagnosed with autism and referred for intervention services," Feigin said, noting that the reported incidence of autism was rising steadily nationally. "Autistic spectrum disorder, or ASD, is associated with severe developmental consequences. The incidence is estimated to be 1 in 166 children, a level of incidence greater than that of pediatric cancer, diabetes, Down syndrome, and other significant childhood disorders."[29]

Feigin was determined to create an optimal intervention program for these children, one that was comprehensive, intensive, and individualized. Assisted by a group comprising pediatric neurologists, an educational psychologist, geneticists, neuropsychologists, psychiatrists, developmental pediatricians, speech/language pathologists, and occupational and physical therapists, Feigin created the evaluation protocol for a multidisciplinary clinic specifically for children with ASD.[30]

Previously, as cochief of the clinic for the diagnosis of autistic spectrum disorders in 2001, Feigin collaborated with Dr. Diane Treadwell-Deering to initiate the clinic's first multidisciplinary evaluation of children exhibiting behaviors associated with autism. A team of highly experienced clinicians met with each child to perform the various components of the comprehensive evaluation. "In addition to the administration of the Autism Diagnosis Interview-Revised and the Autism Diagnostic Observation Scale, a medical evaluation is conducted to identify signs of coexisting genetic or medical disorders," Feigin explained. "Moreover, each child receives a speech/language evaluation, a sensory-integration occupational/physical therapy evaluation, a neuropsychological evaluation, and an audiology evaluation."

To serve the needs of this growing patient population in 2003, Feigin analyzed the various intervention programs available for children with ASD. When initially identified in 1943, ASD was thought to be a psychological disorder, but it later became recognized as a developmental disorder with neurologic origin. Over the decades, perplexed physicians, psychologists, and educators had developed a wide variety of different approaches to treat the core characteristics of ASD—specifically, the deficits in social interaction and in verbal and nonverbal communication, as well as restricted patterns of interests and behaviors.

One such program was the developmental, individualized, and relationship-based model (DIR) for diagnosis and intervention pioneered by psychologist Dr. Stanley Greenspan and psychologist Dr. Serena Wieder. The result of more than 20 years of clinical research in child development, DIR was a comprehensive treatment approach tailored to the individual needs of a child. In the 2001 report titled *Educating Children with Autism,* issued by the Committee on Educational Interventions for Children with Autism and published by the National Research Council, DIR was included as one of the ten comprehensive, intensive, individualized intervention programs that appear to be an effective therapeutic approach to the care of children with autism. However, there were no definitive clinical trial studies supporting any one approach and no comparative studies between any of the recognized approaches.

As Feigin learned more about the DIR model, she became convinced that it was worthy of endorsement. "Each child's profile of developmental, cognitive, language, motor, and sensory processing strengths and weaknesses are identified and used to create a unique and individualized therapeutic program," she said. "The model may be characterized as including all aspects of developmentally appropriate practice and accommodating to the special challenges of children with autism."

The guiding principle of the DIR approach is to follow the child's lead, constantly tailoring interactions to the individual differences in the way the child processes experiences. According to the DIR model, this enables the child to master successfully the emotional stages of development—namely, relating, thinking, and communicating. Moreover, a subgroup of these children are able to master levels of creative and reflective thinking including high levels of empathy thought to be unattainable by children with autism.

"The DIR model views children with autism as possessing the capacity to learn through emotionally meaningful relationships, the fundamentals of relating to others, communicating with others, and thinking, thereby providing a path to independence and problem solving," Feigin said. "Utilizing this philosophic approach to intervention, the information gathered during the initial evaluation is used to develop a comprehensive treatment plan and the resulting therapeutic plan for each child focused on strengthening developmental weaknesses, solving medical problems and limiting the impact of family and environmental complexities."[31]

In order to implement a comprehensive intervention program for children diagnosed with ASD and other developmental disabilities, Feigin created the Bridges therapeutic preschool program, a multidisciplinary therapeutic program housed in a separate facility designed and created for the program. Opened in 2002 as a component of the Learning Support Center at Texas Children's Hospital, the program included speech/language therapy, sensory integration occupational and physical therapy, and floor time therapy, the interactive experience between child and adult that permits the child to practice continually the process of attaching affect and intent to behavior and language. "You actually get on the floor and follow the child's lead," Feigin said. "DIR focuses on creating opportunities for learning interactions that build on the child's natural emotional interests and harnesses their capacities to interact, problem-solve, and engage in creative and reflective thinking. The Bridges program goes from 8:30 a.m. until 2:30 p.m. and it includes adaptive behavior skills, as well as preschool cognitive skills. Lunch becomes a time to learn communication skills and feeding skills. It also has an extensive parent education program, provides a parent support group, and creates home programs for the children, to guide parents in the skills that will permit them to serve as their child's most effective therapists."[32]

The necessity of active parental involvement was underscored by the report, *Educating Children with Autism*. Among the findings of the multidisciplinary committee—which was charged "to integrate the scientific, theoretical, and policy literature and create a framework for evaluating the scientific evidence concerning the effects and features of educational interventions for young children and adults"[33]—was the conclusion that children with autism required a minimum of 25 hours a week of instruction in academic and social skills. "The implication of that finding compels parents to actively participate in therapy because therapy cannot take place only at school," Feigin explained. "Parents have to be actively engaged in the therapeutic process."[34]

Families of children with autism embraced the Bridges therapeutic program enthusiastically in its first two years of operation. The future growth of the program was a certainty. Originally built as a 6,000-square-foot facility, Bridges was projected to expand to more than 15,000 square feet in 2007. By 2004, Bridges provided intensive intervention for 14 children and had an additional 14 children on its waiting list. Plans called for the implementation of separate classes for children ages two, three, four, and five.[35]

In the meantime, Feigin continually fine-tuned various details of the intervention program at Bridges. Aware that the parents of children diagnosed with ASD were often distraught, she developed an intervention questionnaire to ascertain additional services the multidisciplinary intervention team at Bridges might provide to families.

This willingness to listen to the patient population and adapt to changing needs was a trademark of the Learning Support Center at Texas Children's Hospital. Also ingrained in Feigin's leadership style was an ability to alter programs deemed outdated or ineffective in the field. "We realized our group programs at the Learning Support Center had not been subjected to rigorous examination, so as data became available about evidence-based programs we modified our modes of intervention," Feigin said. "The data suggested that children with aggressive behavior required one type of intervention, whereas those with anxiety and mood disorders required a different therapeutic approach as did children with attachment disorders."[36]

Another new program, the health psychology program, was introduced in 2004. Throughout the 20-year existence of the Learning Support Center at Texas Children's Hospital, medicine recognized the emotional and cognitive effects of a chronic illness or modes of treatment on children, and psychologists received specific training to care for children with chronic medical disorders. The health psychology program was created to respond to the needs of the patients of Texas Children's Hospital and to the interests of the clinical psychologists at the Learning Support Center. Affiliated with a growing number of medical subspecialty clinics at Texas Children's Hospital, the health psychology program included inpatient psychological consultation services within the hospital setting, as well as outpatient therapy in the Learning Support Center's space in the Clinical Care Center.

Neuropsychological evaluations were performed on patients with chronic medical illnesses such as leukemia, brain tumors, sickle cell disease, HIV, cochlear implantation, organ failure, and transplantation. In addition, the neuropsychologists in the Learning Support Center evaluated the children who were assessed in the clinic for attention problems and the children with autistic spectrum disorders. As clinical investigators on research projects funded by the National Institutes of Health and designed to identify the cognitive sequelae of various treatments for cancer, bone marrow transplantation, organ transplants, genetic disorders, diabetes, lupus erythematosus, traumatic brain injury, Tourette syndrome, and other neurological or systemic medical conditions, the neuropsychologists at the Learning Support

Center performed neuropsychological evaluations in both outpatient and inpatient settings.

Also introduced in 2004 were modifications to intervention programs related to anxiety and mood disorders, AD/HD, and disruptive behavior disorders, each redesigned to reflect new information regarding the efficacy of treatment modalities. "We are using an evidence-based, validated early childhood intervention program called PCIT, parent-child interaction therapy," Feigin said. "Our staff of psychologists had formal training to develop expertise in this mode of therapy."

With a growing staff of clinical child psychologists and pediatric neuropsychologists, the Learning Support Center emphasized the development of certified training programs for psychologists and neuropsychologists. Feigin announced in 2004: "We have altered the name of our department to the 'Learning Support Center for Neurobehavioral Psychology' in acknowledgement of our change in focus from special education to psychology."[37]

The new name reflected not only the changes made in the recent past, but also those planned for the future. Offering the only comprehensive predoctoral psychology internship and postdoctoral psychology and neuropsychology fellowship training programs in child psychology and child neuropsychology in a pediatric hospital at a major medical school in Texas, the Learning Support Center for Neurobehavioral Psychology at Texas Children's Hospital gained accreditation from the Association of Postdoctoral Programs in Clinical Neuropsychology and from the Association of Post-Doctoral and Pre-doctoral Internship Programs (APPIC). Applications for certification of its predoctoral and postdoctoral training programs were submitted to the American Psychological Association.

With these training programs in place, Feigin predicted unlimited growth. "The accredited training programs in the Learning Support Center at Texas Children's Hospital will be the new child psychology program in the School of Allied Health Sciences at Baylor College of Medicine," she said.

Plans also included specialized certification programs for AD/HD coaching services and a training program in DIR therapy as part of the Learning Support Center's child psychology program in the School of Allied Health Sciences, making it the first such center in the Southwest to offer this specialized training. "There is a scarcity of these specialized certification programs in child psychology," Feigin explained. "Only seven other centers in the country offer training for AD/HD coaches and training for DIR therapy is available at only five other sites in the United States at this time."

As for the ability to cope with unexpected changes in healthcare, Feigin anticipated that the future of the Learning Support Center for Neurobehavioral Psychology at Texas Children's Hospital always would adapt to the varied needs of the patient population at Texas Children's Hospital. "We continue to learn about the cognitive and emotional sequelae of chronic illnesses and to identify the multiple cognitive strengths and weaknesses that characterize genetic disorders," she said, pointing out those discoveries might dictate entirely different therapeutic approaches than those currently in use.

With a justifiable sense of pride in the Learning Support Center she had created, modified, and nurtured for almost 20 years, Feigin said: "I think I have put in place the administrative structure and the programs required to serve children with cognitive, emotional, and social disorders." [38]

Whatever the patients and families needed, the Learning Support Center for Neurobehavioral Psychology at Texas Children's Hospital was prepared to deliver it in 2004 and in the decades ahead.

W ithin weeks of first hearing about the clinic for attention problems in the Learning Support Center at Texas Children's Hospital, the mother and son arrived for their first appointment at the multidisciplinary clinic.

Referred, at her request, by their pediatrician, the mother was told to bring her son's school records and medical records to the clinic.

Although expecting her son to undergo a battery of tests, she was somewhat surprised to find herself answering a comprehensive questionnaire before his testing had even begun. When told that parents were considered an integral part not only of the clinic's thorough assessment of children's inability to regulate attention, but also of its resulting treatment plan, she enthusiastically concurred.

After responding to written questions about her son's medical, social, emotional, attention, and cognitive characteristics, the mother was interviewed formally and informally by the clinic's psychologists and physicians. These interviews took place before, during, and after her son's two-day medical and neuropsychological assessment conducted by the clinic's team of professionals.

The team, consisting of psychologists, educators, and physicians with expertise in neurology, psychiatry, and neuropsychology, evaluated the medical and development status of the child. In addition, his academic skills and emotional and environmental status were assessed to identify areas of weakness that may contribute to attention and behavior.

The areas of development assessed included intellectual ability, receptive and expressive language skills, visual perception and visual motor integration, aural perception, phonemic segmentation, memory, executive function, components of attention, and emotional status.

At the completion of these tests, members of the team conferred privately to evaluate the results of each assessment, identify the source of attention fluctuations, and propose an intervention plan.

While waiting to hear her son's diagnosis, the mother worried that such a comprehensive screening process might produce more questions than the answers she sought.

It was a needless concern, she discovered. In addition to the diagnostic conclusion, she was given detailed explanations of the multidisciplinary team's observations and opinions.

When informed by the team that her son had a nonverbal learning disorder (NLD) and did not have ADD, the mother immediately learned what that diagnosis meant and what the Learning Support Center's recommended treatment was.

Described in detail by the team, NLD was a genetic neurological syndrome believed to result from damage to the white matter connections in the right hemisphere of the brain. Often misdiagnosed as ADD, NLD resembled ADD in that children with NLD demonstrated poor attention to visual and tactile input.

These deficits were identified during the assessment of the boy, indicating that there was limited access to the areas of the brain that are linked to these modalities. Affecting the ability of his brain to think, process, and store non-verbal information and to solve visual problems, the child's deficits affected what the team called visual–spatial–organizational skills. The result was a specific weakness in interpreting and organizing visual–spatial information, problems adjusting to transitions and novel situations, deficits in social judgment and social interaction, and poor fine motor skills. Lacking the ability to comprehend nonverbal communications, the boy demonstrated difficulties in reading faces and body language and in adjusting to transitions and novel situations. These difficulties limited his social judgment and positive social interactions, affecting his ability to make and keep friends.

Although he exhibited poor attention to visual and tactile input, the child demonstrated exceptional verbal skills, excellent auditory attention and memory, and the ability to learn primarily through verbal mediation. In essence, what he heard, he remembered, and what he only saw, he did not.

Following a detailed explanation of the boy's learning disability, the team explained to his mother that the behavioral interventions and the educational modifications designed by the Learning Support Center would minimize the effects of her son's non-verbal learning disability on his academic and social performance. She was told that Ritalin generally did not improve the inattention of children with NLD. Her son's previous experience with the drug suggested to her that the educational and behavioral approach might succeed where medication had not.

To maximize the boy's opportunities for success, the team stressed the importance of his mother's advocacy and the necessity of its continuance. She was told that because students with NLD were just beginning to receive the understanding and appropriate stimuli they require in schools, her involvement was of paramount importance. She was counseled to stress to her son's teachers his inability to process visual–spatial information accurately and to emphasize her son's ability to learn from verbal explanations. She was told that a representative from the Learning Support Center was available to discuss the specifics of her son's learning disability with his classroom teacher, if that proved to be necessary.

After her son's screening and evaluation at the clinic for attention problems at the Learning Support Center at Texas Children's Hospital, the mother found that the experience had been both enlightening and validating—particularly since her son proved to be a brilliant child, maybe even a genius, just as she thought.

That he learned differently from others only made him that much more special to her.

And, with the utmost confidence in the expert guidance received at the Learning Support Center at Texas Children's Hospital, she anticipated that her son soon was going to believe in himself as much as she did.

21

﹌ MEYER CENTER FOR ﹌
DEVELOPMENTAL
PEDIATRICS

S HERRY SELLERS VINSON BELIEVED THAT her true calling was to be a reading lab specialist.

In 1982, while teaching children with learning disabilities how to comprehend heroic adventures in print, Vinson did not realize that she was about to embark on her own heroic adventure in real life.

Unknown to her at the time, the impetus for this life-changing experience was sitting in her reading lab.

"One of my students was dyslexic, and her mother told me she was taking the child to be evaluated at the Meyer Center for Developmental Pediatrics at Texas Children's Hospital," Vinson recalled. "She asked me if I wanted to come with her to hear the Meyer Center's evaluation of her child."[1]

Vinson enthusiastically accepted the offer, eager to learn more about dyslexia from the medical experts' standpoint.

She had become interested in learning disabilities while teaching junior high school history and business. A graduate of Abilene Christian University (ACU), Vinson had earned a bachelor's degree in secondary education with a field in history and secretarial business. While teaching, she became frustrated with the below-average reading skills of some of her junior-high students.

Convinced that early intervention would help improve reading and communication skills, Vinson decided to become a reading lab specialist to provide the intervening measures required. After earning a master's degree in reading at Sam Houston State University, she became a reading lab specialist at Sam Houston Elementary School in Conroe, Texas.

To her dismay, Vinson soon discovered that her education was insufficient to accomplish the goals she set for herself. Eager to learn more—not only about how to teach children to learn, but also about how children learn—she embarked on a quest.

"I taught with Dr. Rita Sawyer, who had her PhD in reading education," Vinson explained. "I knew that I wanted to get more education in the
reading field, so I asked Dr. Sawyer what she recommended."

Thinking that Sawyer would suggest a doctorate in reading education,
Vinson was genuinely surprised by her unexpected response.

"I don't think I was adequately prepared to think about what goes on in
the brain when you learn," Sawyer told her. "What I recommend is that you
find a way to learn about that, and I don't think the education schools are
teaching that right now, but I think we have the science to know about it."

Frustrated by Sawyer's suggestion, Vinson discussed her ambitions
with others. When her student's mother suggested that the solution might
be found at a staffing session at the Meyer Center for Developmental
Pediatrics, Vinson became intrigued with the possibility, although not convinced of the probability. Nonetheless, when she accompanied that mother
and daughter to the Meyer Center, she went with an open mind, ready to
learn whatever she could.

The "staffing," she discovered, was the consultation given by the multidisciplinary staff members of the Meyer Center to the parent of an
evaluated patient. Present in the room were the director of the Meyer Center,
Dr. Murdina M. Desmond; a pediatric developmentalist, Dr. W. Daniel
Williamson; and a number of other professionals in the field of learning disabilities. Each spoke about a specific area of concern, giving recommendations
for habilitative measures available in the community.

What happened next changed Vinson's life.

"When Dr. Desmond and Dr. Williamson explained 'the brain pathways' involved in dyslexia and the Orton Gillingham method taught at the
Neuhaus Center, I said to myself, 'Aha,' that's the answer," she explained. "I
went and talked to them, told them about my ambitions, and asked whether
I should go to the Neuhaus Center to learn more about brain pathways."

The doctors' reply was simple and direct: "What you should do is go
to medical school to become a developmental pediatrician."

The 30-year-old teacher was speechless. This, obviously, was the
answer she had sought, but how could she do such a thing at her age? She
had seriously considered going back to school to get her PhD, but a medical degree? Where would she go? What courses did she have to take?

"I knew I'd have to do about 30 hours of pre-med and I didn't know
if I could pass it because the only science I'd had on a college level was non-
major chemistry at Abilene Christian University," she said. "But I said to

myself, 'If I'm ever going to do it, I'm going to do it now' and decided to give it a try."[2]

Curious to see whether she could pass a pre-med course, Vinson enrolled in summer classes at ACU. Too embarrassed to ask for advice about which courses to take, she looked at the college catalogue and selected the first two courses, biology and botany.

"I saw an older person sitting in this class and I kind of teamed up with her and found out she also was a school teacher who wanted to be a psychiatrist," Vinson recalled. "When we told our teacher, he said, 'Oh, this is the best time in the history of the United States for an older woman to try to get in med school.' That's what he said, exactly. Of course, we were both offended, but happy he said it."

Inspired by her teacher's enthusiastic encouragement, as well as the A's she made in both her summer courses, Vinson began her pre-med curriculum at ACU.

Three years after hearing two powerful words, "brain pathways," at the Meyer Center for Developmental Pediatrics at Texas Children's Hospital, the 33-year-old former reading lab specialist entered her first year of medical school at Texas Tech University Health Sciences Center.

The heroic adventure was just beginning.

How a small clinic evolved over four decades to become a complex multidisciplinary developmental center was attributable to myriad influences—medical, technological, governmental, and personal.

The beginnings of the Meyer Center in 1960 as the mental retardation clinic in the Junior League Diagnostic Clinic of the outpatient department at Texas Children's Hospital were due to the personal influence of Leopold L. Meyer, president of Texas Children's Hospital board of trustees. Also serving as chairman of the board of governors of the Houston Council for Retarded Children, Inc., a nonprofit organization, Meyer was "in search of facilities for the many children in Houston who were in need of special attention." His diligent efforts on the council's behalf led him to recommend the establishment of a new service at Texas Children's Hospital.[3]

"It was apparent to me that there also existed the need for a medical link which would develop patterns of diagnosis and research to cope with the problem of mental retardation," Meyer recalled. "This entity I envisioned as being a part of the Texas Children's Hospital system. Consequently, Dr. Russell

J. Blattner, pursuant to having procured emergency aid through my efforts, proceeded to apply for federal funds to establish such a facility."[4]

Blattner's efforts were successful. Supported by a grant from the Maternal and Child Health Division of the Texas State Department of Health, the mental retardation clinic of the Junior League Diagnostic Clinic of the outpatient department at Texas Children's Hospital became a reality in September 1960. Operated under the joint auspices of the State of Texas and the department of pediatrics at Baylor College of Medicine, the clinic also received financial support from a federal grant-in-aid from the Children's Bureau, the Maternal and Child Health Services of the Department of Health, Education, and Welfare.

The established function of the mental retardation clinic of the Junior League Diagnostic Clinic of the outpatient department at Texas Children's Hospital was to provide diagnostic services to children with overt or suspected mental retardation. Staffed by a pediatrician, a public health nurse, a part-time psychologist, and a social worker, the clinic also provided social services and advised parents concerning educational and habilitative programming, such as they were.[5]

"In 1960, the magnitude of the population of children with developmental disabilities was not known," recalled Dr. Murdina M. Desmond, former director of the Meyer Center. "Relatively few services were available for children with particular educational needs in either public or private school settings. Services for multihandicapped children, those with educationally significant deficits in more than one area, were non-existent in Houston."

The insufficient availability of services in the 1950s and early 1960s was attributed to the general public's indifference to those with developmental disabilities and to the stigma that was commonly attached to mental retardation at the time. With a limited number of places to turn to for help, parents in Houston placed their developmentally impaired children in the Austin State School, which had begun accepting children in 1917.

Institutionalization was the commonly accepted procedure for parents—not only in Houston, but also throughout Texas and the United States, according to Frank Borreca, the first director of the Center for the Retarded, Inc. "If a child was born with a known cause of mental retardation, say Down syndrome, it was called 'mongoloidism' then, the doctor would say to the parents, 'Don't take your child home. Don't even get attached,'" Borreca explained. "The child immediately was placed in a state school. It was as if no one had given birth."[6]

Silence and secrecy also were the accepted norms for those parents who balked at such a drastic remedy and chose to raise their child at home. More often than not, the child was rarely seen in public and never discussed outside of the family. One such closely guarded secret was Rosemary, the sister of President John F. Kennedy. Born mentally retarded during a flu epidemic in 1918, she lived at home until 1941 and then became institutionalized after a prefrontal lobotomy. Like most families at the time with a mentally retarded child, the Kennedys never discussed Rosemary. During John F. Kennedy's campaign for the presidency and after his subsequent election to that office, reporters who asked of Rosemary's whereabouts were told by the family that she was in a convent.[7]

Although universally accepted as being appropriate, this exclusionist behavior towards the mentally retarded was totally unacceptable to at least one member of the Kennedy family. Eunice Kennedy Shriver had been investigating the issue since the mid-1950s. "There was a complete lack of interest in them and lack of knowledge about their capacities," she recalled. "They were isolated because their families were embarrassed and the public was prejudiced."[8]

Convinced that the Kennedy family should set a new standard of behavior, in 1962 Shriver sought and received permission from her father and President Kennedy to reveal their closely guarded family secret. The resulting story about Rosemary appeared in the September 22 issue of the *Saturday Evening Post*. Later hailed "as one of the biggest moments in perhaps the most important contribution the Kennedys made to the nation," the publication of that article significantly and positively influenced the public's perception of mental retardation.[9]

Also influencing the public's perception was the 1962 report from the President's Panel on Mental Retardation, a 26-member group of physicians, scientists, educators, lawyers, psychologists, and social scientists appointed by President Kennedy and charged with conducting an "intensive search for solutions." The panel's published conclusions were that the quality of services in state institutions needed to be upgraded and that the services provided by local communities needed to be comprehensive.

As public opinion slowly began to change during the Kennedy administration in the early 1960s, the mental retardation clinic of the Junior League Diagnostic Clinic of the outpatient department at Texas Children's Hospital also underwent a transformation. With a federal grant issued directly from the Children's Bureau, the clinic discontinued its joint affiliation with the Texas State Department of Health in 1962 and changed its name to the mental evaluation clinic at Texas Children's Hospital.

The expansion of its multidisciplinary services rendered to children with either manifest or suspected retardation occurred in 1967, as did another name change. The mental evaluation clinic became the child development clinic at Texas Children's Hospital. Designated for inclusion in the newly renamed clinic was the Rubella Study Project for victims of the 1964 rubella epidemic.

Inspired by the 1964–65 discovery that congenital rubella could involve a continuing infection of the brain, resulting in a wide range of developmental disabilities, the Rubella Study Project at Texas Children's Hospital opened in 1965 and immediately experienced unexpected growth. "We decided we would start a follow-up clinic, but what we were not counting on was how many babies we would have," explained neonatologist Desmond. "They began to come in great numbers, and suddenly we had more than 200 children."[10]

Initially funded by a limited grant from the Hartford Foundation and $25,000 from Texas Children's Hospital board president Meyer, Desmond's clinic began and flourished in the Junior League Outpatient Department at Texas Children's Hospital. The congenital rubella syndrome anomalies encountered in the infants seen in the Rubella Study Project were eye defects, congenital heart defects, hearing loss, disorders of the blood and blood-forming organs, enlargement of the liver and spleen, and central nervous system involvement with mental retardation. Since these children with multiple handicaps required various kinds of specialized care, the Rubella Study Project at Texas Children's Hospital evolved from a neonatology effort into a multidisciplinary approach to patient care and research.

The development of the Rubella Study Project took place over a short period of time. "It was unique," Desmond said. "It was unique because the speed of the cooperation of Texas Children's Hospital, the Clinical Research Center, and the virology department at Baylor College of Medicine was such that we were really one of the few groups that were able to get much information on these children when they were young. Gradually, all the departments became involved and we began to have a true multidisciplinary clinic. This was the first time that I remember that we had a very large clinical team working on a particular group of babies."

As the number of congenital rubella syndrome cases increased, the funds available to the Rubella Study Project decreased and Desmond's team sought a remedy. "Mr. Meyer's money lasted us a few months, and then we put in for a grant to the Children's Bureau, which took care of us for the next year," she explained. "We then were moved out of the Junior League Outpatient Department into the child development clinic. Drs. Gloria and Winston

Cochran, who were that clinic's director and associate director, both were specifically trained in child development at Philadelphia Children's Hospital and were certified in pediatrics. They had applied for and received a much larger Children's Bureau grant for a program for the multihandicapped."[11]

The Cochrans also established a preschool nursery in the child development clinic at Texas Children's Hospital with the new grant from the Children's Bureau. In cooperation with the Houston Speech and Hearing Center and the Texas Institute of Rehabilitation and Research, the nursery was a therapeutic education program geared to the young Down syndrome child, as well as others with multiple handicaps. Because of limited space in the child development clinic, the nursery was held at the Texas Institute of Rehabilitation and Research in the Texas Medical Center.

With this and other additional programs, the child development clinic outgrew its space in Texas Children's Hospital. In 1968, the clinic moved to larger facilities off-campus in the Kelsey-Seybold Building. Although temporary, the new location permitted additional direct patient services, expansion of the professional staff, and further program development. Also available were training opportunities for students in psychology, social service, physical therapy, and child development.

Four years later, the child development clinic moved temporarily again. With the promise of permanent facilities on the first floor of Texas Children's Hospital, the clinic briefly occupied space on the fourth floor of the hospital in 1972. It was during this time that the idea of a broader function for the child development clinic began to emerge.

The new concept followed the resignation of the Cochrans on July 1, 1972. Appointed as interim clinic director, and also as chairman of the search committee for a new clinic director, was Dr. Thomas E. Zion, assistant professor of pediatrics and neurology at Baylor College of Medicine.

To achieve its mission, the search committee first assessed the overall needs of the child development service at Texas Children's Hospital. Discovering that there were overlapping and uncoordinated services being provided by various child development projects both at Texas Children's Hospital and at the hospitals affiliated with Baylor College of Medicine, the committee stressed the need for centralization in order to avoid the duplication of efforts.

To accomplish this, the committee ascertained the primary concerns of the existing child development projects. At Texas Children's Hospital, the child development clinic was for patients with mental retardation, developmental delays, learning disorders, birth defects, and multiple handicaps.

Also offering diagnostic and genetic counseling for children with birth defects was a separate birth defects clinic at Texas Children's Hospital, as well as a follow-up clinic for birth defects at Jefferson Davis Hospital. In addition to that clinic at Jefferson Davis, there were separate follow-up clinics for high-risk infants, infants on prenatal psychoactive medication, and infants with congenital viral disease. Furthermore, in the Junior League Outpatient Department at Texas Children's Hospital, a one-year pilot clinic for learning disabilities, initiated and supported by the Junior League of Houston, was underway.

Zion's committee proposed that all of these child development activities be combined and placed under the aegis of a single section for coordination within the department of pediatrics. The idea received enthusiastic endorsement from Dr. Russell J. Blattner, chairman of the department of pediatrics and physician-in-chief at Texas Children's Hospital. The search committee also recommended that neonatologist Desmond become head of that new section and director of the child development clinic. Accordingly, the establishment of the section for developmental pediatrics in the department of pediatrics at Baylor College of Medicine occurred on July 26, 1972, with Desmond named as head of the section.

The selection of Desmond for this newly created position was highly favored by Zion, whose professional association with Desmond had been memorable. He was particularly impressed by Desmond's demonstrated belief in the need for pediatric neurology to interact with neonatology. "She was sort of the only one who was interested in this and, by her own bootstraps, was breaking ground in this area," Zion recalled. "We discussed this and she told me, 'I am going to talk to Dr. Blattner about taking a year's sabbatical and coming and doing a year in neurology, so I can have the base for doing some of the things I want to do.' Well, although that never came about, her interest continued to go more and more in the direction of developmental neurology. When there came a need for someone to move into a developmental center which, up to that time, had been a traditional mental retardation center, here was Dr. Desmond with the interest and the experience and the determination."[12]

Although Desmond immediately accepted the position in July, Zion's interim directorship of the child development clinic at Texas Children's Hospital continued for six months. "He assumed responsibility for keeping the clinic running," recalled Blattner. "He literally spent part of his day at Texas Children's Hospital holding that clinic together until Dr. Desmond could wind up her responsibility as head of the newborn section and then take over as head of the developmental pediatrics section."[13]

Having been Baylor College of Medicine's first neonatologist in the late 1940s, Desmond stepped away from that service to become one of the pioneers in the field of developmental pediatrics. Yet to emerge as a new subspecialty in the early 1970s, developmental pediatrics nonetheless had its roots in one of the first sections established in the American Academy of Pediatrics. Known as the 'section on mental growth and development,' it began in 1948, disbanded in 1958 due to lack of focus, and re-emerged in 1960 as the 'section on child development.' Renamed the 'section on developmental and behavioral pediatrics' in 1988, the subspecialty did not come of age officially until November 2002, the date of its first certification board exam. Thirty years earlier, Desmond had begun to make her innovative mark in that new field.[14]

One such innovation spearheaded by Desmond in the child development clinic involved preventative medicine, the primary goal of pediatrics. Named the Good Start program in 1972, it was for the prospective follow-up of very high risk infants—very low birthweight premature infants, infants with congenital infections, and those who experienced birth asphyxia or nursery morbidity involving the central nervous system. It was a continuation and expansion of the high-risk clinic that Desmond had introduced at Jefferson Davis Hospital in 1967. Serving as consultants for diagnosis and intervention, Desmond and her staff worked in partnership with the child's private physician or community clinic.

"The Good Start program evolved gradually because neurodevelopmental disorders occur in accordance with a timetable," Desmond explained. "Anticipatory care and orderly developmental surveillance permit early identification and maximal utilization of community resources for high-risk and developmentally delayed children."[15]

Also begun under Desmond's direction in 1973 were longitudinal studies, often in collaboration with other services at Texas Children's Hospital. The stated goal of these research projects was to apply preventative medicine to child development and attempt to anticipate problems, so that identification and educational habilitation can begin at the earliest possible age.[16] "The aim of the program is to find strengths and weaknesses of a child's development at each key age," Desmond explained. "We see children before the problem is acute, before they fail in school. This is preventative medicine."[17]

With the implementation of these new research studies, along with the incorporation of other existing child development programs such as the Junior League's pilot program for learning disabilities, the child development clinic underwent another name change. Having expanded its service, training, and research roles, it became known as the center for developmental pediatrics in 1973. The new name reflected the service's expanding areas of responsibility. "Since its beginning at Texas Children's Hospital in 1960 and throughout its various names, the Center for Developmental Pediatrics' scope of diagnostic services continuously broadened to serve children with delayed development, multihandicaps, school difficulties, learning difficulties," Desmond explained. "Beginning in 1973, we included high-risk infants in our growing patient population."[18]

Still located in its temporary space on the fourth floor of Texas Children's Hospital in 1973, the rapidly expanding center for developmental pediatrics moved to its new facilities on the first floor of Texas Children's Hospital in 1974. With the move came another name change, one that honored an individual who had been a tireless supporter of children with developmental disabilities, Leopold L. Meyer.

Designated by the board of trustees of Texas Children's Hospital, the official naming of the new center took place November 26, 1974, with the dedication of the Leopold L. Meyer Center for Developmental Pediatrics. This tribute to one of the founding trustees and the president emeritus of Texas Children's Hospital was an emotional one for all who attended. Located within the waiting room of the Meyer Center was a glass case filled with a collection of dolls dressed by Meyer's late wife, Adelena Meyer, and a portrait of his late daughter, Fan Harriet Meyer, to whom the display was dedicated. "If I were not moved by this occasion, I would be less than human," stated Meyer in an eloquent, extemporaneous statement at the dedication.[19]

The honoree remained uncharacteristically speechless when Desmond declared: "Your name is forever part of Texas Children's Hospital, the Houston Center for Retarded Children, the Rubella Study Project, and many other institutions and agencies serving children in the Houston area. In this multidisciplinary clinic for children who must walk uphill to walk ahead, we intend to make you proud."[20]

This was a pledge that Desmond and her team were committed to fulfilling. They were off to a good start in 1974. The multidisciplinary diagnostic approach originated by the Cochrans in 1960 and praised as unique by Desmond in the Rubella Study Project began to flourish in the Meyer Center for Developmental Pediatrics. "It is the unique feature of the Meyer Center," stated Desmond. "In a single setting its multidisciplinary staff carries out a broad, medically based developmental and educational evaluation of the child, consults with the referring pediatrician, and provides guidance to the parents as well as referral to appropriate community resources."[21]

To accomplish these goals, the Meyer Center's multidisciplinary staff included physicians, psychologists, speech pathologists, occupational therapists, physical therapists, public health nurses, and social workers. Because of the complexity of the problems encountered during patient evaluations, the 13 professionals on the Meyer Center's staff began working closely with staff members from neonatology, otolaryngology, audiology, pediatric neurology, child psychiatry, physical medicine, and genetics.[22]

Of utmost importance to the Meyer Center were referrals. "Our closest relationship is with the practicing pediatrician or primary care provider," Desmond explained. "We view ourselves primarily as consultants to them. At the completion of an evaluation, copies of all records are sent back to the referring physician."[23]

In addition to those services, in the late 1970s the Meyer Center began serving as an interface between pediatrics and public education. Directly influencing and expanding the community role of the Meyer Center was the 1978 implementation of the Education of All Handicapped Children Act of 1975. That legislation, Public Law 94-142, later known as the Individuals with Disabilities Education Act (IDEA), ordered school districts to provide education for the handicapped. The law also provided parents of children with developmental disabilities the right to participate in the planning of each child's education.

Having often referred to the multihandicapped children in the Rubella Study Project as "pioneers in modern special education," Desmond credited the successful implementation of that legislation partly to the large population of rubella children in the United States. "They became the wedge to open legally mandated educational opportunities for the handicapped," she stated. "And parents have filled the unaccustomed role of being their child's advocate."[24]

The lengthy delay in implementing the law in Houston rankled Desmond, who told a newspaper reporter: "Since all children, regardless of handicap, are now entitled to a public education, there are many needs in the community that should be met. It is high time for the school board to settle down and stop fighting with one another and become concerned about education."[25]

Such outspoken advocacy for children was to become a Desmond trademark throughout her tenure at the Meyer Center for Developmental Pediatrics at Texas Children's Hospital. In the decade following the IDEA, the Meyer Center began its consulting service to the Children's Lighthouse for the Blind and to area schools, particularly to the Houston Independent School District for its special education programs. Meyer Center staff members also began serving as members of the professional advisory committees to the Harris County Center for the Retarded, the Mental Health-Mental Retardation Authority, the March of Dimes, the Cerebral Palsy Developmental Disabilities Treatment Center, the Orton Dyslexia Society, the Neuhaus Foundation for the Remediation of Learning Disabilities, and the Texas Rehabilitation Commission.

The implementation of IDEA also influenced the day-to-day activities of the Meyer Center. By 1985—the twenty-fifth anniversary of the evolved Meyer Center—there were three basic categories of patients seen by the center: pre-school children referred by their pediatricians because of delays in any field of development; school-aged children and young adolescents who encountered academic difficulties; and infants and young children who were at high risk for later developmental problems. Approximately 800 patients were evaluated yearly, ranging in age from newborn infants to young teenagers, with many under three years of age.

The extensive research program at the Meyer Center included addressing the question of how a mother's illnesses during pregnancy, or a baby's illnesses after birth, influenced the child's development through school age. Among the continuing longitudinal research studies conducted by the Meyer Center were those of babies with asymptomatic and symptomatic congenital cytomegalovirus (CMV) infection, congenital rubella infection, and bacterial/viral meningitis. Also researched were the early neurodevelopmental outcome of low birthweight infants and the anticipatory healthcare and developmental course for the very low birthweight infant after discharge from intensive care. Other research projects involved the behavioral effects of children with meningitis, infants with cerebral hemorrhage, and infants of mothers on narcotics, alcohol, and central nervous system active drugs.

As the largest center of its type in the Houston area in the early 1980s, the Meyer Center for Developmental Pediatrics at Texas Children's Hospital served as a major link to the rapidly growing number of community agencies established to serve children with developmental disabilities. As the Meyer Center became more involved in the community and continued its expansion of services, in 1982 its future became uncertain because of funding. Static since 1964, the grant from Maternal and Child Health Bureau was terminated. "Evaluation procedures have been streamlined and the unit has been able to integrate much more closely with other services within the hospital and other research programs," Desmond announced. "Recently the Meyer Center has been honored and challenged by a matching grant from the Cullen Health Trust Foundation. In order to receive this grant, $200,000 must be raised by October of 1986. This is a singularly important goal for the future of the Meyer Center."[26]

Suddenly thrust into the role of fund-raiser, Desmond began a four-year campaign of writing request letters, attending benefits honoring the Meyer Center, writing thank-you notes, and accompanying volunteers making personal calls on potential donors. "I worked on this almost full-time. I'll never forget it. It was amazing," she recalled. "I would go out with Rabbi Schachtel, whose wife was one of our psychologists. He would start off talking to everybody, asking how their families were, and saying how blessed they were. Then he would work into the conversation our request for contributions. He was marvelous to watch."[27]

In February 1984, in the midst of the endowment campaign, a tragedy occurred involving the most famous patient at the Meyer Center for Developmental Pediatrics at Texas Children's Hospital. David Vetter, the "bubble boy" whose body's inability to fight infection forced him to live inside a series of plastic bubbles, had died at the age of 12. For David's entire life, Desmond was a member of the medical team that treated him and tried to help him live as normally as possible. As the child development expert, she dedicated her attention to anticipating the needs of a child who lived in medically imposed isolation—the only child ever to do so at Texas Children's Hospital. "It stretched the mind," Desmond said. "It really did because you couldn't really imagine what it was like to be in David's place. You had nothing to go on. Everyone's feelings were so wound up with David. It was sometimes hard to keep your equilibrium."[28]

Desmond maintained her balance by working with all her other patients and with the multidisciplinary team at the Meyer Center at Texas Children's Hospital. "It's remarkable what you learn working with a team. You learn to read patients, which I had never done. You learn to be aware of their feelings in a way I had never been," she recalled. "To sit across the table with parents and discuss the future of their children was incredible. It wasn't always good news. It was mostly bad, but our aim was not just to diagnose and tell the parents. Our aim was to work out a program for living and for education. It takes a lot to go from bad news to working out a problem. And that's where a team is so wonderful. One member can lift the other, one can watch the parents for a sense of despair or to see when they have had enough, and one can be the one who says, 'Let's stop for today. Let's do this another time.' I found the Meyer Center to be incredibly marvelous, just what I always thought practicing medicine ideally should be like."[29]

Desmond's enthusiasm was influential in the successful completion of the Meyer Center's $1 million endowment fund campaign in August 1986.

After more than two decades spent helping direct the future of children in the community, the Meyer Center for Developmental Pediatrics received the help needed from the community in order to secure the center's own future. The accomplishment was most attributable to Desmond's trademark nature. "She is the most enthusiastic individual I have ever met," said long-time colleague and fellow neonatologist Rudolph. "She'll develop an area of interest and then really get everyone fired up about it."[30]

Designating the successful campaign as the appropriate end to her medical career, Desmond announced her retirement on August 26, 1986. At a ceremony honoring her contributions to developmental pediatrics, Dr. Ralph D. Feigin, chairman of the department of pediatrics at Baylor College of Medicine and physician-in-chief at Texas Children's Hospital, stated: "Dr. Desmond's interest in developmental pediatrics was a natural extension of her earlier work in neonatology. She was quick to perceive that with the advent of neonatal intensive care nurseries, more babies were surviving, but were also developing handicapping conditions which require comprehensive evaluation and long-term care."[31]

To honor Desmond, the Meyer Center for Developmental Pediatrics established the Desmond Neonatal Developmental Follow-Up Clinic in 1984. Providing referral services for premature infants who were born at 31 weeks or less, the Desmond Clinic also followed those infants who received special therapies and medical interventions. Patients were seen at regular intervals for the first three years of life. "I was thrilled, really. If I were rich, that's what I would endow, believe me," said Desmond of the honor. "I think of premature babies as orchids. They are more complex to raise, but they are well worth it."[32]

Another lasting tribute to Desmond's 13-year tenure as director of the Meyer Center for Developmental Pediatrics was the fact that many of the programs and procedures she introduced and championed at the Meyer Center continued unchanged for more than 15 years after her departure.

One month after Desmond's retirement in 1986, the Meyer Center for Developmental Pediatrics moved into the new Texas Children's Hospital Clinical Care Center on North Stadium Drive. Named as its new director was Dr. W. Daniel Williamson, a pediatric developmentalist who had trained with Desmond. Williamson was to continue in that role through the Meyer Center's thirtieth anniversary in 1990 and its subsequent move the following year into the newly built Clinical Care Center, later known as the Feigin Center at Texas Children's Hospital.

When Williamson decided to go into private practice in 1993, Feigin named Dr. Frank R. Brown as director of the Meyer Center. A developmental pediatrician and former professor of pediatrics at the Medical University of South Carolina in Charleston, Brown served as director until 1998. He was followed by pediatric developmentalist Dr. Geraldine Wilson for one year. Named acting director in July 1999 was Dr. Sherry Sellers Vinson, the former reading specialist whom Desmond had inspired to become a pediatric developmentalist.

Celebrating its fortieth anniversary in 2000, the Meyer Center for Developmental Pediatrics at Texas Children's Hospital continued to thrive under the influence of Desmond's original guidelines. Performing more than 2,000 evaluations each year, the Meyer Center team offered comprehensive diagnostic services for infants and children with suspected developmental disabilities and also provided preventative guidance for infants at risk because of prematurity or congenital infections.

Since its founding in 1960, the Meyer Center at Texas Children's Hospital had helped children with special needs, a patient population that expanded with the emerging identification of congenital conditions that may affect a child's physical or mental development. By the year 2000, conditions such as prematurity, birth defects, infections, accidents, and prenatal exposure to drugs or alcohol were known to cause abnormalities that affected a child's ability to walk, talk, or learn. Some may have visual or hearing impairments and others may have central nervous system disorders. Many had multiple handicaps resulting from birth defects, accidents, and illness.

Such children and their families were being referred to the Meyer Center at Texas Children's Hospital in 2000. "We diagnose and develop management plans for children who have complex problems such as learning disabilities, cerebral palsy, mental retardation, autistic spectrum disorders, and disorders of language, behavior, and attention," Vinson said. "Our approach is interdisciplinary and family-centered. This means that a team of professionals evaluates each child and works with the family on assessments, team meetings, and conferences to develop an individualized treatment program."[33]

Following an initial evaluation of each child by the developmental pediatrician, a neurodevelopmental examination determined if additional assessments were necessary to meet the needs of the child and family. Should other Meyer Center professionals need to be consulted, the developmental pediatrician referred the child. Available for consultation were a neuropsychologist/developmental psychologist, a speech/language pathologist, an occupational therapist, a physical therapist, a social worker, and, if needed, any of the other medical services available at Texas Children's Hospital.

For the neurodevelopmental assessment of pre-term babies and families in the Desmond Neonatal Developmental Follow-Up Clinic, specialists from the neonatology service at Texas Children's Hospital joined forces with the Meyer Center team. Each child was seen at regular intervals, usually every four to six months, for the first three years of life. When determined necessary by the team of physicians, referrals were made to other pediatric specialists at Texas Children's Hospital or to community resources.

Although the patient population of the Meyer Center for Developmental Pediatrics at Texas Children's Hospital incrementally increased through the years, it was expected to grow substantially in the future as neurodevelopmental disabilities and developmental behavioral pediatrics became more clearly defined. Pediatric neurologist Dr. Geoffrey Miller, chief of developmental medicine, was convinced that this clarification was eminent. "In pediatrics, they are asking: What is developmental disabilities? What does it encompass? Who does it? Who does what? There is sort of a general turmoil going on at the moment," he explained. "The spectrum is very broad. It has spread all the way across through learning language and behavior disorders, to chronic neurological disorders and the provision of services for that diagnosis and management. So, it is extremely broad and we would include in all of that the developmental outcomes of various illnesses, medical procedures, and interventions."[34]

Developmental outcome and longitudinal studies remained the focus of research projects in the Meyer Center in the early 2000s. Plans called for investigating the management of neuromuscular disorders and studying the developmental effects of child abuse. "The Meyer Center is also involved in looking at developmental disabilities and its evaluation in various ethnic groups," Miller said. "We might become involved with the management of congenital heart disease, it's what I've done in the past. We will be looking at those disorders that affect the function of the brain which arise before birth or after birth, but once arisen do not worsen, which differentiates it from ongoing infections or tumors."

Miller believed that the Meyer Center for Developmental Pediatrics at Texas Children's Hospital was positioned in 2004 to become one of the major centers of its kind in the United States. With its proven ability to provide education, research, and training in areas that traditionally were called either neurodevelopmental disabilities or developmental behavioral pediatrics, the foundation necessary for expansion was already in place.

The future of the Meyer Center for Developmental Pediatrics at Texas Children's Hospital is sure to be like its past, in that it will be dramatically influenced by medical discoveries, technological advances, and governmental regulations.

What will remain constant at the Meyer Center and at the Desmond Neonatal Developmental Follow-Up Clinic at Texas Children's Hospital is an appreciation of the magnificent contributions to developmental pediatrics made by namesakes Leopold L. Meyer and Dr. Murdina M. Desmond.

Fifteen years after her visit as a reading lab specialist in 1982, developmental pediatrician Dr. Sherry Sellers Vinson returned to the Meyer Center for Developmental Pediatrics as a staff member in 1997.

The heroic adventure inspired by Vinson's first visit had not been an easy one. "I was one of the older students at Texas Tech Health Science Center, so I didn't have that 'youthful stamina,' but my maturity and real-world experience compensated for it," she said. "I knew I was on the right path."[35]

There had also been some unexpected twists and turns on that path. During her lengthy quest to learn all there was to know about learning disabilities, Vinson discovered that she had a learning disability of her own. Diagnosed at the age of 35 with visual–spatial problems that limited her ability to understand in three dimensions, she began regular therapy to allow her to function professionally.

"When they would teach a three-dimensional subject using flat slides, the only way I could learn it was to build it. I would take pencils, paper, whatever I could find," she said. "I would go home, get my textbook, and design what they were talking about in three dimensions. I couldn't just look at a picture of the brain, I had to buy one of the puzzles with brain parts you can take apart to see where everything is located."[36]

Utilizing the appropriate compensation skills, Vinson excelled both in the classroom and in clinical training. Accepted for her pediatric residency at Chicago's Cook County Hospital, the tough inner-city hospital portrayed in the television series *ER*, she felt that the hospital's "hands-on" approach to tough problems provided her with the best education in developmental pediatrics.

Following her residency, Vinson was awarded a fellowship at Johns Hopkins University School of Medicine. While training at that school's Kennedy Krieger Institute, she worked with world-renowned developmental pediatrician Dr. Arnold Capute, who had been one of the esteemed members of President Kennedy's President's Panel on Mental Retardation in 1962. "Kennedy Krieger Institute is a multidisciplinary center for children who have any kind of neurodevelopmental disability," Vinson explained.

"The developmental pediatric fellowship at Johns Hopkins is connected with the institute. Dr. Frank Brown, the director of the Meyer Center, had done his fellowship there so my mentors got me in touch with Dr. Brown and that is how I got hired at the Meyer Center, exactly where I wanted to be."[37]

Although the doctors who had inspired her to become a developmental pediatrician were no longer at the Meyer Center, Vinson retained the initial excitement of her "Aha!" moment there. "This is more than what I always hoped," she explained after joining the staff at the Meyer Center. "I can say that despite the fact that I think Johns Hopkins and the Kennedy Krieger Institute are top-notch places; I have never worked with a staff like the one at the Meyer Center. Each of them are the best I ever worked with and I worked with plenty of really good ones at Johns Hopkins."

Vinson believed that one of the reasons why the Meyer Center was such a loved place was "because we specialize in helping parents who just received bad news about their child's cognitive or motor ability. We specialize in making that diagnosis and helping the parents deal with it. We have social workers here that are specifically trained to help parents think through what they need to be thinking through at the appropriate times. The Meyer Center is not one in which you can hurry in and out. We take the time to look at the whole child, everything that's going on, everything that possibly could be involved in that child's development."

One important component in every child's development was education. Because the Meyer Center at Texas Children's Hospital worked so closely with Houston-area schools, Vinson relied on her background experiences to communicate successfully with teachers. "I am realistic about what the classroom teacher can do," she explained. "I don't think I ask for things that are impossible. I understand what it is like to be a teacher in a school district with limited funds to help children with various challenges."

Such empathy produced results. "Teachers are more apt to open up to her since she has been in their shoes," said Carmen Dickerson, social worker at the Meyer Center. "The school districts really respond to her."

Vinson also established empathetic relationships with the parents of her patients. Having been diagnosed with a developmental disability of her own, she drew upon that experience when talking to parents about the results of their child's evaluation. She shared other success stories as well, including that of a friend who was mildly autistic but had earned a master's degree and, with regular therapy, functioned professionally.

Attributing her seasoned approach to maturity, Vinson admitted: "I am old enough now. I'm still idealistic, but I realize that people have so many problems in their lives that they can't gear toward the solution I am suggesting. I think I'm tolerant, understanding. I have had enough failures in my life. I don't know all the answers either, so I am not as dogmatic."

Vinson was, however, steadfast in her opinions about the Meyer Center for Developmental Pediatrics at Texas Children's Hospital. "The Meyer Center has helped people get to their highest potential, and we have helped families function despite horrible circumstances," Vinson said. "We are a place of comfort for families who have worries about their children's development."[38]

The Meyer Center for Developmental Pediatrics at Texas Children's Hospital also was a place where a reading lab specialist discovered her true calling and began a new chapter in her life.

22

♨ NEONATOLOGY ♨

HOUSTONIANS SANDY AND JACK BABER thought that their 1981 Christmas-week holiday was going to be a tranquil respite.

More than 820 miles away from Houston at the beautiful Angel Fire resort in the Sangre de Cristo Range of the Rocky Mountains in New Mexico, the seven-months-pregnant Sandy was content just to bypass the hectic holidays at home. It was their last trip as a two-person family, both able to do whatever pleased them. It was idyllic until, suddenly, on December 28, Sandy discovered that her amniotic fluid was leaking. Soon after she went into premature labor.

Since it was the holidays, the Babers knew that it would be almost impossible to reach her obstetrician—or any other Houston physician—on the phone. Their only option was to go to the emergency room at the Taos Hospital, 30 miles away. After undergoing an evaluation in that hospital, the Babers were told to go to the Albuquerque hospital, where there was a level III neonatal intensive care unit (NICU) for premature babies.

The Albuquerque hospital was a 150-mile drive from Taos. The Babers left immediately. "We were just moving; I don't know how we did it," Sandy said. "This whole sequence of events was bizarre. We didn't check out of the Taos Hospital, we walked out, got in the car, and drove to Albuquerque."[1]

During that drive, the Babers were filled with apprehension. "We were prepared for a normal birth—Lamaze," Jack said, remembering their uncertainty about what might happen next. "What we went through was an abrupt change and it was a vertical learning curve. It was immediate and it was that way for months. We really went from a standing start to a radical change in a matter of moments."[2]

At the Albuquerque hospital, Sandy was examined and the Babers were advised to return to Houston as soon as possible. "They could tell by the ultra-sound that the baby's birthweight was probably not going to be much over three pounds," Sandy said. "They told us if the baby was born in Albuquerque and survived, we would be there for a long time. They also said there was a big chance the baby would not survive."

The Babers were anxious to leave immediately. Jack wanted Life Flight to send the jet from Houston and pick them up, but a series of thunder-storms prevented the plane from flying until the next morning. Unable to find a commercial flight to Houston that night, they checked into a hotel. "We got on the first plane out the next morning and came to Houston," Sandy said, recalling how she did not mention she was in labor to the tick-et agent for fear of not being allowed to fly. "We changed planes in Dallas and the contractions really started then."

When the Babers arrived in Houston on December 29, they went straight to Woman's Hospital of Texas, where John L. Baber IV was born the following day. Weighing only 1,020 grams (two pounds and four ounces) and born at 28 weeks, baby "Jack" could not breathe on his own and was intubated and stabilized by neonatologist Dr. Charleta Guillory in the deliv-ery room at Woman's Hospital.

Within moments, the Babers' ride on an emotional roller coaster esca-lated to full throttle. "Someone came in my room and said, 'Oh, by the way, we need to tell you something. One ear was not developed,'" Sandy said. "That was the least of the worries at the time. We knew he was small and that development of the ear did not have anything to do with his survival. It was not life-threatening. So, at that point, we said, 'We'll deal with that later.' But they had to tell us that he was not the perfect baby."

They soon learned that their newborn son was to be transferred to the newborn center at Texas Children's Hospital. As the ambulance transported the baby, his bewildered father followed closely behind in his own car. "The idea that they weren't going to keep the baby at Woman's probably never crossed our mind," he said. "But it didn't strike me as unusual that they were going to take him to Texas Children's, because he was a very sick child."

The distraught father checked his son into the Texas Children's Hospital admissions office and then went to the neonatal intensive care unit (NICU). His first impressions were indelible. "There were 20 or 30 isolettes with all kinds of noise and alarms," he remembered. "Looking back on it now, that process now is probably so low-tech it's laughable, but to us it was extremely high-tech. They had monitors for each of the babies. All of them had all sorts of tubes and each one of them had a nurse very close by. I think it was one nurse per two, at that point in time, who was there all of the time."

From that very first moment in NICU, Jack realized that the vertical learning curve had begun in earnest. "'We learned everything out of necessity," he said. "One of the first things we learned were the numbers—how critical those oxygen numbers are to survival and to progress. He was on a ventilator for so long. We would call in shorthand to the nurses. What is this? What is that? What's his weight? And by the time you knew the numbers, you knew that there had been problems or there hadn't been problems."

Advised in the first week that baby Jack had hyaline membrane disease, the same lung disease responsible for the death of President John F. Kennedy's premature son in 1961, Sandy and Jack asked their church pastor, Larry Hall, to come to the hospital and baptize him. "We didn't know if the baby was going to make it," Jack said. "You just don't know."

In the first ten days in the Texas Children's Hospital NICU, the Babers learned more and more. They were told by the team of specialists that their very low birthweight baby had patent ductus arteriosus, a hole in the heart; intraventricular cranial hemorrhaging, bleeding in the brain; hydrocephalus, water on the brain; apnea of prematurity, sudden stops and starts of breathing; and congenital aural atresia, a craniofacial malformation of the external and inner ear. "They put a team together, a wonderful support group of medical professionals who, more often than not, worked together," Jack said. "This group included a lot of specialty practices who gave us a high degree of comfort that we were getting excellent and cutting-edge kind of medical thought."

With each new diagnosis, the Babers asked the neonatologists, specialists, therapists, nurses, and fellow parents of preemies in the NICU, "What does that mean?" With each new treatment prescribed, they would ask, "What is that?" Jack soon learned that "you get information from all sources in this kind of environment. Because you bond in that environment, you get information from the other parents. And, of course, from the specialists and neonatologists, from the residents on that service to the doctors who are running it, and the nurses, who are incredibly committed to that service."

The Babers developed a close relationship with most of the nurses in the NICU at Texas Children's Hospital. "We would usually be there a couple of times of day in the morning and the evening, and when we were not there we could call in," Jack said. "Or they would call us. I never had the feeling someone wasn't watching and responsible for Jack. They really encouraged us to call in, and we could call in the middle of the night. In fact, they would suggest, 'If you wake up in the middle of the night and you're worried, call us and we'll tell you what's going on.' And somebody was also close enough, it wasn't, like, 'Could you hold the phone and I'll check?' They could pretty much tell you the minute they picked up the phone. The care was constant."

Such care was extended to both the babies and the parents. Encouraged by the nurses to touch, stroke, and caress her son, at first Sandy was unable to pick up the baby and hold him because he was still on a ventilator. Finally, after six weeks, the ventilator was removed and Sandy could, at long last, hold her baby in her arms—and, like all new mothers, rock him to sleep. "They had rocking chairs and everything necessary to make us feel comfortable," Sandy recalled. "He was still hooked up to a feeding tube that gave him a high-protein, high-calorie feeding so he could gain weight."

Sandy also remembered the sympathetic care she often received from the nurses. "For somebody to be in that rotation and be a neonatal nurse, I don't know how long they emotionally could do it," Sandy said. "You have to be a special person to be able to do that for any length of time."

Also impressed with the neonatal nursing staff at Texas Children's Hospital was Jack, who observed their interaction with other families in the NICU with admiration. "It was tough for us, since it was our child," he said. "But the nurses dealt with a lot of death, and a lot of real, real sickness, and a lot of heartbreak."

With the Babers, the nurses dealt instead with unbridled joy and gratitude. On April 9, 1982, after spending nine and a half weeks in the NICU and three and a half weeks in the preemie nursery, the six-pound John L. Baber IV went home. "Our experience at Texas Children's Hospital," Jack stated, "was way beyond just a positive experience. It was family."

The words "neonatology" and "neonatologist" first appeared in print in 1960.

Pediatrician Dr. A. J. Schaffer introduced the nomenclature in his 1960 book *Diseases of the Newborn* with this apology: "We trust we shall be forgiven for coining the words 'neonatology' and 'neonatologist.' The one designates the art and science of diagnosis and treatment of disorders of the newborn infant, and the other, the physician whose primary concern lies in this specialty"[3]

In 1971, 11 years after Schaffer's book was published, one of the first neonatology services in Texas was created at Texas Children's Hospital. Responsible for laying the foundation for this service was one of the pioneers in the field of newborn medicine, Baylor College of Medicine pediatrician Dr. Murdina MacFarquahar Desmond. Having begun her groundbreaking work with newborns 12 years before the words to describe that subspecialty and its practitioners were coined, Desmond became known among her peers as "the first neonatologist in Texas."[4]

Born in 1916 on the Isle of Lewis in Scotland, Desmond moved to the United States with her mother, brother, and sister in 1924. She graduated from Smith College and received her medical training at the Temple University School of Medicine in Philadelphia, specializing in pediatrics. After interning in New York and serving in the Navy, she began a fellowship at the George Washington University School of Medicine. Her mentor at George Washington, Dr. L. K. Sweet, "had a fellowship for research work in newborn infants and he gave it to me and I worked it that way and I loved it."[5]

During the war years, Desmond met, fell in love with and married a Texan, Jim Desmond. Her husband's plans to enter dental school in Houston precipitated the newlyweds' move there in 1948. Once in Houston, Desmond's search for employment led her to the newly constructed Baylor College of Medicine in the Texas Medical Center.

Desmond vividly recalled her first interview with Dr. Russell J. Blattner, the newly appointed chairman of the department of pediatrics at Baylor College of Medicine. When he asked about her area of interest, Desmond replied: "Working with the newborn." This was most unusual at the time, and "he was very surprised," Desmond remembered. "But he was game. He said, 'Fine.' So, that's what happened. I joined with that understanding."[6]

As an instructor at Baylor College of Medicine, Desmond began her work with newborns in 1948. In the early 1950s, the midst of the postwar Baby Boom era, she worked in the nursery at Jefferson Davis Hospital, the Baylor-affiliated teaching hospital in Houston. Desmond supervised newborn and premature care, kept mortality statistics, conducted follow-up care, and maintained close communication with state and local health departments.[7] "A distinct change in direction of delivery room procedure occurred in 1953, when Virginia Apgar, obstetrical anesthesiologist, introduced an objective scoring method for assessing the overall condition of the newborn at one minute after delivery," Desmond said.[8]

While instituting the Apgar scoring system and observing the vast number of newborns at Jefferson Davis Hospital, Desmond realized that the babies were acting just like patients coming out of surgery. "We began to realize they were recovering patients. They were recovering from the experience of birth," she said. "I had an idea for transitional care research and applied to the John A. Hartford Foundation, Inc., of New York for a grant."[9]

With the opening of Texas Children's Hospital in February 1954,

Desmond became a charter staff member, seeing infants there when called in for a consultation. But because there wasn't a department of obstetrics or a nursery at the new hospital, she continued clinical work and teaching staff and students at Jefferson Davis. Anxious to learn more about advances in the field of newborn care, Desmond told Blattner of her quest. He arranged a Jesse H. Jones Scholarship for her in 1957, allowing her to spend four months at Children's Hospital Boston working with the renowned physiologist Dr. Clement Smith, a pioneer in the care of newborns. While there, Desmond met Dr. Arnold Jack Rudolph, a pediatrician from South Africa who had practiced privately for ten years before spending three years in fellowship training with Dr. Smith. It was a chance meeting that proved to be pivotal.

Returning to Houston in 1957, Desmond was chosen to head the newly created newborn section in the department of pediatrics at Baylor College of Medicine. Awarded in 1959 with the $172,000 grant she had requested from the Hartford Foundation, she began her clinical research for a transitional care nursery at Jefferson Davis. The diagnostic study of the infant's crucial period of adjustment—the transitional time between birth and the first feeding—was "to evaluate children before they got sick, hoping to pick them up early, rather than picking up the problem after the crisis had come."[10]

Knowing that this funded research would involve processing the clinical behavior of more than 700 infants, Desmond decided that she needed additional help on the project—preferably someone who had trained in newborn medicine. Her first choice was the dedicated pediatrician from South Africa whom she had met in Boston. "I recruited Dr. Rudolph," Desmond said. "I wrote and asked if he would consider coming to Texas and he said, 'Yes.' But it took two years to get him here."

The delay in Rudolph's arrival was due to a requirement of the United States Immigration Service. After three years of fellowship training with Smith in Boston, in 1959 Rudolph returned to Johannesburg, South Africa, for the required two years of residency outside of the United States. He then came to Houston. "I arrived here in 1961, and I'll never forget it," Rudolph recalled. "It was on a Saturday, two days before Hurricane Carla. I say, to this day, if my wife had come with me with the kids, we wouldn't be in Houston today."[11]

During the storm that wreaked havoc in Houston, causing electrical outages, fallen trees, and flooding, Rudolph drove to Jefferson Davis Hospital. "I was compulsive," he said, remembering the horror with which the staff at the hospital greeted his arrival during the storm.[12] "I was surprised to see him there," Desmond remembered. "He stayed at the hospital and told me to go home, and I did. I came home. And he didn't leave the hospital for three days, I believe."[13]

Rudolph weathered his introduction to Jefferson Davis and immediately joined Desmond's grant project. Together, they observed the clinical behavior of high-risk newborn infants. The work furthered the theory that newborns should be observed and clinically monitored in the same way as were post-op patients, rather than being placed in a nursery and casually observed.

In 1963, Desmond wrote her trademark article, "Clinical Behavior of the Newly Born," which described in detail the recovery and reactive periods of newborns. Also published in peer-review journals were her observations on the effect on infant recovery from low Apgar scores in 1964. "It was Dr. Desmond who proposed the name 'transition' to this series of recovery events and encouraged the identification of a nursery in hospitals to closely observe infants as they passed through the transition," said Dr. Reba Michels Hill. "I dare say that the majority of hospitals in the United States now have a Transition Nursery today as a result of her careful observations and writing."[14]

Hill had received her newborn training under Desmond at Jefferson Davis as a medical student and resident at Baylor College of Medicine. She returned for a one-year fellowship following a year of postdoctoral training in newborn medicine with Dr. John Kennel and Dr. Benjamin Spock at Case Western Reserve in Ohio. "I was really interested in the effect of maternal drugs early on," Hill said. "When I was a resident, I saw a child one time who had been delivered to a mother who was on Dilantin, and the baby had hypertrophied gums. I took the child to Dr. Desmond and said, 'Do you think this baby could have this hypertrophy of the gums because the mother is on Dilantin?' And she said, 'Well, Reba, I don't know. As far as I know, it's never been published before, but maybe no one has ever looked.'"[15]

Desmond was proud of Hill's resulting accomplishments. "Reba took this as her fellowship project, and she's been working with drugs ever since," Desmond said. "Her work has been magnificent. When they opened the premature nursery at St. Luke's, she went over there to become director of research. She's done a magnificent job."[16]

Hill remembered that when she arrived at St. Luke's Episcopal Hospital in 1961 as the first full-time pediatrician assigned to the Linda Fay Halbouty Nursery, "nobody had the foggiest idea of what newborn research was. Dr. Desmond, I think, spearheaded that there was a need for that type of person. But my charge was to take the Halbouty Nursery and make a research unit out of it."[17]

The Linda Fay Halbouty Nursery had been donated to St. Luke's

Episcopal Hospital in 1956 by Mr. and Mrs. Michel T. Halbouty. It was named in honor of their daughter, who had been born prematurely at St. Joseph's Hospital. Originally housing 20 cribs, the nursery expanded in 1960 to include 50 cribs. "The concept of the Linda Fay Halbouty Nursery was to provide specialized medical care for any neonate, delivered at Methodist Hospital and St. Luke's Episcopal Hospital, and infants born within a 100-mile radius of Houston, who were experiencing problems in transition from an intrauterine to an extrauterine life," said Hill.[18]

With the establishment of the Linda Fay Halbouty Nursery at St. Luke's Episcopal Hospital, Desmond's transitional care concept of taking care of not just premature infants, but any infant who had difficulty at the moment of birth, had become a reality. It was a completely new idea in newborn care in the United States, predating the concept of neonatal intensive care units by a decade. "Dr. Desmond's concept was so new in the late 1950s and early 1960s, nobody wanted to believe it," Hill said. "It took a long time to get her paper published. I think it took something like eight years to get it published. And St. Luke's was not accustomed to research being done. And it wasn't so much research. It was, actually, if you think about it now, it was essentially establishing some of the things we do now. I was doing things that were beginning the field of neonatology."[19]

While Hill continued her research activities at St. Luke's Episcopal Hospital, Rudolph and Desmond were continuing their breakthrough research in newborn care and laying more groundwork for neonatology specialization at Jefferson Davis. "We started doing transition of premature babies, transition of babies with low Apgar scores, transition of babies with problems, and that type of thing. And we were watching these babies very carefully," Rudolph recalled. "And around about 1964–65, people started talking about neonatal intensive care. And we established, Dr. Desmond and myself, established the first neonatal intensive care unit in the whole of the southwest at Jefferson Davis."[20]

With the invention of infant respirators in 1970, Desmond and Rudolph were able to abandon the hand-administered respiration techniques and mechanically aid the infants' breathing, draw blood to monitor how much oxygen there was in the infants' blood, and monitor the variability of heart rates in newborns. Their methods were firsts for Houston hospitals.[21] "I remember Dr. Desmond's and my hand bagging, giving a baby positive pressure breathing. Dr. Desmond, one nurse, and myself took it in shifts, 24 hours around the clock, to do that baby with hyaline membrane disease. The baby survived," Rudolph said, recalling the days before respirators.

While continuing to monitor closely the transition of all newborns at Jefferson Davis, Rudolph and Desmond made a noteworthy discovery during the rubella epidemic of the early 1960s. "We had known for years, since the studies of Gregg in Australia, that if the mother had rubella during pregnancy, the babies could be born with heart disease, patent ductus arteriosus, and other much less common types of heart disease," Rudolph said. "We also knew that those babies could be born with small heads, microcephaly. We also knew that those babies could have congenital deafness from the rubella infection. And we also knew that those babies could have eye problems, such as glaucoma or cataracts of the eye, or a small eyes condition called microphthalmia."

What they didn't know and soon discovered "by sheer serendipity," Rudolph explained, were the changes in the long bones, the femur and the humerus, caused by congenital rubella. While examining a newborn with lesions on the skin, whose mother reported no history of illness, Rudolph first thought that it was congenital syphilis. He ordered an X-ray of the long bones to confirm the diagnosis, a method still practiced today. The test for syphilis was negative, but Rudolph observed changes in the long bones that he had never before seen. The baby had a low platelet count as well. Desmond and Rudolph were somewhat puzzled by this; they didn't know what the baby had.

When another baby was born the next day with the same type of symptoms, Rudolph and Desmond realized that they were on the brink of a new discovery. "We got X-rays of the long bones, and there were the changes again," Rudolph said. "And this baby also had these lesions that we called the 'blueberry muffin lesions.' And we thought that these lesions were areas of purpura in the skin. But this mother gave a history of having German measles while pregnant. And after that, we just saw a whole bunch of cases. We saw over 250 cases of congenital rubella. But that was how we picked up the bone change, by sheer serendipity. And we were the first to report that throughout the United States."[22]

In an editorial written by Blattner in the *Journal of the American Medical Association,* published within three months of Rudolph and Desmond's long bone discoveries, the findings—which had never before been described in rubella—were given the name of "expanded rubella syndrome."[23]

At Jefferson Davis, an overwhelming influx of victims of the rubella epidemic necessitated the opening of a large follow-up clinic in a central location. Ultimately, these patients also changed the path of Desmond's career. "These babies were hit in so many different areas. Some of them had cardiac problems. A lot of them had eye problems. And most of them had hearing problems. A lot were sent to Dr. McNamara and cardiology. A lot were sent to neurology. A lot were sent to otolaryngology. They were all at Texas Children's. The multidisciplinary idea grew." Desmond said. "So, I decided to set up a clinic at Texas Children's Hospital in the Junior League Outpatient Department with Dr. Martha Yow."

In order to establish the new clinic, Desmond needed funding. She called the Hartford Foundation and asked if she could switch the money still available in the transitional nursery grant to this new challenge. The foundation agreed. "But that wouldn't begin to take care of it," Desmond said. "So, I talked to Dr. Blattner and Mr. Newell France, the administrator of the hospital, and presented our problem. Mr. France talked to Mr. Leopold Meyer, who gave us $25,000 with the proviso that no family be charged a dime. At the same time, we were writing a grant to the Children's Bureau. We got that grant and started to follow rubella in the clinic at Texas Children's."[24]

Because the infants were contagious and required separate staffing in the outpatient clinic, Desmond brought the nurses from the rubella clinic at Jefferson Davis over to Texas Children's Hospital. "It was just multiple consultants, our nurses, ourselves, and our patients," Desmond recalls. "It was a very successful clinic. I actually followed those kids until they were 18."

In addition to the rubella clinic at Texas Children's Hospital, Desmond and Rudolph continued their newborn work together at Jefferson Davis. In 1970, Blattner offered Rudolph the opportunity to take over the Junior League Outpatient Department at Texas Children's Hospital from Yow, who wanted to conduct further studies in infectious diseases. "I was pushing Blattner for a promotion," Rudolph said. "So, he came up with the idea that if I would take over the Junior League clinic, he would put me up for full professorship. I told him I would consider it, provided he also let me develop a neonatology service at Texas Children's Hospital."[25]

Blattner, in turn, spoke with Desmond about Rudolph's move to Texas Children's Hospital. She enthusiastically agreed to the plan. "He was ready," she said. "He was more than ready to have a big operation of his own."[26]

Before Rudolph arrived at Texas Children's Hospital, he discussed his ideas for the neonatology service and its needs with director of nursing Opal M. Benage and hospital administrator France. Rudolph wanted to develop a neonatal intensive care unit with its own separate nurses, the prime purpose being to reduce infant mortality and morbidity. Benage and France agreed to provide the necessary equipment and staffing to achieve the advantages evident at Desmond and Rudolph's infant care facilities at Jefferson Davis.

Rudolph was appointed director of the Junior League Outpatient Department in 1970. One year later, Blattner announced the creation of the neonatology service at Texas Children's Hospital and Rudolph's appointment as chief. The service began with four NICU beds at Texas Children's Hospital and the 25-crib nursery at St. Luke's Episcopal Hospital. "Dr. Hill was taking care of the babies in the Halbouty Clinic, and I took care of babies in the Texas Children's Hospital pediatric intensive care unit," Rudolph said. "And, within a matter of a few months, we were running a census there of five, six, seven, eight babies. And were getting a lot of referrals. We actually were taking care of most of the babies in infant care."

To his surprise and consternation, right after he started the newborn service, Rudolph discovered that his approved plans for the NICU at Texas Children's Hospital were in jeopardy. "After previously agreeing to all my plans, Mrs. Benage came to me and said, 'You don't think we're going to put separate nurses there and run a separate unit, do you?'" Rudolph recalled. "Within a few months, and just as spontaneously, she came to me and said, 'I'm going to let you have that one area of four beds for neo.' And I said, 'What about the nurses?' 'No, we can't do that,' she said. Well, within another four or five months, we were getting nine, ten babies, so she gave me another four-bed area. And then she started complaining that we were taking all the beds away from pediatrics."

The success of the NICU at Texas Children's Hospital could be measured in the number of referrals, which steadily increased month after month. And then, out of the blue, Benage said to Rudolph: "I'm going to let you have your own neo nurses for the babies."[27]

As Rudolph's newborn service at Texas Children's Hospital was "just exploding," Blattner offered Desmond the opportunity to head the child development center at Texas Children's Hospital. After devoting the first 23 years of her career at Baylor College of Medicine to newborns, in 1972 Desmond decided to undertake a new career. She was named chief of the child development center at Texas Children's Hospital and head of the newly established section for developmental pediatrics at Baylor College of Medicine.

Before accepting her new positions, Desmond asked for and received approval to provide anticipatory or forward care for very high-risk infants, in addition to children with developmental delay and learning disabilities who were referred to developmental pediatrics. "The link between neonatology and developmental pediatrics was the rubella epidemic. We needed to continue the follow-up," Desmond explained. "In my training as a newborn person, I was taught that you had to follow your own patients, so I was accustomed to doing that. We had clinics all the time at Jefferson Davis. And so, developmental pediatrics was not new to me. I didn't know too much about kids over 18 months, but it was a learning thing for me."[28]

With Desmond's move to another section, in 1972 Blattner appointed Rudolph as head of the newborn section of the department of pediatrics at Baylor College of Medicine. "I was still in charge of the Junior League Outpatient Department and running between Jeff Davis and here and just driving myself crazy," Rudolph recalled, thinking of how the NICU and newborn service continued to outgrow its space. "We were filling all the beds and spilling over into the pediatric beds at Texas Children's Hospital. Mr. France went to Dr. Blattner and said, 'It's ridiculous having NICU over there and infant I and II someplace else, and the Halbouty Premature Nursery someplace else.' He wanted it all unified."[29]

In 1974, the Linda Fay Halbouty Newborn-Premature Nursery became a joint facility of Texas Children's Hospital and St. Luke's Episcopal Hospital. The nursery was remodeled to form an intermediate care nursery and low birthweight nursery. With this consolidation, Texas Children's Hospital had 69 beds for the care of newborn infants.

Because of the increasing need for infants to receive specialized nursing and medical supervision during their early natal days, and with increasing demand from the community, the NICU was expanded to include 14 beds in 1976. The growth was funded by proceeds from the National Foundation-March of Dimes charity ball in Houston.

As the number of cribs assigned for neonatal beds grew, the number of faculty members also increased. At its inception in 1971, the Baylor College of Medicine neonatology faculty consisted of Rudolph and Hill. In 1973, Dr. Anthony Corbet and Dr. Gilbert Duritz joined the staff. The first neonatology fellows, Dr. James Adams and Dr. John Kenny, came in 1975. Dr. Michael Speer and Dr. Joseph Garcia-Prats joined the faculty in 1976 and 1977, respectively, and Dr. Zvi Friedman became a member of the staff in January 1979. Dr. Winifred Gorman joined the full-time staff in July 1979.

In January 1979, a completely new 20-bed NICU opened at Texas Children's Hospital under the directorship of Adams. The new facility incorporated all the latest concepts and developments in the care of sick neonates. "Let me tell you a statement Mrs. Benage made one day in 1979, after we both were in the new NICU," Rudolph said. "I said, 'You know, Mrs. Benage, you promised me that we could do everything, and once I came, you ...,' and she's a very blunt sort of person. She interrupted and said, 'You know, before you came here, when these babies came in, they just died. And when you told me you were going to do this and you're going to save the babies, I'd seen so many babies die, I just didn't think there was anything to it. After you came here and I saw these babies going home alive and doing well, then I decided that it's time to do something for it.'"

Benage's observations were a matter of record. In the early 1970s, according to March of Dimes statistics, 50 percent of all pediatric deaths occurred in the neonatal period—the first 28 days of life. In the eight years since Rudolph's arrival at Texas Children's Hospital, Benage had witnessed, firsthand, the introduction and use of the amazing technology and medical procedures necessary to save babies. Along with the machines to help babies breathe, regulate temperatures, drip fluids into tiny blood vessels, and monitor physiologic functions, and the close and constant supervision by the NICU staff, there had been significant changes in medical procedures and medications. "If you went back to the 1960s, if a baby weighed less than 1,000 grams, less than 2.5 pounds, nearly every one of them died. In the 1970s, about 10 to 15 percent of those low birthweight babies survived. In the 1980s, you come to a survival of 50 percent," Rudolph said. "If a baby weighed less than 750 grams, you didn't do anything."[30]

Such improvements in the neonatal mortality and morbidity statistics were attributed not only to vast technological advances, but also to research, an integral function of the neonatology service at Texas Children's Hospital in the 1970s. As a result of her ongoing research on the adverse effects of maternal drugs on the fetus, Hill published numerous articles on the epidemiology of drugs ingested by pregnant women. In many of these articles, she described a grouping of malformations in infants exposed to anticonvulsant drugs in utero. Hill also published a book, *Breast Feeding: A Passage in Life,* to instruct mothers on breast-feeding their infants and warn them about the dangers of drugs that cross into breast milk.[31]

During the early 1970s, Texas Children's Hospital neonatologist and cardiorespiratory physiologist Corbet gained recognition for his work at Texas Children's Hospital on surfactant activity and the drugs that may inhibit or induce production of surfactant in infants with respiratory disease. Corbet worked on the clinical development of the first commercially available exogenous surfactant, Exosurf, and the second, Survanta, for the treatment and prevention of hyaline membrane disease in newborn infants. Neonatologist Speer devoted his research activities to those infections peculiar to newborns, such as meningitis and group B streptococcal infections, and in monitoring antibiotic blood levels in the treatment of disease.

While Rudolph's work in many areas of neonatal care was published widely during the 1970s, his research on the cardiodynamic function in the neonatal period had a significant impact on the field of neonatology. Researching the lack of beat-to-beat variation in the heart rate of severely ill newborn infants, particularly those with hyaline membrane disease, he recommended fetal monitoring to detect alerts of possible problems in the fetus, a practice that has since been adopted by obstetricians.[32]

Because most infants who required neonatal intensive care had problems with either their heart or their lungs, research efforts in the Texas Children's Hospital NICU in the late 1970s and early 1980s were directed to those areas. Three projects were designed to study the various heart and lung disorders in the fetus and newborn infant: a study of heart failure in the fetus, a study of oxygen toxicity in the newborn, and a study of the cause of high altitude pulmonary edema.[33]

The advances made in technology, research, and medicine were vitally important at Texas Children's Hospital—as were those made in patient care, a philosophy Rudolph instilled in his fellows and staff. "He was a physician whose patients always came first," neonatologist Dr. Charleta Guillory said. "He trained us, his fellows, well, not only in the clinical setting, but for life. For Dr. Rudolph, his babies always came first."[34]

Concern about the care of sick neonates who required transportation to Texas Children's Hospital inspired the development of an effective neonatal transportation program. Established by neonatologist Adams in 1978, the neonatal transport team consisted of specially trained neonatology nurses and fellows. The team would later be known as the Kangaroo Crew at Texas Children's Hospital.

The implementation of Adams' neonatal transport team personified the philosophy of the neonatology service at Texas Children's Hospital. "Dr. Rudolph taught us to think of the patient first; then, to think of medicine as a whole and then medicine within the context of a community," said former fellow Speer, associate professor of pediatrics at Baylor College of Medicine and director of nurseries at The Methodist Hospital in 1999.[35]

Insisting that parents be allowed to visit their babies at any time, Rudolph let parents in to touch and become involved with their babies in NICU, a practice that had never before been allowed in premature nurseries. Rudolph's revised visitation rights enhanced and encouraged parental involvement in the physical care of infants. Along with a specially trained neonatal nurse, two pediatric residents, a neonatology fellow, and a faculty neonatologist supervising the medical care of the infants at all times, the parents became an integral part of the team devoted to their baby's survival.

Furthermore, as residents, interns, and fellows rotated through NICU to learn skills in stabilizing the vital functions, assessing the metabolic needs, and acquiring knowledge about long-term ventilatory management and the diagnosis and treatment of diseases in neonates, parents often were drawn into the process rather than being excluded from it, as in the past.

The effective utilization of family interaction became a vital teaching tool in the neonatology fellowship program in the section of neonatology in the department of pediatrics at Baylor College of Medicine. Originated by Rudolph in 1975, this became one of the largest neonatology fellowship training programs in the United States. Graduates of the program, which numbered more than 120 in 1999, went on to practice neonatology at Texas Children's Hospital and other Houston hospitals, as well as hospitals in California, Pennsylvania, Ohio, Canada, Brazil, and throughout the world.

By 1980, more than 1,000 infants were receiving medical care each year in the NICU at Texas Children's Hospital. The neonatal transport team organized by Adams was transporting 200 infants per year from St. Luke's Episcopal Hospital and other hospitals in the Houston area. Studies indicated that intensive care reduced the mortality rate of infants by 30 percent. Rudolph celebrated the successes at Texas Children's Hospital with a reunion of neonatal graduates March 23, 1980.

More than 200 families from all over the United States returned to Texas Children's Hospital for the reunion. Suggested by Frances Heyck, coordinator of community affairs, and planned by a committee with representatives from seven departments, the three-hour celebration in the lobby of Texas Children's Hospital was a huge success. So popular was the event that it was repeated annually thereafter for an ever-increasing number of neonatal graduates.

Stepping down from his administrative duties as head of the neonatology section in 1986, Rudolph remained on the neonatology staff for ten more years, until his death in 1995. Named to replace him as head of the section was Dr. Thomas N. Hansen, a 1980 graduate of his neonatology fellowship program. Hansen would hold the position until 1995, when he left to become chairman of the pediatrics department at Ohio State College of Medicine.

When Desmond also stepped down in 1987, she had served for 15 years as head of the Leopold L. Meyer Center for Developmental Pediatrics, named in 1984 to honor Meyer. During her career, Desmond had witnessed many changes in the causes of children's developmental problems. Some causative agents, such as rubella and syphilis, had been eradicated or greatly reduced through medical advances. "Other factors, such as prematurity, cytomegalovirus, alcohol, cocaine, and HIV assumed prominent places as potentially devastating causes of developmental problems," Desmond said. "The Meyer Center will continue its mission of promoting children's development through clinical service, research, and teaching of health and education professionals."[36]

Also continuing was Desmond's practice of seeing premature and low-birthweight infants for follow-up and providing counseling to their families. Low birthweight affected one in every 13 babies born each year in the United States, with a low birthweight baby reportedly being born every two minutes. Developmental pediatric programs for follow-up, such as Desmond's at the Meyer Center at Texas Children's Hospital, began to be established at hospitals across the country.[37]

This national explosion of low birthweight infants also affected the newborn center at Texas Children's Hospital. The center's average daily census in 1990 exceeded 90 patients, even though it only contained 80 beds. Plans to meet the need for additional beds were approved and, on September 24, 1991, the NICU moved to its newly expanded location in the West Tower and doubled in size to 40 beds. With 60 beds available in intermediate care, the Texas Children's newborn center now totaled 100 beds. The full-time faculty numbered 27, with an additional 20 postdoctoral fellows, 19 full-time nurses, and 32 healthcare employees on the staff.[38]

Since its inception in 1978, the transport team established by Adams to take infants born outside the Texas Medical Center to Texas Children's Hospital had transported more than 3,800 critically ill neonates. In 1980, Adams instigated a specific course for the training of neonatal nurse clinicians. The bulk of the transport activities, originally consisting of a specially trained transport nurse and a Baylor College of Medicine neonatologist, passed into the hands of this group of expanded-role neonatal nurse clinicians.

Also designed by Adams in 1990 was a new program to teach neonatal nurse clinicians the skills necessary to carry out primary patient management in the NICU and in the intermediate care units at Texas Children's Hospital, as well as respond to delivery room emergencies at St. Luke's and The Methodist Hospital. "The goal of this program was to use these specially trained individuals to carry out the duties of pediatric residents in the special care units so that future growth of these units would not be dependent on increasing the size of the residency program," Hansen said. "This program has been extraordinarily successful."[39]

Other successes were achieved in some of the new therapies practiced in the Texas Children's newborn center in the early 1990s. These therapies included extracorporeal membrane oxygenation (ECMO), the therapy of putting infants with respiratory failure on cardiopulmonary bypass; a heart–lung machine; and nitric oxide therapy, the therapy utilizing nitric oxide gas to relax tightly constricted blood vessels in the lungs of infants with respiratory failure. "In 1975, less than one-half of the infants weighing less than 1,000 grams at Texas Children's newborn center survived. In 1990, the survival rates for infants weighing less than 1,000 was 75 percent," Hansen explained. "By 1990, the survival rate for infants weighing more than 750 grams was similar. More importantly, the morbidity, especially the neurological morbidity, has decreased parallel to the decreased mortality in all weight groups."[40]

With more than 700 infants admitted to the Texas Children's Hospital NICU on an annual basis in the late 1980s, Hansen and his staff of 18 faculty members and 15 postdoctoral fellows achieved a 90 percent survival rate among all neonates born at Texas Children's Hospital. During 1986, the NICU at Texas Children's Hospital was one of the few centers in the country chosen to administer surfactants on a trial basis to premature babies whose lungs lacked that crucial material needed for breathing. That clinical trial and other research efforts propelled Texas Children's Hospital to the forefront of neonatology research. "We do not have all the answers," Hansen said in 1988. "But with continued research and improved treatment techniques, we are confident that tremendous advances will continue to be made."[41]

Approximately 200 of the 700 babies admitted in the early 1990s were very low birthweight infants, weighing less than 1,250 grams. With a major clinical thrust directed at those babies, NICU director Adams explained: "We set about to gear our care specifically for the very low birthweight baby, and particularly to take into account a couple of things that some basic research suggested might play a role in the cause of intraventricular hemorrhage. One of those is birth asphyxia, having oxygen levels too low at the time of birth."[42]

An inability to predict which very low birthweight infants were susceptible to intraventricular hemorrhaging and which were not led to an aggressive approach. Adams sent his transport team of physicians and nurses over to the delivery rooms at The Methodist Hospital and St. Luke's Episcopal Hospital to attend the delivery of all very low birthweight infants. To provide specialized care to high-risk mothers and their babies, the neonatology service at Texas Children's Hospital, in conjunction with St. Luke's Episcopal Hospital, established the perinatal center in 1993.

"We have sort of developed a one-bed, intensive care unit in the delivery room, one of the first in the nation," Adams said. "If the baby is not breathing well, we can immediately take over and support his breathing and stabilize him. In fact, what we aggressively do with all the babies under 1,500 grams is assume they are going to have insufficiency of breathing. We put them on respirator support, stabilize their breathing, and keep them in the delivery room, where we do all the things we normally do in NICU. Take some measurements of their oxygen levels and their blood and adjust the respirator. Get them good and warm. Give them some IV glucose and make sure they are stable before we move them to NICU. In other words, we try to prevent the consequences of respiratory failure."

The procedure to transport an inborn infant to the NICU at Texas Children's Hospital was the same as that of an outborn. In the transport incubator with its own respirator, oxygen supply and temperature control, the infant was monitored by Adams' transport team throughout the journey. "What we do is bring those babies to the nursery, and for the first five days of life we place them in minimal stimulation. We do as few things as possible to them which would agitate them, that wake them up, that cause increments in their blood pressure. We literally keep them in an environment where they just lie there and everything stays as stable as possible," Adams said. "It's during the first three to five days that they're the most vulnerable, and during that period we try to do as few things as possible. And we think we've influenced outcomes with this method."

Incidences of intraventricular hemorrhaging among transported inborn babies of very low birthweight fell to 28 percent in 1992. The occurrence among infants transported from the outside, however, remained at 48 percent. "The factor we can't control with the children under 1,500 grams who are born outside of the hospitals here is how long it takes for us to get the baby," Adams explained. "The overall mortality, however, is low. For those born here it is about 18 percent, and for outside it is 25 percent. The chance of survival in a low birthweight baby here is very good these days."[43]

With approximately $80,000 worth of specialized technology and equipment at each bedside in the NICU at Texas Children's Hospital, the neonatologists and other subspecialists could perform diagnostic studies and complicated procedures without moving the infant out of the NICU and into the operating room. Because of this innovation in design, one of the first bedside surgeries—a ligation of patent ductus arteriosus—in an intensive care unit was performed there. Between 1983 and 1991, more than 700 surgical procedures were performed in the Texas Children's Hospital NICU.

Pointing out the floors that were carpeted to deaden the sound and the lights in each cubicle that could be dimmed, Adams said: "This NICU was built to manage the environment, to make it as low stress and as noninvasive as possible. We think that being able to keep the babies in a real quiet, stabilized environment is important. The nurses are all trained in how to avoid stress in premature babies and to offer constant and consistent care."

Although often perceived by outsiders as a high-tech center, the Texas Children's Hospital NICU was "really a people place," said Dr. Leonard E. Weisman, appointed head of the neonatology section in the department of pediatrics at Baylor College of Medicine and chief of the newborn service at Texas Children's Hospital in 1995.[44] Despite the amount of technology, the key factor was still the people who were taking care of the baby and operating the equipment. "They're still the most important piece in the whole equation; their attitude is outstanding," said Adams. "They're proud of what they do. They should be. They do a very good job."[45]

The parents of sick neonates in the NICU at Texas Children's Hospital also deserved praise for their efforts. To enhance the outcome of their babies, parents were encouraged to interact with the infants and to be involved in their care from the beginning. Holding and caressing the babies, communicating with whispered words of encouragement, and offering skin-to-skin contact, parents become an integral part of Texas Children's team approach to patient care. The bonding process produced optimal results in each infant's progress. "It's our overall resources that we can bring together as an overall healthcare team which enable us to do the miraculous things that we are able to do for children," Adams said. "This nursery has been a research center in neonatology for a long time. That's given us the opportunity to offer some of these breakthroughs to our patients. And it has allowed us to always be on the forefront of new developments in our field."

In December 1998, Weisman, Adams, and the 123 members of the neonatology service at Texas Children's newborn center were catapulted onto the front pages of newspapers worldwide. The attention was due to the birth of the Chukwu children, the world's first set of octuplets to be born alive. Within hours of the announcement of their birth at St. Luke's Episcopal Hospital, the octuplets became the focus of the electronic media. *CBS Evening News, ABC World News Tonight, NBC Nightly News,* and CNN all led their broadcasts with reports on the babies. Updated information about the octuplets was regularly posted on the website of Texas Children's Hospital, garnering more than one and a half million visits in the month following the birth.

Amid the media frenzy at Texas Children's Hospital, the doctors, nurses, respiratory therapists, nutritionists, and other healthcare workers in the NICU team continued, uninterrupted, with their efforts to stabilize and save the lives of the newest patients in their care.[46] According to Weisman, those last two weeks of 1998 proved to be the busiest since the NICU was founded.[47] Obscured by the publicity surrounding the Chukwu octuplets was the fact that on New Year's Eve 1998, the staff of Texas Children's newborn center was treating a total of 119 infants—56 of whom were also in the NICU with the octuplets—including a set of five surviving sextuplets from an earlier multiple birth. Addressing the media, Weisman stated that while all the patients in the NICU are tiny, "these patients don't have little problems—they have big problems."[48]

At birth, the Chukwu octuplets ranged in weight from 810 grams (28.6 ounces) to 320 grams (11.3 ounces). The first baby, born 15 weeks premature, and her seven brothers and sisters, delivered two weeks later and 13 weeks premature, had been conceived with the help of fertility drugs. Transferred by Adams' transport team from the delivery room at St. Luke's Episcopal, the babies were all in critical condition when they arrived in the Texas Children's Hospital NICU. Given the extremely low birthweights and the prematurity of the octuplets, medical statistics suggested that they had barely a 50–50 chance of surviving.[49] Weisman was "cautiously optimistic" that the babies would survive and grow up to be normal.

After a weeklong battle for life, the smallest of the octuplets succumbed to heart and lung failure, despite the NICU staff's heroic efforts to save her. After employing the NICU's sophisticated technology, bedside surgeries, and proven medical treatments, the neonatology team of specialists at Texas Children's Hospital were able to save the remaining seven babies, sending all home to their parents within six months of their birth.

Weisman credited the survival of the seven babies to developments in neonatology over the past two decades, rather than to any radical new discovery. The use of the commercially available exogenous surfactant, the drug application researched at Texas Children's in the 1980s, was "the No. 1 reason that these kids are doing as well as they are. Their survival wasn't a medical miracle," Weisman said. "The success is the result of dedicated teams involving several hundred pediatricians, nurses, nutritionists, pharmacologists, respiratory and other technicians, experts in developmental biology, and other workers."[50]

Indeed, such dramatic advances in the care of neonates were envisioned by Rudolph when he established the newborn service at Texas Children's Hospital. In a tribute to Rudolph's accomplishments in the field of neonatology during his 40-year career, former Baylor College of Medicine colleagues Dr. Gerardo Cabrera-Meza and Virginia Schneider compiled *Atlas of the Newborn,* a five-volume collection of Rudolph's photographs of virtually every disease, disorder, and condition affecting the newborn. When it was published in 1998, Weisman said, "*Atlas of the Newborn* is a great collection and will provide a wonderful reference tool for all physicians who take care of babies and students who are studying to do so. It should become a standard reference before too long."[51]

In 1999, the newborn center at Texas Children's Hospital was another example of the cumulative advances that had been made in the field of neonatology. Weisman, who was a student at Baylor College of Medicine in the 1970s, remembered when neonatologists did not even go to the delivery of babies who were extremely low in birthweight, less than 1,000 grams, because their outcome was uniformly poor. "In a span of 25 years, we've gone from 100 percent mortality to 90–95 percent survival in that extremely low birthweight population of patients, which count for 1 percent of the births in the United States," he said. "That's a substantial change. In 1999, just about every infant in the nursery is under 1,000 grams. It's amazing."[52]

As to whether newborns weighing less than 500 grams would also experience an extended survival rate, Weisman predicted that this was a possibility with future improvements in technology and in the quality of patient care. "We don't want to experiment, so we really need to have a new service to offer, a new technique to extend survival much below 500 grams at this point," he said. "But, then again, 25 years ago 1,000 grams was unimaginable."

Another unforeseen development in the section of neonatology at Baylor College of Medicine was the impact of the neonatal-perinatal medicine fellowship program instituted by Rudolph in 1975. By 2003, more than 150 fellows had graduated from the program, accounting for more than four percent of the practicing neonatologists in the United States. One of the first programs to be accredited by the Accreditation Council for Graduate Medical Education in 1984, the fellowship program had more than 15 full-time fellows in training at any given time. With the maximum allowable accreditation granted continuously through 2008, the neonatal–perinatal medicine fellowship program at Baylor College of Medicine and Texas Children's Hospital was poised for the future.

What could not continue as part of the fellowship program was a tradition first introduced by Weisman in 1995. Annually, until her death in 2003, Desmond had been a special guest of honor at each graduation ceremony for fellows. "Dr. Murdina Desmond was a renowned and respected leader in neonatology worldwide," said Weisman. "Her research accomplishments were extensive, but none more than her work on the newborn's transition from fetal to neonatal life. This work was a major milestone in neonatology and continues to enhance the care of all babies today. Murdina was an outstanding medical educator and everyone enjoyed spending time with her because of her friendly and outgoing personality. She gave birth to neonatology at Baylor College of Medicine, blazed the trail for those who followed, and was an inspiration to everyone who knew her. She was a brilliant scientist, a thought-provoking teacher, a wonderful leader, and a fabulous friend. We all are going to miss her, but were blessed to have known her."[53]

In the five decades since Blattner had first granted Desmond's wish to work with the newborn, the section of neonatology at Baylor College of Medicine she established had grown to become the one of the largest academic neonatology divisions in the United States. The section had 40 full-time faculty members who receive in excess of $2.5 million annually in extramural funding. Inspired by Desmond, developed by Rudolph, enhanced by Hansen, and led by Weisman, the neonatology section at Baylor College of Medicine represented in 2004 the successful culmination of 50 years of tireless efforts to advance the treatment and care of newborns.

Having grown to become one of the largest and busiest neonatal care centers in the United States, the newborn center at Texas Children's Hospital had maintained since 1999 an 82 percent survival rate for infants weighing less than 1,000 grams—one of the highest in the nation. "Texas Children's Newborn Center routinely cares for the smallest, most fragile infants while maintaining tremendous outcomes,"[54] Weisman said, noting how outcomes improved as knowledge expanded through ongoing research.

One such research effort was the outcomes database, a complex computer-based system established at Texas Children's Hospital in 1986. "It is a unique and valuable resource that has grown since its inception," Weisman said. "After collecting, maintaining, and reporting on neonatal outcomes, the database director provides clinicians with detailed analyses, feedback on the quality of care, data for clinical research. It is a basis for changes in many management strategies."[55]

With a constant goal of improving clinical practice at Texas Children's Hospital, the dedication of the neonatology service to state-of-the-art basic and clinical research had not wavered since 1971. In addition to its accomplishments in developing artificial surfactant for the prevention and treatment of hyaline membrane disease, nitric oxide for the treatment of neonates with pulmonary hypertension, and Respigam and Synergis for the prevention of RSV hospitalization in high-risk infants, the service also established other extensive research programs. Among these were programs dedicated to the molecular biology and biochemistry of the developing lung, gene therapy, pharmacology and experimental therapeutics, neurophysiology and neurobiology, pulmonary physiology, nutrition, and immunotherapy in the neonate.

Under the direction of Weisman, the neonatology service at Texas Children's Hospital had expanded in every aspect into an extremely professional academic entity that performed uniform and highly effective perinatal–neonatal care. By 2004, the medical education program instigated by Rudolph in 1975 had grown to include more than 160 medical students, 160 pediatric residents, 18 neonatology fellows, and numerous nursing students, nurses, respiratory therapists, allied health professionals, and community and academic physicians. "The section produces numerous educational materials for professionals, including the thirteenth edition of our *Acute Care Guidelines Booklet* and the fourth edition of the *Care of Respiratory Diseases in the Neonate* manual," Weisman said. "We also produce materials for members of the community, which includes a newsletter, books on the post-discharge care of the preterm infant, and brochures on feeding techniques for babies. We are developing, in conjunction with Texas Children's Hospital, the capability to rebroadcast the section's many lectures for access by physicians in the community with CME provided by Baylor College of Medicine."[56]

The always-expanding neonatology service at Texas Children's Hospital developed and operated several clinical programs that were unique, attracting referral patients and producing outstanding results. In 2004, these programs included the ECMO, nitric oxide, chronic lung disease, neonatal nutritional support, lactation support, pain management, oral feeding, short bowel, pain management, international neonatology, neonatal and community health, and developmental care programs. In addition, the neonatology service collaborated extensively with the general pediatric surgery service and the maternal fetal medicine service in the fetal surgery program at Texas Children's Hospital.

Also under Weisman's direction in 2004 was the center for acute and chronic neonatal respiratory therapy at Texas Children's Hospital. Established by the neonatology service in conjunction with Baylor College of Medicine in 1996, the center was dedicated to the development and implementation of new strategies and technologies to improve the outcome of neonates with severe acute and chronic lung disease.

To provide primary and consultative outpatient follow-up services for the growing number of complex patients discharged from Texas Children's

Hospital, the neonatology service implemented a neonatology graduate clinic in 2002. "This clinic is a community resource and provides patient care for referring physicians and families; a mechanism to train others to provide this care and to investigate problems specific to the patient and to develop risk intervention strategies and is the source of outcomes reporting to national databases and media inquiries," Weisman said. "The service also developed a Virtual Visitation program where families at remote facilities can visit with their child who was transferred for care at Texas Children's Hospital and their care providers in a live audio and video connection."[57]

Such advances in the treatment and care of newborns at Texas Children's Hospital would have astounded pioneering physicians. Unfortunately, Desmond, Hill, and Rudolph did not live to see the culmination of their collective efforts in the 2004 opening of the new 138-crib nursery and NICU featuring state-of-the-art medical technology in the Texas Children's newborn center.

With more than 2,900 critically ill newborns treated in 2004, what had begun at Texas Children's Hospital in 1971 as Rudolph's four-crib NICU had become one of the largest and most sophisticated neonatal care centers in the United States. Bedside workstations included a computer and mobile physiologic monitoring system, while partial walls between each patient increased privacy for families. The 50 percent increase in the amount of space per patient was larger than the recommended standard and allowed more technology at the bedside, a necessity for bedside surgeries. "The increased space and design of each bed improves the efficiency with which care is provided, decreases the stress of the patient and family, and improves the comfort of the baby and encourages the family to spend more time at the bedside," said Weisman. "It is a more efficient, less stressful, less intrusive, high-technology environment that will meet the needs for several years to come and improve the outcomes of our patients."[58]

Future expansion of the neonatology service at Texas Children's Hospital was a certainty, given its past accomplishments. "We envision continued growth of patient admissions, complexity, and acuity," Weisman said. "Likewise, the range and scope of the Kangaroo Crew Transport Team will continue to expand across Texas and to adjacent states. We are poised for the future and our mission to extend the lives and improve the quality of life of our newborn patients through education, research, and patient care."[59]

When the new Texas Children's newborn center opened in 2004, it had been 45 years since the coining of "neonatology" and "neonatologist." That both terms were being continually redefined at Texas Children's

Hospital and Baylor College of Medicine was an undisputed fact.

W hen four-month-old John L. Baber IV came home from Texas Children's Hospital on April 9, 1982, his health was fragile and his future uncertain.

Diagnosed while he was still in the NICU with hydrocephalus attributed to the "severe bleed" of the intraventricular cranial hemorrhaging, baby Jack had to undergo countless spinal taps. "They just take the fluids out before it makes the head big," his father said. "There was a chance the bleeding would arrest by itself and it eventually did."

Uncertain about whether there would be long-term effects of his son's severe bleed, Jack began to learn more about this condition. "They number the bleeds sequentially, 1 to 4," he said. "Many kids that were diagnosed with learning difficulties may have had bleeds at 1, so it's a much more common event than most people, most doctors, even knew. In preemies, they do a CAT scan to determine how severe the bleeds were and Jack's was a 3–4, which meant 3 on one side, 4 on the other side—4 being worst, 3 being next-to-worst."[60]

When Sandy and Jack both asked the doctors at Texas Children's Hospital what their son's 3–4 rating meant, they were told it could mean severe retardation or it could mean nothing at all. "They didn't know," Jack said. "They said babies have a way of changing dramatically, especially little babies, and compensating. If there's been damage, then maybe the brain will compensate."

To prepare themselves for their baby's future, Sandy and Jack devoted their time and energies to guaranteeing its best possible outcome. Beginning at the age of six months and continuing twice a year for seven years, Jack was taken to the Leopold L. Meyer Center for Developmental Pediatrics at Texas Children's Hospital to have his developmental skills tested. "In the first two or three years, he was developing pretty much within normal range except for his speech and language," Sandy recalled. "The Meyer Center recommended some type of speech pathology. That's when Robbin Parish was starting The Parish School. So, literally, Jack was carried in the door at The Parish School when he was 18 months. The Parish School gave him the early intervention for the speech and language development, which I feel is so important for all children."[61]

A teacher by education, Sandy had quit her job when the baby came home. She remembered rocking him and reading to him all the time. "He was getting constant stimulation," she said. "Wherever we went I was always talking to him, explaining things to him. I can remember a person came up to us outside one of the doctor's offices and said, 'Gosh, you talk to that baby all the time.' And then, thankfully, The Parish School could continue that constant stimulation. They do so much, every step of the developmental process, and really making sure the brain is going to regenerate."

As Jack grew older, his parents always encouraged him to do his best. "You're fine. You can do it. Yes, you have to work harder at things, but you can do it," they repeatedly said. Another source of encouragement for both Jack and his parents were the neonatal reunions at Texas Children's Hospital. "They were really neat, from our standpoint," his father said. "You got a chance to go to see the kids you knew and to see older kids. And we thought it was good, 'cause Jack was a pretty normal kid by then, thanks to The Parish School, and we could show the nurses this was a success."

With his parents' proud and unwavering support, Jack became a very good student who worked very hard. "He's a fighter," his mother said. "He was one of the babies who pulled his tube out in NICU, so the indications early on were this kid was a fighter."

One ongoing problem Jack wrestled with was the atresia of his right ear. He not only developed chronic hearing problems, but also had major otitis, fluid of the middle ear, in his left ear. After undergoing numerous surgeries to insert tubes in his ears while an infant at Texas Children's Hospital, when he was in the fifth grade Jack underwent surgery to have his eardrums rebuilt to save his hearing.

The timing of the plastic surgery to reconstruct his outer ear was left up to Jack. Having endured so many surgeries, Jack was not eager to volunteer for another one. "It had been on the back burner for some time," Sandy recalled. "When he was about six years old, we heard about this doctor in California, the one who had started the procedure of reconstructing outer ears. We decided he was the one we would go to. But we left it up to Jack as to when he would have it done."

Jack decided that the summer before his first year in high school was the time to begin the three necessary operations. The ear surgery was performed successfully. Following his recuperation, Jack attended Episcopal High School, where he was an excellent student. Always working and studying very hard, the pattern he had formed as a younger student, he made all A's and was in the honors classes. His parents knew he would achieve whatever goal he set for himself.

Their prediction was based not just on parental pride, but also on one of Jack's most recent accomplishments. He earned 21 Boy Scout merit badges, exhibited leadership and outdoor survival skills, and performed more than 50 hours in a community service project that he had planned, organized, and executed. After submitting the required written report of his completed project in hopes of achieving the honor of becoming an Eagle Scout, Jack and his parents waited to hear the results from the national headquarters of Boy Scouts of America.

More than 17 years after their emotional roller-coaster ride had begun, Sandy and Jack Baber reached its pinnacle in the spring of 1999. The occasion was a ceremony at the Eagle Court of Honor, where John "Jack" Baber was awarded the rank of Eagle Scout.

The former two-pound-four-ounce preemie whose future had been uncertain had grown up exceptionally well, attaining an honor that only 2 percent of all boys who enter the national Scouting program achieve.

Overtly proud of his son's many accomplishments, Jack's father said: "His mother and I frankly believe a miracle occurred. Beside the care and attention he received at Texas Children's Hospital, we think there was a little of God's work involved."

23

⚘ NEUROLOGY ⚘

Y ASMINE BALLANTYNE AND HER HUSBAND, Dr. Christie Ballantyne, expected the birth of their first child to be routine.

"We were very at ease about it," Yasmine explained. "I had gone for whatever needed to be done and everything was just perfect. It was a perfect pregnancy and a perfectly healthy baby."[1]

This pattern of perfection continued when Yasmine's water broke on the baby's precise due date in September 1985. When they arrived at The Methodist Hospital, the Ballantynes thought that a perfect delivery would soon follow. They were mistaken.

After six hours at the hospital, the Ballantynes were still waiting for Yasmine's contractions to begin. "I already had my IV and there was a monitor on the baby," she said. "We were just sitting there and chatting and waiting. I did not have contractions and baby was not moving. Dr. Terry Simon came in and said, 'Well, we might have to do a C-section. We don't want to wait too long. Things are OK, but we need to make a decision. You are healthy. The baby is healthy. Everything looks fine.' He then said he was making rounds and that he would come back in and see me."

Noticing that Yasmine was growing increasingly uncomfortable, the nurses offered to refresh the linens on her bed. "All of a sudden, the monitor started acting funny and I said, 'Oh, I feel just drenched,' and I lifted up the sheet and there was blood everywhere," Yasmine recalled. "The nurses called a 'code blue' and began to run. It was kind of like you are in a movie because things are happening so fast. I knew enough to know it was a disaster, but not enough to panic. Things happened so fast, there was no time to panic."

Yasmine's husband, who at the time was a fellow in cardiology at Baylor College of Medicine, instinctively knew what was wrong. "My wife had a velamentous insertion of the umbilical cord, so there was basically a complicated delivery and she hemorrhaged," he said, explaining the rare condition that occurs when the veins of the baby are outside instead of within the umbilical cord. The condition is often fatal to the baby at birth.[2]

Aware that the situation required an emergency cesarean section, Christie joined the nurses as they rushed Yasmine to the operating room. "We basically went as fast as we could over to the OR, and Terry Simon was there with a knife, ready to get that baby out," he said. "We had to wait a minute or two for the anesthesiologist, but the neonatology fellow from Texas Children's Hospital, Steve Welty, was already there. Within probably a minute or two, Terry got the baby out."[3]

Born in shock, eight-pound newborn Leyla Ballantyne had no vital signs and received an Apgar score of zero at birth, an indication of severe asphyxia. The neonatologists whisked her away, intubated her, and began resuscitating her. Christie observed those heroic measures with mounting pessimism. "I peeked in the room and saw they were doing compressions on her chest," he said. "I didn't think she was going to make it because they were in there forever."

More accustomed to resuscitation efforts performed on adult patients, where there was a narrow window of opportunity to succeed, Christie was skeptical of the outcome of such prolonged efforts. Countless minutes passed before his own father, who was also a physician, arrived and immediately went into the operating room for an update on his granddaughter's condition. "When he came out, he said they were making some progress and she was doing better," Christie said, recalling his surprise. "I guessed kids were more resistant than adults, because the neonatologists ended up transfusing her and basically got her back. Then they took Leyla immediately to the neonatal intensive care unit at Texas Children's Hospital."

It had taken approximately ten minutes to revive Leyla. Her father feared that the extended period of oxygen deprivation would cause either irreversible brain damage, cerebral palsy, epilepsy, or other mental and motor disabilities. When told that Leyla had an abnormal EEG, Christie discussed her prognosis with the neonatologists. They advised him that the baby had a one-third chance of dying that day, a one-third chance of being severely developmentally retarded, and a one-third chance of being more or less normal.

This was the discouraging news awaiting Yasmine when she recovered from the emergency C-section at The Methodist Hospital. The first time she ever saw her daughter was in the neonatal intensive care unit (NICU) at Texas Children's Hospital, where the baby spent the first week of her life. It was there that the Ballantynes first met Dr. Marvin A. Fishman, chief of child neurology. "He saw her in the neonatal unit and mentioned that we were lucky she was a girl, because girls tend to be able to be more resistant to shock and hypothermia," Christie recalled. "We talked about some of the issues in regards to the potential for motor abnormalities or mental retardation, and Dr. Fishman was reassuring, explaining what we would be looking for."

As Yasmine listened to Fishman speak about the uncertainties in her daughter's future, she was numbed by the possibilities. "You just don't know what will happen because there were so many things that were short-circuited in her brain," she said. "So we took her home and I just thought I would take it one day at a time, but I was just numb."

Once home, Yasmine discovered that she had "no motherly feelings" at that time. It was Christie who became both mother and father to Leyla. "He hovered over her and worried about her day and night; he was terrified she would die," she said. "He worked seven days a week and would come home to see Leyla, have dinner, and read Leyla a story. He would fall asleep on the floor in her bedroom. At 10 p.m., he would wake up, say 'I have so much to do,' and go back to the office. Then he would come home again, go to sleep, and start all over again at 6 a.m. the next morning."

As a physician, Christie was acutely aware of his daughter's progress. Always anxious about her development, he concentrated his efforts on stimulation. "We did everything we could to try and stimulate development in terms of reading, numbers, and signs," he said, knowing the impact of such efforts could not be measured immediately. "You don't really know until the child is three or four years old."

Christie also accompanied Yasmine and Leyla to their first appointment, as well as all subsequent ones, with Fishman at Texas Children's Hospital. "It was always reassuring to see him," he said. "We would ask him question after question. It's an extremely anxious period. You want the facts; you don't want false information. He had the balance of giving the facts to people, and being calming and being reassuring at the same time. Not everybody can do that well. The facts are disturbing, and yet there is hope and there is the issue that it could be worse."

What disturbed the Ballantynes most during that first visit to Texas Children's Hospital was the fact that Leyla again had an abnormal EEG. Although Fishman found that the test did not reveal any precise impairment, they knew what their only recourse was. They would have to wait years to see if the first ten minutes of their daughter's life would severely impact the rest of all of theirs.

When Texas Children's Hospital opened in 1954, the pediatric sub-specialty of child neurology was in its formative stages.

Although Dr. Bernard Sachs had published the first definitive textbook of child neurology in New York in 1895, the actual development of a separate discipline from adult neurology was slow to evolve over the following five decades. Substantial progress in its development occurred in the 1950s, when leading figures in neurology and pediatrics formed a movement to determine the parameters of the new subspecialty.

After this prominent group concluded that child neurologists must be trained both in pediatrics and in adult neurology, the first formalized child neurology training programs were established in the mid-1950s in Boston, Philadelphia, and New York. Less than a decade later, when the American Board of Psychiatry and Neurology (ABPN) formally recognized child neurology as a special area of expertise in 1959, the independent specialty was officially born.

From its inception, child neurology experienced rapid growth in tandem with an explosion of knowledge in both basic and clinical neurosciences—including a better understanding of developmental neurochemistry, metabolic diseases, molecular genetics, and neurotransmitters.[4] When the ABPN initiated the issuance of special certificates in child neurology in 1969, 30 candidates received certificates and no fewer than 30 received certificates in each subsequent year, totaling more than 1,000 by the mid-1990s.

Texas Children's Hospital was to benefit immensely from this evolution, as well as contribute to it measurably. The roots of this unforeseen eventuality were firmly planted in the early years of the specialty, when one of the earliest board-certified child neurologists in the United States was Dr. Marvin A. Fishman, who received his ABPN certificate in 1972.

To achieve this goal, Fishman pursued a definitive plan. After receiving his medical degree from the University of Illinois in 1961, he completed his pediatric residency at Michael Reese Hospital in Chicago in 1964. Fishman then joined the military and spent the following two years as a captain in the U.S. Army Medical Corps, where he served as chief of the outpatient clinic at William Beaumont General Hospital in El Paso, Texas. He then began a fellowship in child neurology.

Fishman chose his subsequent career path during the first months of his pediatric residency in Chicago. "I decided that I wanted to do child neurology," he recalled. "At that time, there were perhaps a half dozen noted child neurology training programs, and one of which was at the Massachusetts General Hospital. I had applied there based upon recommendations of people and had interviewed with my subsequent mentor, Philip Dodge. After I finished my military service, I went to Boston to start training with him in 1966. When he left Boston to go to St. Louis, I followed him there."[5]

The reasons for Fishman's loyalty were obvious. A prominent member of the child neurology movement of the 1950s, Dr. Philip R. Dodge was heralded as one of the modern founders of child neurology. Having established and presided over one of the first training programs for the new specialty at Harvard Medical School and Massachusetts General Hospital, he made lengthy and noteworthy contributions to the neurologic care of children. After Dodge departed Boston in 1967 to become chairman of the department of pediatrics at Washington University School of Medicine and St. Louis Children's Hospital, Fishman—along with other medical professionals who were also Dodge's loyal followers—joined him there.

One such medical professional was Dr. Ralph D. Feigin, a pediatric infectious diseases expert who had "spent some time in Boston associated with Dr. Dodge, as well, but I did not know him there," said Fishman. "I met him when we were both on the faculty in the department of pediatrics at Washington University. We both had been recruited by Dr. Dodge."[6]

For the next 12 years, Fishman excelled in his chosen career path in St. Louis, eventually achieving full professorship in pediatrics, neurology, and preventative medicine at Washington University School of Medicine. He also served as director of the Irene and Walter Johnson Institute of Rehabilitation at Barnes Hospital. Interested in eventually developing his own child neurology training program, he knew that this goal was not realistic for St. Louis. "The section of neurology was actually a superb section with a lot of talented people, all of about the same age," Fishman explained. "I was looking for other opportunities."[7]

In his search for the perfect environment necessary to fulfill his goals, Fishman questioned friends who were departing St. Louis for other medical schools and hospitals. When Feigin accepted the offer to become chairman of the department of pediatrics at Baylor College of Medicine and physician-in-chief of Texas Children's Hospital in 1977, Fishman recalled saying to him, partly in jest, "Ralph, scout it out and see how it looks and what the opportunities are."[8]

When Feigin arrived at Texas Children's Hospital in 1977, he observed patients—including very ill inpatients—who required pediatric neurology services, but only "a couple of pediatric neurologists in private practice," and

only one person on the full-time faculty at the hospital. "There was no training program in pediatric neurology and there was no research," Feigin said. "In
a completely separate operation in an adult hospital, The Methodist Hospital,
was The Blue Bird Circle Clinic, established predominantly for children with
seizure disorders. There was no coordination between that program and the
neurology services at Texas Children's Hospital."[9]

What Feigin observed was steeped in Houston history. The Blue Bird
Circle, one of the oldest women's charity groups in the city, had been affiliated with The Methodist Hospital since its inception. Established in 1923
by 15 young women of the First Methodist church, the circle had one major
philanthropic endeavor between 1924 and 1945: the continual support of
the Arabia Temple Shrine ward for crippled children at The Methodist
Hospital on the corner of San Jacinto and Rosalie in downtown Houston.
After raising and donating funds for the "Little Hospital" in 1934, members
of the circle served in the ward as volunteers while the Arabia Temple
Shrine maintained the building. When The Methodist Hospital announced
plans for the building of a new hospital in the Texas Medical Center in
1945, the Arabia Temple Shrine decided not to continue its relationship
with the hospital. Instead, the organization announced its own plans for a
new facility for the care of crippled children.

Subsequently, when the crippled children in the Little Hospital moved
away in 1949, the 300 members of The Blue Bird Circle found themselves
with no continuing project to support at The Methodist Hospital. During a
meeting with hospital administrator Josie Roberts in 1949 to discuss possible future projects in the new facility, circle members encountered Dr. Russell
J. Blattner, the professor of pediatrics at Baylor College of Medicine who later
became the first physician-in-chief at Texas Children's Hospital. "They wanted to work with children, and since Texas Children's Hospital was only in
the planning stages at the time and there already was a Junior League pediatric clinic at Hermann Hospital, a group of physicians from Baylor College
of Medicine and I suggested they work with neurologic disorders," recalled
Blattner, who also pointed out that such a clinic would be the first of its kind
in the South and one of only three in the nation.[10]

When presented to the circle's entire membership, the idea of supporting this new community service was approved. The Blue Bird Seizure Clinic
in the recently vacated Little Hospital opened in 1949. With an unpaid
administrative head and an annual budget of less than $12,000, the clinic
was run in association with Baylor College of Medicine and was managed by
the circle. With a limited professional staff, supplemented with volunteers,

the clinic began slowly, seeing only between ten and 20 patients monthly. Within two years, the operating budget grew to $35,000 and the number of patients doubled, then tripled, dictating a need for expanded facilities at The Methodist Hospital under construction in the Texas Medical Center.

When the need for expansion required additional funding, The Blue Bird Circle established a foundation. Initially, funds to support The Blue Bird Seizure Clinic were raised mostly by members of the circle. They created and sold embroidered tea towels and handmade Easter eggs and baskets, and also hosted various fund-raising events. With the establishment of a foundation, the circle began receiving sizeable donations that relieved the financial strains experienced by its rapidly growing clinic.

The $400,000 financial obligation for constructing the fourth floor of The Methodist Hospital in the Texas Medical Center was met and The Blue Bird Clinic for Children's Neurological Disorders opened there in 1951. Expanding rapidly, the clinic saw 1,897 patients in 1955. It soon gained national recognition as one of the country's only clinical units that operated on a daily basis and was devoted exclusively to the neurological disorders of children.

Throughout the next two decades, The Blue Bird Clinic for Children's Neurological Disorders continued to grow in both size and stature. Additional space in The Methodist Hospital was acquired in 1965. By 1972, more than 3,365 patients were seen. To support the annual budget of more than $183,000, the circle opened a resale shop, instigated numerous other fund-raising projects, and continued to create and sell its trademark tea towels and Easter creations.

Financial support also came from individuals in the Houston community. In 1973, Baylor College of Medicine and The Methodist Hospital announced plans for three new buildings to house the Neurosensory Center. Longtime Blue Bird Circle benefactors Alice and David C. Bintliff made a generous gift of $2 million, allowing the clinic to move into the new structure in 1977, shortly before Feigin's arrival at Texas Children's Hospital.

When the Bintliff Blue Bird Clinic in the Neurosensory Center opened in 1977, members of the professional staff were full-time faculty of the Baylor College of Medicine with dual appointments in the departments of pediatrics and neurology. However, none were board-certified child neurologists, a requisite for establishing a training program. Most were clinicians involved with patient care and clinical research at three institutions affiliated with Baylor College of Medicine, but all readily admitted that they did not have the skills or the background necessary for basic research endeavors.[11]

As members of a three-person team, these child neurologists found themselves to be "spread extraordinarily thin throughout the affiliated hospitals." Increased demand for their services created major logistical problems, progressively affecting the quality of patient care. "We first established a regularly scheduled pediatric neurology clinic in the Junior League Outpatient Department at Texas Children's in 1972 that met for a half day a week, on a weekly basis, and we also did the same thing at the Ben Taub Hospital," recalled Dr. Thomas E. Zion, medical director of The Blue Bird Circle Clinic from 1965 to 1991. "We were having formally scheduled clinics for children with neurologic problems at all three of the major hospitals."[12]

In order to alleviate the overall administrative responsibilities of such an expansive program, the child neurologists each had a specific area to supervise. With Zion as director of The Blue Bird Clinic, the other two members of the pediatric neurology section at Baylor College of Medicine assumed responsibility for services at other hospitals. Dr. Fabio Fernandez, a former neurology fellow, was appointed chief of pediatric neurology at Ben Taub in 1975 and Dr. Robert Zeller, the only child neurologist on the faculty at Texas Children's Hospital, was appointed that hospital's chief of pediatric neurology in 1975. As the demand for neurological services continued to expand at each hospital, the three physicians were overwhelmed. In an overview of their section written in 1978, they stressed that the "pressing need is the recruitment of additional faculty to share the service commitment."[13]

Such a request came as no surprise to Feigin, who had been acutely aware of the problem since his arrival in 1977. He seized the opportunity and in 1978 made a rather ambitious presentation to the board of trustees at Texas Children's Hospital. Feigin proposed a five-year plan for the development of a pediatric neurology service, which was designated as a priority among his long-range planning goals. Along with the recruitment of qualified faculty and the establishment of a program to train future child neurologists, the service would require a board-certified child neurologist as both chief of the service at Texas Children's Hospital and head of the department of pediatric neurology at Baylor College of Medicine. Feigin's plan called for the continuation of The Blue Bird Clinic at The Methodist Hospital, "a great program for seizure disorders," with the addition of rotating child neurologists from Texas Children's Hospital for training purposes. Once the plan had been approved, Feigin wasted no time in taking the next step. "I needed to have someone who would develop a real program," he said. "So I recruited Marvin Fishman."[14]

The recruitment process was not lengthy. At Texas Children's Hospital,

Feigin had found precisely what Fishman had been hoping for when the two discussed the matter in St. Louis. During his first visits to Texas Children's Hospital, Fishman was intrigued with all he learned. The existing service performed well, but conformed to no defined structure and had no established traditions in need of modification. Fishman saw limitless possibilities and his decision to accept Feigin's offer was influenced mostly by the possibility of developing an exemplary child neurology section.

"I think having known Dr. Feigin in St. Louis gave me some degree of comfort, in that I knew whom I would be working with and I knew his capabilities," Fishman said, recalling his decision to come to Texas Children's Hospital. "I knew of his vision to expand the hospital and that the board of trustees were of the same philosophy. With that type of background and with his support, it provided an opportunity for me to accomplish what I wanted at that point in my career."[15]

Within months of his arrival in 1979, Fishman embarked on his five-year plan to recruit new faculty and develop a certified training program in child neurology. While focused on program development, Fishman also exemplified his career-long reputation as a superb clinician and teacher. "I think that one of the characteristics of a good teacher is to be a good role model," he said. "I think that one's own practice and approach to children with neurological problems, or any other problems, has to be one of concern, empathy, intellectual curiosity, and honesty. I think that residents and trainees perceive their teacher's attitudes and they respond and develop those type of attitudes."[16]

This compassionate and inquisitive role model for future child neurologists also personified the importance of having both a knowledge base and the ability to implement it. Of utmost importance to Fishman was the fact that children with neurological problems were not small adults, especially since many of the neurological diseases in children were unique to the pediatric population. "Examples of these conditions would include certain types of epilepsy and seizures such as those seen in newborn infants with febrile illnesses, and a very unusual form of epilepsy called infantile spasms in which lightning-fast jerks of the extremities and trunk occur in very small infants," he explained. "Certain types of brain tumors are more common in children than adults, particularly those that involve the cerebellum, the balance organ of the brain. Among birth defects, congenital malformations of the brain, including hydrocephalus and spina bifida, are relatively common and insults to the brain of the newborn baby and young infant may result in life-long conditions such as epilepsy, mental retardation, and cerebral palsy."[17]

Since the central nervous system could be affected by the complications from diseases affecting other organs, children with congenital heart disease, leukemia, and liver problems often developed neurological problems. Although migraine headaches and strokes occurred in children as well as adults, the causes often were different in children. "The needs of these children and their families are special," Fishman said. "The neurological problems they encounter may affect the developing and immature brain differently than the fully developed nervous system of an adult. They may affect the child's ability to perform and participate in school, extracurricular activities, and social activities. To fully meet these needs, the services of a multidisciplinary team, including other sub-specialists, pediatricians, and related health personnel, are necessary. Fortunately, all of these resources are available at Texas Children's Hospital where we can provide exemplary care to children with neurological problems."[18]

The depth and scope of that exemplary care continued to expand. During the following five years, Fishman and his steadily growing staff evaluated and treated an increasing number of children with a wide variety of nervous system disorders. By 1984, in addition to providing services to inpatients, the pediatric neurology service at Texas Children's Hospital evaluated more than 1,300 outpatients per year in the Junior League Outpatient Department.

Key members of the pediatric neurology service in 1984 were six fellows, two on each level of a three-year training program leading to board certification by the American Board of Psychiatry and Neurology with special competence in child neurology. Officially established in 1981 by Fishman and Dr. Stanley Appel, chief of adult neurology at Baylor College of Medicine, this child neurology program had already become the largest of its type in Texas and one of the largest in the United States.

To enter the neurology program, each participant had to have completed two or three years of pediatric training. At first, half of the trainees were graduates of the Texas Children's Hospital pediatric residency program. In the program's fledgling year, each fellow received training in adult clinical neurology, as well as broad background in the related neurosciences such as neuroanatomy, neurochemistry, and neuropharmacology. "It was hoped that this would accommodate trainees who may have had an early interest in adult neurology but became enlightened during their training and wanted to transfer to child neurology," Fishman explained.[19]

In the second and third years, each child neurology fellow attended activities in The Blue Bird Clinic for Children's Neurological Disorders and the muscular dystrophy clinic and received training in clinical pediatric neurology, as well as neuroradiology, neuropathology, and clinical neuro-physiology. For an aspiring academic neurologist who was planning a career in research, training in the clinical neurophysiology service at Texas Children's Hospital offered a unique opportunity.

One of the first such services established in the United States, the neu-rophysiology service at Texas Children's Hospital was founded in 1973 by renowned neurophysiologist and epileptologist Peter Kellaway, PhD. One of the pioneers in the establishment of the field of neonatal and pediatric elec-troencephalography (EEG), Kellaway gained international recognition as an expert in the clinical use of EEG and its application in the evaluation and management of patients with suspected neurological conditions.

Kellaway had arrived at Baylor College of Medicine in 1948 after earn-ing his doctoral degree in neurophysiology at McGill University in Montreal. "I really wanted to do basic research in neurophysiology," he recalled. "I was interested in the electrical activity of the brain, where it was coming from, what was its origin, what role did it play. I also was interest-ed in sleep and the mechanisms of sleep. When I arrived, Dr. Greenwood had given the first EEG machine to Baylor and I thought this was going to be tremendously valuable for children, as opposed to adults."[20]

Having begun his career at Baylor College of Medicine at a time when studies of children with epilepsy were limited, Kellaway pioneered exten-sive research studies of neonatal seizures and infantile spasms; the characterization of normal and abnormal patterns in neonates, infants, chil-dren, and adults; the identification of genetic contributions to EEG activity and seizure disorders in children; and descriptions of intrinsic biorhythms that influence seizure occurrence.

An advocate for a comprehensive approach to care for children with epilepsy, Kellaway was instrumental in the establishment of The Blue Bird Clinic for Children's Neurological Disorders at The Methodist Hospital in 1949 and served as its director until 1960. "When the clinic opened, the only other major clinic for neurological disorders in children at that time was in Boston and The Blue Bird Clinic grew to become regarded as the top epilep-sy program for children in the country," Kellaway said. "Epilepsy is one of the most common neurological disorders, and there was always this antipathy that people had towards epilepsy. The larger part of seizures in children is rel-atively a benign disorder, but they have terrible symptoms. There were all kinds of theories as to what was going on, but until the EEG came along, no one knew that these electrical storms took place in the brain."[21]

It was his avid interest in epilepsy research that led Kellaway to establish the Epilepsy Research Center at Baylor College of Medicine in 1973. Kellaway also served as director of the center, which was funded by the National Institutes of Health (NIH). He was to continue serving in that capacity until 1998, stepping down at the age of 78. Throughout his 55-year career, his research resulted in more than 200 scientific publications, the last of which was published several months before his death in 2004. In his lifetime, Kellaway's illustrious efforts produced advancements in the care of children with epilepsy, the development of EEG use in the everyday diagnosis of children with seizure disorders, and countless contributions to the field of electrophysiology research.[22]

"Peter Kellaway derived great pleasure from teaching students at Baylor and he left a living legacy of innovative and creative neuroscientists and neurophysiologists," said Dr. Eli M. Mizrahi, a former fellow who ultimately became chief of the neurophysiology service at Texas Children's Hospital, director of the Baylor Comprehensive Epilepsy Center at The Methodist Hospital, and director of the NIH-funded Clinical Research Center for Neonatal Seizures. "These scientific children and grandchildren now carry on the many programs of excellence he fostered."[23]

One such research program began shortly after Fishman's arrival in 1979. With many members of the neurology staff actively involved in clinical research projects in an effort to learn more about the diseases that affect the developing nervous system, Mizrahi concentrated his efforts on neonatal seizures, often the first indication of neurological dysfunction in a baby. "Seizures in the neonate often take different forms than those seen in older children because of the immaturity of the nervous system in these babies," explained Fishman. "With the cooperation of the neonatology service at Texas Children's Hospital, Dr. Mizrahi undertook a comprehensive study of this important problem."[24]

To ascertain whether the movements observed in premature babies were due to seizures, normal activity, or a non-epileptic abnormality of the brain, Mizrahi designed and fabricated a cribside-monitoring unit in the neonatal intensive care unit at Texas Children's Hospital. This portable system allowed synchronized EEG and video monitoring and produced simultaneous recording of multiple physiological parameters such as eye movements, respiratory efforts, airway flow, and measurements of oxygen, carbon dioxide, and blood pressure.

Over a period of several years, Mizrahi and Kellaway studied 349 neonates at Texas Children's Hospital and recorded 415 clinical seizures in 71 infants. In 11 other infants, they recorded seizures that were not accompanied by EEG activity and therefore not epileptic in nature. It was a landmark finding.[25] Published in 1987, these pioneering investigations served as the foundation for the detailed characterization and classification of neonatal seizures, a better understanding of the function of the immature nervous system, and the design and implementation of therapeutic intervention for central nervous system dysfunction in neonates.

Another neurophysiology research program instigated in the early 1980s was a collaborative effort with the pulmonary service at Texas Children's Hospital. Working with that service's Dr. Carol Rosen, former fellow Dr. Daniel G. Glaze began to study sleep apnea in neonates—specifically, the area of the brain thought to be involved in the control of breathing and sleep. "Utilizing the Clinical Research Center at Texas Children's Hospital, they are studying the control of respiration, as well as the respiratory responses to various stimuli and sleep patterns," Fishman announced in 1984. "Dr. Glaze also is involved in ongoing studies of infantile spasms, a major research interest in the neurophysiology and neurology services at Texas Children's Hospital. The current efforts are directed towards therapeutic trials of drugs which may affect the way impulses are transmitted to the brain."[26]

While most research programs in child neurology involved the study of patients, many required initial laboratory research. At Texas Children's Hospital in the early 1980s, Dr. Jan Goddard-Finegold, a pediatric pathologist in the child neurology service, gained international recognition for the development of the animal model for the study of what may cause or contribute to intraventricular hemorrhage in premature infants. "The baby who is born prematurely is at risk for many problems," Goddard-Finegold stated in 1986. "One of the problems most feared is brain damage, and one of the causes of brain damage, cerebral hemorrhage, is a major focus of research at Texas Children's Hospital."[27]

A collaborative effort with other pathologists and neurophysiologists, these research studies were initiated at the time when this condition of bleeding in the brain was found at death in as many as 50 percent of premature infants who weighed less than 1,500 grams at birth. With the advent of improved treatment of respiratory insufficiency in low birthweight babies, many who suffered cerebral hemorrhages survived but developed major problems such as hydrocephalus and various forms of cerebral palsy. The goal of the research was to provide information that will lead to the prevention of brain damage.

Remarkable progress in evaluating and monitoring cerebral hemorrhages in premature infants was achieved in the late 1980s. Based upon the findings of Goddard-Finegold's studies, the incidence of cerebral hemorrhages in premature newborns at Texas Children's Hospital decreased by half. These studies also shed light on factors that control cerebral blood flow in premature babies, important developmental information that was previously unknown.

"The functions of the developing brain are fascinating," Fishman said when reporting the advances attributable to the collective efforts of the neurology service at Texas Children's Hospital in the 1980s. "These functions control how children learn to smile, crawl, walk, talk, and think. When everything progresses normally, we all enjoy these wonderful experiences. However, when problems arise, facilities and physicians capable of diagnosing and treating the illnesses can help restore functions to as near as normal as possible. This will allow children to function to their maximum capabilities consistent with their abilities. These are the goals of the neurology service at Texas Children's Hospital."[28]

To achieve these goals, Fishman continued to recruit new faculty members and to expand his service. The patient population in the former once-a-week neurology clinic in the Junior League Outpatient Department continued to grow, making it necessary to extend the clinic to four days a week. When a shortage of available space for expansion resulted in the opening of Texas Children's Hospital's first off-campus pediatric facility for outpatient clinical care at 8080 North Stadium Drive in 1986, the neurology clinic moved there. Along with fellow child neurologists Dr. Rita Lee, Dr. Julie Park, and Dr. Fabio Fernandez, Fishman evaluated and treated more than 1,000 children with seizures, epilepsy, neuromuscular diseases, headaches, cerebral palsy, developmental and congenital nervous system disorders, and injuries to the nervous system from trauma, infection, and metabolic diseases.

Also evaluated in the neurology clinic was an array of neurological disorders for which there was no known cure or treatment at the time. The consequences of such disorders varied, but sometimes produced a relentless deterioration of the child's mental and physical faculties—all of which were devastating to both the child and the family. For Fishman and his growing team of child neurologists at Texas Children's Hospital, it "was very difficult to tell parents that we do not yet understand the cause."[29]

To find the elusive answers required further complex research in pediatric neurology. At Texas Children's Hospital and Baylor College of Medicine in 1988, studies to investigate the origins of neurological disorders on the molecular level were in progress. Advances in the techniques of molecular biology enabled neuroscientists to identify and classify the origins of diseases. Many such accomplishments occurred at Texas Children's Hospital.

These achievements garnered national recognition, as well as additional outside funding for other neurological research studies at Texas Children's Hospital during the 1980s. One of these studies involved a recently identified and rare developmental disorder, Rett syndrome, first published in medical literature in 1983.[30] Originally recognized in 1966 by Viennese physician Dr. Andreas Rett, this genetic disorder was thought to occur predominantly in young and previously well girls whose development slows and then plateaus. Those afflicted with the disorder lose the purposeful use of their hands, lose language skills, and develop stereotyped behavior. Additional problems include difficulties with coordination, abnormal breathing patterns, and possible epilepsy. Although less than 1,500 children worldwide had been diagnosed with Rett syndrome in 1988, several were patients of the pediatric neurology service at Texas Children's Hospital. With an NIH-funded five-year study under the direction of Dr. Alan K. Percy in the Baylor College of Medicine Rett Center, Texas Children's Hospital established one of the nation's major centers for studying this puzzling illness.[31]

Such federal support for scientific research began to diminish dramatically during the national budget crisis of the 1980s. A steady decline in the percentage of approved grant proposals that received federal dollars was apparent at Texas Children's Hospital by the end of the decade. Fishman was among many who voiced a growing concern. "Because all this complex research takes such a long time, it is critical that the work be supported by stable sources of funding," he said. "Without that security, there is always the possibility of losing momentum. With it, scientists are able to produce a body of work that attracts other funding and the momentum increases."[32]

Quite unexpectedly, this much-needed funding came to Texas Children's Hospital in 1988 through an act of goodwill from the Houston community: the establishment of the Gordon and Mary Cain Pediatric Neurology Research Foundation at Texas Children's Hospital. Conceived and established by the senior executives of Cain Chemical, Inc., Sterling Chemicals, Inc., and the Sterling Group Inc. and funded by individual charitable donations, the foundation honored founder Gordon Cain and his wife Mary, who had the unique concept of sharing ownership and profits with the employees of these successful companies. "The Cains' generosity and foresight for the welfare of their employees was the spirit with which the foundation was established, so that children with presently incurable neurological diseases and their families may benefit from the same spirit of sharing," said the truly surprised and grateful Fishman. "The foundation will provide a permanent endowment to help support research, laboratories and equipment."[33]

The Gordon and Mary Cain Pediatric Neurology Research Foundation had an immediate and measurable impact on the pediatric neurology service at Texas Children's Hospital. Grants received from the foundation enabled Fishman to support and expand current research projects; recruit John W. Swann, PhD, as the foundation's scientific director; and enlist other accomplished scientists and experienced researchers for future endeavors.

Cain Foundation funds also were used to complete and equip a 4,500-square-foot laboratory space in the new 12-story ambulatory care and research facility, opened in 1991 and named the Feigin Center in 1997. "There, established investigators, promising new scientists, and students will work together to obtain an understanding of how the brain works, what causes its functions to go astray, and hopefully gain insight into treating and preventing currently unapproachable neurologic diseases," Fishman predicted in 1990. "And the generosity inspired by Gordon and Mary Cain will play an important role in all of these achievements."[34]

This enthusiastic prediction for the future was based on a certainty that existed in the field of neurology at the time. More than 90 percent of all advances made in disorders and disabilities involving the brain had been made during the 1980s, and even more productivity was expected in the 1990s. In recognition of these achievements—and the 50 million Americans who suffered from neurologic disorders and disabilities—the United States Congress passed a resolution in 1989 to designate the 1990s as the "Decade of the Brain."

During that promising decade, Fishman's vision of placing Texas Children's Hospital at the forefront of investigations into neurological diseases affecting infants and young children became a reality. Among the many accomplishments made by his service during the 1990s, one outstanding example was the 1999 discovery by Dr. Huda Y. Zoghbi of the defective gene MECP2, which causes Rett syndrome. One of Fishman's first fellows in the early 1980s, Zoghbi later became a specialist in the neurology service at Texas Children's Hospital, a Howard Hughes Medical Institute investigator, and a professor in the departments of pediatrics, neurology, neuroscience, and molecular and human genetics at Baylor College of Medicine.

When she arrived at Baylor College of Medicine as a resident in the early 1980s, Zoghbi had planned to become a pediatric cardiologist. She changed her mind after a rotation with Fishman in child neurology. "I loved it," she said. "Neurology grabbed me because of how logical it is. You observe the patient, analyze her symptoms, and work backward to figure out exactly which part of the brain is responsible for the problem. You solve anatomical riddles by paying attention to details, listening to the patient, and then putting all the information together."[35]

Fascinated by disorders that affect the brain, Zoghbi became a child neurologist at Texas Children's Hospital in 1988. After working with patients with neurological disorders for which there were no known treatments or cures—such as Rett syndrome—she wanted to help find the answers to their problems. Convinced that the possibility of such solutions lay in molecular biology, Zoghbi decided to set aside her clinical work and devote her attention to the laboratory. After three years of training in molecular biology at Baylor College of Medicine, she acquired the skills needed to track down the genes that underlie neurological disorders.

Although initially interested in studying Rett syndrome, Zoghbi was drawn to the study of spinocerebellar ataxia type 1 (SCA1), a hereditary disorder of the nervous system that resulted in the late onset of the deterioration of balance and coordination. Patients with SCA1 are unable to walk or talk clearly. Eventually, years after the onset of the disorder, they become incapable of swallowing or breathing. After identifying a large family in Montgomery, Texas, that was particularly prone to this fatal disorder, Zoghbi learned that another family was participating in a University of Minnesota study under the direction of Dr. Harry T. Orr. When Zoghbi proposed a collaborative study with Orr, he accepted because it made "scientific sense." Their joined efforts resulted in the 1993 locating, mapping, and cloning of the defective gene responsible for SCA1.[36]

As the codiscoverer of the SCA1 gene, Zoghbi quickly gained international recognition in the field of neurology and molecular genetics. She began devoting more of her laboratory time to Rett syndrome, the disorder that had originally inspired her to enter the field of molecular research.

It had been more than a decade since Zoghbi first encountered the puzzling disorder as a fellow at Texas Children's Hospital in 1983. She later participated in the five-year NIH-funded study of Rett syndrome at Texas Children's Hospital and in the diagnosis and care of girls and women with Rett syndrome at The Blue Bird Circle Rett Center. Active in the center since its 1986 inception at The Methodist Hospital, Zoghbi was aware of the increasing number of patients affected by the disorder. In 1999, there were more than 10,000 documented cases of Rett syndrome in the United States. Identified as one of the most common forms of mental retardation in females, Rett syndrome was known to rob previously healthy girls of their language, mental function, and ability to interact with others. There was no known treatment.

Since it was rare for more than one member of a family to be infected, "finding the genetic cause of Rett syndrome has been the most challenging problem I have worked on," Zoghbi said. "Usually we can map the location of a disease gene by studying the way the genetic defect is inherited in families. But Rett syndrome occurs sporadically more than 99 percent of the time, so we had very few families to study where more than one member is affected with this neurologic disorder."[37]

Zoghbi's 1999 landmark discovery of the gene responsible for Rett syndrome played an important role in advancing knowledge about the disease and in allowing early diagnosis. The identification of the defective gene also enhanced the possibility of the development of a cure. "This gene is essential to life, not just for brain development," Zoghbi explained. "We are excited it gives hope for Rett patients and gives us a tool for understanding brain development, which may in turn provide insight into other diseases and ultimately help us unravel the most complex system in the human body."[38]

It was the insight provided by another research effort at Texas Children's Hospital that resulted in the 1992 development of the Texas Children's Sleep Center. One of the nine accredited centers in the country specializing in the diagnostic evaluation and treatment of pediatric sleep disorders, it was established under the medical direction of Glaze, Fishman's former fellow who had enacted studies of sleep apnea in neonates during the 1980s. "Abnormal events of sleep must be properly diagnosed as sleep disorders to differentiate them from other abnormal events such as epileptic seizures." Glaze explained. "The key to managing sleep problems is awareness. Once a sleep disorder is diagnosed, it usually can be managed with medication, lifestyle changes, or surgery in the case of sleep apnea. When sleep is managed properly, both the patient and the family experience a greatly improved quality of life."[39]

As this and other new programs were introduced throughout the 1990s, the child neurology service at Texas Children's Hospital continued to grow at its established steady pace. In less than two decades, Fishman had nurtured child neurology from its small beginnings to its annual patient population of more than 2,000, making it the twelfth-largest clinic at Texas Children's Hospital in 1997. The following year, this status dramatically changed.

In contrast to the previous pattern of gradual growth, in 1998 there was an exponential increase in the number of patients with neurologic disorder. This occurred when The Blue Bird Clinic for Pediatric Neurology and The Blue Bird Circle Rett Center ended its 50-year affiliation with The Methodist Hospital and began an affiliation agreement with Texas Children's Hospital. The immediate combination of both patient populations resulted in a total of more than 6,000 children, catapulting child neurology overnight to its ranking as the fourth-largest clinic at Texas Children's Hospital. "It was a big jump," Fishman said. "I think the major difference, besides the size, is that Texas Children's Hospital now had a dedicated neurology clinic. When that happened, we had the opportunity to get more space because the need was there."[40]

Since the new Clinical Care Center at Texas Children's Hospital was in the planning stages in 1998, Fishman's previously requested space for the child neurology clinic was reconfigured and enlarged to accommodate the needs of the newly combined patient populations. Upon the building's completion in 2001, The Blue Bird Clinic for Pediatric Neurology and The Blue Bird Rett Center moved physically from The Methodist Hospital to the ninth floor of the Clinical Care Center. Remaining at Baylor College of Medicine was The Blue Bird Circle Neurogenetics Laboratory, founded in 1986.

Continuing the tradition of excellence established in 1949, more than 300 members of The Blue Bird Circle began volunteering at The Blue Bird Clinic for Pediatric Neurology and at The Blue Bird Circle Rett Center at Texas Children's Hospital in 2001. Distinguishable by their royal blue uniforms, the volunteers provided invaluable assistance to the physicians, residents, neuropsychologists, nurse practitioners, nine clinical staff, and social worker in the new clinic. Focused on the quality care of patients and their families, volunteers staffed the front desk, worked as clinical aides, and helped with medical records and transcriptions. "We try to provide patients and their families with the best comprehensive service we can," said social worker Ann Alexander, a member of the clinic since 1968. "The volunteers and staff have a mutual respect for each other. It's easy for us to stay committed when you have such dedicated volunteers who support the clinic with a clear vision and mission."[41]

Such steadfast dedication was measurable in both time and money. Each individual member's commitment to provide 150 volunteer hours a year resulted in the organization's annual contribution of more than 100,000 volunteer hours at Texas Children's Hospital. Circle members also donated their time and efforts to the organization's longtime signature fundraising endeavors. Profits from the resale shop, gift shop, embroidered tea towels, Easter eggs, Easter baskets, annual gala, and various other projects benefited Blue Bird Circle programs at Texas Children's Hospital and Baylor College of Medicine.

"Our 53-year-old mission is to support pediatric neurology," said president Annette Moore in 2003. "We help children with a wide variety of conditions that affect the function of the developing brain and we have a million-dollar commitment every year in support of our programs. Over the years, through the work of dedicated circle members and the generous support of circle donors, we have given more than $21 million to the Houston community."[42]

Another valuable result of the successful merger of The Blue Bird Circle Clinic for Pediatric Neurology and Texas Children's Hospital was its expanded ability to provide patients with more intensive and comprehensive care. Specializing in the diagnosis, treatment, and follow-up care of neurological disorders in children from birth to age 17, the clinic addressed the full spectrum of neurological disease from developmental and neuromuscular problems to metabolic and generative disorders.

As the only one of its kind in the Southwest, The Blue Bird Clinic for Pediatric Neurology at Texas Children's Hospital experienced a steady growth in patient population in its first two years. By 2003, more than 8,000 children with epilepsy, motor problems, seizures, static encephalopathies, cerebral palsy, developmental delay, headaches, brain tumors, congenital malformations, weakness, movement disorders, and degenerative diseases received comprehensive treatment and care each year. Because of the complex nature of most neurological conditions, patients often were referred to the clinic's subspecialty programs, the sleep center, the epilepsy center, the Meyer Center for Developmental Pediatrics, and The Blue Bird Circle Rett Center, the largest of its type in the world.

The need for further subspecialization was evident to Fishman as he observed the growing and diverse spectrum of neurological disorders treated in The Blue Bird Clinic for Pediatric Neurology at Texas Children's Hospital. To remain in the forefront of neurological treatment and care, the development of programs for muscular dystrophy, cerebral palsy, and other diseases was an anticipated necessity. Fishman also knew that such an expansion plan would require the implementation of a five- and ten-year vision to take advantage of the opportunities that existed. It was this certainty that motivated his decision to step down from his administrative duties in 2004, relinquishing his responsibilities to the new chief of child neurology, Dr. Gary D. Clark. "At this stage of my career," Fishman said, "I thought I was not the best person to continue the future growth of the program."

Without question, in 1979 Fishman had been the best one to begin it. During his 25-year career as chief of child neurology at Texas Children's Hospital, he achieved what he had hoped in the beginning to accomplish— particularly the growth of the faculty and its success in developing all the components of the child neurology service at Texas Children's Hospital. "It's just been a fine group of people who have provided excellent clinical services, excellent educational experiences for trainees, and an increased knowledge base in neurological diseases through their research activities," he said. "I am proud of what they accomplished."[43]

Always inclined to praise others instead of himself, Fishman found gratification in their successes. The attainment of his own vision—establishing one of the top four child neurology training programs in the field—reaped the kind of rewards for which he had hoped. Making an indelible mark on the field of child neurology, most of the more than 55 child neurologists trained by Fishman went on to head their own child neurology training programs elsewhere.

To all the trainees he inspired and mentored, the thousands of patients he treated with loving and compassionate care, the medical students he educated and nurtured, the medical staff he encouraged and motivated, and the Blue Bird volunteers he welcomed and appreciated, Fishman was more than the chief of child neurology at Texas Children's Hospital for 25 years. He was also the personification of unselfish and dedicated service.

At the age of seven months, Leyla Ballantyne was a fat and happy baby.

Happier still were her parents. Having successfully accomplished her first major developmental milestone at the appropriate age, Leyla had fulfilled their wildest expectations. "It was a big deal when she sat up for the first time," Yasmine Ballantyne said. "We were just ecstatic. She had done everything she was supposed to do."[44]

After sharing this good news with Dr. Marvin Fishman during Leyla's examination at the child neurology clinic at Texas Children's Hospital, Yasmine was surprised by his actions. "He was holding the baby like a doll, and then he acted like he was dropping her on the floor," she said, vividly recalling the moment years later. "I didn't have a clue what he was looking for, but learned later that he wanted to know if she was going to get startled. He told me that at seven months, if their emotions are developing along with their physical traits, babies instinctively realize there is a menace to them and will exhibit fear, which is exactly what Leyla did. It was very interesting to know the things he looked for. We think of physical development and he was looking for everything."

This process of discovery continued during each of Leyla's subsequent appointments. When the Ballantynes returned with Leyla to see Fishman every six months, "he was always very thorough; from head to toe he would look at her and talk to her," Yasmine recalled. "He never rushed us out, and you know, he's very busy. If I had 50 questions, he always answered them and we never felt that any question was not important enough to ask."

In search of answers about every phase of her development, Yasmine had quit her job to stay at home with Leyla. Christie continued his concentrated routine of developmental stimulation, including his nightly routine of reading both his daughter and himself to sleep. Advised by Fishman to look for aberrations in her behavior that might require rehabilitation, the Ballantynes maintained their endless vigil. They reveled each time Leyla achieved a developmental milestone at the appropriate time and were in awe of each accomplishment, no matter how small.

"It really was amazing," Yasmine said. "We never had any trouble with her, but we watched every milestone. The doctors said she could be totally normal, and then certain functions just don't develop at all. She may not have any feelings for others, or she may not have a depth of understanding of certain things. The fact that she was crawling and then walking was just, 'Wow,' as was the fact that she wanted to feed herself and stick her hand in the food. Anything that she would do, we were ecstatic."

Such unbridled bliss was commonplace for the Ballantynes during the first three years of Leyla's life. An avid fan of *Sesame Street* since she was 18 months old, Leyla could recite the alphabet and all the numbers by the time she was 22 months old. Intrigued with books, she could sit for hours and look at pictures on the pages and began reading at the age of three.

In spite of these accomplishments, her father remained vigilant in his observance of every aspect of his daughter's development. "I was always very anxious with it in terms of whether she was moving funny and things like that," he said. "She had normal coordination, normal development, and when she started reading at the age of three it was because I was so overly concerned about her stimulation all the time. Dr. Fishman would call me and say she was doing very well, which was always very reassuring."[45]

Leyla's remarkable progress at the age of three was evident to Fishman, who told the Ballantynes that they no longer needed to bring her to the child neurology clinic at Texas Children's Hospital. Should there be a need for a neurological examination in the future, which Fishman doubted, her pediatrician would be able to recognize it and refer them back. Hearing such an optimistic prognosis had been unfathomable three years earlier, especially "when you look back at how we started and things looked so pessimistic,"

Christie said. "Leyla apparently had some injury, but being a baby and with her growth, her brain was able to overcome it and basically confine it."

For the following 15 years, Leyla never demonstrated the need to see Fishman again. With an insatiable appetite for life, she made friends easily and her determined focus to succeed became evident in sports of every variety. "She was emotionally grounded and a very happy little girl," Yasmine said. "I told Christie the trauma must have removed any genes for unhappiness in this child, because she was always smiling."

This childhood trait, coupled with her ability to excel, had become Leyla's signature by the time she entered high school. At St. John's School in Houston, she became a national merit scholar semifinalist in her junior year and scored 1520 on her SAT. Enthusiastic praise for her accomplishments came not only from her family and friends, but also from her instructors. "Every day, she saunters into class with a smile on her face, but, beneath that casual demeanor, there lurk powers of mind and will and heart that can (and will, I bet) change the world," English instructor John Allman said in 2004. "Leyla is one of the most exciting students we've had the pleasure and privilege to teach. She energized our campus with her intellectual passion, her independence of thought, and her moral courage."[46]

For her justifiably proud parents, Leyla's ever receiving such accolades had been unimaginable at the time of her traumatic birth and early infancy. As they remembered those experiences in 2004, what Yasmine described as a miracle, Christie likened to the equivalent of surviving a natural disaster. "We were fortunate to be in the right place to get the right care; it is when things go wrong that you really need outstanding people around," he explained. "Within a couple of minutes, if the right people did not do the right things, it would have been a disastrous outcome. The brain has a tremendous capacity for tolerating some damage and then recovering, but there is such a narrow window of opportunity. We were very lucky because we were just within that window."

Although she had no personal recollections of these experiences, Leyla was no stranger to the details. She had heard her parents praise Fishman for his attentive and reassuring care during her many visits to the child neurologist at Texas Children's Hospital, but she had no memory of him. When the opportunity came for her to renew their acquaintance, the set of circumstances differed dramatically from that of her initial encounters. The first were a necessity; this was a luxury.

Invited to attend a 2004 seminar in honor of Fishman's 25-year career as chief of child neurology at Texas Children's Hospital, Leyla went with her mother. After being introduced to the gathered crowd of scientists by long-time family friend Dr. Huda Y. Zoghbi—who briefly outlined the details of Leyla's birth and resuscitation, the Apgar score of zero, the fears about her not surviving that first year, the overwhelming possibility of a poor outcome, and then remarkable development and outstanding achievements—Leyla took a bow with her trademark smile.

Eighteen years after being held in his arms as a newborn at Texas Children's Hospital, the perfectly poised high school graduate spoke directly to her child neurologist for the first time in her memory. "I would like to thank you for spending your life doing this, and I guess I am one of the recipients of your knowledge," she said to Fishman. "I just want to thank you on behalf of all the kids you work with."

Since this heartfelt speech was unrehearsed and unexpected, Leyla Ballantyne had once again surprised everyone with a delivery that was not routine.

24

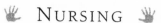 NURSING

M ONA KHEIR USED TO DREAM about what she wanted to be when she
grew up.

She saw herself as a member of the healthcare profession, an area
of expertise that became increasingly familiar to her throughout her
childhood years.

Mona also dreamt about where her chosen career path would ultimately lead. It was to Texas Children's Hospital, the place she affectionately
called "my home away from home" for more than a decade.

"I was born with a urologic birth defect in Tripoli, Lebanon, but my
family moved to Amarillo when I was a baby," Mona explained. "When they
took me to see the doctor there, he referred us to Dr. Gonzales at Texas
Children's Hospital in Houston. I was 16 months old at the time. That, my
first visit, was in 1980, and my last appointment was in 1993."[1]

During those 13 years as a frequent patient, Mona continued to receive
treatment from Dr. Edmund T. Gonzales, Jr., and his nurse, Barbara
Montagnino. One of the first 15 physicians in the United States to practice
pediatric urology full-time, Gonzales was director of the pediatric urology
service and chief of the department of surgery at Texas Children's Hospital.

As a child, Mona underwent 12 surgical procedures at Texas Children's
Hospital. "I have big scars on my stomach and back from all those surgeries,
and little scars on my arms and legs from all the IVs I have had over the
years," she explained.

Mona also had lasting memories. The most vivid were those about the loving care she received at Texas Children's Hospital. Whenever she was bored or
frightened or in pain, someone was always there to ease her anxieties and provide comfort to her. Two such individuals left a particularly strong impression.

One was Gonzales, her doctor and surgeon; the other was Montagnino, his nurse. Throughout Mona's various surgeries, countless days in the hospital, and numerous office visits, they became her role models. "At first, I wanted to become a doctor, just like him," she said. "Then I decided to become a nurse, like her."

That decision, made when Mona was a teenager, was based on her cumulative experiences at Texas Children's Hospital. "I remember the nurses who were nice to me and took really good care of me," she said. "I had great experiences and wanted to give back what my nurses gave me."[2]

After deciding her future, Mona addressed her past. "All my friends used to tease me, calling me 'Mona Lisa' and other names, so I decided to change my name," she said. "So, as a teenager, instead of Mona Kheir, I became Jaimee Kheir."[3]

With her new name, Jaimee graduated from high school and began studying nursing at Galveston College. After completing a two-year program, which was approved by the Board of Nurse Examiners for the State of Texas and accredited by the National League for Nursing Accrediting Commission, she was awarded the associate in applied science degree in associate degree nursing. After successfully completing the National Council Licensure Examination for Registered Nurses, she fulfilled her childhood dream of entering the healthcare profession.

"I was so eager to become a nurse, I opted for the two-year program instead of four years," Jaimee said. "I plan to go back and earn my bachelor degree in the future."[4]

After graduation, Jaimee wanted to complete her career path as planned, but ended up taking a circuitous route back to Texas Children's Hospital. First, she joined a travel nurse program and worked at hospitals throughout the country. Then she returned to Texas, got married, and began looking for a job.

"Every time I drove by Texas Children's Hospital, I said to myself: 'That's where I belong,'" she recalled. "And today, that's where I am."

In 1999, Jaimee Kheir-Westfall, RN, was hired as a nurse in the progressive care unit at Texas Children's Hospital. She had returned to her home away from home.

Jaimee's childhood dream had come true. At the age of 20, she was exactly what and precisely where she had dreamt she would be when she grew up.

T he metamorphosis of the nursing service at Texas Children's Hospital began the first stage of its evolution November 17, 1987.

On that day, the respective presidents of Texas Children's Hospital and St. Luke's Episcopal Hospital signed the new operating agreement that further documented the 1984 separation of joint services. This formalization marked the beginning of myriad changes in the nursing service, but the goals that had been set at the hospital's opening in 1954 remained unchanged. As they had done for more than 33 years, the nurses at Texas Children's Hospital continued to devote all of their time, energy, and clinical expertise to the dedicated care of children and their families.

Fulfilling this mission was particularly challenging in the period immediately after the separation agreement, particularly for those who were adapting to the centralization of hospital facilities and services. "I left a very secure position at St. Luke's to come to a place that was in chaos," remembered Sylvia A. Doyle, MSN, the new director of operating room nurses. "I kind of thrive in chaos."[5]

Doyle's immediate priority was to organize a temporary surgical operating suite exclusively for the pediatric patients at Texas Children's Hospital. To transform disorder into order, she embarked on a plan. "At the time that we separated, there was a lot of activity that had to happen prior to our opening the operating rooms," she said. "We had to pull our team together, get all of our staffing. We had to do all of the policies and procedures, separate out all of the instrumentation, all of the equipment."[6]

Just two months after the November 1987 separation announcement, Texas Children's Hospital opened its first surgical operating suite solely devoted to all pediatric surgical care, with the exception of cardiovascular surgery. Consisting of eight rooms on the fourth floor, the suite opened on January 2, 1988, and included a holding room, an anesthesia induction area, and a recovery room specially designed for pediatric patients.

"It's really the nursing team that did that," explained Doyle. "It was the nurses that took that responsibility and accountability to make sure that everything was in place, so that the surgeon walking in just had to go in and just concentrate on what they had to do and not worry about anything else. I guess that's the way that I've always seen nurses. They are part of the glue that holds the whole thing together."[7]

The cohesive efforts of the nursing service had been evident throughout the unchecked expansion of Texas Children's Hospital in the decade preceding the separation agreement. Outpatient visits during that period had increased from 37,000 to 125,000 per year; the number of day surgery cases had increased 600 percent. With patient care delivered in more than 26 separate locations, the nursing service, under the administrative direction of Ruth Sylvester, MSN, RN, continuously adapted its skills to meet the situation.

Sylvester had been recruited from St. Luke's Episcopal Hospital by Dr. Ralph D. Feigin, physician-in-chief at Texas Children's Hospital. She assumed responsibility for the nursing service in 1978. "Dr. Feigin worked very closely with me that first year," she recalled. "We had our ups and downs, but I was pretty hard on everybody while trying to get things moving."

Sylvester's determination was obvious to all. From her first weeks on the job, she championed the concept of family-centered care and introduced methods to achieve that goal. "We developed a system by which everyone became involved in the care of the patient and the family," she explained. "It was more than just giving medicine, it now became the care of the family. We had to really work and develop an understanding of how people react to their child's illness. We put some nurses in working with the psychologists and the psychiatrists, and we had developed a course that they taught them on how to work with the other nurses in the psychosocial care of the patient."[8]

Along with the escalating number of patients spread across multiple locations, Sylvester encountered another population explosion during the 1980s. "We had residents coming out of our ears!" she exclaimed. "The residency program was so overwhelming. Dr. Feigin, with his ability to bring in all these people, made it the leading pediatric residency in the country. When Dr. Feigin came in 1977, it just exploded. And it had just been hardly anything up to that time. We knew we had to get more involved with the physicians."[9]

To accomplish that objective, Sylvester arranged for nurses to become a part of the medical rounds made by residents, medical students, and pediatricians. "It had to be the manager or the assistant manager or the unit teacher, but somebody of those three had to make rounds every day so that they would know what the doctors were saying about every patient, and they could also have input into it," Sylvester explained. "So, pretty soon, the doctors started letting them talk, because they take care of the patient 24 hours a day when everybody else is gone."[10]

Sylvester and her administrative assistants effectively included the nursing service as a necessary participant in the multidisciplinary care offered at Texas Children's Hospital. At the same time, other opportunities to excel were also addressed.

One program introduced by Sylvester in the late 1970s was the unit teacher, an RN working on the unit who was also in charge of the training program for new pediatric nurses on that unit. This highly effective orientation program was incorporated into nursing education when that department was formally established in 1987. Created and directed by Myrtle Williams, MSN, RN, nursing education at Texas Children's Hospital was to play a pivotal role in the exponential growth of the nursing service.

That growth began with the 1984 decision by the boards of Texas Children's Hospital and St. Luke's Episcopal Hospital to dissolve the joint operating agreement. Working with a progression of short-term hospital administrators in the early 1980s and culminating with Feigin's tenure in that role, Sylvester found herself "taking care of all kinds of different administrative duties and beginning to develop new departments. They wanted to separate everything immediately. That meant administration, pharmacy, central services, admitting, radiology, and medical records. It was just separate, separate, separate."[11]

Developing new ways of delivering quality patient care in the newly independent hospital was a priority for Sylvester and the nursing service. While coping with the problems inherent in an ever-expanding patient population distributed among far-flung and overcrowded facilities, the nursing service never faltered in providing expert care to patients—or in searching for solutions. A breakthrough came with a 1988 announcement from Feigin.

"It has become impossible to provide for efficient services to this number of patients within the current facility," he said. "The separation agreement provides the means for Texas Children's Hospital to embark upon a long anticipated program to expand the facilities to meet the healthcare challenges of the future."[12]

Two new buildings were planned, scheduled for completion in 1991. The first was the Clinical Care Center, a multistory facility later named the Feigin Center, which consolidated the 26 separate facilities used for the rapidly expanding ambulatory and research programs.

The second building was the five-story West Tower, built on a foundation that could support a tower of patient rooms planned for construction at some time in the future. The initial facility would include a large pediatric emergency center, a ten-room pediatric surgical suite, a recovery room area, and a centralized location for anesthesia, radiology, and other support services. On the third level was space for the expansion of intensive care services for newborn children.

The nursing service was asked to participate in the planning stages for the new buildings. "We were very, very involved with the building of that facility, particularly the operating suite," recalled Doyle. "Ruth Sylvester had so much experience. Having helped build the operating rooms at St. Luke's during the 1970s, it was kind of second nature to her."[13]

Doyle applied the lessons she had learned while working for four years in the hastily organized temporary operating suite on the fourth floor. "We knew we had to incorporate more space for the post-anesthesia care unit (PACU), because of our allowing parents into that area," she said. "Because you've got the bed or the crib, the rocking chair, and the nurse and parent, we learned you have to have more square footage."[14]

As construction on the two new buildings began, the nursing service endured a period of upheaval. At the same time, the service began to experience the effects of a national shortage of nurses. The crisis affected more than half of the hospitals in the United States and threatened to disrupt the quality of patient care at Texas Children's Hospital.

To alleviate the impact of the nursing shortage, strategies were devised and implemented. Because the two new buildings and the growing number of patient beds would necessitate increased staffing, an aggressive recruiting campaign began. In its extensive search for additional staff, the nursing service at Texas Children's Hospital defined the special sensitivities required for pediatric nurses in a 1990 WATCH Magazine article. "The rapidity of change in the status of a child's condition requires keen observation and assessment skills," the article stated. "Exceptional interpersonal skills are essential to enable the nurse to relate to the child, the parents, and other family members. The pediatric nurse must be creative and innovative in finding ways of dealing with a sick child who may be frightened."[15]

Advocating nursing as a career choice that offered diverse possibilities, the recruiting material promoted the hospital's commitment to increased opportunities for professional development. Aware that most nurses had no prior pediatric experience, the nursing service at Texas Children's Hospital emphasized its nursing education programs and touted its six-to-12-week on-the-job orientation program.

Such concentrated efforts produced remarkable results. In the first quarter of 1990, Texas Children's Hospital hired almost as many registered nurses (RNs) and licensed vocational nurses (LVNs) as had been hired in all of 1989. Projecting that the nursing service would include more than 1,000 nurses when the two new buildings were completed in 1991, Texas Children's Hospital CEO Mark A. Wallace began steering the service in a new direction.

"As the largest pediatric hospital in the United States, we needed to create an environment and culture here for professional nurses," Wallace said. "We wanted experienced nurses, and the new graduates who wanted to come to work and not just hold a job, but build a career. So, we initiated a search to bring in the right leadership for the nursing service."[16]

Recruited in 1990 as vice president of patient care services and chief nursing officer was Susan M. Distefano, MSN, RN. Charged by Wallace to set the desired tone, environment, and culture for the nursing service, Distefano conceived a plan of action.

Implementing that plan took time and effort. "For the first six months, it was like we were always swimming upstream," recalled special projects coordinator Patti Rogers, RN, who arrived six months after Distefano. "But we were always moving ahead. No place that I have ever worked has ever come close to the continuous rate of change of Texas Children's Hospital. And, silly me, for the first couple of years I kept thinking it was going to slow down. I am starting to think it's not going to happen."[17]

When Rogers arrived, her first impression was that Texas Children's Hospital basically was a little hospital in a single building, named Abercrombie. She explained: "Walking around the nursing units and doing the work studies in 1990, I knew 80 percent of the nurses by name on all the units."

This shared feeling of intimacy belied the fact that Texas Children's Hospital was more than just one building at the time. With the entire nursing service scattered between 26 locations for ambulatory patients and more than 40 subspecialty clinics, the size and scope of Distefano's assigned tasks might have been even more daunting were it not for the existing organizational structure of the nursing service.

"In some hospitals, everyone who is a nurse reports to the chief nursing officer, but we are not exactly like that," said Rogers. "We have nurses parsed out to three different vice presidents. Susie's area includes the inpatient critical care and acute care units, neonatology, and the emergency center, to name a few. The operating room, post-anesthesia care and GI procedure suite, and a couple of others, report to Randy Wright. And Cheryl Stavins has all the ambulatory nurses, pediatric surgery, and the wellness center, among others. But Susie's over policy for all of them. The direction of nursing at Texas Children's Hospital is set by Susie, so she works collaboratively with Cheryl and Randy."[18]

Working to formulate a definitive mission for the future of the entire nursing service, Distefano began by observing what already existed when she arrived in 1990. Having previously worked in a general hospital, where pediatrics often was an afterthought and never an administrative priority, she quickly found the exact opposite to be true at Texas Children's Hospital. "One of the first things I noticed about coming here was that every day, all day, the entire interdisciplinary team focused only on a child," she said. "Totally focused. I never had to create a case for why a specific patient had a particular age-specific need. And I was struck by the fact that I didn't need to describe that to anyone, whether it be personnel, equipment services, or programs. It is all understood, from the board of trustees through medical, administrative, and on down to the frontline caregivers. It's part of the mind-set."[19]

During her initial observations of daily life at Texas Children's Hospital, Distefano witnessed the compassionate care that the nurses gave to each and every child. This first impression was to become a lasting one. More than a decade later, Distefano reflected: "Since I arrived in 1990, I have continued to be impressed with the level of dedication and skill of our nursing staff."[20]

With these attributes as the building blocks of its foundation, Distefano began developing the vision and mission of the nursing service. First, she incorporated the vision of Texas Children's Hospital, dedicated to providing the finest possible pediatric patient care, education, and research. Next, she emphasized how the fulfillment of that vision by the nursing service was ensured by Texas Children's Hospital's commitment to creating and maintaining a work climate where nurses consistently go above and beyond in providing nursing care to children and their families.

For the nursing service's mission, Distefano adopted a philosophy consisting of five specific areas of concentration: nurses must be nurtured from novice to expert; the environment in which nurses practice must support and foster professional growth and career satisfaction; a family-centered approach must be used in delivering nursing care; advanced education is essential to the advancement of nursing; and nurses must be encouraged to participate in nursing research and to incorporate those findings into practice.

Distefano then embarked on a mission to create new programs that would support this philosophy. Noting the lack of a sophisticated and up-to-date system to evaluate the skills of the nursing staff, she collaborated with nursing education to design one.

"It was one of the first things Susie and I did," recalled Myrtle Williams. "We called it the competency-based performance development system. We knew we had to know what competencies each nurse needed to have to provide quality patient care. Once we gathered that information, we then had to know how well they were performing those competencies."

While the identification of each of these skills and the specific criteria required for evaluation took months to assemble, the process became a valuable learning experience for Distefano and Williams. "Once we identified the skills in some of the acute care areas, we realized we had to build specific training programs to support those skills," Williams said. "When we developed these courses to help the nurses in those areas to support their knowledge base and to develop further skills, they were thrilled."[21]

Having initiated an extensive evaluation and education program, Distefano and Williams turned their attention to the existing orientation program for new staff members. To nurture novices into experts and to support their professional growth and career satisfaction, the program needed some fine-tuning.

In particular, a sharper focus on pediatrics was required. "Every group of clinical personnel, nursing, nutritionists, social service, respiratory therapists, all these professions have a degree of emphasis on pediatrics in their baccalaureate training, but not much," Distefano said. "We felt every clinician who comes to Texas Children's Hospital needed extensive orientation in pediatrics to understand a lot of the issues we deal with in our diverse and complex patient population."[22]

To help the nursing staff acclimate to a particular unit, a preceptor program was launched. Supplementing the unit teacher system originated by Sylvester, who retired in 1991, the education of new staff members became the responsibility of individual RNs known as preceptors. Having completed a competency program to validate the skills of other nurses, each preceptor evaluated and trained one newly hired nurse. The preceptor documented the orientation process on a weekly basis, indicating whether or not the new nurse was on target and the issues involved in her work. In turn, the new nurse provided written feedback, allowing the evaluation of both the individual preceptor and the overall program.

"The unit teachers, whom we called unit educators, used to do all the orienting, but their job got too big when we started hiring hordes of people," explained Williams. "We train the preceptors in nursing education, and they have to demonstrate their competencies before they can precept someone."[23]

The resulting preceptor program, dedicated to mastering job skills, served to fortify an existing strength of the nursing service at Texas Children's Hospital: that of delivering exceptional family-centered care. A concept pioneered by Texas Children's Hospital, the inclusion of family members in the care of patients became a national trend in the 1980s.

While other children's hospitals scrambled to formulate philosophies and strategies for this singular approach to pediatric care, Texas Children's Hospital continued to rely on established policies—some of which had been in place before the hospital opened in 1954. Since the hospital's construction—when physician-in-chief Dr. Russell J. Blattner included a designated area in each patient room where a parent could stay overnight with the child—

the family had always played an important role at Texas Children's Hospital.

As hospital services expanded, new strategies reflecting this emphasis on the family evolved. With the introduction of pediatric surgery programs in the late 1950s, nursing director Opal M. Benage initiated the policy of allowing family members to visit a child in the surgical recovery room. A decade later, when Benage helped to create the critical care areas—which in other hospitals allowed families only limited visitation privileges—she insisted that there be open access.

Equally accessible were the nurses themselves. Always available to answer questions and provide information about a patient, the nurses included the family in their care of the child. And, to facilitate the transition of a patient from hospital to home, the nursing service taught parents how to administer medications and treatments.

As the decades progressed, so too did the complexities involved in this task. "We ask some of these parents to become nurses overnight, literally," said Distefano, noting the intricate devices required for some patients. "What we want to do is send them home feeling confident to take care of their kids and our patients. It's fairly intimidating unless there is a thoughtful and comprehensive plan on how to educate them."[24]

The introduction of other family-centered policies proliferated during the 1970s and 80s. When appropriate—often in response to medical and technical breakthroughs—many of these policies were updated or altered. Other policies were enhanced to meet the needs of expanded or newly introduced hospital services. Following the establishment in 1987 of the independent pediatric surgical suite, Ruth Sylvester and Sylvia Doyle extended Benage's access policy to include all pre- and post-surgical areas.

Regardless of the expansion of facilities, staff and services, the family-centered policy that remained unaltered at Texas Children's Hospital was the one regarding visiting hours allotted to parents. From the hospital's opening day, there were few restrictions. Based on the premise that parents were not visitors, this open access applied to a vast majority of patient areas—including those in critical care. The unique policy garnered praise from families and astonishment from administrators of other hospitals.

"We had so many hospitals who looked at our visiting hours several years ago and said, 'Pedi ICU is closed for two hours for rounds but otherwise it's open? What?'" said Debbie D'Ambrosio, pediatric intensive care unit (PICU) assistant director. "They were accustomed to their own critical care area's offering 45 minutes to visit in the morning and 45 minutes to visit at night, and otherwise it was closed to visitation by parents. But it's always been very wide open like that here. Now it is open at all times, except during shift changes."[25]

Although this aspect of family-centered care at Texas Children's Hospital had been constant since the 1950s, what was evolving was the composition of patients' families. No longer headed by a traditional mother and father, the family unit of the 1990s often was an unpredictable assortment of individuals. Whether comprised of single parents, grandparents, siblings, cousins, neighbors, or friends, this new type of family was the child's social support system.

No matter who comprised this support system, the mission of the nursing service remained the same. Distefano explained: "We want it to be very clear to an orientee that these children do not come in unattached. We want them to understand that it is not just the patient, but the entire family we are caring for at Texas Children's Hospital. We want them to focus on the family and include them in every way that we can."[26]

The reason for this focused attention was clearly defined. "The healthcare team knows what's best for the family from a clinical perspective, but the family can tell us what's best for them from their perspective as individuals and families in a foreign environment," Distefano said. "They see things that we don't see. The more we can do to put them at ease and make them feel comfortable, the better prepared and able they are to learn about their child's illness."[27]

Because the composition of each family differed from patient to patient, the nursing services instituted the use of a Family Data Sheet to provide valuable insights at the time of admission. With this in-depth information about the personal likes and dislikes of the patient and family members, nurses were able to create a personalized family-centered plan of care for each patient. "It's probably too many questions for an initial assessment, but we just want to know every single thing," said Distefano. "We get a great deal of information and feed it into the medical record so that we all know the particulars about each child and family."[28]

This new method of garnering all there was to know about a patient and family was effectively integrated into service, with preceptors teaching the system to new members of the nursing staff. Realizing that each preceptor needed to be a font of information about all new policies, as well as medical and technical breakthroughs, Distefano and Williams devised more continuing education classes and implemented a new component of the preceptor program.

"To assure our preceptors are up-to-date, they have to complete a knowledge assessment annually," Williams explained. "In a 2003 telephone survey of other pediatric hospitals, we were the only one to have measures in place to evaluate and update preceptors' performance."[29]

Destined to enhance the performance of every member of the nursing staff in the early 1990s were the emerging opportunities presented by Distefano's concentrated emphasis on education. Keyed to the philosophy that advanced education was essential to the advancement of nursing, the ever-expanding program continued to flourish throughout the decade. By 1999, there were more than 865 training and development programs offered annually at the learning academy at Texas Children's Hospital.

Offered simultaneously with these ongoing educational programs were comprehensive internship programs. Available to both novice and experienced nurses, internships were designed for nurses who wanted to focus their development in acute care, special care, perioperative, and emergency center settings.

For nursing students, a work-study and scholarship program named Students Transitioning Effectively into Practice (STEP) was offered. STEP provided those who were still in school with an opportunity to work in a clinical setting as patient care assistants while receiving a salary and career guidance. Texas Children's Hospital nurses who wished to further their formal education were given time off to attend school and also had their expenses reimbursed. Other programs included pediatric nurse practitioner scholarships and pediatric oncology nurse practitioner fellowships.

"There are many other hospitals with many more nurses than we have that don't have the educational and developmental support that we have," Williams said. "To assist the nursing staff in attaining, maintaining, and advancing their knowledge and skills, we established top-notch programs. Other hospitals may want to have what we have, but they simply don't have the resources to support it like we do."[30]

With such resources, Distefano continued to mold the infrastructure of the nursing staff by actively nurturing the development of research initiatives. An integrated component of the nursing philosophy, the establishment of ongoing projects in which nurses acted as leaders or collaborators, began to unfold. Although initially few in number, nursing research initiatives flourished during the next decade.

Among the more than 20 nursing research projects at Texas Children's Hospital during the 1990s was the first child-fatigue research study in the United States. Spearheaded by the advanced nursing practice group in the Texas Children's Cancer Center and supported by two grants, the study revealed that nurses could play an active role in decreasing fatigue in children with cancer. Clinical documentation illustrated the beneficial effects of nursing interventions that included adding rest times during the day, decreasing sleep interruptions, and structuring nighttime hours.[31]

Other ongoing nursing research projects at Texas Children's Hospital included studies involving the effectiveness and comfort of one breast-pump brand over another in milk volume maintenance for the mothers of hospitalized preterm infants; physiologic outcomes in children under three years of age who are sedated for an echocardiogram; the prevalence of pressure ulcers and skin breakdown on all inpatients and the risk factors associated with those conditions; pain assessment and management for children; and temperature assessment and fever management for children.[32]

The day-to-day developments and clinical outcomes from nursing research and initiatives at Texas Children's Hospital resulted in better healthcare solutions for children all over the world. As the personification of "Nursing brings life to research and research to life," one of the national slogans for nursing research during the 1990s, these efforts reinforced the growing importance of research as an integral part of Distefano's nursing philosophy.[33]

Also gaining momentum in the early 1990s was Distefano's concept of interdisciplinary care to foster optimal productivity and to improve the quality of patient care continually. "What Susie did was start a patient care coordinating council with representatives from all clinical areas," explained Williams. "She recognized that in order for the patient to get the quality of care needed, everybody who touches or has some contact with that patient has to work together. Instead of it being nursing and all the other disciplines, it has become an integrated and complex collaborative effort."[34]

Other concepts initiated by Distefano included a staff nurse council, clinical nurse council, and unit practice council. Once formed, these councils began to assess, plan, implement, and evaluate practice policies, procedures, and standards of care. Although Distefano initially served as chairman of the councils, she stepped down to give other participants that opportunity.

As staff nurses assumed chairmanship roles in councils and committees, the need to enhance their leadership skills became evident. To assist them in managing meetings, controlling discussions, prioritizing issues, and accomplishing goals, Distefano and Williams arranged for each staff nurse to attend a three-day workshop on facilitative leadership.

"What Susie did was elevate the bedside nurse into decision-making roles," said Williams. "She doesn't step in and resolve issues for them. She supports their resolving those issues themselves and helps them maneuver through the system to get it taken care of effectively. The strength that comes out of knowing that they do have voices, that they do have the ability to affect outcome, makes them better advocates for the patients, families, physicians, and all the other disciplines. The end result is that an empowered nurse is a better nurse and the quality of care that is being delivered is of a higher level."[35]

Because of its ability to deliver this elevated level of patient care, the newly empowered nursing service played a strategic role in helping Texas Children's Hospital receive industry recognition throughout the 1990s and early 2000s. Over a 12-year period, four consecutive awards of accreditation with commendation were received from the Joint Commission on Accreditation of Healthcare Organizations (JCAHO), the nation's preeminent organization for healthcare standards and accreditation.

Instead of resting on these laurels, Distefano viewed successive commendations as both a validation of past accomplishments and a motivation for future achievements. "We are better," she said in 1998. "And part of being better is continuing to look for other opportunities to improve ourselves."[36]

One such opportunity presented itself in 1999 with the announcement of the $345 million four-year expansion project at Texas Children's Hospital. As they had during previous expansions, the nurses intimately familiar with each area of the hospital contributed invaluable input. Once again, the designers of the new surgical suites received seasoned advice from nursing director Doyle, who was to retire in 2001.

Determined to "provide an ideal family environment that feels like home," inpatient nurses assisted not only with the placement of beds and medical equipment in patient rooms, but also with the selection of simulated wood flooring, color schemes, and other design elements. Just as involved in the expansion were the outpatient nurses, who shared their insights during the design of each clinic in the new 16-story Clinical Care Center.

With characteristic attention to detail, the nursing service effectively enhanced its own efforts to deliver quality family-centered care throughout the hospital. The positive impact of the nurses' involvement in hospital design was thought to be immeasurable. However, Distefano and her team of directors—Williams, Dana Nicholson Bledsoe, Margaret Jones, Mary Jo Andre, Jody Ayers, and others—embarked on a plan to prove otherwise.

"We applied to the Magnet Recognition Program directed by the American Nurses Credentialing Center (ANCC), the largest nursing accreditation and credentialing organization in the United States," said Williams. "It required our compiling more than five three-inch volumes of information, because there are more than 94 standards and you have to demonstrate how you meet those standards."[37]

Developed by the ANCC in 1994 and coveted as one of the highest honors in nursing, the Magnet Recognition Program was designed to acknowledge the attainment of nursing excellence by a healthcare organization. Of the more than 6,000 hospitals in the United States, only 67—including just three freestanding children's hospitals—received Magnet recognition by the ANCC in 2003. One of those was Texas Children's Hospital.

"We are one of the few hospitals that did not get any recommendations from our Magnet process," said Williams. "Usually, they tell you what your strengths are and where your opportunities for improvement are. They said we had no opportunities for improvement."[38]

Credit for achieving this accolade was shared equally among the more than 1,000 nurses working in 40 pediatric subspecialties at Texas Children's Hospital. Collectively and individually, these nurses experienced the pride of accomplishment, renewing their commitment to the nursing service's vision, mission, and philosophy.

"The achievement of Magnet designation means that Texas Children's is among the elite hospitals that are considered 'magnets,' attracting a reputation that is among the best in the nation," said Distefano, gratified at being so recognized by the most respected nursing group in the nation.

"Hospitals applying for Magnet status must show that their nursing service consistently provides the highest standards of care," she continued. "Excellence in patient care is our highest goal and we are very excited because this recognition of Texas Children's quality patient care and nursing excellence brings national recognition to our nursing staff, which we know is among the best in the country."[39]

For the future of this nationally recognized service, Distefano had plans. While the service remained focused on providing excellent patient care in a family-centered environment, Distefano also wanted to create an ideal work environment for the nursing staff and to foster nursing research aimed at improving pediatric care. And, as they had in the past, she and her nursing staff encouraged others to enter their demanding, fast-paced, and rewarding profession.

In 2003, with its soaring reputation, the nursing service at Texas Children's Hospital took wing in pursuit of new heights. As an essential part of every patient care team, nurses provided children and their families with the highest quality of care. Highly specialized, the advanced practice nurses concentrated on specific areas such as cancer, cardiology, intensive care, pulmonary, neonatology, and transplants. Nurses skilled in acute care could be found in neurology, surgery, renal, pulmonary, adolescent medicine, cardiology, cancer, transplants, and general pediatric medicine. Operating room nurses worked in the specialized surgical suites, coordinating the care of patients in general surgery, heart surgery, plastic surgery, neurosurgery, otolaryngology, urology, ophthalmology, dental surgery, and orthopedic surgery. And, providing care for the more than 190,000 outpatients who came to Texas Children's Hospital in 2003 were the ambulatory care nurses in the 40 pediatric subspecialty clinics.

Another area of specialization for nurses at Texas Children's Hospital was the care of critically ill and post-surgical patients in the neonatal intensive care unit (NICU), the cardiovascular intensive care unit (CVICU), and the pediatric intensive care unit (PICU). For the acutely or chronically ill patients in the progressive care unit (PCU), nurses took the lead in coordinating care for patients in need of continuous monitoring and observation, giving special emphasis to those with respiratory, neurological, and surgical disorders. Since many of the patients were dependent on technological support, nurses also taught families how to operate the often-complicated equipment and how to care for a chronically ill child.

Other nurses at Texas Children's Hospital concentrated their efforts in nephrology, delivering renal replacement therapies, educating patients and families about disease management, and helping end-stage renal disease patients achieve an optimal level of functioning. With expertise in conservative management, peritoneal dialysis, hemodialysis, continuous renal replacement therapies, pheresis, and renal and extra-renal transplantations, nurses delivered this specialized care to patients in various settings, from the intensive care units of Texas Children's Hospital to the patient's home.

Also delivering care to the homes of patients was an entire team of home-health nurses. These specially trained pediatric nurses were on call 24 hours a day to deliver infusion therapy, phototherapy, apnea monitoring, enteral therapy, total parenteral nutrition, rehabilitative services, and respiratory therapy. Should the patient need to see one of the 150 primary care pediatricians who were part of the Texas Children's Pediatric Associates, there were Texas Children's Hospital nurses in the offices to provide care, patient education, and family support.

Texas Children's Hospital nurses were also an integral part of the staff of pediatric specialists at the Texas Children's Health Centers. Established to deliver the quality care synonymous with Texas Children's Hospital, these neighborhood centers for the diagnosis and treatment of children were located in Clear Lake, Cy-Fair, Sugar Land, The Woodlands, and West Houston.

When the metamorphosis of the Texas Children's Hospital nursing service began in 1987, there were so few nurses that they all knew each other's name. As the evolution continued in 2004, the more than 1,000 nurses at Texas Children's Hospital may not have known each other's names, but they did know that every one of them shared a common identity. Each nurse at Texas Children's Hospital was recognized as a consistent deliverer of quality care.

This recognition came not only in the coveted Magnet designation, but also—and more importantly—in the expressions of gratitude and praise from the patients and families who received quality care at Texas Children's Hospital.

From her first day on the job, progressive care unit nurse and former patient Jaimee Kheir-Westfall immediately felt comfortable at Texas Children's Hospital.

Kheir-Westfall was familiar with both her physical surroundings and the demands of her profession. Caring for that unit's acutely or chronically ill patients who required continuous monitoring and observation, she responded with care and compassion to their needs and wants.

Although she had never been a patient in that particular unit, Kheir-Westfall instinctively knew how to bond with each of the children and families in her care. Drawing from her extensive memory bank, she often used her own experiences as a patient to comfort others. "I know this is going to be painful," she said to patients before administering an IV. "I know because I have had many of them, but I am going to try and make this as painless as possible."[40]

To convince those in her care who remained unsure of her good intentions, Kheir-Westfall willingly showed them the tiny IV scars on her arms and wrists. Always reassuring and compassionate, she explained the necessity of the medication and stressed its beneficial effects.

"I am very attentive to pain and empathize with patients who get bored and lonely," she said. "I can relate to what the patients are going through."[41]

Kheir-Westfall also knew from experience the important role that a family can play in the care of the patient, both in and out of the hospital. The loving care she had received from her mother—who was taught the necessary home-care techniques at Texas Children's Hospital and who later became a nurse herself—was an inspiration to her. It was a memory that directly influenced her dedication to teaching parents how to use the complex devices and administer the treatments needed at home.

One night, the ability to apply her experience as a child to the knowledge and skills she now needed every day took on a new dimension. Arriving early to work for the night shift, Kheir-Westfall met the progressive care unit's clinical nurse specialist, who worked the day shift. It was her role model from childhood, Barbara Montagnino, the former urology service nurse.

"I was so surprised to see her," recalled Montagnino. "It had been ten years and I had no idea she was working in the unit. Since she not only had changed her name to Jaimee, but also gotten married, I had not recognized either her first name or her hyphenated last name when I read it on the work charts for months."[42]

Equally astonished was Kheir-Westfall. Having already seen Dr. Gonzales several times since she returned, she knew that Montagnino no longer worked with him and assumed that she had left Texas Children's Hospital. She soon learned that her assumption was only partially correct. "After 18 years in the urology service, I did leave to work in the private sector," Montagnino explained. "When I returned to Texas Children's Hospital, I joined the progressive care unit."

Following their impromptu reunion that night, both took great pride in sharing their story with fellow nurses, families, and patients. "When I enter a room in which Jaimee is with a patient, she will introduce me as her former nurse at Texas Children's Hospital," Montagnino explained. "She serves as a good example to chronically ill children, giving them hope that they will grow up to live normal lives and achieve their dreams like she did."

Kheir-Westfall knew that she might inspire other patients at Texas Children's Hospital to follow in her footsteps and enter the healthcare field. She often asked her patients if they knew what they wanted to be when they grew up. Several, to her delight, indicated a desire to do exactly as she had and become a nurse.

"The best part of nursing is mentoring," said Montagnino "It is so rewarding to know I had a part in restoring Jaimee to good health and also had an impact on her career choice. I was excited to learn she had not only chosen nursing, but chosen to work in the progressive care unit, a unit that offers a variety of clinical experiences for pediatric nurses."[43]

One such experience Kheir-Westfall had not expected was that of working side-by-side with her role model. An opportunity born of happenstance, it was one she embraced with respect. "I looked up to Barbara then," she said. "And I look up to her now on a personal and professional level."

With this continuum in place, Jaimee Kheir-Westfall realized that her dream of becoming a nurse at Texas Children's Hospital had been more than fulfilled. It had been embellished in a way that even she could never have imagined as a child.

25

❦ PULMONARY MEDICINE ❦

W HEN JOHN ROWLAND WAS A CHILD, he was full of mischief.

With a bucket of water perched precariously over the closed door, he would lie in bed waiting for the nurses to enter his booby-trapped room at Texas Children's Hospital.

At other times, he filled syringes with water, ready to give the nurses a shot in return for all the ones he was receiving. Although greeted with good humor by his victims, these particular pranks ended "a long time ago," he said, unable to remember exactly when the truce had occurred.

Also forgotten was an exact count of the number of times Rowland was admitted to Texas Children's Hospital during his childhood. "In a good year, I was there once. In a bad year, three or four times," he said.[1]

What Rowland does vividly recall is the first time he was a patient at Texas Children's Hospital. It was during the Christmas holidays in the early 1970s, when he was seven years old. During his stay, he was presented with an unexpected gift from the Women's Auxiliary to Texas Children's Hospital.

It was a toy Evel Knievel stunt cycle, a miniature version of that colorful daredevil's motorcycle. Although it was the most highly prized toy of the time, Rowland had never even seen one before. Unlike other boys his age, he had not mimicked Knievel's famous death-defying exploits by jumping multiple trashcans on his Schwinn bike in the backyard after school. Instead of playing outside or attending school on a regular basis, he had been inside, performing his own death-defying deeds—those of undergoing daily treatments for cystic fibrosis (CF).

Diagnosed with the disease when he was five years old, Rowland was not expected to live past the age of 12—the median age of all children with CF in the early 1970s.

Although this was a dire prognosis, there was room for optimism nonetheless. By the 1970s, there had been dramatic changes in the treatment and care of children diagnosed with this inherited abnormality capable of destroying the lungs and causing serious impairment of the pancreas, intestines and liver. Two decades earlier, CF had routinely killed children in infancy. However, with medical and clinical advances in the treatment of CF, life spans had begun to increase. At Texas Children's Hospital, the medical professionals were able not only to delay the inevitable outcome, but also to improve the quality of a CF patient's prolonged life.

"They tried to encourage us to do everything," said Rowland. "But a lot of the publications used to say that we had a life span of 12 years old. You know, you look at that, but you can't let that stuff get you down. We'd always all brag, 'We're going to live until we're 50 and all that kind of stuff.' The good thing about the CFs in here, is they encouraged us. They never slowed us down in the least."

Inspired by the encouragement he received at Texas Children's Hospital, Rowland began to believe that he could do just about anything he wanted. He played sports. He went to school whenever he was able. And he learned to enjoy life, taking one day at a time and always remembering that his health was the most important thing.

"Your health dictates how you've got to take care of yourself, or you end up in the hospital all the time," he explained.

Taking care of himself meant a daily routine of multiple antibiotic, enzyme, and vitamin pills; following a prescribed diet; and undergoing various pulmonary therapy treatments at home.

Prescribed by pediatric pulmonologist Dr. Gunyon M. Harrison, the first director of the Cystic Fibrosis Care Center at Baylor College of Medicine and Rowland's physician at Texas Children's Hospital, the treatments were mandatory.

"Dr. Harrison is why I look so good," Rowland said. "He always motivated me to do everything, while everybody else just was real friendly about it and real nice. Harrison's friendly, but it's more of a kind of big brother kind of a way. He's a good doctor and really good with kids. He really knows his stuff and what you're supposed to do. And he yells at you really well if you don't do what he says. He really puts you in line. That's why my parents sent me to him."

With scheduled appointments at the Cystic Fibrosis Care Center, Rowland saw Harrison on a regular basis, whether he was feeling good or bad. But whenever his health seriously deteriorated, he knew that he had to go to Texas Children's Hospital to feel better. This is not to say that he liked undergoing rigorous physical therapy treatments four times a day as a patient at the hospital. In fact, he hated it. Although at first he did not understand why such torturous therapy was necessary, Rowland quickly found the answer: "Once you started breathing easier, you knew why."

Having the disease has been a constant learning process for Rowland. When diagnosed, he learned that CF was characterized by the production of unusually thick and sticky mucus that obstructs the airways of the lungs, the bronchial tubes, and bronchioles. If Rowland was unable to clear the mucus from his respiratory system, bacteria grew and multiplied, causing the airways to become infected and inflamed. He quickly became aware that such life-threatening lung infections caused serious breathing difficulties requiring aggressive treatment in the hospital.

Therefore, each time he had to be admitted for the minimum ten-day stay—as dictated by Harrison—on the CF wing of Texas Children's Hospital, Rowland understood the seriousness of his situation and he knew what to expect. Treatments consisting of strong antibiotics, given both intravenously and orally, as well as strict and vigorous physical therapy procedures, chest percussion, aerosol breathing treatments, and mucus drainage, were standard procedures.

Rowland also knew to expect abundant amounts of food from the Texas Children's Hospital dietitian. The high-fat, high-energy diet was necessary to address his omnipresent digestive problems, caused by thick secretions in the pancreas that hindered the delivery of enzymes to the intestinal track. Supplemented by vitamin pills and enzymes, the prescribed diet also included snacks.

"Eating is a job for me," Rowland explained. "I usually only eat huge meals, consisting of at least 1800 calories and over. But we have some dietitians at Texas Children's who are really good and they send you snacks all day long. You end up with 50 million snacks in the room. They're really good! I don't eat snacks during the day, so I ate them along with my meals."

He also relished the fact that he could tell whenever Harrison was nearby. This was because of Harrison's voice, which Rowland said he "can hear all down the hospital, when he comes in on the floor and when he leaves."

It was an advantage that he no doubt utilized whenever he needed to dismantle a water bucket poised for action over the door to his room.

The catalyst for the development of the pediatric pulmonary medicine service at Texas Children's Hospital was a piece of paper.

Tacked onto a bulletin board at Duke University School of Medicine in 1952, the printed flyer caught the eye of first-year pediatric resident Dr. Gunyon M. Harrison.

Years later, Harrison recalled that the flyer said: "If you want to learn how to be involved with the management of acute poliomyelitis and its multiple complications and early rehabilitation in a one-week program, the National Foundation for Infantile Paralysis will pay your way in transportation and board you and feed you."[2]

Harrison found the offer intriguing. While the number of acute poliomyelitis cases in the United States had escalated to more than 24,000 in the 1940s, most physicians knew little about that "mystery disease" with the unknown cause.

Seemingly unstoppable, the disease generated great fear among Americans in the early 1950s. Those afflicted might develop paralysis of a single joint or become completely immobile, with death occurring when the muscles for breathing and swallowing become paralyzed. To many Americans, there was only one thing worse than dying of paralytic poliomyelitis—and that was contracting the disease and living.[3]

As a pediatric resident, Harrison was keenly aware of these fears—especially among the parents of his patients. He yearned to know how he could keep polio patients alive. Interested in diseases of the lung, Harrison was eager to learn all he could about mechanical ventilation. Of particular interest was the successful use of a negative pressure ventilator, a tank respirator commonly known as the "iron lung," on paralyzed patients.

Only one thing made Harrison hesitate. "To sign up for the program, your institution had to agree to release you in case of an emergency epidemic for a period of not less than four weeks and not more than eight weeks," he recalled.[4]

It was a stipulation worth heeding. The outbreak of an emergency epidemic during the summer months was a virtual certainty in the early 1950s. Knowing this, Harrison hesitantly approached the dean of the Duke University School of Medicine. To his surprise, after requesting not only to attend, but also to be released for duty during an epidemic, Harrison received permission. "We can get along without you for four to eight weeks," the dean said. "You ought to go to that program. Somebody in this organization ought to go to that program."[5]

For Harrison, the seized opportunity was one that he never forgot. As a participant in the weeklong training program, held at the University of

Pittsburgh School of Medicine in April 1952, he studied with the recognized experts in poliomyelitis. Among them was Dr. Jesse Wright, who later introduced the rocking bed to help polio patients breathe at night. Harrison learned about the treatment advances made and the extensive equipment needed to rehabilitate polio patients. He also received an extraordinary glimpse into the future by attending a virology lecture given by Dr. Jonas Salk, who told his audience that he was working on a vaccine to eradicate polio.

"I returned to Duke and, on July 3, 1952, I got a telegram that I was to report to the Southwestern Poliomyelitis Respiratory Center at Jefferson Davis Hospital in Houston, Texas, on July 5," Harrison said. "So, all day July 4, I wrote transfer notes on all the patients I was taking care of at Duke. Then I got on a plane at 9 o'clock at night and got to Jefferson Davis at 6 o'clock the next morning. And that's how I got involved in polio."[6]

Arriving in Houston during the aftermath of a polio epidemic, Harrison immediately set to work. With more than 25 seriously ill patients using iron lungs in the new facility—one of the first polio centers in the United States—the staff of the The Southwestern Poliomyelitis Respiratory Center was inundated.

Funded by a grant from the National Foundation for Infantile Paralysis to Baylor College of Medicine, the Southwestern Poliomyelitis Respiratory Center at Jefferson Davis Hospital opened in 1950. Under the direction of Dr. William A. Spencer and the supervision of Dr. Russell J. Blattner, head of the pediatrics department at Baylor College of Medicine, the regional center was responsible for the care of all seriously ill polio patients in Texas, Arkansas, and Oklahoma. As the number of patients continued to grow, the Southwestern Poliomyelitis Respiratory Center eventually became the second-largest polio center in the United States.

With so many patients who needed care, Harrison extended his stay. He remained at the polio center for more than eight weeks, returning to Duke in September 1952 to complete his second year of pediatric residency and to reformulate his plans.

"I got so involved in polio and the ramifications of polio, the respiratory complications secondary to their acute polio. I was so interested in ventilation, in taking care of people who had respiratory involvement, which was totally new at that time. People who had respiratory involvement just died at that day and time. Polio patients were the only patients who were put in a tank respirator. So, I decided I would come back and take my third year of residency here," Harrison said, explaining how he came to complete his residency at Baylor College of Medicine.[7]

This career-changing decision was also influenced by the announced construction of Texas Children's Hospital, scheduled for completion in 1954. "I was interested in seeing how a hospital specifically for children would work," he recalled.

It was a curiosity satisfied not only firsthand, but also continuously for the next four decades. From the beginning, Harrison became an integral part of the history of Texas Children's Hospital. As the resident on duty the day that Texas Children's Hospital opened in 1954, he admitted the hospital's first patient, three-year-old Lamaina Leigh Van Wagner.

During his residency, Harrison rotated between the various facilities affiliated with Baylor College of Medicine. He continued to pursue his interests—not only in polio, but also in diseases of the lung. After reading an article in the December 1953 issue of *Pediatrics* magazine about a newly devised method by which New York researchers were diagnosing cystic fibrosis, Harrison made a decision. The article, which stated that the sweat of children with CF contained markedly increased levels of chloride, inspired him to try the "sweat test." When presented with an undiagnosed child with CF symptoms, Harrison did just that.[8]

The primary diagnostic test of the time involved an invasive procedure to the gastrointestinal tract, but Harrison opted to experiment with the new test. To his amazement, his own unconventional and unscientific version produced the same convincing results. His experiment involved a little girl, his car, and a typical hot day in Houston. "I took her out and I sat her in my Dodge car in the parking lot, rolled up the damned windows, and she sweated and I sweated. So, I scraped sweat off of her back and put it in a test tube and came back in and got the laboratory to run it and, lo and behold, this girl's got CF."[9]

Harrison's knowledge about diagnosing and treating CF greatly increased after he was named chief resident of Texas Children's Hospital in late 1954. He participated in an exchange program instigated by physician-in-chief Blattner, whereby the chief residents of Texas Children's Hospital and Children's Hospital Boston swapped places for six weeks. During the exchange, Harrison seized the opportunity to work with Dr. Harry Schwachman, whose pioneering work with CF patients was becoming legendary.

"When they asked me what I wanted to do at Children's Hospital Boston, I told them: 'I am interested in lung disease in children. I think we can treat a lot of lung disease differently than we have been doing,'" Harrison recalled. "And they said, 'You may be interested in working with Dr. Schwachman. He has all those CF patients who have lung disease.' So, I spent six weeks with him and that's when I got really interested in CF."[10]

It was an interest fueled by observing and learning about Schwachman's innovative approach to the treatment and care of those afflicted with the disease. Harrison also appreciated Schwachman's total care for the patient as an individual. "Schwachman was the first person who ever really made an effort to do preventative, prophylactic medicine in CF," said Harrison. "He started individuals, as best he could, on a good nutritional program by selecting the type of foods they should have, by getting pancreatic extracts on an every-meal basis. He also treated their infections with antibiotics very, very aggressively."[11]

Returning to Texas Children's Hospital and to his primary interest in polio, Harrison completed his chief residency and began a two-year pulmonary function fellowship with the National Foundation for Infantile Paralysis. He trained for three months at the Cardiovascular Respiratory Pulmonary Institute in San Francisco, for three months at Rancho Los Amigos in Los Angeles, and for the remaining 18 months at the Southwestern Poliomyelitis Respiratory Center in Houston. At the completion of his fellowship in 1956, Harrison joined Baylor College of Medicine as an instructor in polio, dividing his clinical duties between the Southwestern Poliomyelitis Respiratory Center and Texas Children's Hospital.

It was during this early stage in his career that Harrison had an epiphany: "If you could ventilate the polio patient with respiratory muscle paralysis, you ought to be able to ventilate any patient with respiratory muscle paralysis."

At the time, the iron lung was the only way of ventilating patients. The device was used exclusively with patients at the Southwestern Poliomyelitis Respiratory Center, leading Harrison to test his theory there. With Spencer's permission, he admitted a Guillain-Barré patient who had breathing problems, "put him in the tank respirator, and he did fine. It was a totally radical approach. I don't know that other people with Guillain-Barré had not ventilated at that time, but I do know he was the first one in Houston."[12]

Inspired by his success with that patient, Harrison was eager to test this unconventional theory on others. With the introduction of the Salk vaccine in 1955 and the subsequent paucity of polio patients admitted thereafter, in 1956 Harrison approached physician-in-chief Blattner with another revolutionary idea. He wanted to start a cystic fibrosis clinic that would offer aggressive respiratory treatments, similar to those given every day to polio patients with chronic lung disease. The idea had first occurred to him when he was working with Schwachman at Children's Hospital Boston.

"I kept telling Harry these CF kids need some kind of aerosol therapy to loosen that secretion," he said. "They need to be beat on. We do this on polio kids all the time because they can't breathe, and they have thick secretions because they can't cough good, and we pulled an amazing number of them through. He hadn't thought about that."

Harrison's innovative plan received the approval of a somewhat doubtful Blattner, who questioned the productiveness of such a program for a terminal disease. This skepticism was not surprising. Previously, doctors had given no hope to children diagnosed with CF in Houston. They told parents to take their children home and love them, because they were going to die within the next three or four years. Harrison, however, refused to accept the premise of CF patients not getting well enough to survive for longer.

"At that time, you didn't have any way of really reversing an illness that was going to lead to death, like respiratory failure," explained Harrison. "Of course, if the CF child were acutely ill, he was placed in the emergency room or the hospital. But my inclination was that the patient needed to be treated every day, and his family needed to know what this disease really is, and why they are to give him that medication. If they know that, and if they know when to bring him to the emergency room, if they know those three things well, that patient can be well cared for. If you treat them aggressively, you can probably turn them around. But parents have to understand what this disease is."[13]

To Harrison, the fact that Blattner had agreed to his unique plan was not out of character. Rather, the decision was entirely consistent with Harrison's impression of the physician-in-chief, whom he compared favorably to General Dwight D. Eisenhower during World War II. Reasoned Harrison: "When he found somebody that wanted to be a general and who was a good general, he let them run with the ball. He never put any restrictions on him. Every now and then he would say, 'Guy, what are you all doing in pulmonary these days?'"[14]

What Harrison was doing in late 1956 was diagnosing and treating 12 CF patients. Ranging in age from two to ten years, the children came to the newly opened cystic fibrosis clinic in the Junior League Diagnostic Clinic of the outpatient department at Texas Children's Hospital. Local press coverage noted the CF clinic's significance as the first such facility in Houston and also cited a universal fact: "What is actually known about the disease is not likely to fill many pages in a medical textbook."[15]

Undaunted by the lack of published procedures for CF treatment, Harrison instigated his own. In doing so, he drew upon his experiences with polio patients as well as with CF patients at Children's Hospital Boston. Inspired by Schwachman's prophylactic treatment program, Harrison emphasized early diagnosis, aggressive medication, and proper diet. In addition, he introduced the aerosol therapy and chest physical therapy procedures for the respiratory care that he championed with polio patients. He also began monthly injections of gamma globulin to build up the children's general immunity to other infections. In an effort to educate CF patients and their families, Harrison wrote, published, and distributed a small booklet that explained CF and its daily treatment. Working closely with the pediatric cardiologists at Texas Children's Hospital, he began special heart studies and periodic electrocardiograms for CF patients "because the disease obviously produces an undue, backward strain on the heart itself."[16]

Within a year, Harrison's efforts to improve and lengthen the lives of CF patients received recognition from an unlikely source. It came from the once-skeptical Blattner, who stated in 1957: "Special studies of patients with this disease are being done at Texas Children's Hospital. Diagnosis can be made with the newly developed sweat test and optimal methods of treatment can be recommended. By the use of antibiotics, proper diet, and substitution therapy, a child who has been malnourished and chronically ill can be transferred into a reasonably healthy child."[17]

Such pioneering efforts at Texas Children's Hospital also caught the attention of the newly formed national Cystic Fibrosis Foundation (CFF), which was beginning to create regional centers similar to Schwachman's at Children's Hospital Boston. Designating Baylor College of Medicine as the first recipient of a CFF grant for a cystic fibrosis center in 1960, the foundation selected Harrison as the center's medical director. This designation also marked the official beginning of the chest section at Texas Children's Hospital. Harrison's one-person service dedicated to the diagnosis and management of children with CF finally had an official name.

In 1961, the Cystic Fibrosis Care Center opened at the Texas Institute of Rehabilitation and Research (TIRR), a Baylor College of Medicine-affiliated facility established by Spencer in 1959. The center provided comprehensive care to CF patients and also helped their families treat and manage the disease appropriately. Three specific functions were assigned to the Cystic Fibrosis Care Center by the CFF grant: to gain in-depth information about the course of the disease by following a large population of patients; to develop techniques of clinical management to extend life spans and treat life-threatening problems; and to attract researchers to engage in studies that would increase knowledge of the disease.[18]

The similarity of the CFF mission to that of the National Foundation for Infantile Paralysis (NFIP) was not a coincidence. In fact, it had been one of the recommendations from Harrison, who also masterminded the CFF's hiring of the former medical director at the NIPF. Responsible for setting up and maintaining polio centers throughout the United States in the 1950s, the new CFF medical director shared Harrison's vision. Therefore, with the opening of Houston's cystic fibrosis center and ten other CFF centers across the country in 1961, what was once only a local idea had come to fruition nationally.

Just as polio patients and their families benefited from proven methods to ensure the successful management and treatment of a chronic disease, so too did the patients at Houston's Cystic Fibrosis Care Center. Using the team approach, Harrison involved professionals from many disciplines to support the patients by assessing their individual physical, psychological, and social functioning. With staff physicians, fellows, residents, interns, nurses, physical therapists, respiratory care practitioners, dieticians, and social workers, the multidisciplinary support provided a continuity of individualized care based on each patient's needs.

With the introduction of a comprehensive and ongoing educational program, the staff of the Cystic Fibrosis Care Center excelled. The team emphasized that knowledge of one's self, the disease, and therapy eased the patient's dependence on day-to-day assistance from the center. Encouraging autonomy as an achievable goal, members of the team taught families how to administer oxygen or respiratory therapy treatments at home. "We already had developed a great training program for the polio families who were going home in the tank respirator, and that's why it went so well," remembered Harrison. "Now, I think about all this to-do about home healthcare and laugh. We did home healthcare in 1952!"[19]

The success of both the home healthcare program and the Cystic Fibrosis Care Center was evident. By 1966, there were more than 200 patients, including outpatients treated at Texas Children's Hospital, the Cystic Fibrosis Care Center, and an inpatient program at Texas Children's Hospital and other Baylor College of Medicine-affiliated hospitals. Noting the substantial decrease in the percentage of deaths attributed to CF, Harrison confidently stated in 1962: "Rather than being considered terminal, 100 percent fatal, cystic fibrosis has been changed with early diagnosis and proper, individual treatment. It is now a disease that varies from chronic disability to normal activity."[20]

In an effort to train other physicians in the management of CF, Harrison introduced a fellowship program in the early 1960s. The yearlong program eventually grew to three years, becoming one of the largest fellowship training programs for pediatric pulmonary medicine in the United States.

While teaching medical students, interns, residents, fellows, and the attending physicians at Texas Children's Hospital, Harrison emphasized the importance of understanding the basic abnormality of CF, the significance of early diagnosis, and the aggressive treatment of the disease. Indicating the possibility of multiple medical complications, he stressed the need to manage the high incidence of severe pulmonary problems.

As the singular resident expert on assisted ventilation—including negative-pressure tanks, as well as the new positive-pressure endotracheal technique introduced in the 1960s—Harrison was in much demand. He became the one-person pulmonary service at all Baylor College of Medicine-affiliated hospital facilities.

Proving his theory that "what had been learned in the treatment of respiratory problems in polio and CF patients was applicable to other patients," Harrison increasingly worked with other departments at Texas Children's Hospital. When asked to see patients who had developed life-threatening or long-term pulmonary problems, he always accepted the challenge. Whether it was in cardiac surgery, cardiology, infectious diseases, allergy, neurology, neurosurgery, or orthopedics, he was there whenever he was called upon. So too were members of his Cystic Fibrosis Care Center team, "who began working with other patients who had pulmonary physiological problems which were quite similar even though the causes of their problems were quite different."[21]

Subsequently, the center at TIRR became known as the Cystic Fibrosis and Related Pulmonary Disease Center. Although pediatric pulmonology did not become formally recognized as a subspecialty until 1986, in the late 1960s Harrison established himself as one of the first pediatric pulmonologists in the United States. With the diverse patient load of the chest section at Texas Children's Hospital, he also established one of the first pediatric pulmonary medical services in existence at the time. Recalling his unique status, Harrison explained that "before 1970, if you went to any other medical school and met with the chairman of the department of pediatrics and he said, 'What do you do?' and you said, 'I'm a pedi pulmonologist,' he would say, 'What is that?'"[22]

What it was at Texas Children's Hospital in 1970 was clearly due to Harrison. Rather than being narrowly focused, pediatric pulmonology was a broad subspecialty that encompassed any type of pediatric lung problem. Harrison's involvement included everything from critical care to allergy infections, from polio and CF to asthma, from bronchial pulmonary dysplasia to accidental aspirations, and from heart transplants to simple surgeries. The fact that he never said "no" when asked for assistance by other physicians continued to broaden the scope of his self-defined subspecialty of pediatric pulmonary medical care at Texas Children's Hospital.

Harrison also epitomized the role of a dedicated physician, taking responsibility not only for extending the lives of his patients, but also for improving their quality of life. Concerned that CF patients were being denied the fun of a summer camp because of their frequent therapy or the severity of their disease, he devised a solution. Harrison helped organize the Children's Summer Respiratory Camp Foundation to plan and manage the first CF camp in the United States.

Providing a traditional camping experience that also met the medical needs of CF patients, Harrison's camp began in the summer of 1969. Offering CF patients and their families a fun-filled experience and a much-needed respite from their rigid home care and clinic schedule, the camp continued annually for more than two decades. Throughout its existence, it attracted a wide range of volunteers. Nurses, respiratory therapists, and pulmonary function personnel donated their time and services—as did staff physicians and pediatric residents from Texas Children's Hospital and students from Baylor College of Medicine.

One such medical student was Dr. Dan K. Seilheimer, whose chance participation in Harrison's camp later proved integral to the development of the pediatric pulmonary medicine service at Texas Children's Hospital. "Dr. Harrison had asked the dean of students about whether a student could help set up a summer camp for children with CF, so I took that job," he recalled. "Helping to establish the CF camp, I saw all the other things that Dr. Harrison did as well. My primary interest was in CF at that time, but I became interested in pulmonary medicine through CF."[23]

It turned out to be a summer job that determined Seilheimer's future career. After graduating from Baylor College of Medicine, he served his pediatric internship and residency at St. Louis Children's Hospital, Washington University School of Medicine in St. Louis, Missouri. Seilheimer then accepted a two-year postdoctoral clinical fellowship in pediatric pulmonary disease with Harrison at Baylor College of Medicine, sponsored by the CF Foundation. After that fellowship, he studied pulmonary physiology for one year at the Cardiovascular Research Institute at the University of California. He then returned to Baylor College of Medicine in 1977 as an assistant professor in the department of pediatrics and rehabilitation. Named director of the newly established pediatric pulmonary function laboratory and assistant director of the respiratory therapy department at Texas Children's Hospital, Seilheimer became Harrison's first full-time staff member in the chest service.

Seilheimer's arrival at Texas Children's Hospital was heralded by Harrison, who enthusiastically announced his new staff member's involvement in the development of a much-needed pulmonary physiology department. Under the direction of Seilheimer, the pulmonary function laboratory was to be "specially geared to obtaining studies for physiological data on infants and children."[24]

While anticipating the extensive and expansive research projects yet to come, Harrison also paid tribute to the clinical research endeavors of the past. Having directed his efforts towards finding more effective ways of treating patients with acute life-threatening diseases, he reported significant results in 1978. Directly attributed to Texas Children's Hospital was an increase in the average survival age for a CF patient, which had escalated from an average of five years to 18 years.

"This improvement in survival is not only due to the care they receive at Texas Children's Hospital, but also due to the training received by medical students and pediatric residents here," Harrison said. "Once they leave Texas Children's Hospital, these physicians are able to diagnose and institute therapy early in the disease so that permanent lung damage from infection may be minimized. Early treatment and aggressive therapy improve the quality of life and increase longevity."[25]

One of those highly trained doctors who left Texas Children's Hospital to go into private practice was Seilheimer. His departure in 1980 found Harrison, once again, as the only full-time staff member of the chest service, a statistic that remained unchanged for the following four years.

Dramatic changes occurred in 1984, when a Cystic Fibrosis Foundation grant established the Cystic Fibrosis Research Center at Texas Children's Hospital and Baylor College of Medicine. Pioneered by Texas Children's Hospital physician-in-chief Dr. Ralph D. Feigin, the grant presented a three-pronged challenge. The objectives were to localize and isolate the gene responsible for the genetic defect; to develop a simple and reproducible test that can be used to detect carriers of the defective gene; and to study the expression or consequence of the disease in peripheral blood leukocytes.[26]

With the creation of the Cystic Fibrosis Research Center at Texas Children's Hospital, the necessity of moving the Cystic Fibrosis Care Center's physical location from TIRR to Texas Children's Hospital became evident. This centralization of all services for CF patients also marked the end of the chest service, as it existed, and the beginning of the newly named pulmonary medicine service at Texas Children's Hospital.

To make way for the new, Harrison stepped down from the leadership position he had held for more than three decades. Dedicating himself to CF patients, he relinquished his other responsibilities to a new chief of service who also was an old friend—Seilheimer.

Recruited back by Feigin, Seilheimer left private practice in 1985 to become not only chief of the pulmonary medicine service and medical director of the Cystic Fibrosis Care Center at Texas Children's Hospital, but also professor of pediatrics and head of the pediatric pulmonology section at Baylor College of Medicine. "I was recruited to really organize the Texas Children's program," Seilheimer said. "There was no physical presence of pulmonary medicine at Texas Children's at that time because Harrison had been headquartered at the Cystic Fibrosis Care Center at TIRR. There was no room at that time for bronchial rehab service, so we rented office space off campus. We were located physically off campus until the Feigin Center was built in 1991."[27]

During the late 1980s, the pulmonary medicine service at Texas Children's Hospital began providing care for a wide range of respiratory disorders in addition to cystic fibrosis. The quickly growing full-time staff began seeing patients with acute, chronic, or recurring upper or lower respiratory infections; congenital malformations of the respiratory system; acute or chronic lung injury; and breathing disorders. Children with pulmonary complications from immunodeficiency, chemotherapy, or congenital heart disease and those with acute life-threatening episodes also received treatment from the service.

With a special interest in the technology-dependent child, the service began assisting patients and families with the home management of patients requiring ventilation, tracheotomy, oxygen, or apnea/bradycardia monitoring. Helping to establish the Texas Children's Asthma Center in 1993, Seilheimer joined forces with a multidisciplinary team of Texas Children's Hospital physicians to address the treatment, care, prevention, and research of asthma. "Traditionally, asthma treatment has been crisis oriented," Seilheimer explained. "There was often no management of the disease until the child had a breathing crisis requiring emergency care. We can teach both community physicians and patients to manage it and we can usually prevent serious or life-threatening episodes."[28]

While assembling a full-time staff for the pulmonary medicine service staff—including faculty physicians, postdoctoral fellows, nurse practitioners, nurses, administrative staff, and respiratory therapists—Seilheimer was also concentrating on clinical research at Texas Children's Hospital. At the same time, as medical director of the Cystic Fibrosis Care Center and the

Cystic Fibrosis Research Center at Texas Children's Hospital, he capitalized on the newly emphasized research activities supported by the 1984 grant. "The CF Care Center and the CF Research Center provide patients with the unique opportunity to help themselves and others by participating in research," Seilheimer announced in 1985. "As current treatment modalities and research trends and findings are available, CF patients at the center are the primary beneficiaries."[29]

One such finding occurred immediately. In 1985, Dr. Arthur L. Beaudet, professor of pediatrics and cell biology and head of the section of genetics in the department of pediatrics at Baylor College of Medicine, was one of the scientists who pinpointed the location of the CF gene to chromosome seven. In 1989, the newsworthy isolation of the gene itself caused medical experts everywhere to predict that the ultimate and imminent cure for CF was gene therapy. It was a prediction that Beaudet prudently shared, saying: "I think the message is that there is good reason to be optimistic, but we also need to be cautious. It may take longer than we think to find a cure. It's not a simple problem."[30]

After isolating the gene came the challenge of identifying the protein that is abnormal in CF patients. Learning more about the disease, researchers at Baylor College of Medicine and Texas Children's Hospital began work on innovative approaches to the diagnosis, management, and treatment of CF. One research project involved Beaudet's successful use of amniocentesis to test the cells of an unborn child for the disease. "Texas Children's Hospital was the first treatment center in the United States capable of performing prenatal diagnosis of CF," Seilheimer said.

Advances in genetics inspired an array of innovative therapeutic approaches to the treatment of patients with CF, including the introduction of new antibiotics to fight chronic infections. Clinical trials for Pulmozyme, the first new aerosol enzyme treatment in more than 20 years, were introduced at Texas Children's Hospital in 1989. After Pulmozyme received FDA approval in 1994, the astonishing development of more than 20 other antibiotics unfolded over the next decade. Among those developed and clinically tested at the Cystic Fibrosis Care Center at Texas Children's Hospital were TOBI, Meropenem, and Chloramphenicol.

"Beaudet's research efforts brought our CF Care Center into the national spotlight," Seilheimer explained. "We began interacting more with other major CF research programs with collaborative studies. Our CF Care Center has been very involved in doing clinical research to show whether new treatments are clinically effective in patients. It has improved the care of children with cystic fibrosis not just here, but everywhere."[31]

These constantly evolving medical strategies for the care and treatment of CF involved not only new drugs, but also old drugs used in new ways. As the beneficiaries of these medical breakthroughs, CF patients began living longer and fuller lives. The Cystic Fibrosis Care Center at Texas Children's Hospital expanded constantly and soon required two medical directors. After naming Dr. Peter W. Hiatt as medical director in 1996, Seilheimer continued to serve as codirector.

The Cystic Fibrosis Care Center at Texas Children's Hospital eventually grew to become one of the largest such centers in the United States. By 2000, the staff consisted of multiple faculty physicians, postdoctoral fellows, clinical researchers and technicians, nurse practitioners, nurses, respiratory therapists, social workers, and a dietitian, pharmacist, physical therapist, and chaplain.

Also growing was the educational program at the Cystic Fibrosis Care Center at Texas Children's Hospital. To address the multiple problems faced by CF patients and their families, particularly the daily management of the disease at home, Seilheimer began developing an extensive educational program in 1988. Creating a partnership between the department of pediatrics at Baylor College of Medicine and the department of educational resources at Texas Children's Hospital, he instigated the Family Education Project.

Supported by a grant from the Division of Lung Diseases within the National Heart, Lung, and Blood Institute of the National Institutes of Health, and with additional support from the Foundation for the Institute of Research and Rehabilitation, the Family Education Project focused on the practical skills needed to manage CF care.

The easy-to-read program was organized into four subject areas with separate booklets for children and adults. The information provided was helpful not only to the recently diagnosed patients and families, but also to those who were familiar with CF. Dedicated to helping CF families learn everything they needed to know about the disease, the program was all-encompassing. Non-medical information was included, along with a vast array of medical management tasks, such as respiratory therapy, chest physical therapy, and medications. Other booklets covered such diverse areas as "Eating for Energy," "The Amazing Body," and "A Day of Choices."

"The project staff hopes that through this comprehensive educational program, families and children can benefit by extending the life of their child through available therapies and, in turn, achieve a better quality of life," Seilheimer stated in 1988.[32]

Enthusiastically received by both families and physicians, the Family Education Project became an ongoing endeavor. Awarded with the Program Excellence Award by the Society for Public Health Education in 1994, the project also earned Seilheimer the Lay Education Award from the American Academy of Pediatrics in 1996.

Harrison was not surprised that the efforts to educate CF patients and their families at Texas Children's Hospital had become more advanced. From the small pamphlet he had written and published in the 1950s, the education program had evolved into Seilheimer's grant-supported, award-winning, multi-booklet project. "As time goes on and you learn more facts, you begin to put it all together," said Harrison. "If you're going to nip it, you have to admit that you have the disease. You have to take treatment every day and you have to understand the disease. What Dr. Seilheimer and all of us worked on and edited, it's a big notebook thing. In the beginning, my initial one was teeny tiny."[33]

Much had changed in the four decades that Harrison had devoted to the treatment and care of children with CF. He had witnessed countless advances in the field of pulmonary medicine, with patients he treated as children surviving until adulthood because of medical advances. Harrison had great hopes for the breakthroughs yet to come. When he retired from Texas Children's Hospital in 2000, he assessed both the past and the future of his field. "As far as the clinical management of CF, I think we've just about hit the pinnacle," he said. "I think our knowledge of how to use the newer antibiotics and how to give the newer therapies is going to peak. I think what hasn't peaked out is the knowledge of and the perfection of lung transplants."

Established within a year of Harrison's retirement was the pediatric lung transplant program at Texas Children's Hospital—the only one of its kind in the Southwest and one of only six pediatric programs in the United States to treat children with lung diseases. Named as director was pulmonologist Dr. George Mallory, a veteran of pediatric lung transplants who had spent the previous nine years as the medical director of the pediatric lung transplant program at St. Louis Children's Hospital. On October 3, 2002— just one year after his arrival at Texas Children's Hospital—Mallory and surgical director Dr. E. Dean McKenzie performed the first pediatric lung transplant at Texas Children's Hospital.[34]

By 2004, with more than 23 pediatric lung transplants performed during its three-year existence, the pediatric lung transplant program at Texas Children's Hospital was among the largest of its kind in the country. The program garnered worldwide recognition when McKenzie and Dr. John C. Goss, director of the pediatric liver transplant program at Texas Children's Hospital, performed the first pediatric lung–liver transplant in Texas.[35] One of only 20 such procedures ever performed on patients of any age in the world, the procedure took place on January 5, 2004.

The recipient of these lifesaving transplants was 13-year-old Chase McGowen, a CF patient from Austin who had moved to Houston eight months earlier with his mother in order to be closer to Texas Children's Hospital. Although the transplants would not solve all of Chase's medical problems, Mallory said, "the good thing is we are going to move on to a whole new set of issues and, hopefully, much more solvable ones."[36]

Lung transplantation was the only option available for some CF patients, and for others who suffered from pulmonary fibrosis, bronchopulmonary dysplasia, chronic lung disease and heart disease, or heart defects affecting the lungs. Of the world's pediatric lung transplant patients, more than 75 to 80 percent survived for one year while 50 to 60 percent survived for five years. "Those numbers aren't good enough," Mallory said. "We all believe we can do better."[37]

This motivation to excel had been one of the distinctive characteristics of every member of the pulmonary medicine service at Texas Children's Hospital since its inception. Originally inspired by Harrison's interest in the respiratory management of children with polio and by his work with cystic fibrosis, under Seilheimer's direction the pulmonary medicine service had expanded to include diverse acute and chronic respiratory diseases. Since 1985, Seilheimer had developed multiple clinical programs to address the needs of a growing patient population at both Texas Children's Hospital and its neighborhood Health Centers in Sugar Land, West Houston, Northwest Houston, Clear Lake, and The Woodlands.

At Texas Children's Hospital in 2004, in addition to the pulmonary medicine service, the Cystic Fibrosis Care Center, and the Texas Children's Asthma Center, Seilheimer oversaw individual clinics for bronchopulmonary dysphasia, life-threatening asthma, and muscular dystrophy. Along with the pediatric lung transplant program at Texas Children's Hospital, there also was a pulmonary hypertension program. "Program development is one of our strengths," he said. "The next one we are just beginning to work on is for patients with neural muscular disease, muscular dystrophy, and spinal muscular atrophy. We currently are taking care of their pulmonary problems at Texas Children's Hospital, but we are developing an organized program for both prevention and treatment of lung problems."[38]

There had also been evolutionary changes in the pulmonary diagnostic lab where Seilheimer had launched his career at Texas Children's Hospital in 1977. Since its founding that year, the lab had expanded to include pulmonary function tests such as spirometry, bronchodilator response evaluation, lung volumes, body plethysmography, exercise tests, methacholine bronchoprovocation, and infant pulmonary tests. The lab also instigated studies for the control of breathing, including multichannel studies to evaluate patients with cardiorespiratory problems and to interpret apnea monitor data. For outpatients, the lab provided respiratory care therapies and educational instruction in asthma, cystic fibrosis, aerosol therapy, and airway clearance.

In the newly renovated research space in the Feigin Center at Texas Children's Hospital, Seilheimer hoped to ensure a stronger basic science research program. With plans to recruit senior scientists into the service, he aimed to enhance the service's reputation as a major contributor to the field of pediatric pulmonology. Regarding the future, Seilheimer predicted: "We will be as strong in research as we are with clinical and educational matters."

Already having an impact on the future of pediatric pulmonology in 2004 were the more than 54 fellows who had completed the pediatric pulmonology training program at Texas Children's Hospital and Baylor College of Medicine—the program initiated by Harrison in 1971. Many of the former fellows had followed the lead of Seilheimer and joined the faculty of Baylor College of Medicine. Some had gone into private practice and some had accepted academic appointments at other medical institutions.

Whatever accomplishments lay ahead, the pediatric pulmonary medicine service at Texas Children's Hospital was built on a solid foundation. In 2004—56 years after Dr. Gunyon M. Harrison first gained inspiration from the printed flyer on the bulletin board at Duke University, and 27 years after Dr. Dan K. Seilheimer joined forces with him at Texas Children's Hospital—the pediatric pulmonary service had become one of the largest and busiest of its kind in the United States.

I n 1998, when John Rowland was an adult, he explained that his "lungs don't quite do what they're supposed to, but I'm doing pretty good."[39]

For more than 27 years Rowland's daily agenda of countless pills, vitamins and enzymes, high-fat diet and pulmonary therapy had continued. With each new medication, pulmonary procedure, or equipment introduced by Dr. Gunyon M. Harrison at the Cystic Fibrosis Care Center at Texas Children's Hospital, Rowland experienced the latest advancement in the treatment and management of CF. "There was a time when they tried everything, but they really didn't know exactly what would work because the antibiotics weren't as good," he remembered. "Back then, I really didn't get to go to a lot of school. It wasn't until I got older that I actually finished whole years of school. A lot of times I was homebound all the time, being miserable. I wanted to be like everybody else."

As he grew older, Rowland abandoned his unrealistic wish to be normal and began to accept the limitations imposed on him by his sometimes-fragile health. "The realization about what you can do with your life and what you can't do with your life comes in stages," he explained. "Once you get past a lot of that stuff, you do a lot better. I knew that I wouldn't be able to be rich or work 80 hours a week. I learned early on that I just couldn't do that. Whenever you come to the realization of all that, you do much better in life."

This acceptance of the realities of living with CF was shared with other patients in the Cystic Fibrosis Care Center and on the cystic fibrosis wing at Texas Children's Hospital—and also with fellow campers at Harrison's annual summer camp for CF patients and their families, which Rowland participated in for 20 years, beginning when he was seven years old. When he became too old to be a camper, he volunteered as a peer counselor "to be with other CF people and try to embed my warped sense of knowledge on them."

At the camp, "I mainly tell them to do whatever they want and be happy," Rowland explained. "If they want to try something, we let them, within reason. We let them run around, we let them swim, everything. They should enjoy life while they can."

This was not a new philosophy for Rowland. Not being sufficiently active or productive had always been one of his pet peeves. Rather than do nothing else while undergoing daily pulmonary therapy at home, he arranged his physical surroundings so that he could simultaneously work on his computer or surf the Internet. When not involved with technological diversions, he had a voracious appetite for entertaining books, reading at least one every other day. Fascinated by a book about musical instruments, he took a music course at the University of Houston and learned to play the cello.

Always willing to try something new, Rowland felt that active participation in various indoor and outdoor activities was essential to his well-being. He also felt that other CF patients needed the freedom to do whatever they wanted, saying: "Let them play all the sports they want to. Let them try to experience everything they can. Don't hold them back. I've seen a lot of parents not letting them play outside when it's raining. Even Dr. Harrison will tell you I played when I was younger. I tried to play all the sports and everything."

As a teenager, when confined at Texas Children's Hospital and unable to go outside, Rowland had championed the instigation of indoor activities for patients in his age group. "We yelled and screamed there wasn't anything to do, and there wasn't back then. There was a TV and that was it," he recalled. "Then somebody said, 'Maybe we need a teen room and we should write a letter.' So, a couple of my CF buddies and I wrote a letter, and lo and behold, there was a teen room built on the first floor."

It was but one of the many changes that occurred during Rowland's many visits to Texas Children's Hospital over three decades. He was an eyewitness to the hospital's phenomenal growth, renovations, and expansion—not all of which he approved.

As a patient who would bring his telescope and peer out a window of the CF wing, Rowland lamented the erection of each new hospital building. Eventually, his view of the sweeping vistas outside was blocked. The only alternative was looking at the four walls in his room, which Rowland found to be an unacceptable substitute. "The wallpaper was bad. They've changed it about eight times. You sit there and look at candy stripes or pink elephants and you go for two weeks and it's awful," he said, recounting one of his most vivid memories of Texas Children's Hospital.

It was a recurring memory that ended in 1997, when Rowland grew too old to be a CF patient at Texas Children's Hospital. With his advancing age came the possibility of contracting adult diseases, ones that required doctors trained in adult medicine. He was transitioned into the newly established adult CF service at The Methodist Hospital.

For Rowland, bidding farewell to the wallpaper was easy. However, leaving the familiar surroundings and the dedicated physician, nurses, therapists, and medical staff who had taken care of him since the early 1970s was difficult. "Dr. Harrison is the only one I've ever seen over the years, until 1997," he said. "I'm not sure exactly why, but I think we're living longer and he's one of the big things why we're living so long."

Rowland also credited Harrison as being the one who not only encouraged his transition, but also facilitated it. Introducing him to his new doctor, pulmonologist Dr. Kathryn A. Hale, director of the adult CF service at The Methodist Hospital, Harrison eased Rowland's anxieties about leaving Texas Children's Hospital. "She was trained by Dr. Harrison, and when I came in to see him, she was waiting there with him. He approved everything and told me that it's going to work out, and I'm sure it will. So he kind of handed me off and made sure everything was going to go okay."

Although no longer his patient, Rowland continued to acknowledge Harrison's enormous impact—not only in improving his health and extending his life, but also in helping him live that life to its fullest. "You've just got to take it one day at a time and try to take it easy, because your health is your most important thing. I think a lot of CFs, and I can site numerous examples, have just rushed headlong into disaster," he said, recalling countless friends with CF who have not survived.

"I don't mind if I don't leave the house for two days, as long as I'm feeling well," he said. "Sometimes I may not even see the sun, but I don't mind at all."

Available to brighten John Rowland's days as a 33-year old in 2004 were those happy memories of his mischievous activities as a child at Texas Children's Hospital.

26

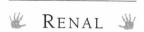 RENAL

Emma Grace Hutchinson was diagnosed at birth with a rare genetic disease, autosomal recessive polycystic kidney disease.

Although most infants born with this rare genetic disease often did not survive the first month of life, Emma was one of the exceptions. Affecting one in 10,000 babies to one in 40,000 babies, autosomal recessive polycystic kidney disease (ARPKD) could be inherited from parents who did not have the disease if both parents carry one copy of the abnormal gene and both pass the gene to the baby. Also known as "infantile PKD" when diagnosed in utero or at birth, the disease had varying degrees of severity, but inevitably caused kidney failure and usually affected the liver, spleen and pancreas. The main complication in newborns was pulmonary distress.

Within moments of Emma's March 21, 1988, delivery at St. Luke's Episcopal Hospital, she was in pulmonary distress. "We knew how bad it was," Emma's mother, Paula Hutchinson, said, recalling the frantic activity surrounding the birth. "We knew she was critically ill. They had a crash cart right there in the delivery room, and they shoved a chest tube in her to inflate her lungs, and everybody from neonatology, nephrology, cardiology, and pulmonology was working on her."[1]

Intubated and rushed over to the neonatology intensive care unit at Texas Children's Hospital, Emma began her valiant struggle to survive. With both kidneys greatly enlarged and covered with fluid-filled cysts, she also suffered from heart problems caused by exceedingly high blood pressure. To deliver the medications Emma needed, neonatologists inserted an umbilical catheter. Although told that their newborn daughter was "holding her own," Paula and her husband, John Hutchinson, knew that the baby's condition was precarious. They began planning for the inevitable.

When they learned that none of Emma's other organs would be suitable for transplant in others, Paula remembered, "It was a very dark point for us."

The distraught Hutchinsons maintained a day-and-night vigil in the neonatal intensive care unit at Texas Children's Hospital as Emma continued to defy the odds against her. "In the midst of all the trauma, Dr. Susan Landers, the neonatologist, got us focused on Emma as a person," Paula said. "I think this was when we realized we were in the right place."[2]

A week after Emma's birth, she continued to exhibit remarkable stamina. Although her kidneys remained nonfunctional, her lungs and blood chemistry showed marked improvement. These were encouraging signs to pediatric nephrologist Dr. Phillip Berry, who transferred her out of neonatal intensive care with cautious optimism. Advising that the future remained uncertain, he discussed what treatment options were available. Because of the severity of Emma's kidney disease, she was a transplant candidate from birth. However, children must reach the weight of ten kilograms, or roughly 22 pounds, before a transplant can be attempted. "Dr. Berry had this phenomenal way about him," Paula said. "He managed to present everything in such a way that he didn't do anything to scare you, he didn't do anything to give you false hopes, but he always seemed to manage the issues."[3]

The Hutchinsons also felt "this affinity" with the entire renal team, Paula explained. "The doctors never treat the nurses or the technicians or anybody else as less than they are. They act as a team. They know how valuable each member of the team is. It's incredible."[4]

The need to increase Emma's minimum food intake was the next challenge undertaken by the renal team. The effort produced a frightening aftermath. With Emma's severely limited urine output, "she blew up like a balloon." As a result, Emma underwent emergency surgery for a nephrectomy and had a catheter inserted for peritoneal dialysis. Within 24 hours of the surgery, three-week-old Emma began peritoneal dialysis. The results astonished her parents. "Miracle of miracles, it was working,' Paula said. "She went from this very swollen baby to this shrunken little baby in a matter of weeks. It took all the fluid off. Helen Currier was her primary dialysis nurse, and she was just phenomenal. She always knew exactly what was going on."[5]

Also knowledgeable about Emma's condition was her father. As a professor of chemistry, John innately understood all the chemical issues involved—all the electrolytes, the balancing, and the calculations necessary for his daughter's survival. Aware of Emma's numbers every moment of the day, he formed a bond with Dr. Berry and was able to communicate easily with the entire renal team. Immediately after the surgery, they all concurred that Emma's numbers were good. But although at first she reacted favorably to dialysis, in the following days and weeks her remaining kidney began to expand rapidly. When a scan revealed that it was four times the size of an adult kidney, the decision was made to return to surgery for another nephrectomy. At the age of five weeks, Emma had her remaining kidney removed.

To stay alive, Emma began a chronic dialysis program consisting of 12 to 14 hours of treatment each night. Trained in the use of the home dialysis equipment by the nephrology nurses at Texas Children's Hospital, Paula and John began making plans in June to take Emma home for the very first time. Anxiously awaiting their arrival was Emma's big sister, seven-year-old Ashlyn, who had been able to visit only briefly with Emma at Texas Children's Hospital. "Our older daughter was going through her own hell," said Paula. "Not only had she looked forward to this baby sister or baby brother, but suddenly she has a sister who might die, who might die again, and you don't know what's going on. At the time, there was a pilot program for visiting siblings in the neonatal ICU and she was able to be in there and visit her."[6]

Emma's long-awaited homecoming was cut short in July, when her vital signs became erratic. Rushing her back to Texas Children's Hospital, Paula and John met Dr. Berry in the emergency room. Within hours, machines were performing every vital function for Emma. Once again, she faced a life-or-death crisis and, once again, she overcame it. Following a month in the pediatric intensive care unit, a reinvigorated Emma returned home in August. "It was as if she had cleared the final hurdle," her mother said.[7]

As they waited for a transplant, every member of the Hutchinson family shared Emma's determination to survive. Together at last, they also shared the beginning of a new life at home—one they knew was certain to become eventful.

The renal-metabolic service was one of the first subspecialty services established at the newly opened Texas Children's Hospital in 1954.

Under the direction of Dr. Charles William Daeschner, Jr., the service was broad in scope. Its responsibilities included the medical care of infants and children with a wide variety of congenital and acquired diseases of the kidney; kidney failure; high blood pressure; abnormalities of salt, water, and acid-base metabolism; and a number of metabolic diseases, including diabetes mellitus and inborn errors of metabolism.

As other subspecialty services emerged at Texas Children's Hospital in subsequent years, the responsibility for many of the diseases originally treated by the renal-metabolic service was assumed by the newly established services of pediatric endocrinology, pediatric nutrition-gastroenterology, pediatric rheumatology, pediatric urology, and genetics. Throughout this process of evolution in the field of pediatrics, the efforts of the renal-metabolic service at Texas Children's Hospital remained heavily concentrated in the treatment and research of renal or kidney conditions in children. The discipline ultimately gained formal recognition in 1974 when the American Board of Pediatrics began certifying physicians as subspecialists in pediatric nephrology. As a result, training programs were evaluated and certified.

In the 1950s, however, the renal-metabolic service at Texas Children's Hospital was in its infancy. Metabolic disorders—specifically diabetes and kidney diseases—were the principal areas of concentration. Daeschner's avid interest in these areas was a passion that he instilled in his first renal-metabolic fellow, Dr. L. Leighton Hill, as well as in those who followed, Dr. Warren Dodge and Dr. Luther Travis.

"I was the chief resident at Jefferson Davis Hospital in 1956, when Dr. Daeschner was chief of the pediatric service there, as well as chief of the renal-metabolic service at Texas Children's Hospital," recalled Hill. "I became his first fellow in 1957. He was all by himself in that service, and it was pretty broad in scope then."[8]

The service also encompassed a wide geographic area. In addition to their patients at Texas Children's Hospital, Daeschner and Hill treated children afflicted with kidney diseases and metabolic disorders at Jefferson Davis Hospital, where Daeschner maintained a renal-metabolic laboratory for research. "We had the first osmometer in Houston and one of the first flame photometers," recalled Hill. "The flame photometer measured sodium and potassium concentrations and the osmometer measured total solute in various body fluids, including plasma. So, we did a lot of things in our research lab in 1957 that are now very routine."[9]

An outstanding example of this pioneering work occurred in 1957, when Daeschner performed one of the first peritoneal dialysis procedures on children. First introduced in 1946 and only rarely used as a treatment for renal failure in adults, peritoneal dialysis involved the use of the peritoneal membranes that line the abdominal cavity as a filter. Special solutions that facilitate the removal of toxins are infused into the peritoneal cavity, where they remain for a time and then are drained out.[10]

"There was little or no dialysis in the late 1950s," explained Hill. "Dr. Daeschner and I did what was called acute peritoneal dialysis in a young child with acute renal failure. There were no solutions available, so we had to make up the solutions in the laboratory; we had to prepare them, filter them, and sterilize them and put them in bottles. There was no equipment made for children, so we had to make our own peritoneal catheters out of the rubber ones used to catheterize the bladder. We used surgical instruments known as 'trocars' to place the rubber catheters in the peritoneal cavities. It was quite an undertaking to do what we believe was the first peritoneal dialysis done in a child."[11]

This improvised treatment began when the two doctors inserted the catheter to transfer the solution into the patient's peritoneal cavity. After leaving the solution in the patient for an hour or two, they removed it and added more fluid, then left it in for another hour or two and took it out again. "The peritoneal cavity is highly vascular, so the fluid is in contact with blood vessels," Hill explained. "The waste products in the body move into this fluid, and if you keep doing this over and over again for six hours or eight hours, 12 hours, 24 hours, or even continuously, you can take waste products out that way. That's peritoneal dialysis. Now we have machines that do the fluid exchanges automatically for as long as necessary, but we did it by hand in 1957."[12]

Daeschner and Hill's pioneering efforts proved to be lifesaving for the child, tiding him over until his own kidneys regained their function. The procedure represented a breakthrough in the treatment of acute renal failure in children. Thereafter, patients with acute renal failure who underwent acute peritoneal dialysis at Texas Children's Hospital survived, when they previously would have died.[13] Both nationally and internationally, the use of this proven treatment for renal failure in adults and children remained limited during the late 1950s and early 1960s. After the introduction in 1964 of a surgically implanted catheter, however, peritoneal dialysis became universally accepted.[14]

Another Daeschner accomplishment in 1957 was the introduction of percutaneous renal biopsies at Texas Children's Hospital, making the hospital one of the first in the country to perform those procedures on children. In an improvised technique, Daeschner used adult-sized liver biopsy needles to pierce through the skin of the child and extract kidney tissue. "Kidney tissues are firmer than liver tissues, so we had to have a little clip in the end of the needle, and we had them made for us," explained Hill. "Now the biopsy needles have progressed tremendously to automatic biopsy devices. You go in with ultrasound and you know exactly where you are, and you just pull the trigger and it takes it for you. Back then, we used adult needles on small children, and it was tough to do."[15]

Although difficult to achieve, the end results of these biopsies were pivotal. Later hailed as one of the six critical discoveries that shaped the evolution of pediatric nephrology, the use of needle biopsies of the kidney provided the first samples of living renal tissue for examination and research.[16] "We started doing them in 1957, and I think the only other place that was doing biopsies at that time was the University of Minnesota in Minneapolis," said Hill. "It was one of the really great advances in clinical nephrology, being able to diagnose and understand renal diseases that you were following while the patients were still alive and could be treated."[17]

Before the advent of percutaneous renal biopsies, the treatment of children with kidney diseases at Texas Children's Hospital and throughout the world was based on clinical observation and criteria. "We would follow them until they developed end stage, but at end stage all kidneys looked the same— scarred and no longer functioning. So, the percutaneous needle biopsy was a tremendous advance in understanding kidney disease at an early point."[18]

Percutaneous renal biopsies became one of the great research tools in the rapidly emerging field of pediatric nephrology. Previously, little was known about the underlying pathophysiology of even the most common kidney diseases, much less about how to treat patients effectively. Many patients did not survive. Those children who developed end-stage renal disease in the 1950s and 60s faced certain death because no proven treatments to prolong life existed. At the time, dialysis for acute renal failure in adults was considered experimental and was available only in select locations in the United States. For children afflicted with other chronic kidney diseases, the introduction of antibiotics, known as "wonder drugs," after World War II had a dramatic impact on survival rates. Until the late 1940s, children afflicted with nephrotic syndrome had a 40 to 50 percent mortality rate. After the introduction of antibiotics to treat life-threatening infections, particularly peritonitis, the mortality rate dropped to 20 to 25 percent.[19] With the introduction of glucocorticoids in the 1950s, the mortality rate for nephrotic syndrome fell to less than 5 percent.[20] Why existing treatments failed in some patients and succeeded in others was a question that only research could answer.

It was Hill's avid interest in research that influenced his decision to seek additional fellowship training at another institution. Daeschner encouraged him to go away for "a year or so of training in a more sophisticated way" and then return to Texas Children's Hospital, because "we weren't very well developed at that time, in the way of research facilities, to train our fellows to do research."[21]

When the opportunity to train with Dr. Bill Wallace presented itself in 1958, Hill left for Western Reserve University in Cleveland, Ohio, to begin a two-year fellowship in renal physiology and water, salt, and acid-base metabolism. The former laboratory director for Harvard's Dr. James Gamble, the most recognized name in water, salt, and acid-base metabolism, Wallace had left Harvard to become chairman of pediatrics at Western Reserve University and chief of pediatrics at Babies and Children's Hospital in Cleveland. "Dr. Daeschner, who trained with Dr. Gamble, spoke so highly of him and Dr. Wallace, who was a very close colleague," said Hill. "I felt it would be good to have some training away from Dr. Daeschner, because all of my training essentially had been with him. I felt, and he agreed, that if I went away for a while and saw how other people did things, that I could gain a different perspective, and when I came back I could bring something with me. In addition to my research interests, that was another motivation to go."[22]

While in training at Western Reserve, Hill participated in the administration of hemodialysis, the recently introduced experimental therapy for acute renal failure. The procedure, which required the use of an artificial kidney apparatus to dialyze the patient's blood, was available at only a few select facilities. Following the success of the first workable machine, developed and implemented before World War II by Dr. William Kolff in Nazi-occupied Holland, similar artificial kidneys were invented. A somewhat different version of Kolff's dialyzer was developed and implemented at Western Reserve by Dr. Leonard Skeggs and Dr. Jack Leonard in 1948. A unique feature of the Skeggs-Leonard "plate kidney" device was the use of countercurrent flow of blood and dialysate or parallel flow. It was a new type of continuous dialyzer for adults with acute renal failure.[23]

Compared with today's highly sophisticated methods of hemodialysis, the procedure at Western Reserve in 1958 and 1959 was "really primitive," Hill recalled. "The Skeggs-Leonard dialysis unit was a big tub that you would pour dialysate in. You would fill buckets of water mixed with measured weights of various salts and pour it in. I remember so well taking a broomstick and mixing it all up. And then, of course, the blood would run through tube membranes in the tub to be cleaned and filtered."[24]

Although unrefined in the late 1950s, hemodialysis was to become a proven method of prolonging life in both children and adults afflicted with chronic renal failure. In its early stages, however, the technique was used only for adults. The necessary advances in equipment and expertise needed for application in children evolved slowly over the following decades.

What was progressing rapidly in the late 1950s was the classification of glomerular disease through percutaneous renal biopsies. When Hill returned to Texas Children's Hospital in 1959, he found that Daeschner and Dr. Warren Dodge, his second fellow, had created and implemented technical advances in the procedure. As one of the few hospitals in which kidney biopsies in children were being perfected, Texas Children's Hospital quickly became the destination for other physicians who wished to learn the procedure.

"We had people coming from all over the United States to learn how to do kidney biopsies in children, and I give Dr. Daeschner most of the credit for really pushing it and making us learn how to do it," said Hill. "We had people from the University of Florida, from Western Reserve, and the University of Texas in Dallas. We even had some people from South America and Belgium come over to learn how to do percutaneous biopsies in children, because they were only being done in two places at the time, at Texas Children's Hospital and the University of Minnesota."[25]

By all accounts—including those from visiting physicians and from students at Baylor College of Medicine—Daeschner was an exceptional teacher. It was a role that he enjoyed immensely and one that ultimately shaped his career. "My thought was that I would stay in the department a year or two and get this bug to teach out of my mind, and then I would join Laura Bickle, George Salmon, and Byron York in practice," he said. "The three of them were practicing together and when they enlarged their facilities, they reserved some space for me. We would talk and, finally, George said to me one day, 'You're not going to give up teaching. I never should have, and I think you're smart enough to where you are not going to do it.' So, I guess I had been there about two or three years before I really made a commitment to stay at Baylor and teach. And I did that for nine years."[26]

Daeschner particularly enjoyed the ability to teach students on a one-on-one basis. Although his method of interactive teaching differed from the formal lecture style of Dr. Russell J. Blattner, chief of pediatrics, there was little conflict between the two. Instead, Daeschner was given "a lot of independence" to run the pediatric service at Jefferson Davis Hospital and the renal-metabolic service at Texas Children's Hospital. His hands-on approach to bedside teaching by involving students in the learning process was contagious, particularly among his fellows. "He felt it was a very important responsibility, and I took to it as a chief resident and then as a fellow," said Hill. "He was certainly one of the first ones to really push this idea of interactive teaching, and he's written a lot about that. And he's best known nationally, I guess, for his efforts and his accomplishments in education and teaching. I think he's been responsible for a lot of the advances in teaching that we've seen in pediatrics."[27]

The chance to implement these teaching concepts on a wider scale was a contributing factor to Daeschner's decision to leave Texas Children's Hospital and Baylor College of Medicine. When he received an offer in 1959 to become chairman of the pediatrics department at the University of Texas Medical Branch (UTMB) in Galveston, Daeschner was at first hesitant to make the move. Saddened to leave his close group of colleagues at Baylor, he nonetheless viewed the UTMB job as an opportunity to pay back his former alma mater by taking on a department that had not had a chairman for three years. "The department was down on its heels, and to do something with it was a real challenge," he said. "There were a lot of subtle factors at work, but I think if I had to point at the one that made me decide to accept the position, it was my desire to try my hand at developing a resident and student teaching program that was along the lines of what I thought was the way to do it."[28]

Daeschner was mulling over the possibility of leaving when Hill returned from Western Reserve in October 1959. Hill was expecting to join Daeschner and become the second member of the renal-metabolic service at Texas Children's Hospital. He planned to spend a limited amount of time involved in clinical work, devoting most of his efforts to research in a renal-metabolic lab of his own design. Several months later, when Daeschner accepted the UTMB job, Hill's once-certain future was in disarray. "I was suddenly offered his job, basically all of the renal-metabolic service and the renal nephrology training program," Hill recalled. "Bill Daeschner wanted me to go to Galveston with him, and it was one of the toughest decisions I ever made because I thought so much of him."[29]

Hill decided to remain in Houston. In spring 1960, he became chief of the renal-metabolic service at Texas Children's Hospital and head of the pediatric renal-metabolic section at Baylor College of Medicine. Hill had inherited from Daeschner the responsibility for a rapidly expanding renal-metabolic service at Texas Children's Hospital that treated children with a wide variety of renal diseases. The medical, as opposed to surgical, diseases included congenital abnormalities of the urinary tract such as cystic diseases; infections of the urinary tract; renal tubular abnormalities; renal disease resulting from diffuse systemic diseases; renal diseases caused by drugs or toxins; various forms of glomerulonephritis, immunological diseases of the kidney; acute renal failure; and many types of nephrotic syndrome.[30] In addition to these patients, the renal-metabolic staff managed a growing number of children with diabetes, genetic inborn errors of metabolism, various types of metabolic bone diseases, hypertension, and severe water, electrolyte, and acid-base disturbances.

Also handed over to Hill was Daeschner's Saturday morning renal-metabolic clinic, held in conjunction with Dr. George W. Clayton's endocrinology clinic, and the endocrine-metabolic-renal conference that followed. Presided over by the two physicians, the luncheon conference lasted several hours, shortened only when there was a Rice University football game to attend. "Dr. Clayton and his fellows presented endocrine patients," recalled Hill. "Then Dr. Daeschner and myself, and later just myself or one of my fellows, would present the renal and metabolic patients. It was very interesting and a lot of interns and residents who were interested in endocrinology and kidney disease, as well as several internist endocrinologists, came to it."[31]

When Daeschner departed in the spring of 1960, Hill became the only trained nephrologist in Houston. It was a distinction he would hold for more than four years and one that affected his workload. In addition to his responsibilities at Texas Children's Hospital, Hill provided consultations and performed kidney biopsies for the medical service at Jefferson Davis Hospital. He also did grand rounds on kidney topics for the internal medicine department at Baylor College of Medicine.

As the only nephrologist in the renal-metabolic service at Texas Children's Hospital between 1960 and 1972, Hill learned to master his demanding 24-hour schedule. In addition to his work at the hospital, he served as chairman of the board of the Kidney Foundation of Houston and the Greater Gulf Coast in the late 1960s and as president of the Southern Society of Pediatric Research in 1967. No matter where he was or what responsibility he was fulfilling, Texas Children's Hospital always remained a priority. "When I was on vacation, when I was off at meetings, wherever I was, I would get calls," he remembered. "The residents or fellows who were taking care of the patients had nobody else to go to, you see. So, I was kind of on call all the time."[32]

Another responsibility became an integral part of Hill's already-crowded schedule. Named chairman of the student education committee of the pediatrics department at Baylor College of Medicine in 1962, he assumed the primary responsibility for supervising the department's medical student teaching program. In this continuing role as a professor of pediatrics, he excelled in teaching, eventually receiving the Baylor Pediatric House Staff Award for Outstanding Full-Time Faculty, the Distinguished Faculty Award from the Baylor College of Medicine Alumni Association, and the Arnold J. Rudolph Baylor Pediatric Award for Lifetime Excellence in Teaching.[33] What was most gratifying to Hill, however, was becoming the first recipient of the

Charles W. Daeschner, Jr., M.D., Lifetime Achievement Award from the Texas Pediatric Society. Presented in 2001, this recognition was "given to an individual whose lifetime accomplishments and contributions to pediatrics best emulate the standards set by Dr. Daeschner."[34]

One such Hill accomplishment occurred at Texas Children's Hospital in the early 1960s. Inspired by his avid interest in research, Hill collaborated with Clayton to seize a monumental opportunity. "Dr. Clayton and I had offices next to each other, and we talked a lot about what we could do if we had a research center," Hill explained. "He convinced Dr. Blattner that we should have a Clinical Research Center (CRC), that the government was supporting these and had announced the intention to some pediatric programs."[35]

With Blattner's approval, Clayton and Hill began their efforts to attain a CRC grant for Texas Children's Hospital. They traveled to the National Institutes of Health (NIH) to attain the necessary grant guidelines and then visited existing units in Boston, Baltimore, Philadelphia, and New York City. For more than six months, Hill and Clayton collaborated on writing the original grant and preparing various protocols at Texas Children's Hospital for the NIH site visit. When the NIH approved the request, it became the first federal grant ever received by Texas Children's Hospital. Hill continued to take great personal pride in the accomplishment. Forty years later, he regarded the work he did with Clayton to acquire the CRC as one of his major contributions to Texas Children's Hospital.[36]

"The CRC opened in 1964, and it allowed us to do a lot of research that had not been possible to do previously," Hill said. "Dr. Clayton was the principal investigator and he tried to talk me into being, I don't know what the titles were back then, but the assistant head, basically. But I had so many things going; I was trying to do my own research and I just felt it was too much."[37]

One of the main research interests of Hill's renal-metabolic service in the 1960s and 70s was the problem of acquired disturbances of the tubular function of the kidney. In collaboration with the nutrition-gastroenterology service at Texas Children's Hospital, Hill performed studies on the effect of malnutrition on tubular functions. A separate study, in cooperation with the pediatric urology service at Texas Children's Hospital, investigated the effect of obstructions of the urinary tract and the relief of obstructions to the urinary flow on these functions.[38]

Of continuing research interest was the correlation of the clinical course of various types of kidney diseases and nephrotic syndrome by microscopic study of tissues obtained by percutaneous needle biopsy. "We were one of the first groups to do immunofluorescent studies on the biopsies,"

Hill said. "We did electron microscopy studies at a fairly early stage. My main interest was in the morphological changes of kidney disease, and I worked very closely with Harvey Rosenberg, who was the first head of pathology at Texas Children's Hospital, and Don Singer, the other pediatric pathologist and a close research collaborator with the renal-metabolic service. We published papers on glomerulonephritis, nephrotic syndrome, hereditary nephritis, and evaluation of patients with hematuria."[39]

This active research program continued to thrive throughout Hill's tenure as chief of the renal-metabolic service, enabling him to train a number of research fellows in pediatric nephrology. Between 1960 and 1994, Hill trained more than 23 fellows in pediatric nephrology—13 of whom became full-time faculty members at medical schools in the United States, Mexico, Costa Rica, Lebanon, and Saudi Arabia. "The things I look back on that I value the most over all those years are all the young people who trained with me, all the fellows and residents," said Hill in 2004. "In the years when we didn't have enough fellows, we used residents. The renal-metabolic service was a very popular resident and medical student elective, the renal service was, and I really valued working with young people and seeing them get ahead."[40]

As he had hoped, a number of fellows who worked with Hill went on to become leading experts in the field of pediatric nephrology. Dr. Steven R. Alexander, a research fellow from 1976 to 1978, became the chief of pediatric nephrology at Stanford University School of Medicine and one of the leading experts on dialysis in children and the treatment of chronic congestive heart failure with continuous hemofiltration. "He and Dr. Edward Kohaut [1971–73] were really the pioneers in much of that," Hill said. "So, you like to see people achieve. Every time they have a national or international dialysis conference, those two are always prominent on the programs. They became much more prominent in the field of dialysis than I."[41]

Dialysis had come of age by the late 1960s. In the decade since Hill had stirred dialysate with a broom handle in the crude beginnings of hemodialysis for acute renal failure, sophisticated refinements in the technique and necessary improvements in Kolff's artificial kidney had taken place. The landmark invention of a Teflon shunt by Dr. Belding H. Scribner at the University of Washington in Seattle enabled repeated circulatory access, making chronic dialysis feasible for the first time. With the Scribner shunt implanted into a patient, doctors could tap into the blood vessels repeatedly and therefore keep the patient on dialysis indefinitely. The introduction of this technical achievement in 1960 permitted patients with end-stage renal disease to live when they otherwise would have died.[42]

In the early 1960s, Scribner's Seattle clinic became the first to provide a center for chronic kidney dialysis and an expanded home-dialysis program. His proven method of extending lives inspired other chronic dialysis centers throughout the United States. The expense of treatment ranged from $15,000 to $20,000 annually, but the success of these programs outweighed the cost. Inevitably, patient demand far exceeded the limited number of dialysis machines and trained treatment teams available at Seattle's popular clinic. The world's first medical ethics committee evaluated who would receive treatment and who would not, thereby deciding who would live and who would die. Similar procedures at other facilities, as well as the spiraling costs of treatment, resulted in public outrage from both doctors and patients. The crisis eventually made its way to Congress.[43]

A congressional committee charged with investigating this escalating dilemma reached a solution after hearing from Bill Litchfield, a Houston engineer, who testified on November 4, 1971, while hooked up to a dialysis machine. Litchfield described "living in constant terror," fearing that his money would run out, that he would be forced to stop treatments, and that "death would come in a matter of weeks." The committee sprang into action.[44] In October 1972, Congress passed legislation requiring Medicare, the federal program for the elderly and disabled, to pay for chronic dialysis and kidney transplantation for any patient, regardless of age, with end-stage renal disease (ESRD). When President Richard M. Nixon signed Public Law 92-601 into law as an amendment to the Medicare Act, ESRD became the only medical condition given that status.

With the commencement of the entitlement program on July 1, 1973, adult dialysis services rapidly expanded. The development of chronic pediatric dialysis services and a growing interest in pediatric transplantation soon followed.[45] "Patients who ordinarily would have died were now supported by Medicare," Hill said. "We had been performing acute peritoneal dialysis for more than ten years at Texas Children's Hospital and, through cooperation with the St. Luke's Episcopal Hospital dialysis unit, hemodialysis became available for the pediatric patient who needed it on an acute basis in the 1970s. The nurses in the St. Luke's adult unit had little experience with dialysis in children, so a pediatric nephrologist had to be in constant attendance during the procedures."[46]

During the 1970s, no end-stage programs for children with fatal kidney disease existed. Although the world's first successful kidney transplant had taken place at Boston's Brigham and Women's Hospital in 1954, attempts to keep children alive with chronic or long-term dialysis in order to perform transplants on them were limited. "Our use of dialysis in the 1960s and in the 1970s was mostly for the treatment of acute renal failure—that is, in patients in whom the recovery of kidney function was expected in three or four weeks," explained Hill. "We also used dialysis to prepare transplant patients for their surgery by correcting the children's chemical imbalances and ridding them of accumulated waste products. The other very useful application of hemodialysis and peritoneal dialysis was to treat certain types of acute poisonings. Some poisons can be removed very rapidly with dialysis, especially hemodialysis."[47]

The eventual evolution into chronic dialysis for children with terminal kidney disease paralleled the advances made in organ transplantation. The first successful human kidney transplant between identical twin boys in 1954 clearly demonstrated that organ transplantation could be lifesaving. The fact that this procedure had circumvented the issue of biological incompatibility stimulated attempts to breach the immunological barrier with immunosuppressant drugs. In 1962, the first successful kidney transplant involving an unrelated donor took place. The transplanted kidney came from a dead donor, making it the world's first successful human cadaveric transplant.[48]

Successful transplantation of other human organs soon followed. Throughout the 1960s and 70s, post-transplant care involved drug-induced immunosuppression and early anti-rejection medications such as prednisone, which offered limited protection from rejection and increased the risks of other complications such as infection. The Food and Drug Administration's approval in 1983 of the drug cyclosporine marked the beginning of a new era for transplantations of kidneys and all other organs. The immunosuppressant medication led to a significant increase in survival of both transplanted grafts and patients.

Kidney transplantation for patients at Texas Children's Hospital became available in the late 1960s through the Baylor Affiliated Hospitals Transplantation Program at The Methodist Hospital. The required management of chronic renal failure in children awaiting transplantation at Texas Children's Hospital was the responsibility of a new member of Hill's renal-metabolic staff, Dr. Carol Wilson, who joined the team in 1972. Trained in pediatric nephrology at the University of California for two and a half years, Wilson was a recognized expert in dialysis. She also served as the Texas Children's Hospital representative in the Baylor Affiliated Hospitals Transplantation Program.[49]

With the arrival of Wilson, Hill was no longer the only pediatric nephrologist at Texas Children's Hospital. Within the following decade the professional staff of the renal-metabolic service continued to grow. Former fellow Kohaut joined the service for two years, from 1974 to 1976, and significantly accelerated research output. Another former fellow, Dr. Sami A. Sanjad, came on board in 1976 to replace Kohaut.

Before the gradual expansion of the service began in 1972, the small service had already made large contributions to the field of pediatric nephrology. Since its inception, research efforts had resulted in more than 60 publications and abstracts, as well as more than 80 scientific presentations at state, national, and international meetings.[50]

Even with all these pluses, there was a major minus, in Hill's opinion. Sorely lacking from the service was a dedicated pediatric dialysis unit at Texas Children's Hospital and Hill was determined to establish one. "We had an acknowledged dialysis expert on staff, but we just couldn't seem to bring it about," Hill explained. "The dialysis unit at St. Luke's lost a lot of money for that hospital, and the administrator of Texas Children's Hospital, Newell France, got it into his mind that dialysis units were losers and we were just not going to have any. It wasn't until Dr. Ralph Feigin came as physician-in-chief in 1977 that we were able to achieve our goal."[51]

The long-awaited Pediatric Dialysis Center at Texas Children's Hospital finally opened in 1979. Located on the hospital's second floor, the center had two pediatric dialysis stations and a staff of two registered nurses with specialized training in pediatric intensive care and pediatric dialysis. Offering both peritoneal dialysis and hemodialysis, it was Houston's only dialysis facility exclusively devoted to the treatment of chronic kidney failure in children. In the early months, three outpatients were treated at the center three times a week. Within one year, there were six outpatients and five nurses. The need for immediate expansion became evident.

The escalating growth also necessitated the 1980 appointment of Dr. Phillip L. Berry as medical director of the Pediatric Dialysis Center at Texas Children's Hospital. A recent addition to the professional staff of the renal-metabolic service, Berry was a graduate of Baylor College of Medicine. He had served his residency in Baylor-affiliated hospitals and his pediatric nephrologist training at the Cincinnati Children's Hospital Medical Center. Hill and Berry foresaw the future of this unique service and began setting long-range objectives in the early 1980s.

Within months of Berry's arrival in 1980, the services of the Pediatric Dialysis Center expanded. Originally responsible for only chronic outpatient dialysis, the center began to offer acute dialysis for inpatients, including those who were too sick to come to the center. "One of the nurses will go to the patient and initiate dialysis using portable equipment," Berry explained. "This is especially useful in the pediatric intensive care unit."[52]

Other innovations introduced at the Pediatric Dialysis Center in the fall of 1980 included the first fully automated peritoneal dialysis machine in Houston. With pre-set pumps and timing devices, this revolutionary machine increased dialysis efficiency, decreased nursing time, and reduced infection. It was a technical marvel—particularly to Hill, who 23 years earlier had helped to pioneer the manual technique of pediatric peritoneal dialysis with Daeschner.

Such ongoing advances in dialysis helped sustain the lives of children who in earlier years would have died following the complete loss of kidney function. For those children undergoing chronic dialysis at Texas Children's Hospital, Berry and Hill instituted a formalized treatment program that included transplantation. "When children with chronic kidney failure reach a point where they need dialysis or a kidney transplant they are said to have end-stage renal disease (ESRD)," Berry explained. "This rather ominous term means that the child's kidneys are at the end of the road, but the child is not."[53]

The continuing road to survival for ESRD dialysis patients at Texas Children's Hospital in the early 1980s included a necessary side trip for kidney transplantation at The Methodist Hospital, where the procedure was the responsibility of surgeons in the Baylor College of Medicine transplantation program. After kidney transplantation, patients received treatment from staff of the renal-metabolic service at Texas Children's Hospital and of the nephrology service at The Methodist Hospital. When Medicare approved Texas Children's Hospital as a renal transplant center in 1987, the patient's trip to another hospital was no longer necessary. Beginning in 1988, Dr. George Noon, a world-renowned surgeon in the Baylor College of Medicine multi-organ transplant program, performed kidney transplants at Texas Children's Hospital.

Other organizational changes in the renal-metabolic service at Texas Children's Hospital preceded Noon's move. When Hill relinquished the service's responsibility for diabetes to pediatric endocrinology in 1985, metabolic was dropped from the service's name. Thereafter known as the renal service at Texas Children's Hospital, the service also boasted an expanded professional staff. Joining Hill and Berry in 1986 was Dr. David Powell, a pediatric nephrologist and endocrinologist trained at the University of California, San Francisco and at Stanford University. "Dr. Powell did very basic bench research on the problem of growth failure in children with renal failure," said Hill, reflecting on Powell's subsequent contributions to Texas

Children's Hospital. "He published many papers and was a frequent invited speaker at national and international research meetings."[54]

Other newcomers to the service in the 1980s included two former Baylor College of Medicine renal fellows, Dr. Seth Kravitz and Dr. Myra Chiang, who came on board in 1988. That same year, Dr. Eileen Doyle Brewer, the former medical director of the Intermountain Pediatric and Adolescent Dialysis Unit at the University of Utah Medical Center in Salt Lake City, Utah, joined the service as director of the Texas Children's Hospital renal transplant program. When Berry subsequently left the service in 1991, Hill appointed Brewer as medical director of the newly named Dialysis and Transplant Center at Texas Children's Hospital.

Relieved of its responsibilities for the care of children with diabetes mellitus, the renal service at Texas Children's Hospital was able to concentrate its efforts on providing diagnosis, treatment, and follow-up care to infants, children, and adolescents with renal conditions and renal failure. These conditions included urinary tract infections, congenital renal disorders, hereditary renal disease, nephritis, renal tubular diseases, nephrotic syndrome, and cystic diseases, as well as patients with proteinuria and hematuria. Another area of responsibility was the management of children with hypertension, which usually was renal in origin during the first ten years of life. "In adults, hypertension is dealt with both in renal and nephrology and in cardiology," explained Hill. "In pediatrics, hypertension is handled by renal or nephrology."[55]

As these and other specific areas of responsibility in the subspecialty of pediatric nephrology at Texas Children's Hospital evolved, the terms 'renal' and 'nephrology' became interchangeable. Aware that this could be somewhat confusing to patients and their families, Brewer often explained: "The Seneca Indian name for kidney is 'okawehna,' the Latin name is 'ren,' the Greek name is 'nephros,' and the English name is 'kidney.' That is why a child comes to the renal clinic to see a pediatric nephrologist for his/her kidney problem."[56]

For those children who developed chronic kidney failure at Texas Children's Hospital, the renal service continued to improve its ongoing ESRD program. The 1980s had ushered in a new era of renal transplantation, and also saw sophisticated developments in the care and treatment of children with ESRD. In 1988, with improved techniques and immunosuppressive drugs such as cyclosporine, the five-year survival rate of transplanted kidneys increased to 90 percent and the patient survival rate approached 100 percent.[57]

"A kidney transplant is the best replacement treatment for all pediatric patients, including teenagers, but especially for growing children," Brewer said in 1992. "A successful kidney transplant is associated with improved physical, psychological, and social health compared to chronic dialysis in all pediatric age groups."[58]

Throughout the evolution of pediatric kidney transplantation, distinct differences from adult kidney transplantation emerged. In both, the source for suitable kidneys for transplants came from living donors and cadavers. Unlike in other solid organ transplants, donor kidneys for pediatric transplantation did not have to be age- and size-matched for pediatric recipients. "Adult kidneys are actually preferable in pediatric transplantation," Brewer said, explaining how a large donor kidney shrinks to adapt to its workload in a child. "A living, related donor can be a healthy parent or grandparent. Children do better with a living, related kidney rather than a cadaver donor kidney transplant."[59]

Concurrent with surgical advances in transplantation were developments in pediatric dialysis modalities. "Pediatric dialysis became more available after the program was developed for adults," Brewer explained. "You have to develop a program for adults, and then you have to redesign the equipment to fit children. So, we had to bastardize and jerry-rig the equipment until we got the equipment that fits children. Advances are being made now because technology caught up with the pediatric market, and we have the needed equipment."[60]

While peritoneal dialysis continued to be the preferred treatment for children at the Dialysis and Transplant Center at Texas Children's Hospital, hemodialysis became a viable alternative following the implementation of improved hemodialysis equipment for children. After tailoring the artificial kidney and adult protocols for hemodialysis treatment to the size of pediatric patients, pediatric hemodialysis was a more efficient treatment—but it required three-to-four-hour sessions, three times a week. Far more convenient for the children and their parents was home peritoneal dialysis, an option introduced at Texas Children's Hospital in the early 1980s.

In order to perform home peritoneal dialysis, parents and children underwent a two-week course with the home-training nurses before they could begin treatments at home with an automated dialysis machine. With 24-hour telephone support from the renal service doctors and nurses, home peritoneal dialysis could take place at any time of the day or night. "These parents and children usually choose to receive dialysis at night so that their days can be free for school or play," Berry said. "They are seen monthly in the renal clinic by members of the ESRD team and have to perform demonstrations of their dialysis skills. Since dietary and psychosocial support are extremely important aspects of the ESRD program, each visit also includes a talk with the renal service dietitian and a representative from social services. It takes a great team effort to keep these children healthy and happy on home dialysis."[61]

An integral member of the team since the late 1970s, nephrology nurse Helen Currier was a clinical specialist in renal dialysis. Having helped recruit and train new nurses for the expanding transplant and dialysis center during the 1980s, she took great pride in her active participation in the center's growth from the original two stations in 1979 to eight in 1988. With 20 chronic dialysis patients and six full-time nurses in 1988, the nursing expertise in the various techniques of dialysis gained a reputation for excellence that led other hospitals to send nurses to Texas Children's Hospital for pediatric dialysis training. "The Texas Children's renal dialysis unit is seen as a leader in pediatric renal issues," Currier said. "Our team is very dynamic and recognized worldwide because of the expertise and research that result from our program."[62]

Research efforts by the renal service at Texas Children's Hospital in the 1980s were inspired by the recent medical and technical advances in dialysis and transplantation. New areas of research included efforts to understand the complications of kidney failure in children and how those complications could be prevented or treated. Having learned much during their clinical efforts to care for children with kidney failure, Berry and Hill knew that the rarity of the disease required collaboration on studies involving a larger group of children with renal disease.

To achieve this goal, the two represented Texas Children's Hospital as charter members of the Southwest Pediatric Nephrology Study Group (SPNSG) in 1980.[63] In collaboration with the University of California, San Francisco and supported by the National Institutes of Health, SPNSG embarked on a long-term study of infants with kidney failure. Further studies included protocols on nephrotic syndrome, chronic renal failure, and dialysis, among others. Within the first few years of operation, the focus of this collaborate effort on the natural history of renal diseases in children was instrumental in providing the basis for the development of therapeutic protocols.[64]

Patients at Texas Children's Hospital participated in one such collaborative study to determine the effect that thorough and aggressive management of kidney failure had on common complications of the disease, particularly growth retardation. "When the kidneys fail, children appear to utilize their own growth hormone poorly and do not grow well," Brewer said, indicating why most children with kidney failure are much shorter than other children their own age. "We may soon be able to 'normalize' growth in children with kidney failure because of recent discoveries about growth hormone."[65]

As clinical and laboratory research in the subspecialty of pediatric nephrology progressed, vast differences emerged between ESRD treatment programs for children and those for adults. "Only about 25 percent of children with ESRD are on dialysis, whereas the vast majority of adults are on dialysis," Brewer explained. "Seventy percent of children with end-stage renal disease have transplants as opposed to adults, where it is about 15 to 20 percent, so it's kind of flipped. We look to transplant everybody, because that's a normal way of life, but you don't stop there. If your transplant fails, you go back to dialysis. You can live on dialysis for years. There are some adults now who started dialysis as children who are still alive."[66]

For those children who required chronic dialysis in 1991, Texas Children's Hospital expanded its Renal Dialysis Unit. Originally envisioned by Berry and Hill in the early 1980s and constantly updated before completion, the state-of-the-art center contained ten dialysis stations and was located in the newly constructed West Tower. The number of patients exceeded expectations. Throughout the 1990s, an average of 50 patients received maintenance dialysis, with an estimated 15 new patients initiating treatment annually. Approximately half of these patients—representing more than 850 hemodialysis treatments per month—came into the hospital for treatment. The other patients received home peritoneal dialysis, an average of 750 to 900 treatments monthly.

With an average of ten kidney transplants performed annually since 1988, by 1994 the renal service at Texas Children's Hospital was on its way to becoming one of the largest and busiest of its kind in the nation. Within the field of pediatric nephrology, Texas Children's Hospital continued to gain recognition for its contributions and Hill was an established leader, serving as chairman of the section on nephrology of the American Academy of Pediatrics from 1987 to 1990. After more than three decades of shepherding the steady growth of the renal service at Texas Children's Hospital, he relinquished his responsibilities to become assistant dean in charge of the office of admissions at Baylor College of Medicine. "Dr. Feigin was becoming dean of education in 1994 and wanted me to go over with him to head the admissions office," recalled Hill. "When I stepped down as chief, I just stayed in the renal section and contributed as much as I could, but I was pretty busy with the admissions at Baylor."[67]

Named chief of the renal service at Texas Children's Hospital in 1994, Brewer assumed leadership of a service dedicated to the comprehensive level of care needed by a child or adolescent with renal disease. "The all-inclusive care we provide helps children and their families better manage the stresses of daily life associated with children who have chronic renal disease," she said. "I believe children and adolescents are better cared for in a pediatric facility designed to meet their specialized needs, both physical and emotional. The appropriate environment greatly improves their outlook for recovery and, in turn, enables us to focus on successful medical outcomes. In order for medicine to advance, we've got to accept change. New ideas and openness to change are two critical ingredients for viable progress."[68]

One therapeutic innovation introduced in the late 1990s was not medical in nature, but proved to be just as effective. It was the introduction of Rena Dee, a 16-inch doll with a dialysis diary designed and created by Currier and a child life specialist. A companion for dialysis patients at Texas Children's Hospital, Rena Dee also traveled to hospitals in England, Virginia, New York, Indiana, California, Missouri, and elsewhere in Texas. Children undergoing dialysis at these hospitals signed their names, wrote notes in Rena Dee's diary, and included their own pictures, souvenirs, and mementos. When the doll was returned to Texas Children's Hospital after each trip, dialysis patients eagerly read each entry in her diary. "Our hope is that Rena Dee will be able to serve as an extended support network for children all over the world on dialysis," Currier said. "Young patients who do not have access to peer support can now connect with other kids going through similar experiences."[69]

For Currier, a clinical specialist in dialysis for more than two decades at Texas Children's Hospital, Rena Dee became symbolic of the rewarding experience gained by working with patients, families, and nursing staff in the Renal Dialysis Unit. "I love working with people who have a great attitude, who say, 'We can do anything, and will try anything, if it makes kids feel better,'" she said. "That's why we are all here."[70]

Sharing this compassionate concern was a professional staff of seven pediatric nephrologists, including Brewer, Hill, Dr. Ewa Elenberg, Dr. Rita D. Sheth, Dr. Daniel I. Feig, Dr. Arundhati S. Kale, and Dr. Stuart L. Goldstein, who became medical director of the Renal Dialysis Unit in 2002. The growing size of the renal service throughout the late 1990s was in direct proportion to the increased number of patients treated. The cumulative results of this established pattern was evident in 2003, when outpatient visits totaled 3,593 and inpatients numbered 284.

With a total of 183 kidney transplants since 1988, Texas Children's Hospital continued to maintain the best pediatric graft survival rate in Texas, treating more than 97 post-transplant patients in 2003. Significant increases occurred in number of dialysis treatments in 2003. More than 67 patients underwent dialysis and the number of treatments exceeded 14,213, representing a 65 percent increase over the number treated in 2000. Included in this figure was a 90 percent increase in home peritoneal dialysis and a 25 percent increase in hemodialysis performed in the unit. Statistics also indicated that Texas Children's Hospital cared for more than one-third of all the children on dialysis in Texas.

This significant increase in dialysis treatments at Texas Children's Hospital reflected the 2002 opening of the new Renal Dialysis Unit. Under the medical direction of Goldstein, the state-of-the-art facility, located on the eighth floor of the newly constructed West Tower, contained 14 dialysis stations and was staffed by 13 certified nephrology nurses. By 2003, the renal dialysis unit also included a pheresis service boasting the latest generation of technology for that process, resulting in more than 234 treatments in its first year. A process of separating unwanted cells or components from a patient's blood and returning the desired components, along with replacement fluids, pheresis treatment was provided by the renal dialysis team. Treatments included plasma exchange for patients with immunological disorders, red cell exchange for patients with sickle cell disease, white cell depletion for patients with leukemia, and stem cell collection for patients in need of a bone marrow transplant. Medical director Dr. Jun Teruya, who partnered with Goldstein and Currier to establish the unit, noted that patients had previously been referred to other facilities to receive this treatment.[71]

For these patients, and all others treated in the Renal Dialysis Unit and throughout Texas Children's Hospital, the renal service team also included two child life specialists and three social workers to help patients and their families cope with the special challenges brought on by chronic illness. "Texas Children's Renal Dialysis Unit is one of the most highly respected in the nation," Goldstein said. "This results from the unique collaborative spirit of the nephrologists, surgeons, nurses, social workers, and child life specialists who care for children receiving dialysis, as well as the numerous cutting-edge medical and nursing research papers generated by the renal dialysis staff."[72]

One major area of research in the 1990s focused on emerging practice patterns involving supportive therapies of critically ill children with acute renal failure at Texas Children's Hospital. Because pediatric patients with acute renal failure required special considerations not commonly encountered in the care of adult patients, Goldstein began efforts to assess both the origins of acute renal failure in children and the outcomes of different renal replacement therapies.

"Pediatric acute renal failure most often results from complications of other systemic diseases, resulting from advancements in congenital heart surgery, neonatal care, and bone marrow and solid organ transplantation," Goldstein said. "In addition, renal replacement therapy modality preferences to treat critically ill children have shifted from peritoneal dialysis to continuous renal replacement therapy (CRRT) as a result of improvements in CRRT technologies."[73]

More than 200 patients in the cardiovascular intensive care unit, pediatric intensive care, and neonatal intensive care stations received CRRT treatment at Texas Children's Hospital in 2003. In addition, more than 300 critically ill patients throughout the hospital received peritoneal dialysis and another 100 to 150 patients received hemodialysis for acute renal failure. Although a significant number of patients were treated for acute renal failure at Texas Children's Hospital, significantly more were needed in order to establish the reliable research criteria required by Goldstein. "No single pediatric center cares for enough CRRT patients annually to analyze the effect of more than a few variables on patient outcome," Goldstein said, explaining his motivation to instigate the formation of a collaborative research effort. "Since January 2001, the Prospective Pediatric CRRT Registry Group has been collecting data from multiple United States pediatric centers to obtain demographic data regarding pediatric patients who receive CRRT, assess the effect of different CRRT prescriptions on circuit function, and evaluate the impact of clinical variables on outcome."[74]

Goldstein's collaborative efforts were not singular in the renal service at Texas Children's Hospital. To focus on various aspects of clinical research in pediatric nephrology, members of the renal service team participated in several other multicenter study groups. A charter member and an associate director of the SPNSG, Brewer also was a member of the Pediatric Peritoneal Dialysis Study Consortium and the North American Pediatric Renal Transplantation Cooperative Study. Having served as president of the American Society of Pediatric Nephrology in 1997–98 and as an elected member to the council of the International Pediatric Nephrology Association, Brewer played a key role in the enrichment of the discipline's research portfolio.

As the knowledge base in pediatric nephrology continued to expand, the renal service at Texas Children's Hospital integrated each new finding to support strong improvements in patient care. With all the medical and technical advances achieved in pediatric nephrology, much had changed in the five-decade history of the renal service at Texas Children's Hospital.

What remained the same throughout its existence was its focus on providing loving care to children with renal diseases at Texas Children's Hospital.

F rom the age of five months to weeks before her second birthday, Emma Grace Hutchinson and her around-the-clock nurses lived in the Hutchinson family's converted living room, surrounded by dialysis machines and equipment.

Because she was immunosuppressed, Emma was not allowed the usual social life of an infant. Careful not to expose her to germs, the Hutchinsons limited Emma's interaction with others, including family members and close friends with the sniffles. "Our very closest friends here had a daughter who was born right before Emma, and we thought they would be the best of friends as they grew up together," Paula said. "We just couldn't be around them, or anybody else for that matter."[75]

This rule of virtual isolation did not apply to Emma's maternal grandmother, Jane Krumboltz, who lived in San Antonio. During Emma's long stays at Texas Children's Hospital following her birth, Jane virtually moved to Houston to help take care of seven-year-old Ashlyn while her parents were not at home. Whenever Emma needed a blood transfusion, a chronic necessity for patients on dialysis, Jane donated hers, routinely alternating as a donor with a nearby neighbor of the Hutchinsons.

"We were just rocking along," said Paula of her family's restructured lifestyle and daily routine. "Emma had to have a couple of hernia surgeries because of abdominal swelling, a common problem with peritoneal dialysis, and a couple of surgeries to reposition the catheter. She continued to thrive, and we just thought life was incredible."[76]

Like most pediatric patients on chronic dialysis, Emma did not grow as rapidly as did other children. During weekly visits to the renal clinic at Texas Children's Hospital, the renal team measured her progress. By the time she was one and a half years old, in October 1989, Emma had finally reached the desired weight of ten kilos, qualifying her for a kidney transplant through the transplant service at Texas Children's Hospital. Before the search for an appropriate donor had officially begun, there was an unexpected volunteer. "From the minute I heard the word 'transplant,' I thought 'Me! Me!'" her grandmother said. "My age, 60, was against me and the fact I had had a heart problem several years ago was another negative factor. But, oh, I prayed they would let me do it."[77]

Jane's enthusiasm was welcomed, but not shared by Paula and John or by the members of the renal team at Texas Children's Hospital. "We kind of laughed and thought it was funny," said Paula. Although she was not surprised by her mother's willingness to donate a kidney, Paula believed that she should not take the risk. "We had a tremendous number of people in our family who said, 'I want to be on the list,'" she said, noting how one by one they became ineligible during a battery of screening tests.[78]

The one person who remained on the list was Jane, whose test results continually surprised the doctors. Another battery of tests followed in which Jane was X-rayed, fluoroscoped, and even psychoanalyzed to determine unequivocally that she was the perfect donor. "They tested parts I didn't know I had," the grandmother exclaimed. "Each time they'd come back shaking their heads, saying I'd passed. I headed into that operating room with pure joy."[79]

The transplant procedure took place on March 7, 1990. The night before, both Emma and her grandmother were admitted as patients to Texas Children's Hospital. On the morning of the surgery, Jane's procedure came first. Refusing the wheelchair provided for her transportation, she happily marched into the operating room. Two hours later, the surgeon began the intricate process of implanting Jane's kidney in Emma. Both procedures totaled more than four hours of anxious waiting for the Hutchinsons. "I can't remember what I felt like, or what I was thinking," said Paula. "Emma had so many incredible things happen in her favor and you vacillate between thinking this is the next miracle or have we had all of our miracles? It was just unbelievable when the transplant coordinator excitedly told us that the transplant was successful. By the time Mom woke up from her anesthesia we knew that her kidney was functioning in Emma and it was the first news she heard."[80]

Having been "split from stem to stern" in surgery, Jane found that her recovery was not as swift as that of her granddaughter. It would be several days before she was able to see Emma again, a much-anticipated event that drew a crowd. This time Jane accepted the offer of a wheelchair. She regally rolled into Emma's room with a crown on her head and a scepter in her hand, accoutrements provided by her grateful family. As the Hutchinsons, their relatives, nurses, and members of the renal team shared Jane's tears of joy, two-year-old Emma was otherwise engaged. Instead of partaking in the festivities, she was voraciously consuming a meal of green beans, the first solid food she had ever eaten.

Post-transplant recovery for Emma was noteworthy in that she did not have a single rejection episode. Prepared for such a complication by the renal team at Texas Children's Hospital, Paula and John waited and waited. But it never happened. "She was back in the hospital with some complications for a week or so, but otherwise it was a remarkably good recovery," Paula said. "Mom had a much more difficult recovery than Emma did."[81]

Paula continued to be overwhelmed by her mother's generosity: "What she did was not something anyone could ask another person to do. She wanted to do it so much, but it was a tough thing to decide to let her risk. It was the most loving gift anyone could ever give."[82]

"I don't feel that I gave; I feel like I received," said Jane, who fully recovered and returned to San Antonio. When reminiscing about how her initial attempts to be Emma's donor were dismissed as foolish, she was particularly proud to have won over the renal team at Texas Children's Hospital—especially pediatric nephrologist Berry. "Jane," she recalled his telling her after the transplant, "that's some kidney."[83]

Following the one-year anniversary of Emma's transplant in 1991, the Hutchinsons were distraught to learn that Berry was leaving Texas Children's Hospital. "We were devastated," said Paula. "We thought we can't deal without him, but the next miracle that came into our life was Dr. Eileen Brewer. We know how fortunate we are that she's right here at Texas Children's. She's not just book smart; she's people smart. She knows how to deal with patients, and she knows how to deal with their families. She trusts her patients. She is just incredible, and we would follow her to the ends of the earth to keep her as Emma's doctor."[84]

For the next 13 years, Emma had monthly appointments with Brewer in the renal clinic at Texas Children's Hospital. Although she continued to have complex medical problems and life-threatening complications, most were attributed to ARPKD and none were related to the kidney transplant. "Dr. Brewer is awesome," Emma said. "She includes my parents and me in on all the decisions so we all know what is going on. She has known me for so long that she can usually know just what to do. I know that one day I will have to get a new kidney, but I also feel the second time will be a lot smoother. Texas Children's Hospital has been a great hospital to be a patient at and I feel safe there even when I am nervous."

As a teenager, Emma had no memory of her struggle for life as an infant, or of the kidney transplant she had endured when she was two— even though she had the scars to prove it. "Sometimes it seems like some dream, it isn't real to me," she said. "I am very grateful that it happened while I was so young so that I didn't miss out on school or the rest of my life. I always feel special knowing that part of my grandmother is inside me. She and I have been the closest buddies ever since the transplant. We do things together all the time and whenever I am sick, she hops on a plane and rides over here to see me."[85]

Emma's exceptional triumphs over the odds were vividly remembered by her grandmother, mother, father, and sister, who would never forget their remarkable experiences at Texas Children's Hospital. "We can't imagine being at any other hospital in the world," Paula said. "We owe everything to the doctors and the nurses who have done so much for Emma and taken care of us as well."[86]

27

⚘ RHEUMATOLOGY ⚘

S EVEN-YEAR-OLD PAMELA STOKES could not bend the middle finger on her left hand.

Her mother, Shirley Stokes, noticed that Pamela was also walking with a limp. She took the child to a doctor, but was not overly concerned. "When your daughter's only seven years old, you never think that anything serious could be wrong with her," she explained.[1]

The sudden realization that serious illness knew no age came to both mother and daughter at the office of Louisiana pediatrician Dr. Patsy Phelps. After examining Pamela's swollen and painful joints, Phelps immediately recognized the symptoms of the chronic inflammatory disease known as juvenile rheumatoid arthritis. "That was in 1964, and a lot of people were not familiar with arthritis in children then," Pamela recalled. "But Dr. Phelps was well-read and she diagnosed it."[2]

This immediate and accurate diagnosis of Pamela's condition was unusual in the 1960s. Juvenile rheumatoid arthritis was thought to be rare at that time, and many health professionals did not even recognize the symptoms. Over the next four decades, juvenile rheumatoid arthritis would become known as the most common form of juvenile arthritis, a rheumatic disease affecting more than 285,000 children in the United States.[3]

Phelps referred Pamela to Children's Hospital in New Orleans, where she received two months of treatment. After returning home, she underwent cortisone and paraffin treatments. She tried to rejuvenate her tired muscles and relieve her sore joints in the whirlpool equipment purchased by her parents. For Pamela, that first year following her diagnosis was "pretty bad," she recalled.[4]

What happened next surprised everyone—most of all, Pamela.

Inexplicably, the symptoms disappeared. "It was the weirdest thing," she said. "All of a sudden, it just went away. I had no symptoms whatsoever from age eight to about age 12. I could run, jump, and play as I did before the onset of the arthritis."

Such joyous activities would not last. "When I was about 12 or 13, it came back," Pamela said. "And when it came back, it came back worse. The pain was excruciating. The slightest movement in bed sent waves of pain throughout my body. It was all over my body. Every joint was affected; I couldn't move."

Wheelchair bound by age 14, Pamela struggled to maintain her studies and remain in school. Suffering from inflamed joints and in severe pain, she was forced to stay home from school. For a while, tutors came to the house. "I couldn't walk. I couldn't get up. It had gotten to the point that I couldn't even take care of my personal hygiene. It was like I couldn't do anything," she remembered. "So Dr. Phelps, this same doctor, the same pediatrician who was taking care of me all these years, found out about Texas Children's Hospital. That's how I came here—it was through her efforts."

Phelps had read medical journal articles about the pioneering studies and research work of Texas Children's Hospital pediatric rheumatologist Dr. Earl J. Brewer, Jr., and Houston orthopedist Dr. W. Malcolm Granberry. Hoping to find some relief to Pamela's suffering, the Stokes family made an appointment, packed up the car, and traveled west for the first of many such trips to Texas Children's Hospital.

Pamela's first meeting with Brewer marked the beginning of months of diagnostic testing, an endless variety of medications, and extensive therapy. She and her parents drove back and forth between Louisiana and Texas, meeting with Brewer and Granberry both before and after each treatment from the various members of their medical team. "They discussed my case, and then I went through therapy," Pamela remembered. "It wasn't getting any better. I was on many different medicines. Some worked, some didn't, and some made me sick."

Nothing provided relief from the pain, and Pamela remained in a wheelchair. Brewer and Granberry discussed the possibility of knee and hip replacements. Since a hip replacement would be one of the first such operations on a teenage patient, Pamela was told to think long and hard about undergoing the surgery. The decision was hers to make, the doctors said. Pamela immediately embraced the idea and chose to have the surgery. "It was hope, a light at the end of my dark tunnel," she said. "It was getting out of the wheelchair and being able to function."

Even though her physical therapist disagreed with her decision to undergo surgery, Pamela was adamant. "I knew my body, and I knew I was in pain, and something had to be done about it," she said. "I think the therapist didn't feel as though I was in that much pain, but I was."

Also skeptical about Pamela's surgery were her parents. In spite of their initial hesitation and some conflicting recommendations from medical professionals elsewhere, they finally agreed to authorize the procedure at Texas Children's Hospital. As an added precaution before undertaking such a drastic course of treatment, Pamela's medical team asked Dr. Richard Pesikoff, a child psychiatrist, to meet and talk with Pamela on several occasions. "He came to visit me a couple of times, just to talk with me. I guess to see how I felt about it, to see if I really was in pain, or if I was putting on," Pamela recalled. "The conclusion was: 'This girl's in pain.'"

With that unassailable confirmation, the surgeries were scheduled and 16-year-old Pamela, along with her mother and her beloved Snoopy doll, checked into Texas Children's Hospital. Granberry replaced Pamela's right hip on October 1, 1973, and her right knee two weeks later. After allowing Pamela time to recuperate at home in Louisiana, Granberry replaced her left hip on January 11, 1974, and her left knee on January 28.[5] "I was afraid," Pamela said. "Of course, I think that's just normal and natural. I didn't like being put to sleep; I didn't like that feeling. I was aware of everything that was going to happen, but still, that doesn't take away the fear, but I remember reading from the Book of Psalms in the Bible the night before the surgery, and that did calm my fears."

Pamela's mother was at Texas Children's Hospital with her at all times, sleeping on the little couch in her room, helping her down the halls as she tried to walk with a walker, and assisting her in therapy. The therapists "showed my mom how to help me, and she did a lot of it," Pamela recalled. "The hips were not as painful as the knees were in the therapy. I did my share of screaming. I became discouraged many times."

Through the long days of painful exercise and frustrating rehabilitation that followed her four surgeries, Pamela persevered. "You've got to do it," she said. "You've got to do one step at a time before you can walk." As an incentive, Pamela's father, John Stokes, promised to give her a $100 shopping spree when she learned to walk again. After achieving that goal, she enjoyed her reward at the Houston Galleria. Nurse Sonia Lucky took the day off from Texas Children's Hospital to accompany Pamela and her mother on the adventure.

Such special attention from one of her caregivers was not unusual,

Pamela remembered. Since all the nurses she knew at Texas Children's Hospital were so personable, she felt like they were her friends. "They made me feel comfortable," she said. "I felt like they were concerned about me. It wasn't just a job to them. It felt like family. They took my mom out to eat. In fact, one of them took her to her house to have supper."[6]

With fond memories of the unexpectedly happy moments that surrounded her surgeries at Texas Children's Hospital, Pamela returned to Louisiana to begin months of physical therapy. Although mostly still confined to her wheelchair, she vowed to walk away from it in the very near future.

The beginning moments of the rheumatology service at Texas Children's Hospital were memorable ones.

"I started my work in rheumatology in a converted bathroom at Texas Children's Hospital in 1958," recalled Dr. Earl J. Brewer, Jr., the hospital's first pediatric rheumatologist. "I ended 30 years later with a rheumatology division comprised of three full-time rheumatologists, four postdoctoral fellows, a research epidemiologist, and a coordinated health team of five health professionals."[7]

Brewer's accomplishments had not gone unnoticed in the emerging field of pediatric rheumatology or at Texas Children's Hospital. "It's really quite fascinating to see how something that started quite small has really developed into a unit that is known all over the United States, really all over the world," said Dr. Russell J. Blattner, Texas Children's Hospital's first physician-in-chief and chief of pediatrics at Baylor College of Medicine.

It was Blattner who assisted Brewer in his early efforts to establish a rheumatology service at Texas Children's Hospital. Searching for space, the two decided to commandeer a bathroom so that they would have the plumbing necessary for the physical therapy equipment. "Dr. Blattner and I looked for a place to put it," Brewer recalled. "We had a yardstick and Mr. Newell France, the hospital's administrator, in tow, and we went into the lady's bathroom at the end of the hall. Leopold Meyer, the president of the hospital's board of trustees, had that bathroom as a fixation. He correctly regarded it as unused, wasted space."

Brewer soon discovered that the space might be wasted, but it indeed was used. "When we were in there measuring, Mrs. Helga Smithson, the hospital's personnel director, apparently was in there, too," Brewer said with a laugh. "She was afraid we were going to measure her cubicle. Then it also happened later that when the three of us were trying to measure it again. By that time, she didn't scream anymore."[8]

Once the space had been appropriated, "Dr. Brewer took the water supply, which was in there, and actually made a very functional physiotherapy unit with all the baths and the Jacuzzi-like things," Blattner remembered.[9]

Converting old ideas into new and better ones became one of Brewer's legacies at Texas Children's Hospital. A 1954 graduate of Baylor College of Medicine, Brewer served his residency at Texas Children's Hospital from 1955 to 1956 before spending a year at Harvard Medical School. He returned to Texas Children's Hospital as chief resident from 1957 to 1958. "At that time, Dr. Blattner had an exchange program with Harvard because the pediatrics program at Baylor College of Medicine was young and he needed the prestige of associating with that institution," Brewer said. "Also, it gave him a way to fulfill his plan to staff his department at the hospital. I think he will never be recognized for it, but I'll recognize him for it. He early on picked bright, young people, sent them away, nurtured their training, and then brought them back to his department. It was the pivotal event in the hospital's history—instead of bringing in, he picked out. The man had a great vision, and an effective one."

Blattner's vision required the financial support provided by fellowship funds. "Through the good offices of Mr. Jesse H. Jones and with the help of Baylor College of Medicine's dean Moursund, we succeeded in getting a Jesse Jones grant to create the Jesse H. Jones and Mary Gibbs Jones Fellowships," Blattner recalled. "We could use this money to give scholarships to qualified medical students, but we used it very effectively in supplementing the travel expenses for members of our house staff to go to Children's Hospital Boston and other hospitals to get specialty training."

Blattner secured one of these scholarships for Brewer, making arrangements for him to work as a Jesse H. Jones fellow with renowned immunologist Dr. Charles A. Janeway, chief of pediatrics at Harvard Medical School. He made similar arrangements at other prestigious hospitals for Baylor College of Medicine graduates in cancer chemotherapy, hematology, neurology, infectious disease, and neonatology. "By using this system, we began to develop our own likely candidates in subspecialties," Blattner explained. "They returned to Texas and established some of the subspecialty facilities which we are now enjoying at the present day. In a sense, the department of pediatrics in Houston, through our selection of these training opportunities, in a sense, inherited the best background from a number of medical centers in the United States."[10]

Living proof of Blattner's theory was Brewer, who returned to Texas

Children's Hospital with newfound knowledge about the care of patients with juvenile rheumatoid arthritis (JRA). "When I was at Harvard as a senior assistant resident at Children's Hospital Boston, we met with Dr. Janeway every Monday morning," he said. "He always was very concerned about the kids over at the House of the Good Samaritan, which was the rheumatic fever institution where a lot of the work in rheumatic fever was done. And they also had the children with arthritis over there. They just kept them there in bed and Dr. Janeway was most distressed about that. He thought what was being done was not proper, so he assigned me to look at all the records of children with rheumatoid arthritis at Children's Hospital, get some sort of an idea of what might be done, and publish it. I reviewed the records and the records were so bad—'Johnny was OK today. Johnny was bad today.'— nothing of medical importance could be published from the data."[11]

After returning to Texas Children Hospital, Brewer told Blattner what he had seen at the House of the Good Samaritan and at Children's Hospital Boston. They discussed Janeway's concern about the totally inadequate care given to arthritic children and the fact that nobody was doing anything about it. "I agree with Dr. Janeway," Blattner told Brewer. "Why don't we establish an arthritis clinic?"

That suggestion resulted in the creation of the arthritis clinic in the Junior League Diagnostic Clinic of the outpatient department at Texas Children's Hospital. The reason for an outpatient clinic rather than an inpatient service was that Blattner and Brewer both believed that children with arthritis should stay at home, not be hospitalized "for months and months at a time where they would be confined to bed without exercise and would become contracted like pretzels."[12]

In the years after he inaugurated his first physiotherapy facilities in Smithson's former restroom, Brewer concentrated on achieving his goals for pediatric rheumatology. "I just wanted to improve care for rheumatic diseases in children," he explained. "Not just for juvenile rheumatoid arthritis, but diseases that were similar, like lupus, polymyositis, dermatomyositis, scleroderma, infectious arthritis, serum sickness, and rheumatic fever."

Brewer's mission to improve the treatment and care of pediatric patients with rheumatic diseases was not limited to Texas Children's Hospital. At a rheumatology conference at Vanderbilt University in 1959, the young and self-assured Brewer publicly challenged the practice of prescribing bed rest for JRA patients. The list of attendees read like a "Who's Who" of rheumatology and included Dr. Joseph Bunim, the director of the National Institutes of Health (NIH) and the head of the Arthritis Institute, and Dr. William Clark, the medical director of the National Foundation-March of Dimes. Participants at the conference, which Blattner had helped organize, compared treatment options and debated whether or not a portion of limited research and treatment funds should be diverted from adults to children.

Brewer was the only pediatrician in attendance. Arguing against extended bed rest for JRA patients, he suggested that range-of-motion exercises, together with appropriate anti-inflammatory medicines, held greater promise. He also urged that more funds be allocated to pediatric arthritis research that might, one day, lead to improved treatments and even a cure for JRA.

Those opposed to diverting funds from adults to children regarded pediatric rheumatoid arthritis patients as "medical curiosities, because they thought there were so few of them," Brewer said. He suggested that the reason his colleagues saw few pediatric rheumatoid arthritis patients was because rheumatoid arthritis was frequently misdiagnosed. And, when the disease was diagnosed correctly, the treatments available at the time were unworthy of the term. Brewer concluded his remarks by saying, "Like anything where no services are available, people don't come."

Unable to convert others to his theory of home care, Brewer set out to prove this premise at Texas Children's Hospital. Soon after the Vanderbilt conference, he and Elizabeth Barkley, the first physical therapist in the rheumatology service, developed a focused program emphasizing exercise, good nutrition, and adequate rest—the time-tested basics of good health—for their young patients. "Elizabeth Barkley, one of the outstanding physical therapists in the state, was very interested in what we were trying to do. She, as much as anyone, taught me about children and exercise and muscles," Brewer said. "And we just developed the whole thing together."

Their innovative program encouraged patients to undertake active exercise programs that would increase their strength, endurance, and flexibility, thereby allowing them to remain ambulatory and stay in school. Central to this program of exercise was the idea that it was best done at home on a regular basis. Parents were educated about what to do to help their children. In 1964, the program was detailed in the booklet *Home Care of the Rheumatoid Arthritis Patient*. Known as "the little orange book," for years the booklet was distributed to the parents of juvenile arthritis patients at Texas Children's Hospital.

Brewer and his associates were convinced that education was a valuable adjunct to their clinical work. The team produced manuals for parents in 1970 and 1976; published the first physician's reference book of its kind, *Juvenile Rheumatoid Arthritis*, in 1970; worked with the University of

Cincinnati to produce two 40-minute films on the diagnosis and management of arthritis in children in 1978; and fostered the development of a coloring book for patients featuring "Wonder Man and Mr. Bone" in 1981.[13]

In 1960, Blattner learned that the tremendous success achieved in the fight against polio was prompting the March of Dimes to find a new focus. He discovered that rheumatologist Dr. William Clark, medical director of the March of Dimes, was interested in working with children. Blattner seized the opportunity, suggesting that the organization direct its attention and support to children with JRA. To launch an aggressive attack on this rheumatic disease, Blattner proposed that the March of Dimes fund a special treatment center at Texas Children's Hospital. His request was honored and the special treatment center opened at Texas Children's Hospital in 1960. "What the March of Dimes gave us was a national presence and recognition, and it gave recognition nationally to children with arthritis," Brewer said. "Ours was the first special-treatment center."[14]

This national recognition helped Brewer play a key role in what he described as "inventing" pediatric rheumatology. In 1961, there was no such thing as a pediatric rheumatologist, even though that was exactly the title that Blattner had given to Brewer several years earlier. It would be 15 or 20 years before such a title was commonly understood, even in medical circles. Much of the credit for that recognition belongs to Brewer.

Asked to undertake the 1964 national effort to help develop pediatric rheumatology as a subspecialty, Brewer served as chairman of the American Rheumatism Association's criteria committee for children. He and his colleagues on the committee worked to formulate criteria that would help doctors accurately diagnose JRA and other rheumatic illnesses and identify the subgroups that vary in clinical course and response to treatment.[15] "The criteria developed and accepted by the American Rheumatism Association in 1972 is still the accepted criterion now," Brewer said in 1992, the year that pediatric rheumatology certification finally began.[16]

In the early 1970s, Brewer and a group of similarly interested and experienced pediatricians also developed a council to have a voice in the affairs of the American Rheumatism Association. A decade later, after he and other pediatric rheumatologists organized the rheumatology section of the American Academy of Pediatrics, Brewer was elected its founding chairman.

In 1972, Brewer founded the Pediatric Rheumatology Collaborative Study Group to identify safe and effective drugs for the treatment of children with arthritis. With Texas Children's Hospital as one of the major participants, the study group was an informal network of 22 academic, medical, and research institutions that conducted research and shared data. The project eventually led to the development of new drugs to treat a variety of rheumatic illnesses in children.

Funded by the Food and Drug Administration (FDA), the NIH, the Arthritis Foundation, and pharmaceutical companies, the study group was based at Texas Children's Hospital from the time of its founding until the late 1980s. In February 1978, after the group published its findings on tolmetin sodium (Tolectin), the FDA approved the non-steroidal anti-inflammatory drug for use by children with arthritis. It was the first drug since aspirin to be so approved.[17]

The study group examined more than 20 other rheumatoid arthritis drugs, developing a methodology that was eventually adopted by the FDA when it formulated its own guidelines for evaluating the safety and efficacy of pediatric drugs.[18] These pioneering efforts at Texas Children's Hospital came to the attention of federal officials at the Maternal and Child Health Bureau, part of the Department of Health and Human Services.

The Maternal and Child Health Bureau was charged by Congress with identifying the unmet medical needs of children and with doing whatever was necessary to address those needs. Years earlier, the bureau had provided leaders in the fields of pediatric cardiology, neonatology, cystic fibrosis, and others with grants under the Special Projects of Regional and National Significance (SPRANS) program to help establish and develop those pediatric subspecialties. When the bureau decided in 1980 that pediatric rheumatology services should be more widely accessible to those who needed them, bureau officials approached Brewer and offered him a $50,000 SPRANS grant to help fund his work in pediatric rheumatology at Texas Children's Hospital. It was the first such pediatric rheumatology grant ever awarded in the United States.

Just as Brewer's modest physical therapy center had begun in a bathroom and expanded into a clinic at the Junior League Outpatient Department at Texas Children's Hospital, that first grant eventually grew beyond expectations. Funding increased to approximately $1 million over the next few years. Brewer used this financial support to establish a program of family-centered and community-based coordinated care for children with rheumatic diseases at Texas Children's Hospital. He also established similar team-care outreach clinics for chronically ill children throughout Texas.

"You must have a focused team helping children with chronic illness, working together, coordinating and planning activities," Brewer explained. "This is why I conceived 'team care,' which includes the doctor, nurse, patient/family educator, nutritionist, social worker, and physical therapist/ occupational therapist. If you just tell the patient to go to the physical therapy department, you don't get a planned program on an ongoing basis. The success comes in assessing the improvement, not just giving a patient a program and pitching them out the door."

Success came for Brewer's efforts to achieve this model of team care at Texas Children's Hospital in the form of subsequent grants from various sources. With additional funds, he was able to fund basic research into the causes and treatment of juvenile arthritis, expand the concept of coordinated team care for all chronic illnesses, and develop subspecialty expertise at clinics across the state.[19]

In retrospect, the initial SPRANS grant of $50,000 had been crucial to the expansion of services for children with arthritis in a way that neither Brewer nor bureau officials could have imagined. Immediately following the 1980 awarding of the grant to Texas Children's Hospital, the assistant secretary of health contacted Vince Hutchins, the head of the bureau at the time, to discuss the decision. Questioning the value of funding pediatric rheumatology services, the bureaucrat felt that the subject was too esoteric and that the illness was too uncommon. The opposite reaction came from state officials, who called Hutchins to ask why juvenile arthritis researchers in their state had not been selected for a grant. The value of the work was established, and "Vince Hutchins told me that when he started getting calls from senators and governors, he knew we were on the right track," Brewer recalled.

Also attracting attention was the rheumatology clinic in the Junior League Outpatient Department at Texas Children's Hospital. A grant from the Fondren Foundation and another from Houston Endowment enabled the building of new and larger facilities to meet the growing demand for clinic services. Contributions also came from the Junior League of Houston, the Gulf Coast Chapter of the Arthritis Foundation, and many concerned citizens. Necessitated by a growing patient population—which numbered more than 500 children stricken with rheumatic diseases in the early 1970s—the expansion was completed in October 1974.

When festivities were being planned for the expanded rheumatology clinic's October 17, 1974, opening at Texas Children's Hospital, an invitation was issued to Texas Governor Dolph Briscoe, the "friend of a friend" of one of the clinic's patients. To nearly everyone's surprise and delight, the governor not only attended, but also agreed to speak. Briscoe used the opportunity to congratulate Texas Children's Hospital on the opening of its state-of-the-art facilities. He also reported on plans to mount a statewide effort to improve care for the more than one million arthritis sufferers in Texas.[20] "It just blew the hospital's mind," Brewer recalled. "Nobody else had the governor open up their offices."[21]

Returning the favor, Brewer served as chairman of the Governor's Conference on Arthritis in Austin during the following week. Praising Briscoe for his personal interest and for providing "a forward thrust at a time when we really need it," Brewer addressed the need for treatment centers. "Frankly, it's a disaster that many patients cannot get the treatment they need," he said. "One of our goals is to encourage more professionals to go into the field and also to attract supportive personnel."[22]

A year and a half later, Brewer was among the few pediatric rheumatology specialists in the United States who helped plan the first national conference to discuss rheumatic diseases in children. On the agenda of that conference held in Park City, Utah, in May 1976 was Houston orthopedist Dr. Malcolm Granberry, who had done pioneering studies with Brewer for more than 15 years. The published results of their studies in synovectomy and joint replacement in children and teenagers with arthritis were already well known in the field. The papers and discussions from the conference were published in *Arthritis and Rheumatism,* at last placing the concerns of pediatricians on the agenda of rheumatologists across the nation.

With this increased awareness of rheumatic diseases in children, pediatricians recognized the importance of early diagnosis. They began referring more and more patients to specialized centers for treatment. By 1976, the medical team in the rheumatology service at Texas Children's Hospital was seeing more than 150 patients with JRA annually and was treating more than 1,000 patients in follow-up programs.

In response to the growing demand for expertise in the field, Brewer established a two-year pediatric rheumatology fellowship program in 1979, one of the first in the United States. The first fellow was Dr. Robert W. Nickeson, Jr., who later became chief of pediatric rheumatology at the University of Florida and All Children's Hospital in St. Petersburg. After the second fellow, Dr. Karyl S. Barron, completed her training, she joined Brewer's expanding team at Texas Children's Hospital—as did the two subsequent fellows, Dr. Andrew P. Wilking and Dr. Daniel J. Lovell.

As the pediatric rheumatology service at Texas Children's Hospital continued to expand in the late 1970s, knowledge about juvenile arthritis was limited to the fact that it was similar to other chronic illnesses in children. Seemingly without geographic boundaries, JRA struck young people the world over. When the United States and the Soviet Union took their first tentative steps towards ending the Cold War in the early 1970s, scientific and medical exchanges were proposed as a way of demonstrating how greater cooperation might benefit both countries. The Soviets, aware that American and Soviet treatment approaches differed significantly, suggested an exchange of information on pediatric rheumatology. The NIH approached Brewer in 1975 and asked him to head the American side of a series of groundbreaking bilateral studies to assess treatment options for children with rheumatic diseases.[23] "Pediatric rheumatology has been a big thing in the Soviet Union," Brewer said. "It was Stalin's influence. Stalin's personal doctor, Professor Nestorov, was a rheumatologist who built an empire of rheumatology, and part of that empire was children's arthritis."

The first joint study undertaken by the Texas Children's Hospital rheumatology service and the Soviets was a relatively small-scale epidemiological study that compared American and Soviet children with JRA. Later joint studies evaluated an oral gold compound for its effectiveness in treating children with JRA and examined the effectiveness of so-called slower-acting antirheumatic drugs in treating children with rheumatic diseases in the two countries.

Although there was skepticism in the American medical community as to whether this collaboration with the Soviets would accomplish anything worthwhile, Brewer remained optimistic. When an October 1983 article in the *Houston Post* stated that "some of Dr. Brewer's colleagues contend he is whistling in the wind for trying to cooperate in clinical drug trials with Soviet medical peers," Brewer responded: "We've already learned a great deal from our mutual work."[24]

Validating Brewer's assessment was a landmark study conducted with the Soviets in the late 1980s. The results, which demonstrated conclusively that methotrexate was the most effective drug developed to date for treating children with severe rheumatoid arthritis, were published in the *New England Journal of Medicine* in 1992. Brewer stated that without the participation of many hundreds of children in the United States and the Soviet Union, these studies—which ended in the early 1990s—would have been impossible.[25]

In total agreement with Brewer was someone who had participated in the studies—Lovell, the former pediatric rheumatology fellow at Texas Children's Hospital. "Our knowledge of the treatment of severe arthritis in children has completely changed as a result of these studies," Lovell said. "They showed what works and what doesn't. They yielded important findings that improved the care young people in each country received."[26]

Brewer felt that one of the most important results of the Soviet/

American studies was more basic than most people realized. Although "the demonstration of the efficacy of methotrexate in JRA revolutionized pediatric rheumatology,"[27] as documented decades later, Brewer also believed that the unprecedented joint effort created a public awareness of the hundreds of thousands of children afflicted with various rheumatic illnesses. "We now have a better understanding of how many children in the world suffer from juvenile arthritis and other rheumatic diseases," he said.[28]

What already was known was that two-thirds of the 285,000 children with rheumatic disease in the United States had never had their disease diagnosed or treated by a pediatric rheumatologist.[29] Although pediatric rheumatic disease was relatively uncommon, the conditions collectively were the most common chronic illnesses in childhood and were known to cause considerable disease burden and disability. The general term for the more than 100 types of arthritis occurring in children was juvenile arthritis, a condition identified by the Arthritis Foundation as being more prevalent than juvenile diabetes and cerebral palsy. As one of the most common forms of juvenile arthritis, JRA consisted of three major types: polyarticular, affecting many joints; pauciarticular, pertaining to only a few joints; and systemic, affecting the entire body. Because the signs and symptoms of JRA varied from child to child and there was no single test that conclusively established a diagnosis of juvenile arthritis, an accurate diagnosis by a non-specialist was complicated and difficult to achieve.[30] Those children who had been accurately diagnosed required ongoing medical care, including physician visits, laboratory work, and physical and occupational therapy.[31]

For the afflicted children who were being treated by a specialist in pediatric rheumatology, the 1992 introduction of low-dose weekly methotrexate to effectively control inflammation was a milestone. Rather than developing significant disabilities from the debilitating joint disease, as in the past, most of these patients did not require surgical joint replacements, intensive rehabilitation for nonambulation, or serial casting or surgery for severe flexion contractures. This ability to medically control joint inflammation with a potent anti-inflammatory drug dramatically improved the outlook for affected children and ushered in a new era in the emerging field of pediatric rheumatology.[32]

The successful outcome of the joint methotrexate study with the Soviets also signaled the end of another era. Having achieved both his personal goals and those he had set for the pediatric rheumatology service at Texas Children's Hospital, Brewer resigned in 1986 in order to devote his time to special projects for the Maternal and Child Health Bureau and for surgeon general Dr. C. Everett Koop. Brewer also worked to develop family-to-family networks to provide support, information, and referrals for families with special needs children. Tapped to serve as cochairman of the 1987 Surgeon General's Conference in Houston, Brewer was among those in attendance who collectively issued the initial call to action for family-centered, community-based, coordinated care for children with special health needs.

Although that 1987 conference marked the debut of the phrase "family-centered care" in medicine, this concept was already a reality in the pediatric rheumatology service Brewer had created at Texas Children's Hospital. The service had grown to become one of the most active in the United States in terms of patient care and clinical and basic research. It included two pediatric rheumatologists, one full-time research associate, two pediatric rheumatology fellows, a drug study coordinator, and a physical therapist. Since the early 1980s, more than 750 patients with rheumatic and related musculoskeletal diseases had received treatment at Texas Children's Hospital.

Diseases of special interest to the pediatric rheumatologists at Texas Children's Hospital included JRA, systemic lupus erythematosus, poly/dermatomyositis, juvenile ankylosing spondylitis, scleroderma, polyarteritis nodosa, rheumatic fever, and a variety of lesser-known conditions. The clinical and basic research in pediatric rheumatology that began with the 1960 March of Dimes grant for the arthritis clinic at Texas Children's Hospital had evolved to become one of only three pediatric research centers for the Arthritis Foundation.

One area of research at Texas Children's Hospital in the 1980s included efforts to learn more about one of the lesser-known diseases, Kawasaki syndrome. Initially described in Japan in 1967 and reported in English in 1974, that distinct condition was identified as the primary cause of acquired heart disease in children in Japan and the United States. "It was thought to be a benign, self-limited febrile illness," said former fellow Barron, named interim chief of the pediatric rheumatology service at Texas Children's Hospital following Brewer's departure in 1986. "It is now known to be a systemic vasculitis occurring predominantly in small and medium-sized muscular arteries, especially the coronary arteries."[33]

Barron pursued her interest in Kawasaki disease throughout the 1980s and early 1990s, becoming the principal investigator for a nationwide collaborative study of intravenous immune globulin in the treatment of that disease. After relinquishing her responsibilities as interim chief of the pediatric rheumatology service in 1988, Barron became actively involved in immunogenetics and immunoregulation. Her work in those areas resulted in the identification of several genetic markers associated with disease susceptibility to both JRA and Kawasaki disease. With the introduction of these newer methods of genetic analysis, Barron was among the scientists who were beginning to cast a new light on the genetic contribution to JRA, Kawasaki disease, and other rheumatic diseases.[34]

When Barron stepped down in 1988, Dr. Robert W. Warren was named chief of the rheumatology service at Texas Children's Hospital and associate professor and chief of the rheumatology section in the department of pediatrics at Baylor College of Medicine. A summa cum laude graduate of Yale University in 1972, Warren earned a medical degree and a doctorate at Washington University in 1978. Following an internship, residency, clinical fellowship, and research fellowship at Duke University in Durham, North Carolina, Warren was named as first chief of the division of pediatric rheumatology and immunology at the University of North Carolina at Chapel Hill in 1983, remaining in that position for five years.

His 1988 arrival as chief of the pediatric rheumatology service at Texas Children's Hospital occurred during a time of transition in the emerging field of pediatric rheumatology. By the mid-1980s, many pharmaceutical companies had significantly reduced their financial support of basic rheumatology research. The decision was based on their belief that the potential market for their drugs was not large enough to justify awarding millions of dollars in research grants every year to academic and medical institutions.

Texas Children's Hospital continued to participate in the Pediatric Rheumatology Collaborative Study Group begun by Brewer. In 1990, however, the study group's chairman, Lovell, and its senior scientist and epidemiologist, Dr. Ed Giannini, moved its headquarters from Texas Children's Hospital to the University of Cincinnati. In the following two decades, the group remained well organized and active, conducting and publishing "a number of important studies on the use of antirheumatic agents in children."[35]

What did continue at Texas Children's Hospital after Warren's arrival were numerous research efforts in pediatric rheumatology, including multiple clinical studies particularly concentrating on the effectiveness of intraarticular steroids in controlling arthritis in children with JRA. Collaborating with Warren in a 1990 study of the role rheumatoid factors play in the pathophysiology of systemic lupus erythematosis (SLE) was the newly arrived Dr. Loren Peterson. Throughout the following decade, Peterson would continue his interest in SLE.

Concentrated efforts to improve medical education began when former fellow Wilking joined the pediatric rheumatology service at Texas Children's

Hospital in the 1980s. Stressing the importance of concepts and imagination over facts, and believing in the value of personal and informal interaction with medical students, Wilking excelled. He received an Educator Leadership Award and a Teaching and Leadership Award at Baylor College of Medicine.

In addition to medical education, Wilking was also committed to providing effective outreach clinic services. A volunteer pediatric rheumatologist at Shriners Hospital for Children in the Texas Medical Center, he conducted clinics twice a month to treat children who sometimes traveled from as far away as Mexico. Easily recognizable to patients by his six-foot, five-inch height and trademark bow tie, Wilking would consult more than 5,000 appointments at Shriners during the following 14 years. "Dr. Wilking's volunteer role is not an issue when it comes to his patients," said Lisa Bermea, rheumatology clinic coordinator. "His holistic approach offers the children his undivided attention and careful assessment of their physical and emotional needs."[36]

To address the educational needs of chronically ill children, Gaye Koenning, who had come to Texas Children's Hospital as a dietitian in the mid-1980s before moving to the rheumatology section, led a $375,000 SPRANS demonstration grant awarded in 1990 from the Maternal and Child Health Bureau. The grant was to expand the school liaison program, launched by the rheumatology service in 1988, which was one of only a handful of such innovative pilot programs for chronically ill children in the United States.[37]

The intention of the school liaison program was to establish a partnership between families, school officials, and healthcare providers. The program was created to integrate children with rheumatic illnesses into everyday life and, more specifically, to help these children overcome the obstacles that threatened their educational success. Those obstacles were many and could be significant. Children with rheumatic diseases may require additional time to walk from class to class; they may not be able to write as quickly as their classmates; they may be unable to climb stairs; and they may need to be excused from physical education classes. From its inception, the school liaison program at Texas Children's Hospital attempted to educate teachers and school administrators about their students' conditions and the obstacles they face, and also to educate the families of children with rheumatic illnesses about their legal rights.

Accomplishing these goals with the JRA patients at Texas Children's Hospital required the expertise of an individual with educational experience. "Our school liaison specialist, Jeff Benjamin, is a special educator who helps parents and school personnel define appropriate school programs for children with juvenile rheumatic arthritis," Warren said in 1990. "Mr.

Benjamin functions in a variety of roles, depending on the severity of the disease, the child's functional capacity, and individual school variables.[38]

Four years later, the success of the Texas Children's Hospital school liaison program became evident when several studies attested to its effectiveness. The program was well received by the Texas Department of Education, school districts, schools, and families, who found that it resulted in more appropriate school programs. More than 530 patients at Texas Children's Hospital requested and received education liaison services in 1994, an indication of the program's importance to school-aged pediatric patients suffering from chronic conditions and to their families.[39]

The rheumatology service at Texas Children's Hospital wanted the school liaison program to provide the maximum possible assistance to every patient who had limited ability to achieve a successful school experience. However, geographic and budgetary constraints hindered this mission. Some patients who lived outside the Houston metropolitan area often had to receive assistance from the program specialist by mail or telephone instead of in person, the ideal methodology. It was a shortcoming exacerbated by the lack of necessary funding after the four-year SPRANS demonstration grant expired. To remedy this situation, Warren and others in the rheumatology service began exploring other ways of funding and expanding the program. Inspired by the documented success of the pilot program, they believed that the services they provided should be extended to all children with chronic diseases at Texas Children's Hospital.

This wish was granted in 1993, when the school liaison program was adopted as a whole by Texas Children's Hospital. The responsibility for administering the program shifted from the rheumatology service to the Learning Support Center, under the direction of Dr. Judith Z. Feigin. Since that time, all patients treated for chronic illnesses at Texas Children's Hospital have had access to the Learning Support Center and, as a result, countless children have received assistance and a better opportunity to maximize their educational opportunities.

Others transitions took place in the pediatric rheumatology service at Texas Children's Hospital in the early 1990s. Barron departed in 1992 to become an associate professor of pediatrics at George Washington University School of Medicine and to serve on the staff of Children's National Medical Center. Through an Intergovernmental Personnel Act appointment, she subsequently worked for four years in the National Institute of Allergy and Infectious Diseases (NIAID) Laboratory of Immunogenetics at the NIH in Washington, D.C. In 1996, that former fellow of pediatric rheumatology at Texas Children's

Hospital was named deputy director of NIAID's Division of Intramural Research at the NIH. In extensively published articles and book chapters on JRA, Kawasaki disease, and other autoimmune diseases, Barron continued to pursue the avid interests she had first developed at Texas Children's Hospital.

Following Barron's departure in 1992, Dr. Maria D. Perez—another former fellow—joined the pediatric rheumatology service at Texas Children's Hospital. Perez's areas of special interest included osteoporosis in children and the study of calcium balance in children with rheumatic disease activity and steroid therapy. She later instituted a two-year longitudinal follow-up study to evaluate calcium metabolism from the onset of newly diagnosed rheumatic disease in children. Actively involved in the ongoing clinical drug studies in the pediatric rheumatology service at Texas Children's Hospital, Perez served as the coordinator representative for the Pediatric Rheumatology Collaborative Study Group.

Also new to Warren's team in 1993 was pediatric rheumatologist and immunologist Dr. Barry L. Myones. Appointed director of research of the pediatric rheumatology service at Texas Children's Hospital, Myones primarily focused his research efforts in the area of pediatric lupus, Kawasaki disease, and juvenile dermatomyositis.

In his new role as director of research of pediatric rheumatology at Texas Children's Hospital, Myones was able to capitalize on a number of advances made in basic and clinical sciences. With the emergence of scientific by-products from the concentrated efforts to sequence the human genome, new technological advances in the field of genetics offered Myones and all pediatric rheumatologists the promise for better future understanding of many crucial factors influencing rheumatic diseases. Advances in understanding human immunology and the identification of immune complex disease as a basic mechanism in rheumatic diseases helped further understanding of tissue damage and enhanced knowledge of the mechanisms of inflammation.[40]

Able to instigate narrowly focused in-depth investigations of the specific aspects of a given scientific or clinical problem, Myones instituted an expanded research program in the pediatric rheumatology service at Texas Children's Hospital. His primary focus was on the structure, expression, and function of complement receptors, proteins in the blood that play a central role in the induction and regulation of immunity. Only identified during the previous two decades, complement receptors were determined by scientists to be of a genetic or familial origin or to be acquired. The emphasis of Myones' research was on the role complement receptors played in immunoregulation and how complement receptors and other genetic factors influence disease outcomes in SLE, JRA, and Kawasaki disease.

"The research program provides a diverse exposure to protein chemistry, biochemistry, cell biology, molecular biology, immunology, lipid chemistry, biological receptors, and cell-cell adhesion," Myones explained. "The ongoing studies have utilized a multidisciplinary approach to many of the projects utilizing most, if not all, of the above skills for each project. We also have an ongoing study of the safety/efficacy of immunization in juvenile arthritis patients on methotrexate that is linked to an in vitro study on lymphocyte responsiveness to vaccine antigens in the presence of immunomodulating agents."[41]

In addition to these research programs under the direction of Myones, Warren continued his advocacy for all chronically ill children at Texas Children's Hospital. After earning a master's degree in public health from the University of Texas School of Public Health in 1995, he devoted his efforts to finding ways of improving communication between parents, subspecialists, and pediatricians regarding the treatment of children with serious illnesses. Warren believed that if such interpersonal communication could be improved, the pediatric patients were more likely to improve as well. Named to serve on and then to chair the state advisory committee of the Texas Department of Health and Human Services, Warren devoted his efforts to improving medical care for children with special healthcare needs. Continuing to serve on the advisory committee for the Texas Health and Human Service Commission in 2004, he also became cochair of the Texas Pediatric Society's committee on children with disabilities.

At Texas Children's Hospital, Warren served on the Family Advisory Board from its inception and gained the reputation for being an exceptional communicator, particularly with his lupus and arthritis patients and their families. "When dealing with children, he will physically get down on their level to talk with them, listening with unusual intensity," said Pat Schwartz, director of nursing research. "Dr. Warren treats all patients, families, and coworkers with respect and as equals."[42]

Warren believed that one of the greatest challenges of healthcare professionals was to care for each child emotionally, as if he or she were their first and only patient. "It's really important that our caring never diminish," he said. "Children have so much potential because they see the world with open eyes and hearts. Helping them overcome illness is an opportunity to help them rediscover that wonder when it's been clouded by disease and pain."[43]

With a growing arsenal of weapons to control arthritis in children and improve the quality of these young patients' lives, Warren also praised the dramatic advances made not only in pediatric rheumatology, but also in immunology and diagnostic imaging. Knowledge gained in the field of immunology enabled pediatric rheumatologists to further their understanding of rheumatic diseases and enhanced their knowledge of the mechanisms of inflammation, inspiring new therapeutic techniques. Advances in imaging techniques such as computer tomography (CT), magnetic resonance imaging (MRI), and ultrasound allowed them to pinpoint organ involvement and tissue damage in patients with rheumatic disease.[44]

In tandem with the introduction of new technology came the advent of modern drug therapies for patients with rheumatic disease. This potent combination of advances at Texas Children's Hospital resulted in unprecedented outcomes among the patient population of the pediatric rheumatology service, a fact that Warren emphasized with great satisfaction. "Of the children I treat now, I don't have a single child in a wheelchair," he said in 2001. "That wasn't the case 15 years ago."[45]

The growing number of such accomplishments in pediatric rheumatology was disproportionate to the size of the subspecialty, one of the smallest in the United States in 2004. Officially recognized by the American Board of Pediatrics as a subspecialty in 1992, when specifically trained pediatric rheumatologists first received board certification, pediatric rheumatology ranked thirteenth in size among the 16 pediatric subspecialties in 2004. Even though there were fewer than 198 board-certified pediatric rheumatologists in the country, there were six in the state of Texas, five of whom were at Texas Children's Hospital.[46]

Of all the pediatric rheumatologists worldwide, more than 19 had received post-graduate training in the pediatric rheumatology service at Texas Children's Hospital and Baylor College of Medicine.[47] Since its inception, the fellowship training program, begun by Brewer and now directed by Perez and Myones, was accredited by the Accreditation Council for Graduate Medical Education in 1996 and remained one of only 27 in the United States in 2004.

Former fellows in the pediatric rheumatology fellowship training program at Texas Children's Hospital could be found not only at Texas Children's Hospital and Baylor College of Medicine, but also throughout the United States, as well as in China, Spain, and Argentina. Following the precedent set by the first fellows in 1979, Dr. Marietta M. DeGuzman achieved board certification and joined the pediatric rheumatology service at Texas Children's Hospital in 2002. The focus of her research efforts involved the treatment of pauciarticular JRA and the hypothesis that intraarticular steroid therapy was clinically superior to nonsteroidal anti-inflammatory drug (NSAID) therapy. In a collaboration with Perez in 2003, DeGuzman also conducted clinical drug studies utilizing COX2 NSAIDS and tumor necrosis factor receptor antibody therapy.

By 2004, the pediatric rheumatology service at Texas Children's Hospital had grown to become one of the largest in the United States. Children from all over the world who suffered from rheumatic diseases visited the rheumatology clinic, totaling more than 3,000 visits per year. Under the leadership of Warren, DeGuzman, Myones, Perez, and Wilking, the pediatric rheumatology team consisted of two fellows, nurse practitioner Martha R. Curry, clinical nurses Valerie Marcott and Lisa Smith, a physical and occupational therapist, and social worker Nicanora C. Cuellar. Together, they provided diagnosis and treatment for pediatric patients with JRA, dermatomyositis, systemic lupus erythematosus, Sjogren syndrome, scleroderma, acute rheumatic fever, and Kawasaki disease.

In addition to the clinical research programs in therapeutic evaluation, intervention, and healthcare services, Warren, Myones, and other members of the pediatric rheumatology service at Texas Children's Hospital continued to pursue laboratory research actively. Research programs in 2004 included in-depth studies of the genetics of SLE and JRA, the etiology and pathogenesis of Kawasaki disease, and the structure and function of antiphospholipid antibodies. Externally, Warren focused his research efforts on improved access to healthcare for children with chronic disease and continued to work with the Texas Department of Health.

In 2004, with dedicated research laboratories and offices in the Feigin Center at Texas Children's Hospital and the rheumatology clinic in the Clinical Care Center, the pediatric rheumatology service at Texas Children's Hospital had come a long way since its beginning in commandeered bathroom space in 1958. "Dr. Brewer was a pioneer," Warren said. "He was on the frontier of making pediatric rheumatology a subspecialty itself, an element of pediatrics, but he also was one of a handful of folks who said, 'Let's make it a science.'"

Warren also praised Brewer's great contribution to the field—promoting both locally and nationally the understanding that kids with rheumatic diseases need team care. "They needed not just doctors, but social workers, physical therapists, occupational therapists, dietitians, and so on," Warren said. "And that team led to better outcomes in the kids. Where that's taken us now, I think, is extraordinary progress in what we can do for kids. Children now are dramatically better with the same diseases, compared to 15 or 20 or 25 years ago. Better recognition and earlier treatment has led to much better outcomes."

While dramatic improvements in the quality of life for children with rheumatic diseases had been achieved, Warren believed that patients would benefit from further advances in the field of pediatric rheumatology in the not-too-distant future. "I expect that with the new therapies that are here, and that are on the horizon, the quality of life for juvenile arthritis patients will continue to improve," he said. "For those children with more rare conditions, I think there are opportunities for research to help discover what causes those conditions. We will make those discoveries. I am sure of it."[48]

The pediatric rheumatology service at Texas Children's Hospital that had begun with some memorable moments was certain to experience countless more in the future.

Three years after her first surgeries at Texas Children's Hospital, following much hard work and many hours of home therapy, Pamela Stokes had made remarkable progress.

Pamela sat in her wheelchair during her 1976 graduation ceremony, but when her name was called the 19-year-old rose and walked across the stage to claim the diploma she had worked so hard to earn. Graduating just one year behind her former classmates, she was justifiably proud of this achievement, given the amount of time that her illness had forced her to be away from school.

Five years later, after attending the University of New Orleans, Pamela graduated from Nicholls State University in 1981 with a degree in elementary education and special education. "I suffered through college, I suffered a lot physically. It was hard for me to get up for classes. It was tough, but I made it through," she recalled. "I just had the will to do it. I guess I was raised that way."[49]

Pamela put her degrees to use for six years as a teacher in private schools. For most of her teaching career, she was generally free of pain, taking medication only after long days on her feet standing in front of her students. Responding to follow-up studies conducted with the former patients of Brewer and Granberry, she noted her 1986 participation in a six-mile walkathon sponsored by the National Federation for the Blind: "I even finished it. It took a while, and I remember being sore afterwards. But I finished."

When Brewer and Granberry invited four former patients, including Pamela, to attend a meeting of the 1990 Clinical Orthopedic Society, she accepted. At the symposium, the doctors discussed the long-term effects of joint replacement surgery on children whose joints and bones were still growing and developing. Pamela agreed to participate in the symposium so that future generations of juvenile rheumatoid arthritis patients, and the doctors who treat them, would benefit from her experience. "He had slides of all of us," Pamela recalled. "Dr. Granberry would call us up by name and we had to go walk in front of this room full of doctors. We had to wear shorts so that they could see the surgery on our knees and hips. It was interesting, because I did get to meet more people with rheumatoid arthritis. Because in my experience, I hadn't met that many people with it."

Only several times before had Pamela seen what she thought was a fellow rheumatoid arthritis patient in public. Once, she and her sisters were at a video store in Louisiana when they saw a girl who resembled Pamela. "She looks just like you," her sisters said. "It was the strangest thing," Pamela recalled. "I had never seen anyone who looked so much like me. The way I walked, the hands, even the jaw line. It was just amazing. I saw this girl another time at a restaurant, and I spoke to her. I told her how interesting it was to meet her because that doesn't happen every day. A couple of months later, I saw her at a church I was visiting. We spoke again, exchanged phone numbers, and developed a friendship."

Pamela experienced a change in her lifestyle after she met Joseph Ferrucci and married him in 1988. She gave birth to their daughter, Hannah Elizabeth, whom Pamela described as the "miracle baby" and "the joy of my life," in 1996. Later divorced and a single mother, Pamela worked as a freelance writer and raised her daughter on her own.

Looking back at her experiences at Texas Children's Hospital and recounting her own long and painful period of recuperation and rehabilitation, Pamela hoped that other young people diagnosed with juvenile rheumatoid arthritis understood how to cope by thinking that "this, too, will pass." She also wanted other sufferers to know that "it's okay to cry, to grieve for a while, but don't make it a lifestyle!"

Because being afflicted with juvenile rheumatoid arthritis is "like losing a part of yourself," Pamela believed that it was okay to grieve. "I saw it with my own eyes," she said. "I was healthy one day and not the next. It was a gradual process, but you noticed it, and you see yourself slowly tearing down, breaking down. The most important advice that I can give to parents of patients with juvenile rheumatoid arthritis is to help them deal with the emotions associated with having a chronic disease by seeking professional counseling."

From being a seven-year-old with a limp and swollen joints, to becoming a teenager recuperating from hip and knee replacements at Texas Children's

Hospital, to suffering through painful days so that she could graduate from college, to becoming a relatively pain-free young mother, Pamela Stokes Ferrucci was, and continued to be, a model of courage and determination.

"You have to keep trying and you have to keep working," was the encouragement her mother always gave her, she said. In turn, it's what she has encouraged in other children afflicted with juvenile rheumatoid arthritis.

28

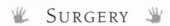
THIRTY-TWO-YEAR-OLD LESLIE DAVIS always had high hopes for her family.
Married to electrical engineer Brad Davis and mother to four-year-old son Thad, she was happily pregnant again in 1991.

Convinced that her second child was going to be as healthy as her first, Leslie decided against taking an alpha-fetoprotein (AFP) test, the screening test that identifies pregnancies at higher-than-average risk of certain serious birth defects. "With my first son, I had the AFP," she recalled. "The tests are often false positive, and I've had several friends who have had scares when they thought something was wrong and it wasn't. So, with my second child, I thought, 'There's nothing wrong with my baby.'"[1]

While undergoing a routine ultrasound examination in her obstetrician's office during the seventh month of her pregnancy, Leslie and her husband received some shocking news. "The doctor said, 'I see something here,'" she recalled. "He was so compassionate. He said, 'You know, you've gained so little weight while you were pregnant that perhaps I can just see through you more clearly, and his brain maybe is not so distended.' He was so sweet. I'm sure he knew all along what he saw."

What the doctor had seen in her unborn son was the most common central nervous system birth defect, spina bifida. In addition to a malformed spinal cord, the doctor also diagnosed myelomeningocele, a skin- or membrane-covered mass on the baby's back that contained the abnormally formed spinal cord tissue, nerves exiting from the spinal cord, and cerebrospinal fluid. There also was a collection of excessive fluid in the cerebral ventricles, indicating hydrocephalus, commonly known as "water on the brain."

Immediately referred to a high-risk fetal expert at St. Luke's Episcopal Hospital, Leslie began having ultrasound examinations every two weeks to follow the progress of the hydrocephalus. She was also referred to a geneticist and a pediatric neurosurgeon at Texas Children's Hospital. Leslie had soon arranged for all the necessary medical expertise to be in place when her son was delivered by cesarean section, the preferred delivery method for high-risk neonates. "It was not the happiest of times," Leslie remembered. "I was real upset, but I didn't want anybody to know because I didn't want everybody to worry for me, or make assumptions about how he was going to turn out."

In spite of such private mental turmoil, Leslie remained maternally optimistic about her soon-to-be-born son, eventually obviating her worries with confident expectations.

"I think this is hard for some people to understand, but when a woman is carrying a baby, you have the highest hopes for your child," she said. "You think they are going to be the brightest, the smartest, the most gifted athlete; you always have high hopes, even when you find out your child has a birth defect. The doctors don't know how it's going to affect your child until he is born, so you still really have high hopes."

Leslie's optimism never waned, although it was severely tested. When Dylan Davis was delivered by cesarean section at St. Luke's Episcopal Hospital, he was immediately transferred to the neonatal intensive care unit at Texas Children's Hospital. With a spinal lesion at the lumbar five region, within 24 hours he had undergone neurosurgery to close the defect. Within 48 hours, neurosurgeons had operated on Dylan again, this time to implant a shunt in his head to relieve the pressure and drain the excess cerebrospinal fluid in and around the brain and spinal cord, a procedure necessitated by hydrocephalus. "I was so glad that I knew to be at St. Luke's," Leslie said, grateful for the hospital's proximity to Texas Children's Hospital.

Even though Dylan was close by, his mother could not be with him during his first two surgeries. As Leslie recuperated from the cesarean surgery in her hospital room, she and her husband waited for the status reports of Dylan's surgeries, both of which were initially successful. In the first six weeks of his life, Dylan had five surgeries for shunt revisions. His parents were always at his side. "Finally, the pediatric neurosurgeon went into the other side of his head and that one worked," Leslie said.

During this time of multiple surgeries, an apparent crisis emerged. Always feeling the top of Dylan's head to see if the soft spot had hardened from excess fluids, Leslie discovered one day that the baby's head was as hard as a rock. Fearing that she had touched him too often and done something to cause brain damage, she frantically rushed her son to the emergency center at Texas Children's Hospital. When an emergency center physician said, "You have done no harm," Leslie was overjoyed. "He was the nicest, most reassuring doctor," she said. "Right then, I needed to hear that more than anything."

Another worry Leslie had concerned her son's malformed feet, which she had first noticed "when he was lifted over my head when he was born." Diagnosed as congenital vertical talus, the rare abnormality was also known as "rocker-bottom foot" because of the rigid deformity. To correct this problem, pediatric orthopedic surgeons at Texas Children's Hospital began putting casts on Dylan when his weight reached 13 pounds. Changing the casts every two weeks until the baby's feet were straight, the surgeons then performed an operation to correct the feet permanently. During that procedure, the pediatric surgeons also performed a hernia repair.

Although his feet were now properly positioned, Dylan was unable to walk due to the lesion in his lower spine and the resulting paralysis. He had some sensation on the front of his thigh, but none on the back or below the knee. With no surgeries available to correct these defects, Dylan was fitted for leg braces. He began physical therapy to enhance his leg muscles. Dylan learned to walk short distances with a child-sized walker and the leg braces, but he needed his wheelchair to travel farther.

Dylan also began making regular visits to the spina bifida clinic at Texas Children's Hospital. There he was able to see all of the members of the spina bifida medical team—neurosurgeon, pediatrician, orthopedic surgeon, urologist, and physical medicine and rehabilitation specialist—in a single setting. It also was the first place where Dylan saw other children with spina bifida.

When he was three years old, the diminutive Dylan was referred by the spina bifida team to the endocrinology service at Texas Children's Hospital. There, endocrinologist Dr. Lefkothea Karaviti diagnosed him as being growth-hormone deficient. She also suspected that Dylan had a tethered cord, scar tissue on the spinal cord from his first back-closing operation. Karaviti ordered a magnetic resonance imaging (MRI) scan, and "it turned out he had a build-up of fluid on his spinal cord called a 'syrinx,'" his mother recalled. "Since he had Chiari malformation, the abnormal development of the lower brain that often accompanies spina bifida, his brain is very low in the back of his head and his brain stem is in this really narrow spot. The neurosurgeons thought they could go in, chip the bone away and loosen it up, and the fluid would dissipate."

The three-year-old veteran of countless surgeries underwent yet another operation at Texas Children's Hospital. For his family, there was a reassuring constant: the nursing staff at Texas Children's Hospital. "The same nurses were there from when Dylan was born," Leslie said. "They remember us and they remember Dylan. They would say, 'Dylan, what are you doing in here again?' That's what is so sweet."

When Texas Children's Hospital opened in 1954, the surgeon-in-chief, Dr. Luke W. Able, was the first and only pediatric surgeon in Houston.

The surgical subspecialty of child surgery was in its infancy in the late 1940s and early 1950s. Formal postgraduate training in this emerging field was available at only a few children's hospitals, the most prominent of which was Children's Hospital Boston. It was there that Able had spent 1947 and 1948 studying and working with Dr. William E. Ladd, acknowledged as the father of pediatric surgery, and Dr. Robert E. Gross, the acclaimed heart surgeon who had operated on the first patent ductus arteriosus in a child. As authors of the first modern American textbook on child surgery in 1941, Ladd and Gross were the recognized pioneers in the new field. Titled *Abdominal Surgery of Infancy and Childhood*, their 1,000-page book stressed the fact that children cannot be treated as though they were diminutive adults. This innovative principle soon guided those known as child surgeons.[2]

As to exactly when the appellation changed from "child surgery" to "pediatric surgery" is unknown. Many credit Dr. C. Everett Koop, who had trained at Children's Hospital Boston at the same time as Able, for the new terminology. Following his training, Koop—who later became surgeon general of the United States—established one of the first academic surgical programs for children at The Children's Hospital of Philadelphia.

Whatever this evolving field was to be called, in 1947 Ladd believed that its highly specialized efforts deserved recognition. With the assistance and support of 11 other surgeons, including Koop, Ladd proposed the establishment of the surgical section of the American Academy of Pediatrics. Accepted as the first section within that organization, it was limited to those surgeons who devoted more than 90 percent of their time to pediatric patients. The success of the surgical section later inspired the formation of more than 70 specialized sections within the academy.[3]

Although formally recognized by pediatricians as a subspecialty, pediatric surgery did not gain immediate acceptance from general surgeons and anatomic specialists in the adult populations. Unable to conceive that children were not small adults, a Boston surgeon once told Ladd, "Anyone who could operate on a bunny rabbit could operate on newborns." Although erroneous, the concept was widely held. Pediatric surgeons were determined to prove that it was not true.[4]

Pediatric surgeons were also eager to dispel the fears of pediatricians who, familiar with the high mortality rate of anesthesia, were reluctant to refer pediatric patients for surgery. Accustomed to working with surgeons who dealt predominantly with adults, many pediatricians felt that it was safe to refer older children for surgery but not young ones. Even after taking such self-prescribed precautions with their referrals, the pediatricians still lacked confidence in surgical procedures for children. Doubting that better results were forthcoming from pediatric surgeons, who claimed to be more familiar with a child's physiology and needs, pediatricians throughout the United States adopted a wait-and-see attitude in the late 1940s.

The pediatricians in Houston who were similarly cautious did not have to wait long for convincing results. "In 1948, I operated on the first surviving patient south of the Mason–Dixon Line with esophageal atresia," Able said, recalling the five-pound infant at St. Joseph's Hospital who later grew up to have a child of her own.[5]

Having returned from his fellowship at Children's Hospital Boston and established the first pediatric surgical practice in southwest Texas, Able had dedicated himself to caring solely for children. Although lacking ancillary professional and nursing support, he soon began receiving patient referrals from pediatricians. Devoted to each child's well-being, Able routinely involved himself in every aspect of patient care. He would arrive the day before surgery to start the IV and often would stay after surgery, sitting by the bed as the child recuperated. "It kept me running," he remembered. "Before surgery, if you couldn't start the IV, you couldn't do the case. In those days, there wasn't a recovery room. You recovered your own patients. The joke around town was I not only operate on them, I nurse them."[6]

Able was also known never to turn away a child who needed his services. Regardless of their ability to pay, all patients were accepted and cared for in his inimitable way. He soon attained legendary status among patients, many of whom were known to say, "You don't forget that kind of treatment."[7]

Since all of Able's surgeries in the late 1940s and early 1950s necessarily took place in adult hospitals, he was acutely aware of the need for a children's hospital, one with infant-sized operating-room equipment and specialized services. An active supporter of Dr. David Greer and the Houston Pediatric Society's efforts to build such a hospital, Able was asked to become its surgeon-in-chief on a part-time basis. Because the arrangement would enable him to remain in private practice, he enthusiastically accepted the offer. "Texas Children's Hospital opened in 1954 and immediately we had surgical patients," said Able. "The first cardiac patient was an infant with pulmonary stenosis in severe failure. The cardiologist, Dan McNamara, assisted me in the right ventriculotomy and a Potts pulmonary valvulotomy with immediate success for the infant heart failure—a first for this geographic area."[8]

After this successful beginning, the caseload for the pediatric surgical program at Texas Children's Hospital slowly but steadily increased over the next two years. Many patients were referred by once-doubting but newly converted pediatricians. Other Houston surgeons, those in private practice who operated on both children and adults, also had privileges to use Texas Children's Hospital's operating facilities for their young patients.

The pediatric surgical service at Texas Children's Hospital included programs in patient care, teaching, and research. In 1956, Able instigated a two-year residency program for pediatric surgery, one of the few in the country at that time. The first resident to complete the program was Dr. Franklin J. Harberg. Appointed as the first American to hold the position of senior surgical registrar to the thoracic unit in London's Hospital for Sick Children, Great Ormond Street, Harberg left Texas Children's Hospital to spend a year in England. When he returned to Houston in 1959, he opened a private practice and joined the surgery department at Texas Children's Hospital on a part-time basis.

Harberg discovered that the pediatric surgery service had grown during his yearlong absence. Dr. Benjy Brooks, the first woman to be trained as a pediatric surgeon at Harvard and Children's Hospital Boston, had joined Able in 1958. Brooks became not only the second practicing pediatric surgeon in Houston, but also the first and only female surgeon in Texas. "I contacted Dr. Able and told him that I was a Texan and wanted to come back; they didn't need me in Boston and they didn't know they needed me here," Brooks said, recalling her decision to join the pioneers at Texas Children's Hospital. "I could have stayed in Boston. But, as I told Dr. Gross, 'In 20 years, I know exactly where I would be and I just can't stand knowing where I'm going to be.'"[9]

Where Brooks found herself in 1958 was "absolutely wonderful. Texas Children's Hospital was a 106-bed hospital, but more like a little hotel," she recalled. "What drew me was the fact that parents could stay with children, something that was not allowed in Boston. Parents there had visiting hours every Thursday and Sunday. They didn't realize how much it helped to have the parents there. And at Texas Children's, Dr. Blattner did."

Brooks was further impressed by the fact that "people were smiling" in Texas Children's Hospital, something she had not experienced before.

Also notable was the number of doctors already on the staff who had completed fellowships at Children's Hospital Boston. "I thought this was just great. We were all on the same wavelength," she said. "You can't imagine how wonderful it was for me to come to that kind of hospital."

Equally unimaginable was what the team of Able, Brooks, and Harberg was able to accomplish over the next decade. Scientific advancements and improvements in operating-room techniques enabled many children who formerly would have been classed as inoperable to undergo life-saving surgery. With a survival rate of more than 75 percent, the newly established surgical program at Texas Children's Hospital compared favorably with medical centers throughout the world.[10] "The attitude that little was lost when a premature baby died with a congenital defect has been replaced by the concept that our goals are 70 year survivals," Brooks reported in "Urgent Surgery of the Newborn," an April 1965 article in the *Journal of American Medical Women's Association*.

The optimism of the revised goal was based on experience. As "surgeons of the skin and its contents," Able, Brooks, and Harberg operated on all parts of the child. They performed surgical procedures that ranged in complexity from simple inguinal hernias to complex neurosurgical problems.

Utilizing a special technique, anesthetists administered minute amounts of anesthesia for tiny newborn infants with congenital birth defects and other correctable anomalies of the alimentary tract and respiratory system. The pediatric surgeons at Texas Children's Hospital were thereby able to perform procedures for intestinal obstruction, incarcerated hernia, tracheo-esophogeal fistula, atresia of the esophagus or lower alimentary canal, and Hirschsprung's disease, the massive impaction of the contents of the bowel.[11]

With new research techniques developed and management routines defined, the pediatric surgeons at Texas Children's Hospital began to address other areas. In the management of burns, they made considerable progress by studying the fluid and electrolyte balance, as well as infection control. They were the first to use the Menghini needle for obtaining a liver biopsy, an innovative technique that required local topical anesthesia, particularly suited to small infants. Shortly after its invention, one of the first Holter valves—the apparatus that was destined to revolutionize the shunt procedures for hydrocephalus—was implanted in an infant's brain in 1958. With the advent of chemotherapeutic agents for children with cancer, the surgical management of tumors began to advance.[12] "From the beginning, we had a wide variety of benign and malignant tumors of the liver, thyroid, adrenals, gonads, kidneys, prostate, peripheral soft tissue, and bone," recalled Able. "In the first few years we had 12 patients with primary tumors of the liver. We became proficient in hepatic lobectomies—a first in the area."[13]

With such achievements, the ten-year-old pediatric surgery department at Texas Children's Hospital had begun to make a name for itself. "We were all young physicians who had been educated in tradition, but had none to follow in our own backyard," Harberg said. "There was a need to care for specific—unique, in many instances—medical problems. And that challenge was met by innovative, tough, uniquely talented, and, in a way, daring young physicians who had to put up or shut up, professionally. And they put the place on the map. And there's no question that the map was local and national and international."[14]

Receiving the lion's share of national and international attention in the 1950s and 60s was the pioneering work of Dr. Denton A. Cooley, chief of cardiovascular surgery at Texas Children's Hospital. Cooley's development of a heart–lung machine in 1957 resulted in more than 550 cardiovascular procedures performed on infants and children less than two years of age over a ten-year period. His innovative surgical procedure for the correction of the heretofore inoperable congenital anomaly known as total anomalous pulmonary venous return was adopted by other heart surgeons and became known as the Cooley procedure.[15] With these and other noteworthy accomplishments, Cooley convincingly established himself as one of the pioneers in the new field of open-heart surgery.

Also garnering recognition for surgical advances were Able, Brooks, and Harberg. In April 1965, they achieved a medical milestone that generated headlines around the world. It was the first successful separation of twins who were conjoined at the liver and pericardium. Detailed in *Conjoined Twins*, a 1967 book published by the National Foundation-March of Dimes, the "Bay City Twins Separation" was touted as being "the successful surgical achievement and the good survival of each is attributed to: selective diagnostic studies with delayed and planned elective separation; the primary use of plastics to fill the pericardial, chest, and abdominal wall defects; the support of adequate monitoring and intensive, total professional care, paramedical as well as medical and nursing."[16]

Able credited the surgical team's previous experience with hepatic lobectomies as being most beneficial in dividing the conjoined livers of the twins. He also shared his team's success with Cooley, who assisted in the procedure and suggested the use of the silastic prosthetic patch for the pericardial cavity, invented by Dr. Michael E. DeBakey. "It was a good suggestion," Able said.

"And it worked. Those twins were the first to survive that type of operation. It was the beginning of the era when both twins survived."[17]

The late 1960s marked the start of dramatic changes in the medical care of children, both locally and nationally. At Texas Children's Hospital, the role of a general hospital was beginning to emerge. The hospital's planned expansion, which included a significant increase in the number of beds available, reflected this trend. At Baylor College of Medicine and other such academic institutions across the country, the development of subspecialties in pediatrics was progressing at a rapid pace. Also growing was the number of programs for pediatric specialists in all of the surgical fields, following the pattern set by general surgery for adults. Collectively, these developments were expected not only to revolutionize the treatment of critically ill children, but also to increase the demand for such services.

In anticipation of that predicted growth in surgical services, Able was appointed in 1970 as head of the surgery department at Texas Children's Hospital. Harberg was appointed chief of the general surgery service, consisting of 63 general surgeons who performed procedures at Texas Children's Hospital.

Soon to be missing from that growing number of pediatric surgeons at Texas Children's Hospital was Brooks. In 1973, she was offered a full professorship and the opportunity to develop the pediatric surgery department at the University of Texas Health Science Center. Unable to resist returning to the kind of academic role she had trained for at Children's Hospital Boston, Brooks accepted the offer with ambivalence. "I hated to leave Texas Children's Hospital when I did," she said. "I just cried when I left."[18]

Brooks was reluctant to leave the steadily growing pediatric surgical service, which was beginning to maintain a caseload of more than 1,000 general surgical cases each year. The caseload steadily increased after the inauguration in 1975 of a new concept in medical care: same-day surgery for outpatients.

Having established itself as an "open service," the newly named general surgery service at Texas Children's Hospital not only performed same-day surgery, but also functioned in many areas of the hospital. In addition to the operating room and outpatient department, activities were carried out in the infant care unit, pediatric intensive care unit, pediatric recovery room, emergency center, and surgical unit for neonates, the precursor of the neonatal intensive care unit.[19] "I didn't want the baby to have to go down in the elevator, lose his IV or endotracheal tube, get cold and jostled around, and get an intraventricular hemorrhage in his head," Harberg said, recalling the first time he operated on a neonate in the infant's bed. "I said, 'Why don't we avoid all that and just do it up there where the nurses have been taking care of him one-on-one?' Neonatology was just beginning then."[20]

While other pediatric subspecialties were just beginning in the early 1970s, pediatric surgery had come of age in 1974 when it was recognized by the American Board of Surgery as a subspecialty with the creation of a special certification in pediatric surgery. Because most pediatric surgical problems involved congenital defects, in the following decade pediatric surgeons developed a close working relationship with an escalating number of subspecialists at Texas Children's Hospital. With colleagues who were neonatologists, pediatric radiologists, pediatric pathologists, pediatric hematologists, pediatric gastroenterologists, pediatric urologists, pediatric endocrinologists, pediatric nephrologists, and pediatric infectious diseases specialists, the general service surgeons became integral to the evolving concept of multidisciplinary care.

Also rapidly developing were the more than 50 subspecialties in pediatric surgery, each with its own sphere of interest. By 1988, in addition to the six pediatric surgeons in the pediatric surgery service, there were more than 11 individual subspecialty pediatric surgical services at Texas Children's Hospital. Those that had formally joined the original pediatric surgery, cardiovascular service, and orthopedic service were ophthalmology in 1972, otolaryngology in 1973, urology in 1974, gynecology in 1977, neurosurgery in 1979, hand surgery in 1983, and plastic surgery in 1986.

When Able retired in 1988, more than 2,000 children were undergoing surgical procedures each year at Texas Children's Hospital. When Dr. Edmond T. Gonzales, chief of pediatric urology at Texas Children's Hospital, was appointed head of the department of surgery at Texas Children's Hospital in 1988, one of his first accomplishments was the establishment of the pediatric anesthesiology service. Spearheaded by its chief, Dr. Burdett S. Dunbar, and Gonzales, the anesthesia service had previously been a combined service for adults and children. "It needed to be reevaluated," Gonzales said. "After some discussion among the surgeons and the physicians in anesthesiology, they ultimately did define a pediatric unit within the service and ultimately established the pediatric anesthesiology service at Texas Children's."[21]

The establishment in 1988 of the pediatric anesthesiology service was of strategic importance to the surgical services at Texas Children's Hospital. Eight dedicated pediatric operating suites were scheduled to open at Texas Children's Hospital after the formal separation from St. Luke's Episcopal Hospital in 1988. These eagerly awaited suites featured advanced pediatric monitoring and anesthesia equipment, temperature regulation, and intravenous equipment with volume control units and mini-droppers to calibrate fluid therapy.

With a designated holding area where parents could remain with their child and a postoperative area where they could stay until the child was stable, the new suites were designed exclusively for pediatric patients. A dedicated pediatric anesthesiology service enhanced the ability of the pediatric surgeons to provide superb care. In 1988, the recipients of these surgical services numbered more than 3,000 inpatients at Texas Children's Hospital and more than 2,500 same-day surgical outpatients annually. "Each service had an opportunity to provide its input into its special service needs, its future vision of growth," Gonzales said.

When planning for the surgical suites was underway, Gonzales had also envisioned the consolidation of the surgical service into one physical area. "In the ideal sense, we wanted a great big space, with a nice mahogany door that said 'Department of Surgical Services at Texas Children's Hospital,' so that you could define surgery as one department, not 11 individual entities," he said. "For practical reasons, that was not possible, but we did try to cluster our services in one area."[22]

Although not combined into a single space, the multiple surgical services at Texas Children's Hospital had garnered a singular reputation as one of the premier pediatric surgery programs in the United States. In June 1989, Baylor College of Medicine was granted approval to become one of only 17 institutions in the country to offer a pediatric surgery residency program. In accordance with the regulations of the American Board of Surgery, the two-year program consisted of rigorous training in all aspects of pediatric surgery and patient management at all the hospitals affiliated with Baylor College of Medicine.[23]

At Texas Children's Hospital, the pediatric surgery residency program was developed and implemented by Harberg and Dr. William J. Pokorny, the first full-time faculty member in pediatric surgery and chief of the pediatric surgery section of the Michael E. DeBakey Department of Surgery at Baylor College of Medicine. Harberg, who retired from private practice, had joined Pokorny as a full-time faculty member at Baylor College of Medicine in 1987. Their two-year training program represented a culmination and refinement of efforts begun by Able and continued by Harberg since the 1970s. "We have come a long way in fulfilling our responsibilities as teachers of pediatric surgery," Harberg said in 1990. "We presently have over 25 applicants for the one residency position in pediatric surgery starting July 1990."[24]

The sharing of knowledge about pediatric surgery was an area in which Pokorny had already excelled. Honored with the Outstanding Teacher Award presented by the Baylor College of Medicine pediatric staff in 1988, he had written numerous scientific articles and textbook chapters and had been active in the training of surgical residents and fellows since joining Baylor College of Medicine in 1985.

While Pokorny's academic interests were strong, his primary area of interest was patient care. "During the past few years, there have been, and we have contributed to, many advances in pediatric surgery: the care of the critically ill premature infant, the development of operative techniques in the neonatal intensive care unit, and the evaluation and care of the injured child have been redefined by new imaging techniques and operative procedures," he said in 1986. "Trauma remains the number one cause of death in childhood and gets special attention at Texas Children's Hospital."[25]

As for educating future pediatric surgery residents about the concept of multidisciplinary patient care, a textbook example was established in 1991: the spina bifida clinic at Texas Children's Hospital. Offering the services of neurosurgery, orthopedics, urology, pediatrics, physical medicine, and rehabilitation, the clinic also made available nutrition, psychiatric, social, and physical therapy and occupational therapy services. Attracting a growing number of patients, it was one of the many surgical clinics in which patients were seen by multidisciplinary services in one designated area. This new clinic was located in the recently built Clinical Care Center, later renamed the Feigin Center.

The chief of the spina bifida clinic was the chief of the pediatric neurosurgery service at Texas Children's Hospital, Dr. John P. Laurent. "Twenty-five years ago, before the introduction of corrective surgery to close the spinal column, many children with spina bifida died shortly after birth and few lived through infancy," he explained. "The prognosis of newborn infants with myelomeningocele, spina bifida, is better at this time than at any time in history. Spina bifida occurs in about 3.2 per 10,000 births in the United States. Parents should be made aware that despite the many problems and potential complications associated with spina bifida, the prognosis for their child is usually far from grim. The potential for a high quality of life has been documented."[26]

Also providing optimal patient care for children with complicated problems requiring multiple medical and surgical needs were several other one-stop clinics established at Texas Children's Hospital in the 1980s. Offering the services of all the subspecialties specifically required for each patient were the craniofacial clinic for children with facial and cranial deformations, and the brachial plexus clinic for children with birth injuries to the nerves of the arms and hands.

In the area of multidisciplinary surgical procedures, a unique opportunity was presented in 1992 when twins who were conjoined at the chest and abdomen were referred to Texas Children's Hospital. After performing extensive tests on the twins, Texas Children's Hospital pediatric cardiologist Dr. Michael R. Nihill, Texas Heart Institute cardiovascular surgeon Dr. David A. Ott, Texas Children's Hospital pediatric plastic surgeon Dr. Samuel Stal, and Pokorny "had a pretty good feeling before we started that this was a very doable kind of procedure for us." The team finalized plans for the separation.[27]

The first step was to make sure that each girl had enough skin to cover her chest after the separation. Stal implanted small silicone balloons under each infant's skin six weeks before the surgery, a procedure that produced the desired results. During the five-and-one-half-hour operation—one of the few successful procedures of its kind—Pokorny divided the twins' liver and Ott separated their conjoined hearts.

As with the conjoined twins who had been separated by Able, Brooks, and Harberg at Texas Children's Hospital in 1965, this multidisciplinary operation by Stal, Ott, and Pokorny garnered local, national, and worldwide attention. The success enhanced the growing reputation of the pediatric surgical services at Texas Children's Hospital in 1992.

Two years later, Harberg stepped down from his longtime position as chief of the general surgery service at Texas Children's Hospital and retired from Baylor College of Medicine. Briefly replacing him at Texas Children's Hospital was Pokorny, who formally changed the name to the pediatric surgery service. Before his sudden death in February 1994, the 51-year-old Pokorny had spent nine years at Baylor College of Medicine as head of the pediatric surgery section and had gained a well-deserved reputation for developing "one of the most active and attractive pediatric surgery programs in the United States."[28]

Following the death of Pokorny, Harberg came out of retirement and resumed his position as a full-time faculty member in the Michael E. DeBakey Department of Surgery at Baylor College of Medicine. His appointment to serve as acting chief of pediatric surgery at Texas Children's Hospital was in accordance with the requirements dictated by a recently established policy. "Each surgical chief represents a specific subspecialty area within the broad field of surgery, is a full faculty member in his or her respective surgical specialty at Baylor College of Medicine, and has a full-time commitment to pediatric surgery," Gonzales explained. "The chief of each surgical service is appointed by Texas Children's Hospital's board of trustees from candidates recommended to the board by the chair of the respective surgical department at Baylor College of Medicine. Each service establishes its own delineation of privileges that define the required training experience necessary for a surgeon in that specialty to practice."[29]

As head of the department of surgery at Texas Children's Hospital, Gonzales oversaw a surgical caseload that had experienced continual growth since the 1991 completion of the surgical suites in the critical care and surgical facility known as the West Tower. With the establishment of the congenital heart surgery service in 1995, the department of surgery at Texas Children's Hospital consisted of 12 individual subspecialty surgical services. By 1997, the number of surgical procedures performed at the hospital had surpassed 11,000 per year and showed no signs of diminishing.

Although this phenomenal growth reflected the development of highly defined subspecialties in the field of pediatric surgery, Harberg also attributed it to the pediatric anesthesia service at Texas Children's Hospital. "We couldn't do our work in the manner we do it without the expertise of the people who give these children their anesthetic," said Harberg. "Their refined techniques are just remarkable."[30]

In his role as acting chief of the pediatric surgery service at Texas Children's Hospital for two years, Harberg was responsible for one of the largest pediatric surgical services in the country in 1997. Along with Dr. Mary L. Brandt, Dr. Tom Jaksic, and Dr. Jed G. Nuchtern, Harberg provided surgical care and comprehensive management for premature infants, children with inadequate intestines, children with cystic fibrosis, children with cancer, and injured children.

These accomplishments, as well as the opportunities for future growth of the pediatric surgery service at Texas Children's Hospital, favorably impressed Dr. David E. Wesson, chief of pediatric surgery at New York Hospital and professor of surgery at Cornell University Medical College. Wesson had received his medical degree and surgical training from the University of Toronto and had completed his training in pediatric surgery at the Hospital for Sick Children in Toronto, where he remained for 13 years before moving to New York. Recruited to become the chief of the division of pediatric surgery of the Michael E. DeBakey Department of Surgery at Baylor College of Medicine and chief of the pediatric surgery service at Texas Children's Hospital, he accepted the challenge in 1997. "One of my observations when I first came here was how outstanding the department of pediatrics was at Baylor and at Texas Children's Hospital, and how more than 150 years in surgical history had been compressed to 50 years," Wesson said.[31]

Wesson also noted that the residency program begun by Pokorny and

Harberg in 1990 remained among the top programs in North America with regard to the quality of training and the volume of clinical experience. "We are pleased to report that all of our former residents successfully have completed the examinations given by the American Board of Surgery and now are certified in pediatric surgery," he stated in 1998, noting that one of the recent chief residents had performed the largest number of surgical cases of any resident in the United States. The following year, Wesson established a pediatric surgery fellowship program and recruited two outstanding doctors as the first international fellows.[32]

With an expanded number of operating suites in the West Tower and a vast array of surgical procedures available for children, Wesson began his search for world-class pediatric surgeons in the oncology, prenatal, and neonatal subspecialties for the pediatric service at Texas Children's Hospital. Within the next few years, he recruited Dr. Darrell L. Cass, Dr. Paul K. Minifee, Dr. Michael A. Helmgrath, and Dr. Oluyinka Olutoye. The service began expanding geographically as well, with pediatric surgeons making visits to Texas Children's Hospital neighborhood Health Centers. While all surgery continued to be performed at Texas Children's Hospital, Wesson believed that delivering maximum care with minimum inconvenience to patients would result in countless more children seeking treatment. "With the recently inaugurated Kangaroo Crew transport service, we already are seeing an increase in trauma patients from across the state," he said in 2000. "And since trauma is the number one killer of children, many critical care situations involving traumatic injuries sustained by children require surgical intervention."[33]

To provide comprehensive care to children with unique surgical problems, as well as those in need of routine outpatient surgery or complex procedures, Wesson increased the availability of minimally invasive surgery, such as laparoscopic and video surgery. By 2000, pediatric surgeons at Texas Children's Hospital were already being recognized for their expertise in procedures such as minimally invasive endoscopic surgery for the treatment of gallbladder disease, gastroesophageal reflux, splenic disorders, appendicitis, and congenital mega-colon. Additional procedures such as lung biopsy, decertification, and wedge resection were being performed thoracoscopically at Texas Children's Hospital by 2003. "The increase in surgical experience, advances in surgical instrumentation, and improvements in videoscopic imaging are leading the way for a promising future for minimally invasive surgery for pediatric surgical diseases," Wesson said.[34]

For those infants with congenital problems that required temporary cardiopulmonary support for survival, pediatric surgeons at Texas Children's

Hospital provided all extracorporeal membrane oxygenation (ECMO) services. Because it was risky and extremely stressful for premature babies to be
transported for surgery, pediatric surgeons at Texas Children's Hospital continued to perform neonatal bedside surgery, the innovative program
introduced by Harberg in the 1970s.

The neonatal bedside surgeries most frequently performed by pediatric surgeons at Texas Children's Hospital corrected respiratory problems
or irregularities of the stomach and bowel. As one of only a handful of hospitals where neonatal bedside surgeries were performed, Texas Children's
Hospital maintained a uniquely high success record. "Surgeries in infants,
many of whom weigh less than 1,500 grams, requires specialists who have
extensive experience with neonates," Harberg said in 2002. "Texas
Children's Newborn Center is the nation's largest, with more than 2,800
critically ill infants treated annually, so the hospital has the experience to
perform these surgeries with impressive outcomes."[35]

Other areas of expertise for the pediatric surgery service at Texas
Children's Hospital were developed into special programs. Four board-certified pediatric surgeons provided 24-hour availability to patients and
referring physicians. In addition to the expanded pediatric transplant services for kidney, liver, and lung established by the subspecialty surgeons who
specialized in those areas, Wesson expanded the pediatric surgery service
by establishing a pediatric minimally invasive center, a pediatric anorectal
and colon specialty clinic, and a pediatric trauma and critical care center at
Texas Children's Hospital. "Trauma is one of the most serious public health
issues we face today," he said. "It is the leading cause of death and long-term
disability for children over the age of one year."[36]

The program instituted by the pediatric surgery service at Texas
Children's Hospital to address complex birth defects—the leading cause of
death and illness in the first year of life—made an auspicious debut in
December 2001. It was a successful ex-utero intrapartum treatment (EXIT)
procedure to ensure an adequate airway in an unborn child who suffered
from a giant neck mass. This procedure marked the origin of the Texas
Center for Fetal Surgery, one of only a few such centers in the world.

Officially opened in 2004 as the first of its kind in the Southwest, the
Texas Center for Fetal Surgery was a unique collaboration of Texas Children's
Hospital, St. Luke's Episcopal Hospital, and Baylor College of Medicine.
Codirected by pediatric surgeons Cass and Olutoye, the dedicated center
offered a full spectrum of fetal surgical services. "New surgical techniques
can reduce the potentially devastating consequences of some birth defects,"

Cass said. "The center offers prenatal evaluation, diagnosis, invasive fetal therapy, and open fetal surgery for many genetic and anatomic birth defects that require therapy before or after birth."[37]

For children of all ages, surgical care and treatment at Texas Children's Hospital experienced dramatic growth in the late 1990s and early 2000s. Pediatric surgeons in the 12 surgical services at Texas Children's Hospital performed more than 13,000 procedures with general anesthesia in 1998. Within four years, after the expansion of Texas Children's Hospital was complete, the number of procedures almost doubled.

Opened in 2001, the expanded West Tower and the new Clinical Care Center at Texas Children's Hospital included eight new operating rooms, bringing the total to 21. Each boasted the most advanced technology and was designed to maximize patient flow. A recovery area with 26 post-anesthesia care beds provided ample space for parents to be at their child's bedside following surgery. Same-day surgery for outpatients at Texas Children's Hospital was performed in two locations in 2002, the third floor of the West Tower and the seventh floor of the Clinical Care Center. By 2004, the pediatric surgeons in the twelve surgical services at Texas Children's Hospital had performed more than 20,000 outpatient and inpatient surgical procedures with general anesthesia.

Also experiencing noticeable growth were the clinical and laboratory research programs in the pediatric surgery service at Texas Children's Hospital. Wesson hoped to equal, if not surpass, the other leading children's hospitals in the country in this area. Concentrating on the most challenging problems and opportunities in the field of pediatric surgery, the research programs continued in such areas as pain management, organ transplantation, gene therapy for gastrointestinal disease, thyroid and parathyroid disease in children, immunotherapy of pediatric malignancies, and neuroblastoma tumor biology.

The only limit Wesson foresaw to the ongoing growth of the pediatric surgery service at Texas Children's Hospital, from pre-operative evaluations to postoperative care, was the number of expert pediatric surgeons available. "And we are working on that," he said, noting that more than 12 of the 934 pediatric surgeons practicing in the United States in 2004 were past graduates of the pediatric surgery residency program and fellowship program at Texas Children's Hospital and Baylor College of Medicine.[38]

Since its inception with a single pediatric surgeon in 1954, the department of surgery at Texas Children's Hospital had provided compassionate state-of-the-art care for a steadily growing number of children in need of surgical care and treatment. In 2004, with a complement of more than 50 board-certified pediatric surgeons in 12 pediatric surgical services, the department of surgery at Texas Children's Hospital had experienced remarkable growth over the previous five decades.

Although the future of pediatric surgery at Texas Children's Hospital was unpredictable, there was one certainty. What Dr. William E. Ladd, the founder of pediatric surgery, wrote about "child surgery" in 1935 seemed just as appropriate for pediatric surgery at Texas Children's Hospital in 2004: "Undoubtedly great strides have been made in this field of surgery in the last few years and I have confidence that greater advances are soon to follow."[39]

Although nine-year-old Dylan Davis could walk with the aid of a walker, he preferred to be in his wheelchair while at school.

Using the articulating brace that encompassed his lower body from his waist to his ankles, the third-grader was able to stand, keep his back straight, and swing his legs from the hip. Although Dylan had an average IQ, he had difficulties in comprehending math and science. When diagnosed with a non-verbal learning disorder, a learning disability common among children with spina bifida, he received tutoring two days a week from his teacher at school and was able to maintain his grades.

Because of Dylan's inability to control his bladder and bowel, another dysfunction associated with spina bifida, he wore diapers and had to be catheterized by either the nurse at school or his mother at home. Motivated by learning that he would be able to spend the night with his school friends once he could independently take care of his private functions, Dylan achieved that goal.

With his engaging and outgoing personality, Dylan was a popular child at school and had many friends. As the only student at his school in a wheelchair, he was the center of attention on the school playground. "All the kids fight over who is going to push him in his wheelchair," his mother Leslie said. "They race him and they pop a wheelie and they spin him around. He's like a little toy."[40]

After-school activities for Dylan were altogether different. Since the parents of his school friends were uncomfortable with the unknowns about Dylan's disability, they were reluctant to invite him over to play or spend the night. Regardless of the circumstances, Dylan was more than content to sit in front of his computer and play games at home alone—unless, of course, big brother Thad invited him to join his friends at ball games and other outside activities. "I've always wondered if there will be an age when he's embarrassed to have a brother in a wheelchair," said Leslie. "But today he's no more embarrassed then any other 13-year-old who is embarrassed of a nine-year-old brother."

The only place where Dylan and his mother ever saw other children with spina bifida was at Texas Children's Hospital, but most of those patients were infants. Because most of the time he spent in the spina bifida clinic was in a private examination room, Dylan had no opportunity to see other children his age who were also at the clinic.

The lack of any interaction with a peer group was also a problem for Leslie. When Dylan was born, she knew no other mothers who had children with the same birth defect. In her search for information, she discovered that there was little, if any, printed material or books about spina bifida, hydro-cephalus, shunts and shunt revisions, paralysis, catheterization for bladder dysfunction, and the myriad surgeries Dylan had experienced or was expect-ed to experience. Leslie decided to remedy that situation immediately.

After learning about and joining the Spina Bifida Association of the Gulf Coast, a support group founded for mothers like Leslie, she soon became a board member. To assist others coping with spina bifida, Leslie helped arrange a weekly luncheon in a conference room at the Feigin Center at Texas Children's Hospital. Held on Tuesday, the day of the spina bifida clinic, the lunch included pizza and drinks provided by the association and underwritten by the Junior League of Houston. Signs posted in the clinic invited others to join the gathering. "I have met so many different people, people who have much more severely impacted lives, and people who, after having one shunt operation, have never been back to a doctor since," said Leslie. "There is a huge difference in patients. And even though Dylan has had so many surgeries, he really has had a pretty smooth life, I think."

Whenever the topic at those Tuesday luncheons turned to pediatric surgery, Leslie commented that it was an area of expertise in which she wished she had not become expert. As a child, Dylan continued to have more surgical procedures at Texas Children's Hospital. Two were to implant ear tubes for ear infections and one was to remove scar tissue on his brain stem, a suspected cause of his low oxygen levels and his inability to breathe well at night when he slept. Although a veteran of countless surgical proce-dures at Texas Children's Hospital as a baby and small child, the nine-year-old did not remember those experiences and was apprehensive about one of the ear-tube implantations. Like all children his age, Dylan had lots of questions about the procedure. "I was forthcoming as I could be with him," said Leslie. "If you explain it to him, he'll be scared and I'll tell him, 'It's OK to be scared, but we have to do it,' and he'll do it."

Unfortunately, the surgery did not improve his breathing and Dylan needed to learn how to use a breathing machine at night. "We were just in Texas Children's Hospital three weeks ago and spent two days in the progressive care unit learning how to use the machine, " Leslie explained. "I think he's better. It would just annoy the fire out of me, but Dylan is an incredibly compliant and good-natured child. That's the blessing."

Even though she "would gladly not know all of this," Leslie often shared what she had learned with other mothers of children with spina bifida. She directed them to the same day surgery registration and waiting room on the third floor of the West Tower; explained the holding area where their child was given a choice of a red wagon, a pedal car, or a bed to be taken to the operating room; advised them of the child life tour of the surgical facilities available for the child and the family; informed them about how their child could choose a favorite flavor of anesthesia; and offered reassurance that they could be at the child's side in the recovery room after the surgery.

While sitting in the waiting room for surgery or talking to someone at the Tuesday lunch, Leslie often thought to herself how lucky she was to be living in Houston and able to take Dylan home to sleep in his own bed. "There's a woman who has been having lunch with us every Tuesday whose daughter was born with incredibly complicated spina bifida two-and-one-half months ago," she said. "She's from Lufkin and has not been home for two-and-one-half months. I feel so lucky and so incredibly fortunate that we have this great medical center and all I have to do is deal with the traffic."

Hating the traffic to and from the Texas Medical Center, as well as the all-too-familiar trip itself, Leslie would often burst into tears at the thought of driving to Texas Children's Hospital one more time. But the melancholy was always short-lived and her trademark optimism always prevailed. "Because of all the advances they've made medically, Dylan should have a normal life span, but he has to be vigilant," she said. "When he's too old to go to Texas Children's Hospital, he'll have to go to separate doctors, not to just one convenient clinic like at Texas Children's. So that will be a bigger challenge."

As for other possible roadblocks in Dylan's future life, his mother was concerned about his going to college. However, she was confident that he would be gainfully employed. Although the nine-year-old thought that he would always live at home with his mother, Leslie believed otherwise. She was certain that her son would want a life of his own, and that he would excel in whatever he chose to do. "I think he can be whatever he wants to be and I think other kids in that clinic can, too," she said.[41]

In the nine years since Dylan's birth, the high hopes Leslie Davis always had for her family had not diminished. In fact, her optimism about the future grew to include all of the children in her extended family at the spina bifida clinic at Texas Children's Hospital.

Her compassion was laudable, as well as understandable. Like so many other parents of children at Texas Children's Hospital, she had become an integral part of its legacy of loving care.

NOTES

INDEX

APPENDIX

ACKNOWLEDGMENTS

NOTES

1. The Founders

1. Marilyn Miller Baker, *Caring for the Children: The History of Pediatrics in Texas* (Dallas: Texas Pediatric Society, Great Impressions), 106–7.
2. Joseph Pratt, "8F and Many More: Business and Civic Leadership in Modern Houston" *Houston Review* 1, no. 2 (Summer 2004).
3. Thomas D. Anderson, "Who Was M. D. Anderson?" October 1996, University of Texas M. D. Anderson Cancer Center website, http://www.mdanderson.org; "Chronology of the Texas Medical Center," *Texas Medical Center 1983 Annual Report,* 2.
4. After separating from Baylor University in 1969, Baylor College of Medicine changed its name and became a freestanding institution. For clarity purposes in this book, Baylor College of Medicine is the identification used from this point onward.
5. Dan G. McNamara, oral history, April 18, 1977.
6. N. Don Macon, *Monroe Dunaway Anderson, His Legacy: A History of the Texas Medical Center* (Houston: Texas Medical Center, 1994), 123.
7. Anonymous, "Experts to Inspect Children's Hospitals," *Houston Post,* August 22, 1948.
8. Byron York, oral history, February 6, 1979; Baker, *Caring for the Children,* 120–23.
9. David Greer, "How It All Began," *WATCH Magazine,* n.d.
10. Raymond Cohen, oral history, September 2, 1987.
11. Marguerite Johnston, *Houston, The Unknown City, 1836–1946* (College Station: Texas A&M University Press, 1991), 393.
12. Ibid.
13. Ed Kilman and Theon Wright, *Hugh Roy Cullen: A Story of American Opportunity* (New York: Prentice-Hall, Inc., 1954), 231.
14. Hugh Roy Cullen, biography, Cullen Foundation website, http://www.cullenfdn.org/founders.htm.
15. Kilman and Wright, *Hugh Roy Cullen,* 225.
16. Ibid., 249.
17. Ibid.
18. Walter H. Moursund, Sr., *Medicine in Greater Houston 1836–1956* (Houston: Gulf Printing Company, 1956), 148.
19. Johnston, *Houston, The Unknown City,* introduction.
20. Patrick Nicholson, *Mr. Jim: The Biography of James Smither Abercrombie* (Houston: Gulf Publishing Company, 1983), 322.
21. James E. Llamas, "Leopold Meyer: Beggar Extraordinary," *Tulanian,* February 1969.
22. Nicholson, *Mr. Jim,* page 337.
23. Ibid., 324.
24. Ibid.
25. Ibid.
26. Anonymous, "Tickets Go on Sale Today for Pin Oak Stables Horse Show," *Houston Post,* May 15, 1947.
27. Nicholson, *Mr. Jim,* 325.
28. Leopold L. Meyer, *The Days of My Years* (Houston: Universal Printers, 1975), 239.

29. Anderson, "Who Was M. D. Anderson?"; "Chronology of the Texas Medical Center," *Texas Medical Center 1983 Annual Report,* 2; George Salmon, oral history, February 13, 1987.
30. Meyer, *Days of My Years,* 239–40.
31. Anonymous, "Children's Foundation Hospital Site Selected," *Houston Magazine,* n.d.
32. Edward Singleton and Russell J. Blattner, oral history, April 30, 1979; Blattner, oral history, April 16, 1992.
33. Blattner, "History of the Development of the Texas Children's Hospital," *WATCH Magazine,* February 1956.
34. Salmon, oral history, August 1, 1987.
35. Anonymous, "Shrine to Open Ten-Day Drive for Hospital," *Houston Post,* August 1, 1946; Moursund, *Medicine in Greater Houston,* 374–79.
36. Texas Children's Foundation meeting minutes, May 10, 1948; May 17, 1948; May 31, 1948; June 18, 1948; July 12, 1948.
37. Anonymous, "Shrine, Foundation Plan Own Hospitals," *Houston Post,* August 9, 1950; Anonymous, "2 Children's Hospitals to Be Built in Medical Center," *Houston Chronicle,* August 9, 1950; Anonymous, "Arabia Temple Clinic Dedication to be Held Saturday," *Texas Medical Center News,* February 1952.
38. Six-page, undated, typed document (presumably the statement distributed to the media on October 26, 1950) announcing that sufficient funds had been raised to begin actual construction of St. Luke's Episcopal Hospital and Texas Children's Hospital.
39. Meyer, oral history, April 8, 1977.
40. Nicholson, *Mr. Jim,* 326.
41. Ibid.
42. Ibid.
43. Ibid.
44. Karen Kane, "Lep Meyer: Professional Beggar," *Houston Chronicle, Texas Magazine,* September 7, 1980.
45. Nicholson, *Mr. Jim,* 327.
46. Meyer, oral history, April 8, 1977.
47. Nicholson, *Mr. Jim,* 339–40.
48. Anonymous, "In Memoriam: James S. Abercrombie, Founder of Texas Children's Hospital," *Intercom,* January 1975.
49. Anonymous, "J. S. Abercrombie, 83, Dies at Home," *Houston Post,* January 8, 1975.
50. Ibid.
51. Josephine E. Abercrombie, telephone interview, January 6, 1999.
52. "Anonymous, "The History of St. Luke's Episcopal Hospital," St. Luke's Episcopal Hospital Auxiliary office.
53. Ibid.
54. Meyer, oral history, April 8, 1977
55. Blattner, letter to Dr. Irene Koeneke, September 17, 1950.
56. Meyer, *Days of My Years,* 241.
57. Anonymous, "Hospital to Aid 'Little People' Is Dedicated," *Houston Chronicle,* May 16, 1953.
58. Adie Marks, Gulf States Advertising letter to Leopold L. Meyer, January 22, 1951.
59. Anonymous, "Children's Hospital Brochure Asks Gifts," *Houston Post,* January 27, 1952; Anonymous, "Texas Children's Hospital Catches Popular Fancy!" *Houston Post, Texas Living Magazine,* March 16, 1952.
60. Moursund, *Medicine in Greater Houston,* 435.
61. Singleton and Blattner, oral history, April 30, 1979.
62. Irvin Kraft, oral history, January 17, 1995.
63. Meyer, *Days of My Years,* 241–42.

2. The Administration

1. Ruth SoRelle, "First Patient Lauds Expansion at Texas Children's," *Houston Chronicle,* November 8, 1991.
2. Elmer Bertelsen, "Cute Tot, 3, First Hospital Patient," *Houston Chronicle,* February 4, 1954.
3. Ibid.
4. See Appendix for listing of charter members of the Texas Children's Hospital board of trustees.
5. Herman Pressler, oral history, May 23, 1979.
6. Ibid.
7. Shoemate contract, August 20, 1951, Leopold L. Meyer Collection, #67, Box 5, File 54 at the

Houston Metropolitan Research Center, Houston Public Library, Houston, Texas (hereinafter cited as LLM #67, HMRC;) Shoemate to JS Abercrombie, April 30, 1954, LLM #67, HMRC; Texas Children's Hospital board of trustees annual meeting, January 26, 1954, Texas Children's Hospital corporate records, microfilm.

8. Gammill to LLM, February 2, 1954, LLM #67, HMRC, Box 5, File 64.
9. Elaine Potts, oral history, July 17, 1992; "Dietary Department for Texas Children's Hospital" WATCH Magazine, July 1957; Lydia Jackson Merritt, "Business Machine Dietitians," Houston Chronicle, February 23, 1958.
10. Joint Operating Committee Minutes, December 7, 1953, TCH Corporate Records, microfilm; "The Department That Touches All Our Lives," Intercom, July 5, 1958.
11. Anonymous, "Lookin' and Listenin'," El Campo Citizen, September 26, 1954; Carolyn Mercer, "Chatterbox," unknown source, n.d., copy in WATCH Scrapbook 1954–1955, McGovern Historical Collections and Research Center, Houston Academy of Medicine-Texas Medical Center Library (hereinafter cited as McGHCRC, HAM-TMC.)
12. Lee Gammill to Mr. and Mrs. H. R. Cullen, February 17, 1954, LLM #67, HMRC, Box 5, File 64; "Dolls Deluxe," Houston Post, June 26, 1955; Zella Maxwell, "The Best-Dressed Women in Houston Are 24 Inches High," Houston Press, September 29, 1958.
13. Russell J. Blattner, oral history, May 18, 1977.
14. Anonymous, "Dr. Maynard W. Martin to Retire May 31," WATCH Magazine, May 1972; Annual Report of Administrator, April 12, 1956, TCH Corporate Records, RM Box 335-664.
15. Emma Foreman, "Emma Foreman's Years at TCH," memoir, August 23, 1990.
16. Ibid.
17. Ibid.
18. Newell E. France, oral history, August 14, 1996.
19. France, oral history, BCM, March 31, 1989; France, oral history, August 14, 1996.
20. France, oral history, August 14, 1996.
21. Ibid.
22. Ibid.
23. Ruth Sylvester, oral history, September 23, 1992.
24. Florence Dickey, oral history, July 2, 1996.
25. Anonymous, "Colorful New Uniforms Make Fashion Debut at TCH," WATCH Magazine, October 1960.
26. Foreman, "Emma Foreman's Years."
27. Ibid.
28. Leopold L. Meyer, The Days of My Years (Houston: Universal Printers, 1975), 248.
29. Ibid., 251.
30. Pressler, oral history, May 23, 1979.
31. Ibid.
32. Meyer, Days of My Years, 253.
33. Stanley W. Olson, personal correspondence to Meyer, LLM #67, HMRC, Box 7, File 87.
34. France, oral history, February 9, 1977.
35. France, oral history, August 13 and 14, 1996.
36. France, oral history, February 9, 1977.
37. France, oral history, August 13 and 14, 1996.
38. Pressler, oral history, May 23, 1979.
39. Meyer, Days of My Years, 243.
40. France, oral history, February 9, 1977.
41. Ibid.
42. France, oral history, August 13 and 14, 1996.
43. Ibid.
44. France, oral history, February 9, 1977.
45. George Peterkin, Jr., oral history, July 10, 1992.
46. Ibid.
47. Ibid.
48. Foreman, "Emma Foreman's Years."
49. Ibid.
50. Ralph D. Feigin, "A Caring Agreement," WATCH Magazine, Winter 1998; Foreman, "Emma Foreman's Years."
51. Feigin, oral history, August 25, 1992.
52. Peterkin, personal correspondence to the Committee on the Hudgens Memorial Award, American College of Healthcare Executives, October 8, 1991.

3. The Leadership

1. Mark A. Wallace, oral history, December 9, 1996.
2. Ibid.
3. Wallace, interview, February 17, 2003.
4. Wallace, interview, July 24, 2003.
5. Wallace, interview, February 17, 2003.
6. Ibid.
7. Sandy Lutz, "A 'Lifetime' of Accomplishments by Age 38," *Modern Healthcare,* March 2, 1992.
8. Wallace, "Leadership Philosophy," speech, October 1989.
9. Wallace, interview, February 17, 2003.
10. Wallace, "Leadership Philosophy."
11. Wallace, interview, July 24, 2003.
12. Lutz, "A 'Lifetime' of Accomplishments."
13. Ibid.
14. George Peterkin, Jr., personal correspondence to the Committee on the Hudgens Memorial Award, American College of Healthcare Executives, October 8, 1991.
15. Ralph D. Feigin, "Mark Wallace Heads TCH Management Team," *WATCH Magazine,* Fall/Winter 1990.
16. Peterkin, personal correspondence to the Committee on the Hudgens Memorial Award.
17. Ibid.
18. Wallace, oral history, December 9, 1996.
19. Peterkin, personal correspondence to the Committee on the Hudgens Memorial Award.
20. Lutz, "A 'Lifetime' of Accomplishments."
21. Wallace, interview, July 24, 2003.
22. Ibid.
23. Ibid.
24. Wallace, "TCH Integrated Delivery System," *Developments,* Spring 1997.
25. Wallace, interview, July 24, 2003.
26. Steve Sievert, "Texas Children's Hospital Launches Largest Building Project in Texas Medical Center History," *Texas Medical Center News,* March 15, 1999.
27. Ibid.
28. Andrew Osterland, "CFOs in Health Care," *CFO Magazine,* January 1, 2002.
29. Wallace, "Texas Children's Flood Protection System," Texas Children's Hospital press release, June 2003.
30. Sally I. Nelson, "Tropical Storm Allison Coverage," *Texas Medical Center News,* July 1, 2001.
31. Wallace, interview, July 24, 2003.

4. The First Physician-in-Chief

1. Russell J. Blattner, oral history, May 24, 1979; Blattner, "What It Was Like in 1948: Faculty's View," *40th Anniversary Colloquium,* Baylor College of Medicine, February 17, 1988, archives, Baylor College of Medicine.
2. Anonymous, "Dr. Russell J. Blattner: Three Fruitful Decades," *Inside Baylor Medicine* 8, no. 4 (April 1977); Blattner, oral history, May 24, 1979.
3. Blattner, oral history, May 24, 1979.
4. Blattner, video interview, August 16, 1988.
5. Ibid.
6. Blattner, "What It Was Like in 1948."
7. Anonymous, "Dr. Russell J. Blattner: Three Fruitful Decades."
8. Blattner, oral history, May 24, 1979.
9. Blattner, "What It Was Like in 1948."
10. Blattner, oral history, May 24, 1979.
11. Murdina Desmond, interview, January 8, 2000.
12. B. L. Ligon and F. Stein, "Russell J. Blattner, MD: A Leader Who Welcomes Challenges," *Seminars in Pediatric Infectious Diseases* 11, no. 1 (2000): 73–86.
13. Blattner, video interview, July 15, 1988.
14. Ligon and Stein, "Russell J. Blattner, MD."
15. Blattner, video interview, July 15, 1988.
16. Blattner, oral history, May 24, 1979.

17. Blattner, oral history, May 18, 1977.
18. Ibid.
19. Ibid.
20. Blattner, video interview, August 16, 1988.
21. Blattner, "What It Was Like in 1948."
22. Ligon and Stein, "Russell J. Blattner, MD." Note: In 1957, the Texas Institute for Rehabilitation and Research (TIRR) was incorporated, assuming the functions of the Southwestern Poliomyelitis Respiratory Center. It officially opened in the Texas Medical Center in 1959 and later changed its name to The Institute for Rehabilitation and Research (TIRR).
23. Martha Yow, oral history, May 29, 1996.
24. Blattner, video interview, August 16, 1988.
25. Murdina Desmond, oral history, June 4, 1992.
26. Walter H. Moursund, Sr., *A History of Baylor University College of Medicine 1900–1953* (Houston: Gulf Printing Company, 1956), 164.
27. Edward Singleton, oral history, April 30, 1979.
28. Blattner, video interview, July 15, 1988.
29. Blattner, "History of the Development of the Texas Children's Hospital," *WATCH Magazine,* February 1956.
30. Blattner, video interview, July 15, 1988.
31. Ibid.
32. Blattner, video interview, August 16, 1988.
33. Mrs. Herbert P. Edmundson, letter to Leopold Meyer, June 17, 1953, TCH corporate records, Box 00754; Martha Lovett, Lida Edmundson, Ann Baker, oral history, August 1, 1977; "The Outpatient Department of Texas Children's Hospital, 1956," TCH corporate records, RM Box 191-678.
34. Blattner, "Research Activities in the Texas Children's Hospital," *WATCH Magazine,* July 1957.
35. Newell E. France and Lois Hill, *Texas Children's Hospital—A Pediatric Research Center,* pamphlet, 1964.
36. Blattner, video interview, July 15, 1988.
37. France and Hill, *Texas Children's Hospital.*
38. Ibid.
39. Anonymous, "Dr. Russell J. Blattner: Three Fruitful Decades."
40. France and Hill, *Texas Children's Hospital.*
41. Anonymous, "Baylor Medical Alumni Association Honors Dr. Russell J. Blattner," *WATCH Magazine,* November 1972.
42. Mary Jane Schier, "Symposium Honors Baylor's Dr. Blattner," *Houston Post,* March 4, 1977.
43. Anonymous, "Dr. Russell J. Blattner: Three Fruitful Decades."
44. Anonymous, "Texas Children's Hospital Celebrates 20th Anniversary," *Intercom,* March 1974.
45. Blattner, video interview, July 15, 1988.

5. The Second Physician-in-Chief

1. Anonymous, "Texas Children's Hospital, Baylor College of Medicine Joint Planning Study," January 1976.
2. Bobby R. Alford, letter from the search committee to Newell E. France, February 24, 1977.
3. Ralph D. Feigin, oral history, August 25, 1992.
4. Feigin, "Reviewing an Extraordinary Journey," *WATCH Magazine* 3 (2002).
5. Feigin, interview, March 4, 2003.
6. Ibid.
7. Alford, letter from the search committee to Newell E. France.
8. Russell J. Blattner, personal correspondence, July 7, 1977.
9. Feigin, oral history, August 25, 1992.
10. Ibid.
11. Feigin, interview, March 4, 2003.
12. Anonymous, "Feigin Takes Pediatrics Chair as New Physician-in-Chief," *Inside Baylor Medicine,* June/July 1977.
13. Feigin, oral history, August 25, 1992.
14. Sheldon L. Kaplan, oral history, November 13, 1996.
15. William T. Shearer, oral history, March 5, 1997.
16. Feigin, interview, March 4, 2003.
17. Martha Dukes Yow, *Balancing Act: Memoir of a Southern Woman Doctor* (Austin: Eakin Press,

1997), p. 186.
18. Ibid.
19. Feigin, oral history, August 25, 1992.
20. Feigin, "Saluting Dr. Lorin," *WATCH Magazine* 2 (1998).
21. Martin I. Lorin, oral history, September 6, 1996.
22. Feigin, oral history, August 25, 1992.
23. Lorin, oral history, September 6, 1996.
24. Leslie Loddeke, "Pediatrics Prof Kind of Kid Stuff," *Houston Post,* December 12, 1992.
25. Feigin, interview, March 4, 2003.
26. Ibid.
27. Feigin, oral history, August 25, 1992.
28. Feigin, interview, March 21, 2003.
29. Gina Seay, "Just What the Doctor Ordered, Clinics Designed with Kids in Mind," *Houston Chronicle,* October 16, 1986.
30. Feigin, interview, March 21, 2003.
31. Feigin, oral history, August 25, 1992.
32. Ibid.
33. Ibid.
34. Feigin, interview, March 21, 2003.
35. Feigin, dedication remarks for Feigin Center, April 23, 2003.
36. Anonymous, "Dr. Feigin Moved by Surprise Accolades," *WATCH Magazine* 3 (1992).
37. Ibid.
38. Ruth SoRelle, "Feigin to Head Baylor College of Medicine," *Houston Chronicle,* January 5, 1996.
39. SoRelle, "Changing, Difficult Era ahead for Baylor's Feigin," *Houston Chronicle,* January 7, 1996.
40. Feigin, "Message from the Physician-in-Chief," *WATCH Magazine* 3 (1993).
41. Anonymous, "Low Immunization Rates Verified by Hospital's Survey," *WATCH Magazine* 4 (1993).
42. Feigin, oral history, August 25, 1992.
43. Anonymous, "Dr. Feigin Moved."
44. Feigin, "Reviewing an Extraordinary Journey," *WATCH Magazine* 3 (2002).
45. Ibid.
46. Feigin, dedication remarks for Feigin Center, April 23, 2003.
47. Ibid.

6. Allergy and Immunology

1. Anonymous patient's grandmother, interview, April 5, 2002.
2. Theresa Aldape, interview, April 3, 2002.
3. C. Everett Koop, *Report of the Surgeon General's Workshop on Children with HIV Infection and Their Families,* DHHS Publication No. HRS-D-MC 87-1.
4. Anonymous patient's grandmother, interview, April 5, 2002.
5. William T. Shearer, oral history, May 9, 1979.
6. Ralph D. Feigin, "Message from the Physician-in-Chief," *WATCH Magazine,* Fall 1978.
7. Shearer, oral history, March 5, 1997.
8. Lois Hill, "The Pediatric Allergy Clinic of Texas Children's Hospital," *WATCH Magazine,* September 1959.
9. Anonymous, "David's Story," *Developments,* Spring 1994.
10. Ibid.
11. Shearer, interview, February 8, 2002.
12. Shearer, "Immunoregulation: Its Importance in Allergic and Immunologic Diseases in Children," *WATCH Magazine,* Summer 1982.
13. Shearer, interview, February 8, 2002.
14. Shearer, "Immunoregulation: Its Importance."
15. I. Celine Guerra Hanson, interview, February 25, 2002.
16. Shearer, interview, March 5, 1997.
17. Ruth SoRelle, "David's Death Linked Cancer with Virus, Doctor Says," *Houston Chronicle,* May 2, 1985.
18. Anonymous, "NCI Scientists Identify New Virus as Highly Probable Cause of AIDS," *NIH Record,* May 8, 1984.

19. Shearer, interview, February 8, 2002.
20. Leslie Hiebert and William T. Shearer, "The David Center Today," *WATCH Magazine,* Summer 1996.
21. Ibid.
22. Shearer, interview, February 8, 2002.
23. Hanson, "Children with AIDS," *WATCH Magazine,* Spring 1988.
24. Hanson, interview, February 25, 2002.
25. Sherry Carter Tuell, "Law Would Encourage AIDS Test," *Houston Chronicle,* February 17, 1995.
26. Shearer, interview, February 8, 2002.
27. Hanson, "Children with AIDS," *WATCH Magazine,* Spring 1988.
28. SoRelle, "AIDS-Hit Kids Due Experimental Drugs," *Houston Chronicle,* October 14, 1988.
29. Hanson, "Children with AIDS," *WATCH Magazine,* Spring 1988.
30. Lynne M. Mofenson, "Can Perinatal HIV Infection Be Eliminated in the United States?" *Journal of the American Medical Association* 282 (August 11, 1999): 577–79.
31. Shearer, interview, February 8, 2002.
32. Hanson, interview, February 25, 2002.
33. Feigin, "Children with Immunodeficiency Viral Infection Are the Focus of Attention of Many Clinician/Investigators in the Department of Pediatrics of the Baylor College of Medicine at Texas Children's Hospital," *WATCH Magazine,* Summer 1990.
34. Shearer, interview, February 8, 2002.
35. Anonymous, "Baylor AIDS Initiative Expands International Training Program," Baylor College of Medicine press release, October 16, 2000.
36. Shearer, interview, March 5, 1997.
37. Shearer, interview, February 8, 2002.
38. SoRelle, "In Spirit of David: A Key Genetic Finding," *Houston Chronicle,* April 9, 1993.
39. Anonymous, "Milestone in Gene Therapy: Doctors First to Save Lives Using Technique," *Houston Chronicle,* April 28, 2000.
40. Shearer, interview, February 8, 2002.
41. Shearer, interview, March 5, 1997.
42. Aldape, interview, April 3, 2002.
43. Anonymous patient, interview, April 5, 2002.
44. Anonymous patient's grandmother, interview, April 5, 2002.

7. Auxiliary

1. George Fuermann, *Houston: The Feast Years, an Illustrated Essay* (Houston: Premier Printing Company, 1962), 18.
2. Ibid., 1.
3. Bill Roberts, "Bill Roberts' Tales of Houston: Times Were Easy in the 50s," *Houston Chronicle,* March 10, 1986.
4. Fuermann, *Houston: The Feast Years,* 10.
5. Ibid., 23.
6. Mary Liz Grose, *History of Women's Auxiliary to Texas Children's Hospital,* Auxiliary archives.
7. Elaine Kuper, interview, February 22, 2000.
8. Helen Blumberg, oral history, July 10, 1992.
9. Kuper, interview, February 22, 2000.
10. Jean Walsh, "Memo Spurs Humane Unit," *Houston Post,* November 22, 1953.
11. Ibid.
12. Nancy Bateman, *Annual Report, 1953–1955, Women's Auxiliary to Texas Children's Hospital,* Auxiliary archives.
13. Bateman, *Annual Report, 1953–1955.*
14. Grose, *History of Women's Auxiliary.*
15. Julie Finger, "A Special Kind of Coffee Shop Celebrates Its 24th Birthday," *WATCH Magazine,* Spring 1978, 16.
16. Ibid., 17.
17. Anonymous, *WATCH Magazine* 1, no. 1 (1955).
18. Grose, *History of Women's Auxiliary.*
19. Ibid.
20. Anonymous, "Bob Hope Came, Was Seen, and Conquered," *Houston Press,* May 23, 1958.
21. Finger, "Special Kind of Coffee Shop," 17.
22. Anonymous, "WATCH General Assembly Bids Farewell to Bess," *WATCH Magazine,* July 1976.

23. Lin Fish, "Texas Children's Auxiliary: Changing Roles, 1954–1995," Auxiliary archives.
24. Anonymous, "Women's Auxiliary to Texas Children's Hospital," *WATCH Magazine*, January 1972.
25. Grose, *History of Women's Auxiliary.*
26. Ibid.
27. Ibid.
28. Gen McClelland, oral history, June 19, 1992.
29. Kuper, interview, February 22, 2000.
30. Pat Dolan, interview, February 17, 2000.
31. Ibid.
32. Anonymous, "Giving in the New Year: Volunteers Help Hurting Children Heal," Texas Children's Hospital press release, December 30, 2004.
33. Kuper, interview, February 22, 2000.

8. Cardiology

1. Jill Tinklepaugh, oral history, April 13, 1999.
2. Scott Tinklepaugh, oral history, April 13, 1999.
3. J. Timothy Bricker, oral history, March 31, 1999.
4. Scott Tinklepaugh, oral history, April 13, 1999.
5. Scott Tinklepaugh, oral history, April 13, 1999.
6. Catherine A. Neill and Edward B. Clark, *The Developing Heart: A History of Pediatric Cardiology* (Dordrecht/Boston/London, 1995), 128.
7. Ibid.
8. Dan G. McNamara, "Helen B. Taussig: The Original Pediatric Cardiologist," *Medical Times,* November 1978.
9. Dan G. McNamara, oral history, April 18, 1977.
10. Irving Schweppe, interview, April 4, 1999.
11. McNamara, oral history, April 18, 1977.
12. McNamara, oral history, April 30, 1979.
13. Ibid.
14. Frances Heyck, oral history, May 3, 1979.
15. Edward B. Singleton, oral history, April 18, 1977.
16. McNamara, oral history, April 18, 1977.
17. Russell Blattner, oral history, April 30, 1979.
18. McNamara, oral history, June 25, 1979.
19. Anonymous, *Twenty-five Years of Excellence: A History of the Texas Heart Institute* (Texas Heart Institute Foundation, Texas Heart Institute, 1989).
20. McNamara, oral history, June 25, 1979.
21. McNamara, oral history, April 30, 1979.
22. Denton A. Cooley, oral history, July 21, 1979.
23. G. Wayne Miller, "Into the Heart: A Medical Odyssey," *Providence Journal,* January 10, 1999.
24. McNamara, memo to fellows and staff of the cardiology service, December 24, 1970.
25. McNamara, "A Mini-Guide to Pediatric Cardiology Research: The Research Programs of the Cardiology Section of Texas Children's Hospital," *WATCH Magazine,* Winter 1979.
26. Ibid.
27. Ibid.
28. Neill and Clark, *The Developing Heart,* 135.
29. Ibid., 74.
30. Bricker, oral history, March 31, 1999.
31. Jeffrey A. Towbin, correspondence, July 5, 2005.
32. Anonymous, "The Lillie Frank Abercrombie Section of Pediatric Cardiology," Baylor College of Medicine website, http://www.bcm.edu/pediatrics.
33. Anonymous, "Genetic Therapy Gives Insight into Children's Congenital Heart Disease," Texas Children's Hospital website, http://www.texaschildrenshospital.org/carecenters/heart/genetic_therapy.aspx.
34. Bricker, "Contributions of the Texas Children's Hospital Pediatric Cardiology Program to the Field of Pediatric Cardiology," *Texas Heart Institute Journal,* November 4, 1997.
35. Bricker, oral history, September 9, 1996.
36. Kate Schweppe McNamara, interview, April 3, 1999.
37. William Clifford Roberts, "Interview with Arthur Garson, Jr., M.D.," *American Journal of*

Cardiology 92, no. 4 (August 15, 2003).
38. Ibid.
39. Arthur Garson, Jr., "Pediatric Cardiology: New Faces, Patient Care and Research," *WATCH Magazine,* Fall 1988.
40. Roberts, "Interview with Arthur Garson, Jr."
41. Bricker and Garson, "The Child with Congenital Heart Disease Grows Up ... Challenges and Opportunities," *WATCH Magazine* 3 (1992).
42. Roberts, "Interview with Arthur Garson."
43. Bricker, oral history, September 9, 1996.
44. Ibid.
45. Roberts, "Interview with Arthur Garson."
46. Bricker, interview, April 1, 2004.
47. Baruch S. Ticho, review of *The Science and Practice of Pediatric Cardiology,* 2 vols., *Journal of the American Medical Association* 281 (1999): 387–88.
48. Bricker, David J. Fisher, Garson, and Neish, *The Science and Practice of Pediatric Cardiology,* 2nd ed. (Baltimore, 1998), v.
49. Bricker, oral history, March 31, 1999.
50. Ibid.
51. Bricker, interview, April 1, 2004.
52. Towbin, correspondence, July 5, 2005.
53. Ibid.
54. Anonymous, "Genetic Therapy Gives Insight."
55. Laura Frnka, "Texas Children's Cardiologist Promoted to Chief, Receives Prestigious DeBakey Award," Texas Children's Hospital press release, December 3, 2003.
56. Bricker, interview, April 1, 2004.
57. Towbin, correspondence, July 5, 2005.
58. Jill Tinklepaugh, oral history, April 13, 1999.
59. Scott Tinklepaugh, oral history, April 13, 1999.
60. Ibid.
61. Charles D. Fraser, Jr., interview, March 31, 1999.
62. Bricker, oral history, March 31, 1999.

9. Child Life

1. Loree Smith, interview, October 28, 2000.
2. Ibid.
3. Bonnie Shoemate, "An Open Letter to Parents," correspondence, Texas Children's Hospital administration archive.
4. Mary Liz Grose, *History of Women's Auxiliary to Texas Children's Hospital,* Auxiliary archives.
5. Anonymous, "Play Therapy," *Intercom,* n.d.
6. Gene Wilburn, "Play Part of Child Therapy," *Houston Chronicle,* June 14, 1959.
7. Ibid.
8. Jackie Vogel, oral history, September 3, 1992.
9. Anonymous, "Child Life," *Developments* 4, no. 1 (First Quarter 1988).
10. Vogel, oral history, September 3, 1992.
11. *Texas Children's Hospital Annual Report 1976.*
12. Stefi Rubin, "What's in a Name? Child Life and the Play Lady Legacy," *CHC* 21, no. 1 (Winter 1982).
13. Anonymous, "Child Life Position Statement," Child Life Council website, http://www.childlife.org.
14. Rubin, "What's in a Name?"
15. Anonymous, "What Is Child Life Certification?" Child Life Council website, http://www.childlife.org.
16. Vogel, oral history, September 3, 1992.
17. Anonymous, "5th Floor Library Opens Its Doors ... and the Minds of TCH Children," *WATCH Magazine,* Spring 1984.
18. Julie Gilbert, "Jackie Vogel, Child Life Specialist, Helps Kids Adjust to Hospital Life," *Houston Post,* July 8, 1985.
19. Vogel, oral history, September 3, 1992.
20. Dana Nicholson, interview, October 26, 2000.
21. Anonymous, "Partnership with Bo's Place Helps Families Heal," *Developments,* Spring 2000.

22. Anonymous, "Child Life Specialists Play Important Role," *Houston Chronicle,* April 3, 2000.
23. Nicholson, interview, October 26, 2000.
24. Smith, interview, October 28, 2000.
25. Ibid.

10. Congenital Heart Surgery

1. Jean Parrish, interview, June 16, 2004.
2. Stephen Paget, *The Surgery of the Chest* (London: Wright, 1896), 121.
3. Denton A. Cooley and O. H. Frazier, "The Past 50 Years of Cardiovascular Surgery," *Circulation* 102 (2000): IV-87–IV-93.
4. Ruth SoRelle, "Eminent Surgeon: Cool Hand, Warm Heart," *Houston Chronicle,* November 8, 1987.
5. Dan G. McNamara, "Denton Cooley's Part in the Evolution of Heart Surgery in the Years 1944–1994," *Texas Heart Institute Journal* 21, no. 4 (1994).
6. Cooley, oral history, July 21, 1979.
7. McNamara, "Denton Cooley's Part in the Evolution of Heart Surgery."
8. Ibid.
9. Thomas J. Takach and David A. Ott, "Congenital Heart Surgery in Houston, the Early Years," *Texas Heart Institute Journal* 24, no. 3 (1997).
10. Cooley and Frazier, "The Past 50 Years of Cardiovascular Surgery."
11. Cooley, oral history, July 21, 1979.
12. Anonymous, *Twenty-five Years of Excellence: A History of the Texas Heart Institute* (Texas Heart Institute Foundation, Texas Heart Institute, 1989), 7.
13. Russell J. Blattner, "Research Activities," *WATCH Magazine,* July 1957.
14. Cooley and Frazier, "The Past 50 Years of Cardiovascular Surgery."
15. Ibid.
16. Cooley, "Early Development of Congenital Heart Surgery: Open Heart Surgeries," *Annals of Thoracic Surgeons,* April 26, 1997.
17. Takach and Ott, "Congenital Heart Surgery in Houston."
18. Ibid.
19. Cooley and A. Ochsner, Jr., "Correction of Total Anomalous Pulmonary Venous Drainage: Technical Considerations," *Surgery* 42 (1957): 1014–21.
20. Cooley, oral history, July 21, 1979.
21. Takach and Ott, "Congenital Heart Surgery in Houston."
22. Anonymous, "TCH & SLEH among Top in Nation in Operations Using Heart–Lung Apparatus," *Intercom,* February 20, 1958.
23. Anonymous, "A Talk with Dr. Cooley," *Texas Medical Center News* 20, no. 3 (February 15, 1988).
24. McNamara, "Denton Cooley's Part in the Evolution of Heart Surgery."
25. Ibid.
26. Cooley, oral history, July 21, 1979.
27. Takach and Ott, "Congenital Heart Surgery in Houston."
28. Cooley and Grady L. Hallman, *Surgical Treatment of Congenital Heart Disease* (Philadelphia: Lea & Febiger, 1966), 33–49.
29. Cooley, "Early Development of Congenital Heart Surgery."
30. Cooley, "Growth of Open Heart Surgery," *Medical Record and Annals* 6, no. 7 (July 1967).
31. Cooley, oral history, July 21, 1979.
32. Hallman and Cooley, *Surgical Treatment of Congenital Heart Disease,* 2nd ed. (Philadelphia: Lea & Febiger, 1975), preface.
33. Anonymous, "History of Transplantation," Living Bank website, http://www.livingbank.org/transplantation.html.
34. Cooley, "Early Development of Congenital Heart Surgery."
35. Charles E. Mullins, "The Pediatric Cardiac Catheterization Laboratory," *WATCH Magazine,* Winter 1982.
36. Anonymous, "Reflections," *Texas Heart Institute Today,* Summer 1987.
37. Cooley, oral history, July 21, 1979.
38. Anonymous, "Reflections."
39. Bruce Goldfarb, "The Heart of the Matter," *Hopkins Medical News,* Fall 1998.
40. Cooley, "Early Development of Congenital Heart Surgery."
41. Associated Press, "Boy Receives Heart Hours after Birth," *Houston Chronicle,* October 17, 1987.

42. Takach and Ott, "Congenital Heart Surgery in Houston."
43. McNamara, "The Section of Cardiology, Texas Children's Hospital," *WATCH Magazine*, May 1972.
44. Cooley, "Early Development of Congenital Heart Surgery."
45. Michael Ruhlman, *Walk on Water: Inside an Elite Pediatric Surgical Unit* (New York: Viking, 2003), 184.
46. J. Timothy Bricker, interview, April 1, 2004.
47. Ibid.
48. Ibid.
49. Charles D. Fraser, Jr., interview, March 6, 2004.
50. Ibid.
51. Ibid.
52. Ibid.
53. Michael Ruhlman, *Walk on Water*, 192.
54. Fraser, interview, March 6, 2004.
55. Ibid.
56. Roger B. B. Mee, Fraser's personal recollection from December 1991.
57. Fraser, interview, March 6, 2004.
58. Ibid.
59. Fraser, interview, March 31, 1999.
60. Bricker, interview, April 1, 2004.
61. Ibid.
62. Ralph D. Feigin, interview, March 15, 2004.
63. Bricker, interview, April 1, 2004.
64. Fraser, "Congenital Heart Surgery in the New Century," Thirteenth Congress of the Michael E. DeBakey International Surgical Society, Houston, November 2000.
65. Anonymous, "Pediatric Cardiac Anesthesiologists," Texas Children's Hospital website, http://texaschildrenshospital.org/carecenters/heart/anesthesiologists.aspx.
66. Fraser, "Congenital Heart Surgery: New Challenges for an Evolving Specialty," *Neonatal News* 4, no. 2 (November 2003).
67. Anonymous, "Perfusionists: Sustaining Life During Surgery," Texas Children's Hospital website, http://texaschildrenshospital.org/carecenters/heart/perfusionists.aspx.
68. Fraser, "Congenital Heart Surgery in the New Century."
69. *Child*, 2001.
70. Deborah Mann Lake, "Change of Heart," *Houston Chronicle*, February 27, 2001.
71. Roger Widmeyer, "Dr. Charles D. Fraser, Jr.: Fixing Tiny Broken Hearts," *Texas Medical Center News* 21, no. 2 (February 1, 1999).
72. Fraser, "Congenital Heart Surgery: New Challenges."
73. Anonymous, "Less-Invasive Heart Surgery Lessens Trauma, May Reduce Recovery Time, Say Texas Children's Specialists," Texas Children's Hospital press release, January 22, 2004.
74. Anonymous, "Catheterization: Diagnosis and Treatment without Surgery," Texas Children's Hospital website, http://www.texaschildrenshospital.org/carecenters/heart/catheterization.
75. Anonymous, "When Volume Saves Lives," Texas Children's Hospital press release, February 18, 2003.
76. Widmeyer, "Dr. Charles D. Fraser."
77. Fraser, "Congenital Heart Surgery: New Challenges."
78. Anonymous, "Fellowships: Congenital Heart Surgery," Michael E. DeBakey Department of Surgery, Baylor College of Medicine website, http://www.debakeydepartmentofsurgery.org/home/content.cfm?menu_id=7.
79. Fraser, interview, March 6, 2004.
80. Widmeyer, "Dr. Charles D. Fraser."
81. Catherine M. Ikemba, Claudia A. Kozinetz, Timothy F. Feltes, Fraser, E. Dean McKenzie, Naeema Shaw, and Antonio R. Mott, "Internet Use in Families with Children Requiring Cardiac Surgery for Congenital Heart Disease," *Pediatrics*, March 2002.
82. Anonymous, "Pediatric Heart Surgery: Beating the Odds," Texas Children's Hospital website, http://texaschildrenshospital.org/carecenters/heart/surgeon.aspx.
83. Fraser, interview, March 31, 1999.
84. Cooley, "Early Development of Congenital Heart Surgery."
85. Fraser, "Congenital Heart Surgery: New Challenges."
86. Parrish, interview, June 16, 2004.
87. Leigh Hopper, "Worth the Risk: Parents Opt for Heart Surgery to Save Their Infant Daughter," *Houston Chronicle*, March 25, 2002.

11. Critical Care

1. Wendy, Jody, and Leslie Meigs, interview, September 18, 2000.
2. Charles E. Mullins, interview, July 6, 2000.
3. Mullins, slide from 1972 presentation to Texas Children's Hospital board of directors.
4. Mullins, interview, July 6, 2000.
5. Ibid.
6. Ibid.
7. Anonymous, "Pediatric ICU: Parents Need Attention, Too," *WATCH Magazine,* Summer 1977.
8. Anonymous, "Prescription: Parental Care," *WATCH Magazine,* Spring 1978.
9. Anonymous, "TCH Pediatric Intensive Care Unit," *WATCH Magazine,* Summer 1979.
10. Mullins, interview, July 6, 2000.
11. John J. Downes, "The Future of Pediatric Critical Care Medicine," *Vignettes of Pediatric World Congress* 21, no. 9 (supplement), 307.
12. Thomas A. Vargo, interview, June 16, 2000.
13. Ibid.
14. Anonymous, "TCH Pediatric Intensive Care Unit."
15. Anonymous, "Commitment to Care," *Developments,* March 1993.
16. Ibid.
17. Anonymous, "TCH Pediatric Intensive Care Unit."
18. Vargo, interview, June 16, 2000.
19. Ibid.
20. Larry S. Jefferson, oral history, December 4, 1996.
21. Ibid.
22. Jefferson, interview, September 28, 2000.
23. Fernando Stein, interview, June 20, 2000.
24. Ibid.
25. Jefferson, interview, September 28, 2000.
26. Jefferson, oral history, December 4, 1996.
27. Ibid.
28. Anonymous, "Pediatric Intensive Care Unit," *WATCH Magazine* 1 (1992).
29. Anonymous, "Meeting of the Minds," *Developments,* Summer 2000.
30. Jefferson, interview, September 28, 2000.
31. Stein, interview, June 20, 2000.
32. Mullins, interview, July 6, 2000.
33. Wendy, Jody, and Leslie Meigs, interview, September 18, 2000.
34. Anonymous, "A Clear Path," *Developments,* Summer 2000.
35. Wendy, Jody, and Leslie Meigs, interview, September 18, 2000.

12. Diabetes Care Center

1. Claire and Elizabeth Conroy, interview, June 22, 2001.
2. Anonymous, "Diabetes in Children," American Diabetes Association website, http://www.diabetes.org.
3. Anonymous, "The History of Diabetes," *Countdown for Kids Magazine,* JDRF Kids Online, Juvenile Diabetes Research Foundation International website, http://www.jdrf.org.
4. Morey W. Haymond, interview, June 6, 2001.
5. Marilyn Miller Baker, *Caring for the Children: The History of Pediatrics in Texas* (Texas Pediatric Society, 1996), 85.
6. Anonymous, Washington University in St. Louis School of Medicine website, http://peds.wustl.edu.
7. Charles William Daeschner, Jr., oral history, August 9, 1995.
8. Ibid.
9. Ibid.
10. Andrea Pappas, "The Best Seller Nobody Knows," *UTMB Quarterly,* Winter 2000, 16.
11. L. Leighton Hill, interview, May 30, 2001.
12. Hill, oral history, January 29, 1992.
13. Hill, correspondence, October 21, 2004.
14. Ibid., June 28, 2005.
15. Hill, "Diabetes Mellitus … It's a Common Disease," *WATCH Magazine,* Spring 1979.
16. Hill, correspondence, October 21, 2004.

17. Hill, interview, May 30, 2001.
18. Ibid.
19. Ibid.
20. Hill, correspondence, October 21, 2004.
21. Hill, interview, May 30, 2001.
22. Kenneth Gabbay, "Pediatric Diabetes: A Day-to-Day Challenge," *WATCH Magazine,* Spring 1986.
23. John L. Kirkland III, interview, May 17, 2001.
24. Anonymous, "American Diabetes Association Milestones," American Diabetes Association website, http://www.diabetes.org.
25. Anonymous, "Diabetes," *Developments,* June 1992.
26. Anonymous, "DCCT," *New England Journal of Medicine* 329, no. 14 (September 30, 1993).
27. Kirkland, interview, May 17, 2001.
28. Ibid.
29. Anonymous, "The Best Way to Manage Disease Is for the Patient to Become Independent," *Developments,* Winter 1995.
30. Barb Schreiner, interview, May 31, 2001.
31. Haymond, interview, June 6, 2001.
32. Haymond, interview, June 6, 2001.
33. Claire and Elizabeth Conroy, interview, June 22, 2001.
34. Anonymous, "Insulin Pumps," Diabetes 123 and Children with Diabetes, http://www.children-withdiabetes.com.

13. Diagnostic Imaging

1. Edward B. Singleton, interview, July 31, 2001.
2. Singleton, interview, April 18, 1977.
3. Singleton, oral history, April 30, 1979.
4. Ibid.
5. Anonymous, "Marguerite Garner Is Hospital Pioneer," *Intercom,* February 5, 1958.
6. Singleton, interview, July 31, 2001.
7. Karl Leif Bates, "The X-ray Century," *Detroit News,* November 6, 1995.
8. Ibid.
9. John Holt, Fred Jenner Hodges, and Isadore Lampe, *Radiology for Medical Students* (Chicago: Year Book Publishers, Inc., 1947), 21.
10. Singleton, interview, July 31, 2001.
11. Ibid.
12. Ibid.
13. Ibid.
14. Singleton, interview, April 18, 1977.
15. Singleton, "Radiology Department, Texas Children's Hospital," *WATCH Magazine,* August 1971.
16. Singleton, oral history, April 30, 1979.
17. Ibid.
18. Singleton, interview, July 31, 2001.
19. John Caffey, "The First Sixty Years of Pediatric Roentgenology in the United States—1896 to 1956," *American Journal of Roentgenology, Radium Therapy, and Nuclear Medicine* 76, no. 3 (September 1956).
20. Singleton, interview, July 31, 2001.
21. Lois Hill, "The Radiology Department," *WATCH Magazine,* April 1965.
22. Singleton, "Radiology Department, Texas Children's Hospital."
23. Singleton, oral history, April 30, 1979.
24. Singleton, "New Radiologic Techniques in the Diagnosis of Pediatric Diseases," *WATCH Magazine,* Spring 1982.
25. Singleton, "Pediatric Radiology," *WATCH Magazine,* Summer 1979.
26. Ruth SoRelle, "Magnets, Not Mirrors, behind Imaging Magic," *Houston Chronicle,* December 16, 1985.
27. Singleton, "New Radiologic Techniques."
28. Bruce R. Parker, interview, July 23, 2001.
29. Parker, "Enterprise-Wide PACS Solution," http://www.ImagingEconomics.com, December 5, 2000.

30. Parker, interview, July 2001.
31. Ibid.
32. Ibid.
33. Ibid.
34. Ibid.
35. Laura Frnka, "Texas Children's Chief of Diagnostic Imaging Receives Kudos as He Steps Down," Texas Children's Hospital press release, July 26, 2004.
36. Ibid.
37. Holt, Hodges, and Lampe, *Radiology for Medical Students,* 21.
38. Singleton, interview, 2001.
39. Singleton, oral history, June 10, 1992.
40. Singleton, interview, 2001.
41. Anonymous, "Dr. Edward B. Singleton, Celebrating 46 Years of Service at Texas Children's Hospital," *Developments,* Winter 1999.

14. Emergency Center

1. Anonymous family, interview, August 29, 1999.
2. Ibid.
3. Allen H. Kline, oral history, August 30, 1995.
4. Ibid.
5. Helen A. Dunn, oral history, September 19, 1996. *Note:* When the three-story Texas Children's Hospital opened in 1954, the ground level was known as the second floor and the third story was known as the fourth floor. All floors in the newly expanded seven-story hospital were renumbered on April 14, 1979, making the ground level entrance the first floor and the two lower levels B1 and B2. "No Fooling - On April 14 Everyone Will Be Working on a Different Floor," *Grapevine,* March 23, 1979.
6. Ibid.
7. Anonymous, "All through the Night," *WATCH Magazine,* April 1959, 4–7.
8. Anonymous, "STAT," *WATCH Magazine,* November 1964, 10–12.
9. Anonymous, "New Emergency Center Opens," *Intercom,* June 1972, 2.
10. Ibid.
11. Anonymous, "TCH Emergency Center," *WATCH Magazine,* Winter 1979, 4.
12. Joan E. Shook, oral history, August 17, 1999.
13. Anonymous, "The Meyer and Ida Gordon Emergency Center," *Developments,* 1991, 13–17.
14. Shook, oral history, August 17, 1999.
15. Anonymous, "Emergency Center's Acute Treatment Area," *Developments,* Spring 1994, Hospital Highlights, 3.
16. Shook, oral history, August 17, 1999.
17. Paul Gerson, "Child Abuse—It Is a Monstrous Problem/Horror Isn't Going Away until We Help," *Houston Chronicle,* July 16, 1989.
18. Anonymous, "Child Abuse," *Developments* 5, no. 1 (1989): 6.
19. Shook, oral history, August 17, 1999.
20. Bonnie Britt, "Hospital Team Has Kept Watch over Abused Children for 9 Years," *Houston Chronicle,* April 28, 1985.
21. Anonymous, "Child Abuse," 6.
22. Britt, "Hospital Team Has Kept Watch."
23. Anonymous, "10 Years and 1,000 Children Later," *Developments* 2, no. 2 (Second Quarter 1986).
24. Laura Frnka, "Texas Children's Emergency Specialist Offers Child Abuse Prevention Tactics," Texas Children's Hospital press release, April 20, 2004.
25. Shook, oral history, August 17, 1999.
26. Ibid.
27. Anonymous, "Art Complements Healing at Texas Children's Hospital," *Developments,* Spring 1999.
28. Staci Bonner, "The ER Hazard You Must Know About," *Redbook* 191 (August 1, 1998): 114.
29. Shook, oral history, August 17, 1999.
30. Norma Martin, "Child Injuries Preventable, Houston Coalition Teaches/Wrecks, Burns, and Drownings Lead Causes of Death for about 8,000 Children Yearly," *Houston Chronicle,* April 4, 1993.
31. Shook, oral history, August 17, 1999.

32. Barbara Boughton, "Texas Children's Hospital Emergency Room Exclusively for Kids," *Houston Chronicle,* November 29, 1987.
33. Anonymous, "The Children's Asthma Center," *Developments,* November 1993, 3.
34. Anonymous family, interview, August 29, 1999.
35. Ibid.

15. Gastroenterology, Hepatology and Nutrition

1. Benjamin Sellers, interview, June 19, 2002.
2. Roberta Sellers, interview, June 19, 2002.
3. Benjamin Sellers, interview, June 19, 2002.
4. Roberta Sellers, interview, June 19, 2002.
5. David Baty, interview, June 23, 2002.
6. William J. Klish, interview, May 31, 2002.
7. George W. Clayton, "Clinical Research, Just for Children," *WATCH Magazine,* Fall 1981.
8. Ibid.
9. Clayton, oral history, April 30, 1979.
10. Buford L. Nichols, Jr., oral history, March 11, 1991.
11. Nichols, oral history, September 25, 1992.
12. Ibid.
13. Elaine Potts, oral history, July 17, 1992.
14. Nichols, oral history, September 25, 1992.
15. George D. Ferry, "Pediatric Nutrition and Gastroenterology—A New Subspecialty at Texas Children's Hospital," *WATCH Magazine,* August 1974.
16. Ann M. Petit and Nichols, "Ten Years of Total Parenteral Nutrition at Texas Children's Hospital ... Perfection of the Artificial Umbilical Cord," *WATCH Magazine,* 1978.
17. Klish, interview, May 31, 2002.
18. Ferry, "Pediatric Nutrition and Gastroenterology."
19. Miriam Kass, "Starvation in Houston?" *Houston Post,* March 28, 1971.
20. Klish, interview, May 31, 2002.
21. Ferry, "Pediatric Nutrition and Gastroenterology."
22. Nichols, oral history, March 11, 1991.
23. Mary Jane Schier, "Plans for Nutrition Center Unveiled," *Houston Post,* November 2, 1978.
24. M. E. Ament and D. L. Christie, "Upper Gastrointestinal Fiberoptic Endoscopy in Pediatric Patients," *Gastroenterology* 72 (1977): 1244–48.
25. David V. Graham, Klish, Ferry, and John S. Sabel, "Value of Fiberoptic Gastrointestinal Endoscopy in Infants and Children," *Southern Medical Journal* 71, no. 5 (May 1978).
26. Klish, interview, May 31, 2002.
27. Klish, oral history, January 8, 1997.
28. Klish, "Gastroenterology Section Expands to Meet New Challenges," *WATCH Magazine,* Fall 1984.
29. Klish, interview, May 31, 2002.
30. Ferry, interview, May 8, 2002.
31. Hilary Metherell, "Liver Transplant Program Off to a Healthy Start," *WATCH Magazine,* Summer 1986.
32. Ruth SoRelle, "Children No Longer Need to Leave Houston to Obtain Liver Transplants," *Houston Chronicle,* February 17, 1986.
33. Ferry, "Inflammatory Bowel Disease in Children," *WATCH Magazine,* Spring 1990.
34. Klish, interview, May 31, 2002.
35. Anonymous, "Texas Children's Hospital Announces New Liver Disease Center," *Texas Medical Center News* 22, no. 13 (July 15, 2000).
36. Anonymous, "Types of Liver Transplant," Texas Children's Hospital Parent Resource Center, Texas Children's Hospital website, http://texaschildrenshospital.org/Parents/TipsArticles/ArticleDisplay/aspx.
37. Ferry, interview, May 8, 2002.
38. Klish, oral history, January 8, 1997.
39. Klish, interview, May 31, 2002.
40. Vernisha Shepard, interview, June 19, 2002.
41. Roberta Sellers, interview, June 19, 2002
42. Ben Sellers, interview, June 19, 2002.
43. Vernisha Shepard, interview, June 19, 2002.

44. Roberta Sellers, interview, June 19, 2002.
45. Ben Sellers, interview, June 19, 2002.
46. Roberta Sellers, interview, June 19, 2002.
47. Ben Sellers, interview, June 19, 2002.
48. Baty, interview, June 23, 2002.

16. Genetics

1. Vi Guerrero, interview, December 12, 2001.
2. Eugene Guerrero, interview, December 12, 2001.
3. Harry Angelman, "Puppet Children: A Report on Three Cases," *Developmental Medicine and Child Neurology* 7 (Oxford, 1965): 681–88; B. D. Bower and P. M. Jeavons, "The 'Happy Puppet' Syndrome," *Archives of Disease in Childhood* 42 (London, 1967): 298–301.
4. C. A. Williams and J. L. Frias, "The Angelman ('Happy Puppet') Syndrome," *American Journal of Medical Genetics* 11 (New York, 1982): 453–60; H. Pashayan, W. Singer, C. Dove, E. Eisenberg, and B. Seto, "The Angelman Syndrome in Two Brothers," *American Journal of Medical Genetics* 13 (1982): 295–98.
5. Anonymous, "Molecular Genetic Testing in Pediatric Practice: A Subject Review," *Pediatrics,* December 2000.
6. Vi Guerrero, interview, December 12, 2001.
7. Eugene Guerrero, interview, December 12, 2001.
8. Vi Guerrero, interview, December 12, 2001.
9. Eugene Guerrero, interview, December 12, 2001.
10. Vi Guerrero, interview, December 12, 2001.
11. Arthur L. Beaudet, oral history, September 10, 1992.
12. Russell J. Blattner, oral history, May 18, 1977.
13. F. Clarke Fraser and James J. Nora, *Genetics of Man* (Philadelphia: Lea & Febiger, 1975), 160.
14. Anonymous, "Houston Birth Defects Center," March of Dimes brochure, personal collection of Nan O'Keeffe.
15. Anonymous, *Baylor College of Medicine Pediatrics Department Report 1967–1968.*
16. Nan O'Keeffe, interview, November 7, 2001.
17. Ibid.
18. Beaudet, interview, October 30, 2001.
19. Anonymous, "Career Profile, Art Beaudet," Federation of American Societies for Experimental Biology website, http://www.faseb.org/genetics/gsa/careers/bro-10htm.
20. Anonymous, "The Genetics Revolution Timeline," *Time* magazine website, http://www.time.com.
21. O'Keeffe, interview, November 7, 2001.
22. Beaudet, interview, October 30, 2001.
23. Kleberg Genetics Clinic brochure, personal collection of Nan O'Keeffe.
24. Beaudet, "Genetics and the Birth Defects Center," *WATCH Magazine,* October 1975.
25. Anonymous, "Will My Child Be Healthy?" *Inside Baylor Medicine,* May–June 1974.
26. Beaudet, "Why Risk the Birth of an Abnormal Child?" *WATCH Magazine,* Fall 1978.
27. Ibid.
28. Beaudet, "Rapid Changes in Human Genetics," *WATCH Magazine,* Winter 1981.
29. Ibid.
30. Anonymous, "Genetics Revolution Timeline."
31. Beaudet, oral history, September 10, 1992.
32. Beaudet, "Gene Cloning: Its Use in the Diagnosis and Treatment of Genetic Disease," *WATCH Magazine,* Winter 1984.
33. Beaudet, "Rapid Changes in Human Genetics."
34. Anonymous, "Baylor Founds Genetics Institute, Names Head," *Houston Chronicle,* November 17, 1985.
35. Beaudet, oral history, September 10, 1992.
36. Maya Pines, "Finding the Faulty Gene's Fellow Travelers," Howard Hughes Medical Institute website, http:www.hhmi.org.
37. Spence, C. L. Rosenblum, W. E. O'Brien, D. K. Seilheimer, S. Cole, R. E. Ferrell, R. C. Stern, and Beaudet, "Linkage of DNA Markers to Cystic Fibrosis in 26 Families," *American Journal of Human Genetics,* December 1986.
38. Ruth SoRelle, "DNA Dreams/Gene Replacements Could Turn 'Fantasy Land' into Reality," *Houston Chronicle,* February 10, 1986.

39. Beaudet, oral history, September 10, 1992.
40. SoRelle, "DNA Dreams/Gene Replacements."
41. Beaudet, oral history, September 10, 1992.
42. J. E. Spence, R. G. Perciaccante, G. M. Greig, H. F. Willard, D. H. Ledbetter, J. F. Hejtmancik, M. S. Pollack, O'Brien, and Beaudet, "Uniparental Disomy as a Mechanism for Human Genetic Disease," *American Journal of Human Genetics* 42, no. 2 (February 1988): 217–26.
43. M. D. Clericuzio, "Uniparental Disomy and Genomic Imprinting," *Genetic Drift* (University of New Mexico) 10 (Winter 1994).
44. SoRelle, "Test Closes in on Cystic Fibrosis," *Houston Chronicle,* October 15, 1993.
45. SoRelle, "Baylor Lab Wins $10 Million Grant for Gene Research," *Houston Chronicle,* December 22, 1990.
46. Beaudet, interview, October 30, 2001.
47. Beaudet, "The Future for Somatic Gene Therapy," *WATCH Magazine* 1 (1992).
48. Anonymous, "Human Genome Sequencing Center," Baylor College of Medicine website, http://www.hgsc.bcm.tmc.edu/docs/HGSC_info.html.
49. Anonymous, "Baylor Researcher Discovers Genetic Cause of Angelman Syndrome," *Inside Baylor Medicine,* February 2000.
50. Anonymous, "Cancer Center Welcomes Famed Researcher Malcolm Brenner," *Developments,* Spring 1998.
51. Anonymous, "Gene Discoveries Pave the Way for Research on Treatments," Baylor College of Medicine press release, April 1998.
52. Beaudet, interview, October 30, 2001.
53. Ibid.
54. Ibid.
55. Eugene Guerrero, interview, December 12, 2001.
56. Vi Guerrero, interview, December 12, 2001.
57. Eugene Guerrero, interview, December 12, 2001.
58. Vi Guerrero, interview, December 12, 2001.
59. Eugene Guerrero, interview, December 12, 2001.
60. Vi Guerrero, interview, December 12, 2001.
61. Eugene Guerrero, interview, December 12, 2001.

17. Hematology-Oncology

1. Lindy Neuhaus, interview, October 26, 1999.
2. Bo Neuhaus with Lindy Neuhaus, *It's Okay, God, We Can Take It* (Austin: Eakin Press, 1986), 2.
3. Larry Neuhaus, interview, October 26, 1999.
4. Lindy Neuhaus, interview, October 26, 1999.
5. Larry Neuhaus, interview, October 26, 1999.
6. Lindy Neuhaus, interview, October 26, 1999.
7. Bo Neuhaus with Lindy Neuhaus, *It's Okay, God,* 10.
8. Larry Neuhaus, interview, October 26, 1999.
9. David G. Poplack, interview, October 29, 1999.
10. Poplack, Texas Children's Cancer Center and Hematology Service website, http://www.txcc.org/about-us.htm.
11. Donald J. Fernbach, interview, October 7, 1999.
12. Fernbach, oral history, 1979.
13. Fernbach, interview, October 7, 1999.
14. Ibid.
15. Douglas Starr, *Blood: An Epic History of Medicine and Commerce* (New York: Alfred A. Knopf, 1991), 181.
16. American Association of Blood Banks website, http://www.aabb.org.
17. Anonymous, "New Blood Banking System," *WATCH Magazine,* January 1958.
18. Fernbach, interview, October 7, 1999.
19. Fernbach, oral history, 1979.
20. Fernbach, interview, October 7, 1999.
21. Ibid.
22. Fernbach, interview, October 7, 1999; oral history, 1979.
23. Fernbach, oral history, 1979.
24. Ibid.

25. Fernbach, "Research Hematology Laboratory: Past, Present, & Future," *WATCH Magazine,* 1983.
26. Fernbach, correspondence, June 15, 2005.
27. Fernbach, interview, October 7, 1999.
28. Anonymous, "Fernbach Named to Elise C. Young Chair," *Baylor Medicine,* June/July 1989, 3.
29. Anonymous, "Conquering Childhood Cancer," *Developments* 3, no. 1 (First Quarter, 1987).
30. Ralph D. Feigin, "Message from the Physician-in-Chief," *WATCH Magazine,* 1989.
31. Ibid.
32. Anonymous, "Fernbach Named to Elise C. Young Chair."
33. Fernbach, interview, October 7, 1999.
34. Lisa Davis, "Cancer Survivors Celebrate for the Long Term/Seeing So Many ... Is So Encouraging," *Houston Chronicle,* June 7, 1999.
35. Arlene Nisson Lassin, "Loving What She Does, Who She Works With/Dynamic Dr. Dreyer Makes a Difference in Lives of Young Cancer Patients," *Houston Chronicle,* November 27, 2003.
36. Anonymous, "The Late Effects of Childhood Cancer Therapy," *Developments* 6, no. 2, 1990.
37. Fernbach, interview, October 7, 1999.
38. Anonymous, "Dr. Philip Pizzo," *WATCH Magazine* 1 (1993).
39. Poplack, interview, October 29, 1999.
40. Ibid.
41. Poplack, correspondence, August 15, 2005.
42. Poplack, interview, October 29, 1999.
43. Poplack, correspondence, August 15, 2005.
44. Todd Ackerman, "Center to Offer Cell-and-Gene Therapy Here/New Treatment Option Expected to Become the Future of Medicine," *Houston Chronicle,* July 27, 1999.
45. Poplack, interview, October 29, 1999.
46. Janette Rodrigues, "New Cancer Center to Focus on the Disease in Children," *Houston Chronicle,* January 13, 2001.
47. Poplack, interview, October 29, 1999.
48. Ibid.
49. Tina Foster, "What Does Cancer Look Like?" Texas Children's Hospital press release, n.d.
50. Poplack, correspondence, August 15, 2005.
51. Lindy Neuhaus, interview, October 26, 1999.
52. Bo Neuhaus with Lindy Neuhaus, *It's Okay, God,* 12.
53. Lindy Neuhaus, interview, October 26, 1999.
54. Bo Neuhaus with Lindy Neuhaus, *It's Okay, God,* 46.
55. Larry Neuhaus, interview, October 26, 1999.
56. Lindy Neuhaus, interview, October 26, 1999.
57. Bo Neuhaus with Lindy Neuhaus, *It's Okay, God,* 104.

18. Infectious Diseases

1. Kathy Ykema, email interview, March 26, 2006.
2. Matthew Ykema, email interview, March 26, 2006.
3. CNN transcript, aired March 30, 2005, http://transcripts.cnn.com/TRANSCRIPTS/0503/30/l01.01.html.
4. Stanford T. Shulman, "The History of Pediatric Infectious Diseases," *Pediatric Research* 55, no. 1 (2004).
5. Marilyn Miller Baker, *Caring for the Children: The History of Pediatrics in Texas* (Texas Pediatric Society, Dallas: Great Impressions, 1996), 60.
6. Bernard Guyer, Mary Anne Freedman, Donna M. Strobino, and Edward J. Sondik, "Annual Summary of Vital Statistics: Trends in the Health of Americans during the 20th Century," *Pediatrics* 106, no. 6 (December 2000).
7. R. A. Hoekelman and I. B. Pless, "Decline in Mortality among Young Americans during the 20th Century: Prospects for Reaching National Mortality Reduction Goals for 1990," *Pediatrics* 82 (1988): 582–95.
8. Shulman, "History of Pediatric Infectious Diseases."
9. B. L. Ligon and F. Stein, "Russell J. Blattner, MD: A Leader Who Welcomes Challenges," *Seminars in Pediatric Infectious Diseases* 11, no. 11 (2001): 73–86.
10. Ralph D. Feigin, "Farewell to a Founding Father," *WATCH Magazine* 1 (2003): 1.
11. Anonymous, "History of the National Institutes of Health," NIH website, http://history.nih.gov/exhibits/history/docs/page_06.html.

12. Anonymous, *Advancing the Nation's Health Needs: NIH Research Training Programs* (Washington, D.C.: National Academies Press, 2005), 6.

13. Baker, *Caring for the Children,* 122.

14. Ligon and Stein, "Russell J. Blattner."

15. Beth Sokol, "Fear of Polio in the 1950s," HONR 269J—"The Beat Begins: America in the 1950s," 1997, http://www.honors.umd.edu/HONR269J/projects/sokol.html.

16. Carol Rust, "The Shot Heard Round the World/Race for Polio Vaccine: United Nation Determined to End Disease's Rule of Terror," *Houston Chronicle,* October 7, 1990.

17. Ligon and Stein, "Russell J. Blattner."

18. Martha Dukes Yow, *Balancing Act, Memoir of a Southern Woman Doctor* (Austin: Eakin Press, 1997), 81.

19. Ibid., 108.

20. Yow, oral history, May 29, 1996.

21. Rust, "Shot Heard Round the World."

22. Baker, *Caring for the Children,* 134.

23. Rust, "Shot Heard Round the World."

24. Yow, *Balancing Act,* 105.

25. Rust, "Shot Heard Round the World."

26. Howard Markel, "April 12, 1955—Tommy Francis and the Salk Vaccine," *New England Journal of Medicine* 352, no. 1 (April 7, 2005): 1408–10.

27. Eric Berger, "The Polio Vaccine/50 Years Later/Fight to End a Medical Menace," *Houston Chronicle,* April 10, 2005.

28. Yow, *Balancing Act,* 108.

29. Shulman, "History of Pediatric Infectious Diseases."

30. Yow, *Balancing Act,* 116.

31. Ibid., 120.

32. Ibid., 135.

33. Ibid., 136.

34. Ibid., 139.

35. Yow, oral history, May 29, 1996.

36. Yow, *Balancing Act,* 159.

37. Ibid., 162.

38. Yow, oral history, May 29, 1996.

39. Yow, *Balancing Act,* 163.

40. Ibid., 182.

41. Yow, oral history, May 29, 1996.

42. Ibid.

43. Carolyn Edwards, "'Boy in the Bubble' Doctor Is ENMU Grad," Eastern New Mexico University press release, November 5, 2003.

44. Yow, *Balancing Act,* 167.

45. Ibid., 185.

46. Ibid., 183.

47. Yow, oral history, May 29, 1996.

48. Sheldon L. Kaplan, oral history, November 13, 1996.

49. Feigin, "Message for the Physician-in-Chief," *WATCH Magazine,* Spring 1978.

50. Ibid.

51. Yow, "Old Diseases, New Faces," *WATCH Magazine,* Fall 1979.

52. Ibid.

53. Yow, *Balancing Act,* 168.

54. Yow, "Old Diseases, New Faces."

55. Ibid.

56. Kaplan, "The Infectious Disease Service: More than Just Bugs and Drugs," *WATCH Magazine,* Fall 1978.

57. Yow, "Old Diseases, New Faces."

58. Yow, *Balancing Act,* 187.

59. Yow, "What Is a Diagnostic Virus Laboratory?" *WATCH Magazine,* Summer 1982.

60. Yow, *Balancing Act,* 194.

61. Ibid., 196.

62. Yow, oral history, May 29, 1996.

63. Feigin, "Hemophilus Influenzae: It Infects almost All Children before They Reach the Age of Six," *WATCH Magazine,* Spring 1981.

64. Kaplan, oral history, November 13, 1996.

65. Feigin, "The Future of Children's Health Care," *Junior League of Houston News,* September 1994.
66. Kaplan, oral history, November 13, 1996.
67. Kaplan, interview, September 20, 2005.
68. Ibid.
69. Kaplan, oral history, November 13, 1996.
70. Kaplan, interview, September 20, 2005.
71. Ibid.
72. Anonymous, "Clinical Trials for New Vaccines," *Developments,* Winter 1995.
73. Yow, "Congenital Cytomegalovirus Disease: A NOW Problem," *Journal of Infectious Diseases* 159, no. 2 (February 1989).
74. Anonymous, National Congenital CMV Disease Registry website, http://www.bcm.edu/pedi/infect/dmv/cu1-1-95.htm.
75. Kaplan, oral history, November 13, 1996.
76. Kaplan, interview, September 20, 2005.
77. Ibid.
78. Lori Williams, "New Type of Antibiotic Tackles Hard-to-Treat Pediatric Infections," Baylor College of Medicine press release, October 26, 2002.
79. Kaplan, interview, September 20, 2005.
80. Ibid.
81. Feigin, "Prospects for the Future of Child Health through Research," *Journal of the American Medical Association* 296, no. 11 (September 21, 2005): 1373–79.
82. Matthew Ykema, email interview, March 26, 2006.
83. Kathy Ykema, email interview, March 26, 2006.
84. CNN transcript.
85. Ibid.
86. Kathy Ykema, email interview, March 26, 2006.

19. Junior League of Houston

1. Virginia Holt McFarland, interview, March 21, 2000.
2. Ibid.
3. Charles William Daeschner, Sr., oral history, August 9, 1995.
4. Adele Peden, interview, September 19, 1977.
5. Anonymous, "The Evolution of a Clinic," manuscript, Junior League of Houston, 1933.
6. Anonymous, "A Brief History of Junior League of Houston Health Program," manuscript, Junior League of Houston, 1977.
7. Peden, interview, September 19, 1977.
8. Frances M. Heyck, oral history, 1992.
9. Ibid.
10. Anonymous, "Frances Heyck 'Kind of Eased into' Work," *Houston Post,* November 5, 1958.
11. Heyck, "The Story of the Junior League Diagnostic Clinic and Outpatient Department of TCH," *WATCH Magazine* 1, no. 4 (January 1957).
12. Mrs. Herbert P. Edmundson, letter to Leopold L. Meyer, June 17, 1953, TCH Corporate Records, Box 00754; Anne Baker, Lida Edmundson, and Martha Lovett, oral history, August 1, 1977, Texas Children's Hospital Archives.
13. Anonymous, *The Outpatient Department of Texas Children's Hospital,* manual, 1956, Texas Children's Hospital Corporate Records, RM Box 191-678.
14. Fred M. Taylor, "The Junior League Diagnostic Clinic of the Outpatient Department," *WATCH Magazine,* January 1957.
15. Heyck, oral history, 1992.
16. Taylor, "Junior League Diagnostic."
17. McFarland, interview, March 21, 2000.
18. Ibid.
19. Betty Ewing, "Frances Heyck's Work Speaks Well for Children's Health Care," *Houston Chronicle,* April 14, 1985.
20. Ralph D. Feigin, oral history, February 8, 1979; Feigin, oral history, August 25, 1992.
21. Anonymous, "Texas Children's Hospital Preliminary Feasibility Analysis for Bates Ambulatory/Research Building," December 1985, Texas Children's Hospital Records Archives.
22. Mary Kana, interview, March 24, 2000.
23. Rebecca T. Kirkland, "Ambulatory Services on the Move," speech, November 9, 1989, Texas Children's Hospital Archives.

24. Ibid.
25. Anonymous, "A History of the League's Fundraising," *Houston News,* Winter 1999, 16.
26. Leah Eknoyan, interview, April 4, 2000.
27. Anonymous, "75 years of Women Volunteering to Make a Difference," *Houston News,* Fall 1999, 6.
28. Eknoyan, interview, April 4, 2000.
29. Anonymous, "League Delivers $1 Million Commitment to Help Needy Children in Houston," *Houston News,* Winter 1999, 6.
30. Ibid.
31. Ibid.
32. Marty Racine, "Three Public Servants earn SAVVY honors," *Houston Chronicle,* April 11, 1999.
33. McFarland, interview, March 21, 2000.
34. Feigin, interview, March 4, 2003.
35. Racine, "Three Public Servants."
36. McFarland, interview, March 21, 2000.

20. Learning Support Center

1. Judith Z. Feigin, interview, January 24, 2001.
2. Feigin, interview, July 22, 1996.
3. Anonymous, "Learning Support Center," *Developments* 7, no. 2 (September 1991).
4. Feigin, "The Learning Support Center," *WATCH Magazine,* Winter 1987.
5. Feigin, interview, July 22, 1996.
6. Feigin, interview, April 25, 2005.
7. Allen F. Tinkler, "College Transition Services for Students with Special Needs," *North Shore Today,* December 22, 1993.
8. The definition appears in Public Law 94-142, as amended by Public Law 101-76 (Individuals with Disabilities Education Act-IDEA).
9. Lee Mitgang, "Many Students Don't Comprehend What They Read, Specialists Say," Associated Press, *Houston Chronicle,* September 7, 1986.
10. Dianna Hunt, "HISD Virtually Fills Teaching Vacancies," *Houston Chronicle,* August 28, 1985.
11. Feigin, oral history, July 22, 1996.
12. Feigin, "Learning Support Center."
13. Anonymous, "Learning Support Center."
14. Feigin, interview, January 24, 2001.
15. Ibid.
16. Ibid.
17. Anonymous, *A Report to the President and Congress of the United States,* National Council on Disability, September 1989.
18. Feigin, interview, January 24, 2001.
19. Robert G. Voigt, "Resolving the ADD Riddle," *WATCH Magazine* 3 (1994).
20. Feigin, interview, January 24, 2001.
21. Ibid.
22. Feigin, oral history, July 22, 1996.
23. Feigin, interview, January 24, 2001.
24. David Monroe, "Intervention Program Helps Children with Learning Disabilities," *Texas Medical Center News,* August 1, 1996.
25. Ibid.
26. Feigin, interview, January 24, 2001.
27. Ibid.
28. Anonymous, "Forward Progress," *Developments,* Spring 2001.
29. Anonymous, "Early Intervention Is Key to Easing Autism's Effects," *National Academies in Focus* 1, no. 2 (Fall/Winter 2001).
30. Feigin, interview, April 25, 2005.
31. Stanley Greenspan, "A Developmental Approach to Problems in Relating and Communicating in Autistic Spectrum Disorders and Related Syndromes," *Spotlight on Topics in Developmental Disabilities* 1, no. 4 (1998): 1–6.
32. Ibid.
33. Edward Goldson, review of *Educating Children with Autism,* issued by the Committee on Educational Interventions for Children with Autism, *Developmental and Behavioral Pediatrics* 25, no. 6 (December 2004).

34. Feigin, interview, April 25, 2005.
35. Ibid.
36. Ibid.
37. Ibid.
38. Ibid.

21. Meyer Center for Developmental Pediatrics

1. Sherry Sellers Vinson, interview, November 17, 2000.
2. Cheryl M. Bacon, "Teacher-Turned-Pediatrician Empathizes with Challenges Her Young Patients Face," *ACU Today,* Winter 2000.
3. Leopold L. Meyer and Newell E. France, *The Days of My Years* (Houston: Universal Printers, 1975), 109.
4. Ibid.
5. Anonymous, "Brief History of the L. L. Meyer Center for Developmental Pediatrics," n.d.
6. Allan Turner, "Hall Mark of Success," *Houston Chronicle,* May 28, 2000.
7. Harrison Rainie and Katia Hetter, "The Most Lasting Kennedy Legacy," *US News and World Report,* November 15, 1993.
8. Ibid.
9. Ibid.
10. Murdina M. Desmond, oral history, April 30, 1979.
11. Ibid.
12. Thomas Zion, interview, June 15, 1979.
13. Ibid.
14. Henry L. Shapiro, "AAP Section Looks at Its Past, Future on 40th Anniversary," *AAP News* 17, no. 4 (October 2000): 170.
15. Desmond, "The Good Start Program at Texas Children's Hospital," *Focus: The Medical Newsletter of Texas Children's Hospital,* Spring 1983.
16. Desmond, "Meyer Center Celebrates 25 Years," *WATCH Magazine,* 1985.
17. Julie Gilbert, "Growing Up Premature," *Houston Post,* January 20, 1985.
18. Desmond, "Meyer Center Celebrates 25 Years."
19. Anonymous, "Leopold L. Meyer Center for Developmental Pediatrics Dedicated at Texas Children's Hospital," *Intercom,* December 1974.
20. Ibid.
21. Desmond, "Meyer Center Celebrates 25 Years."
22. Desmond, interview, April 30, 1979.
23. Desmond, "Meyer Center Celebrates 25 Years."
24. Bonnie Ganglehoff, "The Aftermath of an Epidemic," *Houston Post,* June 9, 1985.
25. Connie K. Shafer, "Pediatric Center Aids Children," *Community Topics,* July–August 1974.
26. Desmond, "Meyer Center Celebrates 25 Years."
27. Desmond, interview, September 22, 1992.
28. Rebecca Trounson, "Physicians Pay Tribute to Retiring Pediatrician," *Houston Chronicle,* January 5, 1987.
29. Desmond, interview, September 22, 1992.
30. Trounson, "Physicians Pay Tribute to Retiring Pediatrician."
31. E. Kelly Merritt and Joan London, "Dr. Murdina Desmond Honored for Work in Developmental Pediatrics," *Texas Medical Center News,* January 1987.
32. Desmond, interview, July 10, 1999.
33. Vinson, interview, November 17, 2000.
34. Geoffrey Miller, interview, November 21, 2000.
35. Anonymous, "A Shining Star at Texas Children's, Helping Kids through Tough Times," *Developments,* Spring 1999.
36. Bacon, "Teacher-Turned-Pediatrician."
37. Ibid.
38. Vinson, interview, November 17, 2000.

22. Neonatology

1. Sandy Baber, interview, July 9, 1999.
2. Jack Baber, interview, July 9, 1999.

3. A. J. Schaffer, *Diseases of Newborn* (Philadelphia: Saunders, 1960), introduction.
4. Reba Michels Hill and A. J. Rudolph, "The Evolution of Neonatology at Texas Children's Hospital," *Watch Magazine,* Fall 1979.
5. Rebecca Trounson, "Physicians Pay Tribute to Retiring Pediatrician," *Houston Chronicle,* January 5, 1987.
6. Murdina M. Desmond, oral history, September 22, 1992.
7. Desmond, *Newborn Medicine and Society: European Background and American Practice (1750–1975)* (Austin: Eakin Press, 1998), 169.
8. Ibid., 176.
9. Trounson, "Physicians Pay Tribute."
10. Desmond, oral history, April 30, 1979.
11. A. J. Rudolph, oral history, July 28, 1992.
12. Ruth SoRelle, "Doctor Pioneers Newborn Care," *Houston Chronicle,* April 7, 1986.
13. Desmond, oral history, September 22, 1992.
14. Hill, letter to Virginia Apgar Award committee, February 25, 1988.
15. Hill, oral history, September 8, 1992.
16. Desmond, oral history, June 4, 1992.
17. Hill, oral history, September 8, 1992.
18. Hill and Rudolph, "Evolution of Neonatology."
19. Hill, oral history, September 8, 1992.
20. Rudolph, oral history, July 28, 1992.
21. SoRelle, "Doctor Pioneers Newborn Care."
22. Rudolph, oral history, July 28, 1992.
23. Ibid.
24. Desmond, interview, July 10, 1999.
25. Rudolph, oral history, July 28, 1992.
26. Desmond, interview, July 10, 1999.
27. Rudolph, oral history, July 28, 1992.
28. Desmond, interview, July 10, 1999.
29. Rudolph, oral history, July 28, 1992.
30. Ibid.
31. Hill and Rudolph, "Evolution of Neonatology."
32. Ibid.
33. Thomas N. Hansen, "A Laboratory for Neonatal Research," *WATCH Magazine,* Winter 1983.
34. Anonymous, "The Section That Jack Built," Section of Neonatology, Baylor College of Medicine website, 1999.
35. Ibid.
36. Desmond, interview, July 10, 1999.
37. Anonymous, "Quick Reference: Low Birthweight," March of Dimes website, http://www.marchofdimes.com/professionals/14332_1153.asp.
38. Anonymous, minutes, Texas Children's Hospital board of trustees meeting, December 30, 1992.
3 39. Hansen, "Section of Neonatology Texas Children's Hospital and Baylor College of Medicine," presentation to Board of Trustees, December 3, 1992
40. Ibid.
41. Anonymous, "The Smallest Survivors," *WATCH Magazine* 4, no. 2 (1988).
42. James Adams, interview and tour of the NICU, 1992.
43. Ibid.
44. Leonard E. Weisman, interview, July 7, 1999.
45. Adams, interview and tour of the NICU, 1992.
46. Anonymous, "A Special Delivery: Media Coverage of the Chukwu Octuplets," Texas Children's Hospital press release, January 7, 1999.
47. Leigh Hopper, "Neonatal ICU Working with Record Numbers," *Houston Chronicle,* January 3, 1999.
48. Ibid.
49. Timothy Cooper, Carol Berseth, Adams, and Weisman, "Actuarial Survival in the Premature Infant Less Than 30 Weeks' Gestation," *Pediatrics* 101, no. 6 (June 1998): 975–78.
50. Hopper, "Neonatal ICU Working with Record Numbers."
51. Anonymous, "Section That Jack Built."
52. Weisman, interview, July 7, 1999.
53. Michael E. Speer, "In Memoriam," *NeonatalNews.Net* 4, no. 2 (November 2003), http://www.neonatalnews.net/Nov-03/Memoriam.htm.

54. Weisman, "2004 and Beyond," *NeonatalNews.Net* 5, no. 1 (July 2004) http://www.neonatalnews.net/July-04/front.htm.
55. Weisman, correspondence, July 22, 2005.
56. Ibid.
57. Ibid.
58. Speer, "The Front Line," *NeonatalNews.Net* 5, no. 1 (July 2004), http://www.neonatalnews.net/July-04/front.htm.
59. Weisman, "2004 and Beyond."
60. Jack Baber, interview, July 9, 1999.
61. Sandy Baber, interview, July 9, 1999.

23. Neurology

1. Yasmine Ballantyne, interview, January 11, 2005.
2. Christie Ballantyne, interview, December 17, 2004.
3. Ibid.
4. Marvin A. Fishman, "Child Neurology: Past, Present, and Future," *Journal of Child Neurology* 11, no. 4 (July 1996).
5. Fishman, oral history, October 31, 1996.
6. Ibid.
7. Ibid.
8. Ibid.
9. Ralph D. Feigin, interview, March 15, 2004.
10. Russell J. Blattner, oral history, May 18, 1977.
11. Anonymous, "Section of Pediatric Neurology Department of Pediatrics," internal overview, March 21, 1978.
12. Thomas Zion, oral history, January 15, 1979.
13. Anonymous, "Section of Pediatric Neurology."
14. Feigin, interview, March 15, 2004.
15. Fishman, oral history, October 31, 1996.
16. Ibid.
17. Fishman, "Children's Special Neurological Problems," *WATCH Magazine,* Summer 1984.
18. Ibid.
19. Fishman, "Child Neurology: Past, Present, and Future."
20. Peter Kellaway, oral history, September 2, 1992.
21. Ibid.
22. Eli M. Mizrahi, Timothy A. Pedley, and Stanley H. Appel, "In Memoriam, Peter Kellaway, PhD, 1920–2003," *Neurology* 62, no. 3 (February 10, 2004).
23. Ibid.
24. Fishman, "Children's Special Neurological Problems."
25. Mizrahi and Kellaway, "Characterization and Classification of Neonatal Seizures," *Neurology* 37, no. 12 (December 1987): 1837–44.
26. Fishman, "Children's Special Neurological Problems."
27. Jan Goddard-Finegold, "Prevention of Brain Damage Is the Goal," *WATCH Magazine,* Fall 1986.
28. Fishman, "Children's Special Neurological Problems."
29. Anonymous, "Hope Where the Answers Are So Few," *Developments* 4, no. 3 (Fall/Winter 1988).
30. Judy Siegel-Itzkovich, "Autism or Cerebral Palsy? No, It's Rett," *Jerusalem Post,* July 8, 2001.
31. Anonymous, "Hope Where the Answers Are So Few."
32. Ibid.
33. Fishman, "Neurology in the 1990s at Texas Children's Hospital," *WATCH Magazine,* Fall/Winter 1990.
34. Ibid.
35. Karen Hopkin and Huda Y. Zoghbi, "Howard Hughes Medical Institute," Howard Hughes Medical Institute website, http://hhmi.org.biointeractive/neuroscience/zoghbi.html.
36. Harry T. Orr and Zoghbi, "SCA1 Molecular Genetics: A History of a 13 Year Collaboration against Glutamines," *Human Molecular Genetics* 10, no. 20 (2001): 2307–11.
37. Anonymous, "Genetic Cause of Rett Syndrome Discovered," *Baylor Medicine,* October 1999.

38. Todd Ackerman, "After 16 Years, Scientists Identify Defective Gene in Rett Syndrome," *Houston Chronicle,* October 1, 1999.
39. Anonymous, "School, Behavioral Problems May Indicate Sleep Disorder," Texas Children's Hospital press release, n.d.
40. Fishman, interview, October 20, 2004.
41. Anonymous, "Blue Bird Clinic," Texas Children's Hospital website, http://www.texaschildrenshospital.org/CareCenters/Neuro/Neurology/Bluebirdclinic.aspx.
42. Maurice Bobb, "Circle Keeps Giving," *Houston Chronicle,* April 10, 2003.
43. Fishman, interview, October 20, 2004.
44. Yasmine Ballantyne, interview, January 11, 2005.
45. Christie Ballantyne, interview, December 17, 2004.
46. John Allman, correspondence, January 12, 2005.

24. Nursing

1. Jaimee Kheir-Westfall, interview, April 9, 2003.
2. Maria Cramer, "First a Patient, Now a Nurse," *Texas Medical Center News,* May 1, 2002.
3. Kheir-Westfall, interview, April 9, 2003.
4. Ibid.
5. Sylvia A. Doyle, oral history, November 25, 1996.
6. Ibid.
7. Ibid.
8. Ruth Sylvester, oral history, September 23, 1992.
9. Ibid.
10. Ibid.
11. Ibid.
12. Ralph D. Feigin, "A Caring Agreement," *WATCH Magazine,* Winter 1988.
13. Doyle, oral history, November 25, 1996.
14. Ibid.
15. Anonymous, "Nursing: A Topnotch Career Choice," *WATCH Magazine* 6, no. 1 (1990).
16. Mark Wallace, oral history, December 9, 1996.
17. Patti J. Rogers, interview, March 18, 2003.
18. Ibid.
19. Susie Distefano, interview, July 22, 1998.
20. Distefano, Texas Children's Hospital nursing brochure, 2001.
21. Myrtle Williams, interview, March 18, 2003.
22. Distefano, interview, July 22, 1998.
23. Williams, interview, March 18, 2003.
24. Distefano, interview, July 22, 1998.
25. Rogers, interview, March 18, 2003.
26. Distefano, interview, July 22, 1998.
27. Anonymous, "Family-Centered Care Emphasizes a Team Approach to Patient Care at Texas Children's Hospital," Texas Children's Hospital press release, March 23, 1999.
28. Distefano, interview, July 22, 1998.
29. Williams, interview, March 18, 2003.
30. Ibid.
31. Distefano, Texas Children's Hospital nursing brochure, 2001.
32. Anonymous, "Nursing at Texas Children's Hospital: Research and Innovation," Texas Children's Hospital website, http://texaschildrenshospital.org/Professionals/Nursing/Research.aspx.
33. Kristina Van Arsdale, "Technology Has Taken the Repetitive Task Focus away from Nursing," *Texas Medical Center News* 20, no. 8 (May 1, 1998).
34. Rogers, interview, March 18, 2003.
35. Williams, interview, March 18, 2003.
36. Distefano, interview, July 22, 1998.
37. Williams, interview, March 18, 2003.
38. Ibid.
39. Anonymous, "Texas Children's Hospital Receives Coveted Magnet Nursing Recognition," Texas Children's Hospital press release, January 2003.
40. Kheir-Westfall, interview, April 9, 2003.
41. Cramer, "First a Patient, Now a Nurse."

42. Barbara Montagnino, interview, April 9, 2003.
43. Cramer, "First a Patient, Now a Nurse."

25. Pulmonary Medicine

1. John Rowland, interview, April 27, 1998.
2. Gunyon M. Harrison, interview, July 19, 2000.
3. Jane Smith, *Patenting the Sun: Polio and the Salk Vaccine* (New York: William Morrow and Co., Inc., 1990), 37.
4. Harrison, interview, July 19, 2000.
5. Ibid.
6. Ibid.
7. Harrison, oral history, July 15, 1992.
8. P. A. Di Sant' Agnese, R. C. Darling, G. A. Perera, and E. Shea, "Abnormal Electrolyte Composition of Sweat in Cystic Fibrosis of the Pancreas," *Pediatrics* 12 (1953): 549–63.
9. Harrison, oral history, July 15, 1992.
10. Harrison, interview, July 19, 2000.
11. Ibid.
12. Harrison, oral history, July 15, 1992.
13. Harrison, interview, July 19, 2000.
14. Ibid.
15. Joan Walsh, "Other Diseases Given Blame for Many Cystic Fibrosis Deaths," *Houston Post*, November 1, 1956.
16. Ibid.
17. Russell J. Blattner, "Research Activities in the Texas Children's Hospital," *WATCH Magazine*, 1957.
18. Dan K. Seilheimer and Anna K. Paridon, "The Cystic Fibrosis Center," *WATCH Magazine*, Winter 1987.
19. Harrison, interview, July 19, 2000.
20. Anonymous, "Researchers Closing on Cystic Fibrosis Mystery," *Houston Post*, April 22, 1962.
21. Harrison and Seilheimer, "Problems of the Chest," *WATCH Magazine,* Fall 1978.
22. Harrison, interview, July 19, 2000.
23. Seilheimer, interview, June 16, 2000.
24. Harrison and Seilheimer, "Problems of the Chest."
25. Ibid.
26. Arthur L. Beaudet and William T. Shearer, "The Cystic Fibrosis Research Center," *WATCH Magazine,* Winter 1987.
27. Seilheimer, interview, June 16, 2000.
28. Anonymous, "Asthma Education Prevents Crises," Texas Children's Hospital press release, February 15, 2000.
29. Seilheimer and Paridon, "Cystic Fibrosis Center."
30. Deborah Mann Lake, "Cystic Fibrosis: Today's Patients Are Beating the Odds. New Treatments Are Prolonging the Lives of Those with the Genetic Disease," *Houston Chronicle,* December 12, 1999.
31. Seilheimer, interview, June 16, 2000.
32. Seilheimer and Brenda Congdon, "Helping Families Manage Cystic Fibrosis," *WATCH Magazine,* Summer 1988.
33. Harrison, interview, July 19, 2000.
34. Anonymous, "First Pediatric Lung Transplant Performed at Texas Children's Hospital," Michael E. DeBakey Department of Surgery, Baylor College of Medicine website, http://www.debakeydepartmentof surgery.org/home/content.cfm?menu_id=44&pageview=news&article =118.
35. Anonymous, "First Pediatric Double Lung–Liver Transplant Performed in Texas," Michael E. DeBakey Department of Surgery, Baylor College of Medicine website, http://www.debakeydepartmentofsurgery.org/home/content.cfm?menu_id=44&pageview=news&article=161.
36. Jeannie Kever, "Gift of Life, Times Two/Houston Teen First in State to Get a Double Lung–Liver Transplant," *Houston Chronicle,* January 7, 2004.
37. Leigh Hopper, "New Lungs a Sigh of Relief/A Louisiana Girl Is Proving to Be a Success Story following Her Double-Lung Transplant at Texas Children's Hospital," *Houston Chronicle,* October 25, 2002.
38. Seilheimer, interview, June 16, 2000.
39. Rowland, interview, April 27, 1998.

26. Renal

1. Paula Hutchinson, interview, August 31, 2004.
2. Anonymous, "Who Gave You Your Kidney, Emma?" *WATCH Magazine* 2 (1992).
3. Paula Hutchinson, interview, August 31, 2004.
4. Ibid.
5. Ibid.
6. Ibid.
7. Anonymous, "Who Gave You Your Kidney, Emma?"
8. L. Leighton Hill, interview, July 16, 2004.
9. Hill, oral history, January 29, 1992.
10. Anonymous, "Dialysis Access," Thomas E. Starzl Transplantation Institute website, http://www.sti.upmc.edu/STI_Patient_web/sti/2dialysis.asp.
11. Hill, oral history, January 29, 1992.
12. Hill, interview, July 16, 2004.
13. Hill, oral history, January 29, 1992.
14. Anonymous, "Dialysis Access."
15. Hill, interview, July 16, 2004.
16. Russell W. Chesney, "The Development of Pediatric Nephrology," *Pediatric Research Magazine* (International Pediatric Research Foundation, Inc.) 52, no. 5 (2002).
17. Hill, interview, July 16, 2004.
18. Hill, oral history, January 29, 1992.
19. Chesney, "Development of Pediatric Nephrology."
20. Stuart L. Goldstein, email correspondence, September 16, 2004.
21. Charles William Daeschner, Jr., oral history, August 9, 1995.
22. Hill, interview, July 16, 2004.
23. William R. Clark, "Hemodialyzer Membranes and Configurations: A Historical Perspective," *Seminars in Dialysis* 13, no. 5 (September–October 2000).
24. Hill, oral history, January 29, 1992.
25. Hill, interview, July 16, 2004.
26. Daeschner, oral history, August 9, 1995.
27. Hill, oral history, January 29, 1992.
28. Daeschner, oral history, August 9, 1995.
29. Hill, oral history, January 29, 1992.
30. Hill, "Renal-Metabolic Service Encounters Wide Range of Conditions in Children," *WATCH Magazine,* Fall 1976.
31. Hill, interview, July 16, 2004.
32. Hill, oral history, January 29, 1992.
33. Hill, "Renal-Metabolic Service."
34. Anonymous, *Journal of the American Medical Association* 287, no. 10 (March 13, 2002).
35. Hill, oral history, January 29, 1992.
36. Hill, interview, July 16, 2004.
37. Hill, oral history, January 29, 1992.
38. Hill, "Renal-Metabolic Service."
39. Hill, oral history, January 29, 1992.
40. Hill, interview, July 16, 2004.
41. Ibid.
42. Polly Anderson, "Dialysis Pioneer Scribner Dies," Associated Press, June 20, 2003.
43. Peter Landers, "Filtering Process: Longer Dialysis Raises Hopes, but Poses Dilemma," *Wall Street Journal,* October 2, 2003.
44. Ibid.
45. Chesney, "Development of Pediatric Nephrology."
46. Hill, interview, August 6, 2004.
47. Hill, oral history, January 29, 1992.
48. Joseph E. Murray, "Nobel Prize Lecture: The First Successful Transplants in Man," in *Nobel Lectures in Physiology or Medicine 1981–1990,* ed. Jan Lindsten (Singapore: World Scientific Publishing Co., 1993).
49. Hill, "Renal-Metabolic Service."
50. Ibid.
51. Hill, oral history, January 29, 1992.
52. Phillip L. Berry, "The Pediatric Dialysis Center: It's Exclusively for Children," *WATCH Magazine,* Summer 1981.

53. Ibid.
54. Hill, interview, November 29, 2004.
55. Hill, interview, July 16, 2004.
56. Eileen Doyle Brewer, interview, August 6, 2004.
57. Ken Kolnacki, "Pediatric End-Stage Renal Disease," *Renal Life* (American Association of Kidney Patients, Inc.) 19, no. 5 (March 2004).
58. Brewer, "Renal Transplantation at Texas Children's Hospital," *WATCH Magazine* 2 (1992).
59. Ibid.
60. Brewer, interview, August 6, 2004.
61. Berry, "Pediatric Nephrology: From Newborns to New Kidneys," *WATCH Magazine,* Winter 1988.
62. Anonymous, "Texas Children's Renal Dialysis Unit Makes the Grade in Federal, State Surveys," Texas Children's Hospital press release, January 1, 2002.
63. David Powell, "Pediatric Nephrology," *WATCH Magazine,* Winter 1988.
64. Anonymous, Southwest Pediatric Nephrology Study Group website, http://medicalcityhospital.com/custompage.asp?PageName=spnsghome.
65. Brewer, "Renal Transplantation at Texas Children's Hospital."
66. Brewer, interview, August 6, 2004.
67. Hill, interview, July 16, 2004.
68. April Renberg and Anne Lupton, "Champions of the Children," *Texas Medical Center News,* September 15, 1996.
69. Melissa Quiroz, "TCH Nurse and Companion Comfort Kids Far and Wide," *Texas Medical Center News,* May 1, 1999.
70. Ibid.
71. Anonymous, "Texas Children's Offers Most Advanced Pheresis Service," Texas Children's Hospital press release, May 9, 2003.
72. Anonymous, "Texas Children's Names New Medical Director," Texas Children's Hospital press release, July 30, 2002.
73. Stuart L. Goldstein, "Overview of Pediatric Renal Replacement Therapy in Acute Renal Failure," *Artificial Organs* 27, no. 9 (2003): 781–85.
74. Goldstein, "The Prospective Pediatric Continuous Renal Replacement Therapy Registry: Design, Development, and Data Assessed," *International Journal of Artificial Organs* 27, no. 1 (January 2004): 9–14.
75. Paula Hutchinson, interview, August 31, 2004.
76. Ibid.
77. Ann Cain Tibbets, "The Fruits of a Grandmother's Love," *San Antonio Express-News Magazine,* July 8, 1990.
78. Paula Hutchinson, interview, August 31, 2004.
79. Anonymous, "Who Gave You Your Kidney, Emma?"
80. Ibid.
81. Paula Hutchinson, interview, August 31, 2004.
82. Tibbets, "Fruits of a Grandmother's Love."
83. Anonymous, "Who Gave You Your Kidney, Emma?"
84. Paula Hutchinson, interview, August 31, 2004.
85. Emma Hutchinson, email correspondence, September 8, 2004.
86. Anonymous, "Transplant Services, Emma, Diagnosed at Birth, Infantile Polycystic Kidney Disease (PKD)," Texas Children's Hospital website, http://texaschildrenshospital.org/CareCenters.

27. Rheumatology

1. Shirley Stokes, interview, November 12, 1998.
2. Pamela Stokes Ferrucci, oral history, September 5, 1996.
3. Michelle L. Mayer, Christi I. Sandborg, and Elizabeth D. Mellins, "Role of Pediatric and Internist Rheumatologists in Treating Children with Rheumatic Diseases," *Pediatrics* 113, no. 3 (March 2004).
4. Ferrucci, interview, November 12, 1998.
5. Records, office of Dr. W. Malcolm Granberry.
6. Ferrucci, interview, November 12, 1998.
7. Earl J. Brewer, interview, June 3, 1999.
8. Ibid.

9. Russell J. Blattner, oral history, March 9, 1979.
10. Blattner, oral history, May 24, 1979.
11. Brewer, interview, June 3, 1999.
12. Brewer, interview, January 13, 1999.
13. Anonymous, "Coloring Book: Rx for Juvenile Rheumatoid Arthritis," *Intercom,* October 1981, 12.
14. Anonymous, *Texas Children's Hospital: A Pediatric Research Center* (1964), 6.
15. Brewer, Edward H. Giannini, and Donald A. Person, *Juvenile Rheumatoid Arthritis* (Philadelphia: W. B. Saunders Company, 1982).
16. Brewer, interview, September 16, 1992.
17. Anonymous, *Arthritis and Rheumatism* 24, no. 10 (October 1981): 1318.
18. Brewer, interview, January 13, 1999.
19. Ibid.
20. Mary Jane Schier, "Briscoe to Dedicate Arthritis Clinic at Texas Children's Hospital," *Houston Post,* October 15, 1974.
21. Brewer, interview, January 13, 1999.
22. Schier, "Briscoe to Dedicate Arthritis Clinic."
23. Philippa Maister, "Building Bridges," *Arthritis Today,* July–August 1992, 18–19.
24. Schier, "U.S., Soviets Begin Study of Arthritis," *Houston Post,* October 16, 1983.
25. Brewer, interview, January 13, 1999.
26. Maister, "Building Bridges."
27. James N. Jarvis, "Pediatric Rheumatology: The Future Is Now, or … The Future's So Bright, I Gotta Wear Shades," *Current Problems in Pediatrics Adolescent Health Care,* March 2006.
28. Schier, "U.S., Soviets Begin Study"; Maister, "Building Bridges."
29. Anonymous, "Juvenile Arthritis," American College of Rheumatology website, http://www.rheumatology.org/public/factsheets/arth_in_children.asp?aud=pat.
30. Anonymous, "Arthritis: Timely Treatments for an Ageless Disease," *FDA Consumer Magazine,* May–June 2000, U.S. Food and Drug Administration website, http://www.fda.gov/fdac/features/2000/300_arth.html.
31. Michelle L. Mayer, Christy I. Sandborg, and Elizabeth D. Mellins, "Role of Pediatric and Internist Rheumatologists in Treating Children with Rheumatic Diseases," *Pediatrics* 113, no. 3 (March 2004).
32. Helen Emery, "Pediatric Rheumatology: What Does the Future Hold?" *Archives of Physical Medicine and Rehabilitation* 85 (August 2004).
33. Karyl S. Barron, "Kawasaki Disease: Etiology, Pathogenesis, and Treatment," *Cleveland Clinic Journal of Medicine* 69, Supplement II.
34. Jarvis, "Pediatric Rheumatology: The Future Is Now."
35. Jane G. Schaller, "The History of Pediatric Rheumatology," *Pediatric Research* 58, no. 5 (2005).
36. Raquel Espinoza-Williams, "The Guy with the Tie: Bow-Tie Wearing Doctor Volunteers to Help Kids in Need," *Texas Medical Center News* 25, no. 4 (March 1, 2003).
37. Robert W. Warren and Jeffrey E. Benjamin, "Children with Arthritis: What about School?" *WATCH Magazine,* 1990.
38. Ibid.
39. Gaye Koenning, Warren, and others, *Bridging the Med-Ed Gap for Students with Special Health Care Needs: A Model School Liaison Program,* n.d.
40. Schaller, "History of Pediatric Rheumatology."
41. Barry L. Myones, "Barry L. Myones, M.D.," Baylor College of Medicine website, http://www.bcm.edu/immuno/?pmid=2011.
42. Anonymous, "Making a Difference in the Lives of Children," *Check It Out,* April 24, 1998.
43. Ibid.
44. Schaller, "History of Pediatric Rheumatology."
45. Deborah Mann Lake, "Focus: Juvenile Arthritis/Battling a Childhood Crippler/Arsenal of Tools Offers Improved Care of Children," *Houston Chronicle,* May 22, 2001.
46. Anonymous, "2005 Geographic Distribution of Diplomats by Subspecialty Certificate," American Board of Medical Specialties website, http://www.abms.org/dounloads/statistics/table8.
47. Mayer, Sandborg, and Mellins, "Role of Pediatric and Internist Rheumatologists."
48. Warren, interview, November 1998.
49. Ferrucci, oral history, September 5, 1996.

28. Surgery

1. Leslie Davis, interview, April 28, 2000.
2. C. Everett Koop, "A Perspective on the Early Days of Pediatric Surgery," *Journal of Pediatric Surgery* 33, no. 7 (July 1988).
3. Ibid.
4. Ibid.
5. Kenneth L. Mattox, *The History of Surgery in Houston* (Austin: Houston Surgical Society/Eakin Press, 1998), 297.
6. Luke W. Able, oral history, June 18, 1979.
7. Anonymous, "Second Generation Surgery," *Intercom,* December 1980.
8. Mattox, *History of Surgery in Houston,* 298.
9. Benjy Brooks, oral history, 1992.
10. Lois Hill, "The Pediatric Surgery Service at TCH," *WATCH Magazine,* May 1966.
11. Ibid.
12. Newell France, *Texas Children's Hospital, a Pediatric Research Center* (1964).
13. Mattox, *History of Surgery in Houston,* 299.
14. Franklin J. Harberg, oral history, 1979.
15. France, *Texas Children's Hospital.*
16. Able, E. S. Allin, and P. A. de Vries, "Conjoined Twins," *Birth Defects: Original Article Series* 3, no. 1 (April 1967).
17. Able, oral history, June 18, 1979.
18. Brooks, oral history, 1992.
19. Franklin J. Harberg, "The General Surgery Service," *WATCH Magazine,* January 1975.
20. Harberg, oral history, 1992.
21. Edmund Gonzales, oral history, January 9, 1997.
22. Ibid.
23. Harberg, "New Pediatric Surgery Residency at TCH," *WATCH Magazine,* Winter 1989.
24. Ibid.
25. William J. Pokorny, "The Growth of Pediatric Surgery at Texas Children's Hospital," *WATCH Magazine,* Fall 1986.
26. John P. Laurent, "Spina Bifida," June 18, 1997, Baylor College of Medicine website, http://www.bcm.edu.
27. Leslie Loddeke, "Doctors Separate Conjoined Twins," *Houston Post,* June 10, 1992.
28. Mattox, *History of Surgery in Houston,* 177.
29. Gonzales, "Texas Children's Hospital Department of Surgery," *Developments,* Spring 1977.
30. Harberg, oral history, 1979.
31. David E. Wesson, interview, May 4, 2000.
32. Mattox, *History of Surgery in Houston,* 317.
33. Wesson, interview, May 4, 2000.
34. Wesson, "Pediatric Minimally Invasive Surgery Center," Michael E. DeBakey Department of Surgery, Baylor College of Medicine website, http://www.debakeydepartmentofsurgery.org/home/content.cfm?content_id=274&clinic_pk=8.
35. Anonymous, "Specialists at Texas Children's Hospital Bring Surgery to the Bedside of the Tiniest Infants," Texas Children's Hospital press release, July 15, 2002.
36. Wesson, "Pediatric Trauma and Critical Care Center," Michael E. DeBakey Department of Surgery, Baylor College of Medicine website, http://www.debakeydepartmentofsurgery.org/home/content.cfm?content_id=273&clinic_pk=7.
37. Jennifer Hart, "Texas Center for Fetal Surgery Debuts as First Fetal Diagnosis and Surgery Center in the Southwest," Texas Children's Hospital press release, April 28, 2004.
38. Anonymous, "Summary of Diplomate Statistics," American Board of Surgery website, http://home.absurgery.org/default.jsp?statsummary.
39. William Hardy Hendren, "Pediatric Surgery," *Pediatrics* 102, no. 1 (1998).
40. Davis, interview, April 28, 2000.
41. Ibid.

INDEX

Page references in bold indicate illustrations.

ABC World News Tonight, 496
Abdominal Surgery of Infancy and Childhood, 623
Abercrombie, James (Jim) Smither, 10–12,
    16–21, 23, 26, 48, **99, 102, 105,** 113, 143,
    144, 152, 178
Abercrombie, Josephine E., 11, 18, **113,** 177–78,
    181
Abercrombie, Lillie F., 17, 48, **105,** 113, 144,
    153, 178
Abercrombie, R. H., **99**
Abercrombie Arena, 107
Abercrombie Building, 48, 113, 120, 154, 157,
    162, 430, 535
Abercrombie Chair in Pediatrics at Baylor College
    of Medicine, J. S., 71, 152, 155
Abilene Christian University, 459, 460–61
Able, Luke W., 173, 623–30, 632
Ables, Dorothy Mathias, 432–33
Accreditation Council for Graduate Medical
    Education, 498, 615
Acute Care Guidelines Booklet, 500
Adams, Bud, 368
Adams, James, 489, 491–97
Adkins, A. Thomas, 364
Æsclepius, 5
Agricultural Research Service (ARS), 118, 271,
    325
Air Force, 261, 283
Aldape, Theresa, 124, 138–40
Alexander, Ann, 523
Alexander, Steven R., 580
Alexander Learning Center, Joan and Stanford,
    378
Alford, Bobby R., 74, 77
Alford, Charles, 405
All Children's Hospital (St. Petersburg), 606
Allison, Julia D., **111**
Allman, John, 527
American Academy of Pediatrics, 61, 75, 388,
    401, 402, 413, 467, 563, 588, 603, 623
American Association for the Advancement of
    Science, 75
American Association of Blood Banks, 360
American Board of Pediatrics, 178, 572, 615

American Board of Psychiatry and Neurology
    (ABPN), 508, 514
American Board of Radiology, 289
American Board of Surgery, 629, 630, 634
American Cancer Society, 370
American College of Cardiology, 177
American College of Healthcare Executives, 44,
    50
American College of Obstetrics and Gynecology,
    401
American College of Surgeons, 306
American Diabetes Association (ADA), 270, 274
American Federation for Clinical Research, 75
American Heart Association, 178, 179, 232
American Hospital Association, 147
American Institute for Public Service, 402
American Journal of Human Genetics, 344
American Journal of Roentgenology, 283
American Medical Association, 72
American Medical Society, 396
American Nurses Credentialing Center, 542
American Pediatric Society, 75, 402, 413
American Psychological Association, 455
American Rheumatism Association, 603
American Society of Microbiology, 75
American Society of Pediatric Nephrology, 591
Anderson, Donald, 403, 407
Anderson, Monroe Dunaway, 4
Andre, Mary Jo, 542
Andrew (janitor), 278
Andropoulos, Dean B., 231
Angelman, Harry, 334
Apgar, Virginia, 482
Appel, Stanley, 514
Arabia Temple Crippled Children's Clinic, 16
Arabia Temple Shrine, 16, 19, 510
Army, 211
Army Medical Corps, 208
Arthritis and Rheumatism, 606
Arthritis Foundation, 604, 605, 608–9
Arthritis Foundation, Gulf Coast Chapter, 605
Arthritis Institute, 601
Ashford, Gerald, 143

Association for the Care of Children's Health (ACCH), 197
Association of Junior League International, 435
Association of Post-Doctoral and Pre-Doctoral Internship Programs, 455
Association of Postdoctoral Programs in Clinical Neuropsychology, 455
Atlas of Pediatric Echocardiography, 179
Atlas of the Newborn, 498
Attwell, Kirby, 41
Austin State School, 462
Auxiliary, The, 110, 116, 142–62, 183, 193, 196–97, 199, 436
Ayers, Jody, 542

Baber, Jack, 478–81, 502–4
Baber, John L., IV, 479–81, 502–4
Baber, Sandy, 478–81, 502–4
Babies and Children's Hospital (Cleveland), 575
Babies Hospital (New York City), 82
Bailey, Leonard, 223
Baker, Carol J., 401, 403, 406, 411, 413, 414
Ballantyne, Christie, 505–7, 525–27
Ballantyne, Leyla, 506–7, 525–28
Ballantyne, Yasmine, 505–7, 525–28
Banting, Frederick G., 258
Baptist Hospital, 3
Baptist Memorial Hospital, 8
Barkley, Elizabeth, 602
Barkley, Howard, 424
Barnes Hospital, 509
Barrett, Fred, 400
Barron, Karyl S., 606, 609–10, 612–13
Bartholomew, Kay, 266
Bateman, Nancy, 147–48
Bates, W. B., 35
Baty, David, 316, 333
Baum, Ed, 365
Baumgartner, Bill, 226
Baylor Affiliated Hospitals Transplantation Program, 582
Baylor Collaborative Study Group, 397–98
Baylor College of Medicine, 5–6, 9, 13, 14, 19, 22–23, 37, 57–61, 63–73, 74, 76–83, 88–90, 92, 93, **98**, 118, 126–27, 133–36, 148, 152, 153, 154, 164, 168, 178, 179, 180, 182, 183, 185, 187, 212, 215, 219, 222, 226, 231, 245, 246, 247, 248, 249, 260–64, 268, 271, 283, 285, 298, 318, 320, 321, 322, 323, 324, 326, 327, 328, 335, 337, 339, 340, 342, 344, 346, 347, 348, 349, 350, 358, 359, 361, 363, 365, 366, 369, 370, 373, 374, 375, 376, 388, 390–93, 395–99, 402, 406, 409, 411, 412, 419, 423–29, 433, 436–37, 462, 464–66, 472, 481–84, 488–89, 491–93, 496, 498–500, 502, 505, 509, 510–12, 514–16, 518, 519, 520, 521, 523, 548, 551–53, 555–62, 565, 576–78, 582, 583, 584, 585, 588, 599, 600, 610, 611, 615, 628, 630–33, 635, 636
Baylor College of Medicine Rett Center, 519
Baylor Comprehensive Epilepsy Center, 516

Baylor International Pediatric AIDS Initiative (BIPAI), 136
Baylor Medical Alumni Association, 71, 578
Baylor Pediatric Alumni Association, 111
Baylor Pediatric House Staff Award for Outstanding Full-Time Faculty, 578
Baylor University College of Medicine. *See* Baylor College of Medicine
Beard, Earl, 172
Beaudet, Arthur L., 337, 339–50, 352, 561
Belmont, John, 187
Belmonte, Benjamin, 214
Ben Taub General Hospital, 71, 138, 306, 399, 512
Benage, Opal M., 31–32, 35, 37, 487–90, 538
Benjamin, Jeff, 611–12
Benyesh-Melnick, Matilda, 363
Bermea, Lisa, 611
Berry, Phillip L., 570–71, 583–88, 594
Bertner, E. W., 14
Bertuch, Alison A., 154
Best, Charles Herbert, 259
Bezold, Louis I., 239
Bickle, Laura, 576
Biles, E. W. 'Wiley,' 283, 284
Bill Williams (restaurant), 60
Biltmore Hotel (Phoenix), 17
Bintliff, Alice, 511
Bintliff, David C., 511
Bintliff Blue Bird Clinic, 511
Black, Dorothy, 304
Black, Mrs. George H., 12
Black, Nellie, 422
Blalock, Alfred, 167, 174, 211–12, 216
Blattner, Russell J., 13–15, 19, 22–23, 29, 37–39, 57–73, 74, 77, 78, 80, 81, **98, 108, 111, 112, 113,** 145, 148, 154, 168–69, 171, 261–63, 317–19, 321, 338, 358, 359, 361–62, 388, 390–93, 396–99, 403, 419, 425, 428–29, 461–62, 466, 482–83, 486–89, 499, 510, 537, 551, 552–55, 576, 579, 599–603, 625
Blattner Conference Room, 15
Blattner Fellowship, Russell J., M.D., 154
Blattner Lectureship, Russell J., 111
Bledsoe, Dana Nicholson, 542 *See* Dana Nicholson
Blue Bird Circle, The, 510–11, 523, 525
Blue Bird Circle Neurogenetics Laboratory, The, 523
Blue Bird Circle Rett Center, The, 521, 522–24
Blue Bird Clinic for Children's Neurological Disorders, The, 1, 511–12, 514–15
Blue Bird Clinic for Pediatric Neurology at The Methodist Hospital, The, 510, 512, 522–24
Blue Bird Seizure Clinic, The, 510–11
Blum, Morton, 145
Blumberg, Helen, **114,** 145–46, 148, 159
Bo's Place, 202, 382
Board of Nurse Examiners (Texas), 530
Bob and Vivian Smith Foundation, 327
Boca Ortiz Hospital, 156
Bock, Hans-Georg, 342

Boland, F. James, 305
Borreca, Frank, 462
Boston City Hospital, 75
Boston University School of Medicine, 75, 372
Bowman Gray School of Medicine, 391
Bowser, Barry L., 196
Boy in the Plastic Bubble, The, 400
Boy Scouts of America, 145, 259, 504
Brady, Michael, 153
Brandt, Mary L., 633
Branson, Julie, 198
Breast Feeding: A Passage in Life, 490
Brenner, Malcolm K., 348, 374
Brewer, Earl J., Jr., 448, 597, 599–610, 615–17
Brewer, Eileen Doyle, 585–89, 591, 594
Bricker, J. Timothy, 164–67, 178, 180–88, 190, 225–26, 229–30
Brigham and Women's Hospital, 581
Briscoe, Dolph, 605–6
Brock, Russell, 211–12
Brollier, Ben, 48
Brompton Hospital (London), 212
Brooke Army Medical Center, 64, 390, 393
Brooks, Benjy, 625–28, 632
Brown, Frank R., 472–73, 475–76
Brown, George, 10–11
Brown, Herman, 11, 16
Bruskotter, Jo Anne, 166, 188
Bruskotter, John, 166, 188–89
"Bubble Boy." *See* Vetter, David Phillip
Bunim, Joseph, 601
Bunk, Elizabeth Orsini, 431
Burgher Foundation, 179
Butler, George, 13, **97**

Cabrera-Meza, Gerardo, 498
Caffey, John, 281, 283
Cain, Gordon, 519–20
Cain, Mary, 519–20
Cain Chemical, Inc., 519
Cameron, Harry S., 11
Cameron Iron Works, Inc., 11
Camp Rainbow, 274
Cancer Counseling, 377
Cancer League, 377
Candlelighters, 377
Cantor, Eddie, 391
Capute, Arnold, 475
Cardiovascular Research Institute (University of California), 558
Cardiovascular Respiratory Pulmonary Institute (San Francisco), 553
Care of Respiratory Diseases in the Neonate, 500
Carter, Jim, 145
Case Western Reserve, 484
Casey, Bob, 323
Cass, Darrell L., 634–36
Caskey, C. Thomas, 339–41, 343–47, 349
Castañeda, Aldo R., 223, 224, 227–28
CBS Evening News, 496
Center for the Retarded, Inc., 462
Centers for Disease Control (CDC), 124, 129–30,

135, 242, 395, 411
Cerebral Palsy Developmental Disabilities Treatment Center, 470
Chapman, Don, 424
Charles Thomas Parker Memorial Laboratory, 400
Cherry, James D., 84, 407
Chiang, Myra, 585
Chicago Bears, 368
Child, 55, 90, 236
Child Life Certifying Commission, 198
Child Life Council, 197–98, 203
Children's Bureau of the Department of Health, Education, and Welfare, 70, 462, 463–65
Children's Cancer Foundation, 362
Children's Hospital Boston, 26, 37, 63, 211, 223, 224, 227, 236, 262, 264, 277, 358–59, 419, 483, 552–55, 600–1, 623–24, 625, 626, 628
Children's Hospital, New Orleans, 596
Children's Hospital of Philadelphia, 124, 179, 208, 220, 236, 318, 464, 623.
Children's Hospital San Diego, 181
Children's Lighthouse for the Blind, 469
Children's Medical Center of Dallas, 170
Children's National Cancer Research Foundation, 66
Children's National Medical Center, 612
Children's Nutrition Research Center, **118**, 271, 324
Children's Oncology Group (COG), 362
Children's Protective Services (CPS), 305
Children's Summer Respiratory Camp Foundation, 558
Chukwu octuplets, 496–97
Chung, Taylor, 290
Cincinnati Children's Hospital Medical Center, 583
City and County Health Clinics and Health Department, 366
Clark, Gary D., 524
Clark, William A., 601, 603
Clayton, George W., 69, 72, 176, 263, 268, 317–19, 420, 578–79
Clemens, Roger, **117**
Cleveland (janitor), 278
Cleveland Clinic, 181
Cleveland Clinic Foundation, 229
Clinical Care Center, 48, 50, 53, 86, 91, 111, **117, 118, 119, 120,** 289, 369, 378, 431, 441, 445, 450, 454, 472, 523, 533, 542, 616, 631, 636
Clinical Orthopedic Society, 617
Clinical Pediatric Oncology, 365, 371
Clinical Research Center (CRC), 38, 79–70, 72, 75, 126, 127, 128, 132, 133, 138, 176, 317–21, 325, 329, 396–400, 464, 517, 579
Clinical Research Center for Neonatal Seizures, 516
CNN, 496
Cochran, Gloria, 464–65, 468
Cochran, Winston, 464–65, 468
Cody, Jim, 145

Cohen, Raymond, 7, 9, 13, 65, **97**
Cold War, 607
Columbia College, 75
Columbia University College of Physicians and
   Surgeons, 82
Columbus Children's Hospital, 178
Committee on Educational Interventions for
   Children with Autism, 452
Congenital Malformations of the Heart, 167
Congregation Beth Israel, 10, 145
Congress, 389, 520, 581, 604
Conjoined Twins, 627
Connally, John, 35
Conroy, Claire, 257–59, 272–75
Conroy, Clint, 274–75
Conroy, Kate, 274–75
Conroy, Liz, 257–59, 272–75
Conroy, Tim, 258
Cook County Hospital, 475
Cooley, Denton A., 33, 36, **103**, 171, 174–76,
   183, 211–28, 236, 627
Cooley, Helen, 226, 229
Cooley, Louise, 216
Copeland, Kenneth L., 269–72
Corbet, Anthony, 489–90
Cornell University Medical College, 633
Crafoord, Clarence, 211
Craigen, William, 187
Creighton, John E., 37
Crick, Francis, 337
Crittenden Home for Unwed Mothers, Florence,
   60
Crosswell, Holcombe, 48
Cuellar, Nicanora C., 616
Cullen, Hugh Roy, 8–10, 28
Cullen, Lillie, 8–9
Cullen Building, Roy and Lillie, 9
Cullen Cardiovascular Surgical Research
   Laboratories (Texas Heart Institute), 222
Cullen Foundation, The, 9
Cullen Health Trust Foundation, 470
Cullinan, Nina, 13, **97**
Cummings, Morrow, 17
Current Therapy in Pediatric Infectious Diseases,
   413
Currier, Helen, 570, 587, 589–90
Curry, Martha R., 616
Cystic Fibrosis and Related Pulmonary Disease
   Center, 557. *See also* Cystic Fibrosis Care
   Center
Cystic Fibrosis Care Center, 548, 555–57,
   559–62, 564, 565–66
Cystic Fibrosis Foundation, 555–56, 558–59
Cystic Fibrosis Research Center, 561
Czyzewski, Danita, 266

D'Ambrosio, Debbie, 538
Daeschner, Charles William (Bill), Jr., 260–66,
   288, 395, 419–20, 436, 571–79, 584
Daeschner, Jr. M.D. Lifetime Achievement Award,
   Charles W., 579
Daily, Clarence, 280

David Center, 137
Davis, Brad, 620–21
Davis, Dylan, 621–23, 637–39
Davis, Leslie, 620–23, 637–40
Davis, Thad, 620, 637–38
DeBakey, M.D., Excellence in Research Award,
   Michael E., 187
DeBakey, Michael E., 627
DeBakey Department of Surgery at Baylor
   College, Michael E., 231, 630, 632, 633
DeGuzman, Marietta M., 615–16
Delaney, Mrs. Andrew, 150
deLeon, Jim, **107**
Delta Phi Epsilon, 147
Demmler, Gail, 406, 410–11, 413–14
Department of Education (Texas), 612
Department of Health (Texas), 462, 616. *See also*
   Texas State Department of Health
Department of Health and Human Services
   (Texas), 604, 614
Department of Health, Education, and Welfare
   (federal), 462
DePelchin Faith Home, 60
Desmond, Jim, 482
Desmond, Murdina MacFarquahar, 59–60, 65,
   98, 110, 395, 397–98, 460, 462, 464,
   466–75, 481–89, 492–93, 498–99, 501
Desmond Neonatal Developmental Follow-Up
   Clinic, 472–73
Destiny's Child, **116**
Developments, 269
DeWall, Richard, 214
Diabetes Care Center, 261–72
Diabetes Conrol and Complications Trial
   (DCCT), 269
Dialysis and Transport Center, 585–86
Diamond, Louis, 359
Dickerson, Carmen, 476
Dickey, Florence, 32
Diseases of the Newborn, 481
Disney, Walt, 100. *See also* Walt Disney
   Productions
Distefano, Susan M., 46, 535–43
Dodge, Philip R., 509
Dodge, Warren, 572, 576
Dolan, Pat, 157–59
Dompier, Mimi, 327
Dompier, Tom, 327
Doyle, Sylvia A., 531, 533–34, 538, 542
Dreyer, ZoAnn Rightmire, 369–71, 373
Drucker, Peter, 47
Dudrick, Stanley, 320
Duke University, 182, 183, 550–51, 565, 610
Dunbar, Burdett S., 629
Dunn, Helen A., 297
Dunn, John S., 369
Dunn Research Foundation, John S., 369
Duritz, Gilbert, 489
Dutton, Robert, 284, 287, 288
Dynamic Orthotics, 316

Eastern Virginia Medical College, 181

Edison, Thomas Alva, 280
Edmundson, Lida, 68, 426
Educating Children with Autism, 452, 453
Education for All Handicapped Children Act of 1975, 443, 469. *See also* Public Law 94-142
Edwards, George, 267
Edwards, Morven, 403, 411
Ehlers, Jack (H. J.), 10, 12, 13, 17, **97**
Eisenhower, Dwight D., 554
Eknoyan, Leah, 432–33
El Khoury, Bashar, 195
Elenberg, Ewa, 589
Elkins, James (Jim) A., Jr., 11, 16
EMI Laboratories, 286
Enders, John, 392
Episcopal High School, 503
ER, 296, 475
Evans, Dale, **105**

Fallon, Sarah, 202
Family Advisory Board, 614
Farber, Sidney, 66, 358–59
Fashena, Gladys, 4, 170
Federal Drug Administration (FDA), 326
Federal Register, The, 444
Federated, 10
Feig, Daniel I., 589
Feigin, Judith Z., 53, 91, 92, 441–56, 612
Feigin, Ralph D., 38–40, 45–46, 53, 55, 56, 75–93, **108, 111, 112, 113,** 127, 132, 135, 154, 184–87, 226, 251, 269, 323, 324–25, 369–70, 372–73, 375, 402–3, 407–8, 413–14, 429–30, 433, 435, 472, 509–13, 520, 532–33, 559–60, 565, 583, 588
Feigin Center, 53, 91, **112, 117, 118,** 120, 186, 369, 375, 432, 445, 448, 472, 520, 533, 560, 565, 616, 631, 638
Feigin Fellowship, Ralph D., M.D., 154
Ferber, Edna, 143
Fernandez, Fabio, 512, 518
Fernbach, Donald J., 114, 358–72, 374, 375, 381
Fernbach, Susan, 187
Ferrucci, Hannah Elizabeth, 618
Ferrucci, Joseph, 618
Ferrucci, Pamela Stokes, 619. *See also* Stokes, Pamela
Ferry, George D., 321, 322, 324, 326–29
Finger, Julie, 149, 161
First Methodist, 510
Fisher, David J., 185
Fishman, Marvin A., 507–9, 512–14, 516–20, 522–28
Fitch, Edward Oliphant, 260, 390
Fitch IBCA, 54
Fleming, Alexander, 387
Fleming, Lamar, 11, 16
Florence Crittenden Home for Unwed Mothers, 60
Foley Brothers Dry Goods Company, 10
Fondren Foundation, 605
Food and Drug Administration (FDA), 179, 582, 604
Forbes, Andrea, 266
Forbes, Gilbert, 324
Foreman, Emma Moody, 30, 32–33, 39, 40
Foundation for the Institute of Research and Rehabilitation, 562
France, Newell E., 30–31, 35–38, 39, 429, 487, 489, 492, 583, 599
Frank, Arthur, 403
Fraser, Charles D., Jr., 184, 189–90, 209, 226–39
Fraser, F. Clarke, 339
Frazier, O. Howard, 222–23, 226
Friedman, Richard A., 179
Friedman, Zvi, 489
Friends of the Library at the University of Houston, 10
Frizzell, Dean, 277–78
Fuerrmann, George, 143

Gabbay, Kenneth H., 268
Galveston College, 530
Gamble, James L., 262–64, 575
Gammill, Lee C, 26–27, 29, **99,** 146–47, 276, 278
Garcia, Amelia, 351
Garcia-Prats, Joseph, 489
Gardner, Timothy J., 226, 227
Garner, Marguerite, 278, 291
Garson, Arthur, Jr., 181–83, 185, 188, 222
Gellis, Sydney, 262
General Electric, 280
George Washington University School of Medicine, 482, 612
Giannini, Ed, 610
Giant, 143
Gibbon, John Heysham, 213–14
Gibbs, Richard A., 347
Gillette, Paul, 177, 182
Girl Scouts, 259
Gladu, Donald, 27
Glaze, Daniel G., 517, 522
Glezen, Paul, 403
Glenn, John K., 7, 13, **97**
Goddard-Finegold, Jan, 517–18
Goldstein, Stuart L., 589–91
Goldston, W. J., 16
Gonzales, Edmund T., Jr., 529–30, 546, 629–30, 632–33
Gordon and Mary Cain Pediatric Neurology Research Foundation, 519, 520
Gordon Emergency Center, Meyer and Ida, **115,** 301, 310
Gorman, Winifred, 489
Goss, John C., 328, 563
Governor's Conference on Arthritis (Austin), 606
Grafton, Mike, 39
Graham, David, 324
Granberry, W. Malcolm, 597–98, 606, 617–18
Greene, James A., 58
Greenspan, Stanley, 452
Greenwood (Dr.), 515
Greenwood, Mary Owen, 393

Greer, David, 3, 6–7, 9–10, 12–15, 20, 22, 23, 65, **97,** 142, 150, 425, 624
Gregg, Norman, 486
Griffin, John, 358
Grifka, Ronald G., 179, 234
Grose, Mary Liz, 155
Gross, Robert E., 211, 221, 236, 623, 625
Guerrero, Eugene, 334–37, 350–53
Guerrero, Gina, 334–37, 350–53
Guerrero, Michael, 351
Guerrero, Vi, 334–37, 350–53
Guillory, Charleta, 479, 491
Gulf State Advertising Agency, 21
Gutgesell, Howard, 177, 179
Gutgesell, Margaret E., 429

Halbouty, Michel T., 485
Halbouty, Mrs. Michel T., 485
Halbouty Clinic, 488
Halbouty Nursery, Linda Fay, 584–85
Halbouty Premature Nursery, 489
Hale, Kathryn A., 567
Hall, Larry, 480
Hallman, Grady L., 219–20
Hammill, Hunter, 134
Hansen, Thomas N., 492–94, 499
Hanson, I. Celine Guerra, 125, 130, 133–35, 138–40
Harberg, Franklin J. (Jim), **108,** 354–55, 625–28, 630, 632–35
Harken, Dwight, 211
Harriet Lane Pediatric Service, 337
Harris County Center for the Retarded, 469
Harris County Hospital District, 366, 433
Harris County Medical Society, 25
Harrison, Gunyon M., 248, 548–60, 563–68
Harrop, Mrs. James, 150
Hartford Foundation, John A., 482–83, 487
Hartmann, Alexis F., 260–61, 263–64
Harvard, 66, 69, 75, 262, 340, 509, 575, 600–1, 625
Haymond, Morey H., 271–72
Hazlewood, Carlton, 319
Health and Human Services Department (City of Houston), 433
Hedgecroft Clinic, 15–16
Heinle, Jeffrey S., 232, 233
Helmgrath, Michael A., 634
Henie, Sonja, 143
Henning, Susan, 330
Hermann Hospital, 3, 5, 8, 16, 19, 46, 58–60, 68, 147, 168, 212, 260, 306, 421–26, 510
Hermann Park, 58
Heyck, Frances M., 59, 170–71, 418, 420, 424–27, 429, 492
Heys, Florence M., 59–60, 62, 68, **98,** 388, 391
Hiatt, Peter W., 562
Hill, L. Leighton, 264–68, 270, 317, 572–85, 587–89
Hill, Reba Michels, **111,** 484–85, 488–90, 501
Hippocrates, 386
Hobby, Oveta Culp, 7, 11, 394

Hodges, Fred, 280
Hogg, Ima, 9
Holiday, 142
Holt, Jack, 279, 280
Holy Cross, 337
Home Care of the Rheumatoid Arthritis Patient, 602
Hope, Bob, **104,** 151
Horlock, Frank P., 153
Horlock, Mrs. Frank P., 153
Horlock, Frank Prescott III, 153
Horlock Fellowship, Frank Prescott III, 153, 183
Horowitz, Marc, 374
Hospital for Sick Children, Great Ormond Street (London), 625
Hospital for Sick Children (Toronto), 633
Hounsfield, Godfrey, 286
House of the Good Samaritan, 601
Houston Area Angelman Syndrome Association (HAASA), 352–53
Houston Astros, 117
Houston Center for Retarded Children, 468
Houston Chronicle, 25, **99,** 169, 363
Houston Civic Music Association, 10
Houston Community Chest, 10
Houston Community College, 160
Houston Council for Retarded Children, Inc., 461
Houston Endowment, 605
Houston Fat Stock Show, 10
Houston Galleria, 598
Houston Horse Show Association, 11–13, 16
Houston Independent School District (HISD), 193, 433, 444, 469
Houston Junior Women's Club, 364, 377
Houston Livestock Show and Rodeo, 10, 105
Houston Northwest Medical Center, 385
Houston Oilers, 368
Houston Pediatric Society, 3, 6, 7, 9, 10, 12, 13, 16, 20, 22, 23, 59, 65–67, 142, 425, 624
Houston Post, 18, 21, 72, 100, 142, 143, 607
Houston Retail Merchants Association, 10
Houston Ronald McDonald House, 155, 367–70, 377, 382
Houston Speech and Hearing Center, 465
Houston Symphony Society, 10
Howard Hughes Medical Institute, 520
Hudgens Memorial Award, Robert S., 50
Human Genome Project, 346, 347–48
Human Genome Sequencing Center (Baylor), 347
Humble Oil, 34
Hurricane Carla, 483
Hutchins, Vince, 605
Hutchinson, Ashlyn, 571, 592
Hutchinson, Emma Grace, 569–71, 592–95
Hutchinson, John, 569–71, 592–95
Hutchinson, Paula, 569–71, 592–95

Individuals with Disabilities Education Act (IDEA), 469–70
Infectious Diseases Society of America, 75, 402, 411, 413

Institute for Molecular Genetics (Baylor College of Medicine), 344–47
Institute for Rehabilitation and Research (TIRR), The, 64, 248. *See also* Texas Institute for Rehabilitation and Research (TIRR)
Intercom, 18, 27
Intergovernmental Personnel Act, 612
Intermountain Pediatric and Adolescent Dialysis Unit, 585
International Pediatric Conference (Montreal), 396
International Pediatric Nephrology Association, 591
Irene and Walter Johnson Institute of Rehabilitation, 509
It's Okay, God, We Can Take It, 382

Jacobi Award, Abraham, 72
Jaksic, Tom, 633
James, Marie, **114**
Janeway, Charles A., 262, 264, 419, 600–1
Jarrell, Gammon, 29
Jefferson, Larry S., 245, 248–53
Jefferson Award, 402
Jefferson Davis Hospital, 60, 64, 212, 262, 263, 267, 361, 393, 395–97, 399, 466–67, 482–87, 489, 551, 572, 576, 578
Jefferson Medical College (Philadelphia), 213
John Caffey Society, 284
John S. Dunn Research Foundation, 369
John Welsh Cardiovascular Diagnostic Laboratory, 187
Johns Hopkins, 63, 64, 69, 165, 167, 168, 169, 172, 173, 174, 211, 212, 215, 226–29, 263, 317, 318, 321, 324, 337, 390, 393, 475
Johnson, Phillip, 16
Johnson Foundation, Robert Wood, 90
Johnson Institute of Rehabilitation, Irene and Walter, 509
Joint Commission on Accreditation of Healthcare Organizations (JCAHO), 32, 50, 542
Jones, Jesse H., 11, 63, **99**, 600
Jones, Margaret, 542
Jones Fellowships, Jesse H. Jones and Mary Gibbs, 63, 359, 600
Jones Foundation, 63
Jones Scholarship, Jesse H., 483
Journal of American Medical Women's Association, 626
Journal of Infectious Diseases, 402, 410
Journal of Pediatrics, 61
Journal of the American Medical Association, 185, 362, 397, 486
Journeay, George B., 19
Junior League Children's Clinic at Hermann Hospital, 59, 60, 68, 147, 423–25
Junior League Children's Health Care Center, 432
Junior League Children's Health Clinic, 421–23
Junior League Diagnostic Clinic, 29, 68, 70, 72, **106**, 170, 263, 321, 418, 420, 426–27, 434, 461-63, 554, 601
Junior League Memorial Fund, 422–24, 426, 431

Junior League of Houston, Inc., 12, 16, 68, 71, **106**, 147, 170, 197, 299, 399, 409, 418–37, 466, 467, 510, 605, 638
Junior League Outpatient Department, 73, 79, **106**, 128, 263, 285, 338, 364, 399, 428–30, 432, 461–64, 466, 487-89, 512, 514-18, 604–5
Juvenile Rheumatoid Arthritis, 602

Kale, Arundhati S., 589
Kana, Mary, 430
Kangaroo Crew Transport Team, 253, 385–86, 491, 501, 634
Kaplan, Sheldon L., 79, 81, 84, 90, 402–4, 406–15
Kappa Kappa Gamma, 145
Karaviti, Lefkothea, 622
Karpen, Saul, 328
Keats, Arthur, 175, 215
Kellaway, Peter, 515–16
Kelley, Liz, 368
Kelsey-Seybold Building, 465
Kennedy (Dr.), 416
Kennedy, John F., 463, 475, 480
Kennedy, Rosemary, 463
Kennedy family, 463
Kennedy Krieger Institute, 475–76
Kennel, John, 484
Kenny, John, 489
Kheir, Jaimee, 530. *See also* Kheir, Mona *and* Kheir-Westfall, Jaimee
Kheir, Mona, 529–30. *See also* Kheir, Jaimee *and* Kheir-Westfall, Jaimee
Kheir-Westfall, Jaimee, 530, 545–46. *See also* Kheir, Jaimee *and* Kheir, Mona
Kidney Foundation of Houston and the Greater Gulf Coast, 578
Kirk, Samuel A., 433
Kirkland, John L., III, 268–69, 271
Kirkland, Rebecca, 430–32, 434
Kirklin, John W., 175, 214
Kleberg family, 340
Kleberg Genetics Clinic, 335–36, 340, 346, 349, 351–52
Klein Oak High School, 384, 417
Klevenhagen Family Education Room, Johnny, 378
Kline, Allen H., 297
Kline, Mark, 135–36, 140, 154, 297
Klish, William J., 316, 317, 320, 322–30
Knievel, Evel, 547
Knowles, Beyoncé, **116**
Koenning, Gaye, 611
Kohaut, Edward, 267, 580, 583
Kolff, William, 575, 580
Koop, C. Everett, 124, 609, 623
Kostrewski, Joseph, 277
Kostrewski, Josephine, 277
Kovalchin, John, 209
Krafka, Roxanna, 248
Kraft, Irwin, 22–23
Kravitz, Seth, 584

Krull, Kevin R., 450
Krumboltz, Jane, 592–95
Kuper, Elaine, **114**, 144–46, 148, 157, 158, 159–62
Kuper, Harry, 146
Kuper, Laurie, 145

Laboratory for Genetic Therapeutics, 347
Ladd, William E., 623, 637
Laine, Laura, 332
Lamar Hotel, 11
Lamour, Dorothy, 143
Landa Fellowship, Adeline B., 154
Landers, Susan, 570
Latson, Joseph R., 172, 213, 214
Laurent, John P., 631
Lay Education Award, 563
Leachman, Robert D., 172, 213, 214
Learning Support Center, 91, 439–58, 612
Learning Support Center for Neurobehavioral Psychology, 455–56
Lee, Rita, 518
Lemke, Dea, **102**
Leonard, Jack, 575
Leukemia and Lymphoma Society, 377
Leukocyte Function Laboratory, 154
Life Flight, 479
Lifschitz, Carlos, 153
Lillehei, C. Walton, 175, 213–14
Lillie Frank Abercrombie Section of Cardiology (Baylor), 164, 178, 183
Linda Fay Halbouty Newborn-Premature Nursery, 489
Lion's Camp, 274
Lipinski, Tara, **115**
Lipinski Exercise Room, Tara, 115
Litchfield, Bill, 581
"Little Hospital," 510
Lomas, Robert, 59
London Times, 142
Long, Jane, 278
Lorin, Martin I., 82–83
Lovell, Daniel J., 606–7, 610
Lovett, Martha (Mrs H. Malcolm), 13, **97**
Lucky, Sonia, 598
Lynn, Donald, **102**

M. D. Anderson Cancer Center, 134, 376
M. D. Anderson Foundation, 4–6, 8
M. D. Anderson Hospital for Cancer Research of the University of Texas, 4, 277, 285, 365
Macey, Gene, **116**
Macey Information Desk, 116
Magic of Play: A Guide for Parents of Babies and Children in the Hospital, The, 200
Magnuson, Freda, 146–47
Mahar, Jennifer, **115**
Mahoney, Donald H., 373, 416
Malcolmson, Lee, 149
Mallory, George, 563–64
Manhattan Project, 389
Manual of Women's Auxiliaries, 147

March of Dimes, 60, 337, 339, 349, 391, 394, 470, 490, 603, 609. *See also* National Foundation-March of Dimes
Marcott, Valerie, 616
Marine Corps, 165, 166
Mariscalco, Michele, 154
Marquis, Pamela, 307–8
Marshall, Douglas B., 16
Martin, Mary, 215
Martin, Maynard W., 29–31, 35, 36–37, 150
Martin, Milton Foy, 14–15, 65, **99**
Martinez, Lorien, 415
Mason, Ed, 400, 403–4, 407
Massachusetts General Hospital, 75, 509
Massachusetts Institute of Technology, 291
Maternal and Child Health Bureau (federal), 462, 604–5, 608, 611
Maternal and Child Health Division (Texas), 462
Maternal and Child Health Services (federal), 462, 470
Mayo Clinic, 153, 172, 175, 181, 214
McCabe, Edward, 180
McCarthy, Glenn, 142–43
McClain, Ken, 373
McClelland, Gen., 155–57
McCloskey General Hospital, 11, 12
McCullough, Ralph, 17
McDonald's, 140, 155, 158, 241, 367
McFarland, Russell, 437
McFarland, Scott, 418–19, 436
McFarland, Virginia Holt, **111**, 418–21, 428, 434–38
McGee, William (Bill) K., Jr., 44, 89
McGill University, 515
McGovern, John P., 127
McGowen, Chase, 564
McKeemie, Jack, 59
McKenzie, E. Dean, 231, 233, 236, 563
McNamara, Dan Goodrich, **103, 111**, 168–84, 185–86, 188, 212–15, 217, 224, 339, 487, 625
Medicaid, 34, 38, 139
Medical Genetics: Principles and Practice, 339
Medical University of South Carolina, 472–73
Medicare, 34, 581, 584
Medicare Act, 581
Mee, Roger B. B., 227–30, 234–35
Meigs, Jody, 241, 243, 254–55
Meigs, Leslie, 241–43, 254–56
Meigs, Wendy, 241–43, 254–56
Melnick, Joseph, 363, 397
Memorial Hospital, 283
Memorial Sloan-Kettering, 362
Mental Health-Mental Retardation Authority, 469–70
Methodist Hospital, The, 3, 8, 19, 35, 43, 45, 60, 212, 216, 222, 326, 374, 406, 485, 491, 493, 494, 505, 506, 510–12, 515, 516, 521, 522–23, 567, 582, 584
Mewhinney, Hubert, 143
Meyer, Adelena, 17, 29, 152, 282, 468
Meyer, Fan Harriet, 29, 152, 468

Meyer, Leopold L., 10–13, 16–18, 20–21, 23, 26, 29, 33–35, 37–38, 51, **97, 98, 102, 104, 105, 110,** 151, 152, 282, 435, 461, 464, 468, 475, 487, 492, 599
Meyer and Ida Gordon Emergency Center, **115,** 301, 310
Meyer Brothers, Inc., 10
Meyer Building, Leopold L., 51
Meyer Center for Developmental Pediatrics, 110, 334, 459–77, 492–93, 502, 524
Michael Reese Hospital, 508
Michels, Virginia, 153
Midwest Society for Pediatric Research, 75
Mikhail, Carmen, 331
Miller, Geoffrey, 474
Minifee, Paul K., 634
Mitchell, A. Lane, 7, 13, **97,** 418–19
Mizrahi, Eli M., 516
Montagnino, Barbara, 529–30, 546
Montandon, Corinne, 321
Montgomery, John R., 126, 398–401
Moody, Maxine, 278
Moody's Investor Service, 54
Moore, Annette, 523–24
Mosby Company, 61
Mothers Against Cancer, 377
Moursund, Walter H., 9, 57, 63, 600
Mullins, Charles E., 176, 179, 220–21, 244–46, 248, 254
Mullins, Don R., 367–68
Mullins, Troy, 367
Munoz, Flor, 411
Mustard, William Thornton, 221
Myones, Barry L., 613–16

Nagai, Mary, 361
National Advisory Committee for McDonald's, 367
National Association of Children's Hospitals and Related Institutions (NACHRI), 38, 436
National Cancer Institute (NCI), 360, 361–63, 367, 371, 372
National Children's Nutrition Center, 323
National Congenital CMV Disease Registry, 411
National Council of Jewish Women, 147
National Federation for the Blind, 617
National Foundation for Infantile Paralysis (NFIP), 391, 393, 394, 550–51, 553
National Foundation-March of Dimes, 489, 602, 627. *See also* March of Dimes
National Heart Institute, 171
National Heart, Lung, and Blood Institute, 176, 562
National Human Genome Research Institute, 347
National IBD Consortium, 329
National Infantile Paralysis Foundation (NIPF), 555–56
National Institute of Allergy and Infectious Disease (NIAID), 133, 402, 612–13
National Institute of Allergy and Infectious Disease (NIAID), Division of Intramural Research, 613

National Institute of Allergy and Infectious Diseases (NIAID), Laboratory of Immunogenetics, 612
National Institute of Child Health and Human Development (NICHD), 133, 405
National Institute of Diabetes and Digestive and Kidney Diseases, 265
National Institute of Neurologic Disease and Blindness, 71
National Institute of Neurologic Disease and Stroke, 71
National Institutes of Health (NIH), 38, 68, 69, 71, 81, 92, 118, 126, 131–37, 317, 319, 322, 323, 339, 342, 346, 349, 372, 389, 396, 401, 402, 454, 516, 519, 521, 562, 579, 587, 601, 604, 607, 612, 613
National League for Nursing Accrediting Commission, 530
National Research Council, 452
National Wilms' Tumor Committee, 364
Navy, 482
NBC Nightly News, 240, 496
Neish, Steven R., 185
Nelson, Sally I., 40–41, 54, 55
Nestorov (Professor), 607
Neuhaus, Alexandra, 355
Neuhaus, Charlie, 355
Neuhaus, Larry, 355–56, 380–83
Neuhaus, Laurence Bosworth (Bo), Jr., 207, 354–56, 379–83
Neuhaus, Lindy Wyatt-Brown, 354–56, 379–83
Neuhaus, Mary Kessler, 355
Neuhaus Center, 460
Neuhaus Foundation for the Remediation of Learning Disabilities, 470
Neuhauser, Edward B. D., 277
Neurosensory Center, 511
New England Journal of Medicine, 362, 607
New York Academy of Sciences, 396
New York University, 398
Newman, Lillian, 148, 150
Nicholls State University, 617
Nichols, Buford L., 81, **109,** 127, 128, 317–25, 327, 329–30
Nicholson, Dana, 201–3, 542
Nickeson, Robert W., Jr., 606
Nihill, Michael R., 179, 189, 632
Nirenberg, Marshall W., 339
Nixon, Richard M., 581
Nobel Prize, 280, 339, 349, 365, 392
Noel, Virginia, 147
Noon, George, 584
Nora, James J., 337–39
North American Pediatric Renal Transplantation Cooperative Study, 591
North Carolina Baptist Hospital, 391
Northwest Medical Center (Houston), 163
Nuchtern, Jed G., 633
Nursery Nurses' Association (London), 195
Nussbaum, Robert, 342
Nutrition and the Developing Nervous System, 413

O'Hara, Maureen, 143
O'Keeffe, Nan, 338–40
Oakland Children's Hospital, 231
Ogden, Angela Kent, 369
Ohio State College of Medicine, 492
Ohio State University, 154, 178
Oklahoma Baptist University, 44
Olutoye, Oluyinka, 634–35
Oncology Services of Texas, Inc., 368
Orr, Harry T., 521
Orton Dyslexia Society, 470
Oski's Pediatrics: Principles and Practice, 413
Ott, David A., 165, 222, 225, 226, 632

Paget, James, 210
Pan American Health Organization, 321
Parents Against Cancer, 377
Parish, Robbin, 502
Parish School, The, 502–3
Park, James, 3, 58–59
Park, Julie, 518
Parker, Bruce R., 287–90
Parker Memorial Laboratory, Charles Thomas, 400, 401, 404
Parks, Mabel, 147, 149–51
Parrish, Jean, 207–10, 237–40
Parrish, Rachel, 207–10, 237–40
Parrish, Scott, 207–10, 237–40
Patton, Mary Elizabeth (Bess), 150, 153
Patton Fellowship in Pediatric Subspecialties, Mary Elizabeth, 153, 154, 183
Paul (Dr.), 140
Pauline Sterne Wolf Memorial Foundation Rheumatic Fever Hospital, 60
Peabody College, 150
Pearland School District, 351
Pediatric AIDS Clinical Trials Group (PACTG), 133–36
Pediatric Consultants, 429
Pediatric Dialysis Center, 583–84
Pediatric Gastroenterology Collaborative Research Group (PGCRG), 327
Pediatric Infectious Diseases Journal, 413
Pediatric Infectious Diseases Society, 413
Pediatric Oncology Group (POG), 362
Pediatric Oncology Radiology, 287
Pediatric Peritoneal Dialysis Study Consortium, 591
Pediatric Rheumatology Collaborative Study Group, 603, 610, 613
Pediatric X-Ray Diagnosis, 281
Pediatrics, 235, 413, 552
Pentax Corporation, 329
Percy, Alan K., 519
Perez, Maria D., 316, 613, 615–16
Pesikoff, Richard, 598
Peter Bent Brigham Hospital, 227
Peterkin, George A., Jr., 38–39, 41, 44, 48–51, **113**
Peterson, Loren, 610
Phelps, Patsy, 596–97
Philadelphia Eagles, 368

Phoebe Willingham Muzzy Pediatric Molecular Cardiology Laboratory, 180, 187
Pi Beta Phi Alumnae Club of Houston, 111, 199, 435–36
Pi Beta Phi Patient/Family Library, **111,** 158, 198, 199, 203, 431, 436
Pin Oak Charity Horse Show, 11–14, 17, 21, 28, **105, 107,** 147, 150, 152, 425
Pin Oak Stables, 11, **105**
Pizzo, Philip A., 371
Pokorny, William J., 630–33
Poplack, David G., 114, **117,** 357–58, 371–79
Potts, Elaine, 138, 319
Potts, Willis, 216
Powell, David, 584
Presbyterian School, 307
President's Panel on Mental Retardation, 463, 475
Pressler, Herman, 16, 26, 34, 36, 38, 39
Principles and Practice of Pediatric Oncology, 371
Prospective Pediatric CRRT Registry Group, 591
Prudential Girls, 147–48, 151, 157
Prudential Insurance Company of America, 146
Public Health Services Act, 389
Public Law 92-601, 581
Public Law 94-142, 443–44, 469

Radio Lollipop, **116,** 158, 201–2
Radiology for Medical Students, 279, 280, 290
Rancho Los Amigos, 553
Rashkind, William, 179, 220
Red Book, 402
Red Cross, 425
Rehn, Ludwig, 210
Reinholds, Dace, 51
Reitz, Bruce, 226
Remington, Sara, 223
Renal Dialysis Unit, 587–99
Rett, Andreas, 519
Reul, George J., 222, 225, 226, 314
Reuther, Joan, 156
Rice University, 291, 578
River Oaks Baptist Church School, 356
Robert Wood Johnson Foundation, 90
Robbins, Frederick, 392
Robert J. Kleberg, Jr. Center for Human Genetics at Baylor College of Medicine, 340
Roberts, Bill, 142
Roberts, Clara, 277
Roberts, Josie, 510
Robinson, Ann, 361
Rochester School of Medicine, 324
Roentgen, Wilhelm Conrad, 279–80
Rogers, Ginger, 143
Rogers, Patti, 535
Rogers, Roy, **105**
Ronald McDonald House, 155, 367–70, 377, 382
Roosevelt, Franklin Delano, 391
Rosen, Carol, 517
Rosenberg, Harvey, 359–61, 580
Rosenthal, Gary, 92
Rowland, John, 547–49, 565–68

Rowland, Kelly, **116**
Royal Children's Hospital (Melbourne), 227
Rubella Study Project, 464, 468–69
Rudolph, Arnold Jack, 428–29, 483–92, 497–99, 501
Rudolph Baylor Pediatric Award for Lifetime Excellence in Teaching, Arnold J., 578

Sabin, Albert, 394
Sachs, Bernard, 508
Sakowitz, 28, 146
Salk, Jonas, 394, 551, 553
Salmon, George W., 7, 13, 15, 58–59, **97**, 167–68, 170, 260–61, 264, 423–25, 576
Salvation Army, 8
Sam Houston Elementary School, 459
Sam Houston State University, 149, 459
Sanjad, Sami A., 583
Saturday Evening Post, 463
Sawyer, Rita, 460
Schachtel, Hyman Judah, 10, 20, **99,** 471
Schaffer, A. J., 481
Schneider, Virginia, 498
School of Allied Health Sciences (Baylor), 455
Schreiner, Barb, 270–71
Schwachman, Harry, 552–55
Schwartz, Pat, 614
Science and Education Administration (USDA), 323
Science and Practice of Pediatric Cardiology, The, 182, 185
Scott, Gwendolyn B., 125
Scribner, Belding H., 580–81
Sears, Roebuck & Company, 5, 57
Seilheimer, Dan K., 138, 558–65
Sellers, Benjamin, 314–16, 330–33
Sellers, Roberta, 314–16, 331–33
Seminars in Pediatric Infectious Diseases, 413
Senning, Ake, 221
Sesame Street, 526
Seu, Philip, 328
Shamrock Hotel, 27, 142–44, 146, 159
Shearer, William T., 80, **109**, 125, 126–41, 400
Shelp, Earl, 249
Shepard, Vernisha, 330–31
Sherman, Lori, 269
Sheth, Rita D., 589
Shoemate, Bonnie, 26, 278
Shook, Joan E., **115,** 298–310
Shriners Hospital for Children, 611
Shriver, Eunice Kennedy, 463
Shulman, Robert, 153, 325
Sigma Delta Tau, 147
Simmons, L. E., 92
Simon, Terry, 505–6
Simpson, O. J., 349
Singer, Don, 580
Singleton, Albert Olin, 279
Singleton, Edward B., 66, **103,** 171, 276–87, 289–93
Singleton, Joan, 282
Singleton Diagnostic Imaging Services, Edward

B., 292
Sinha, Anil K., 338
Sisterhood of Temple Beth Israel, 147
Skeggs, Leonard, 575
Smith, Bill, 16
Smith, Clement, 483
Smith, David, 324
Smith, Lisa, 616
Smith, Loree, 191–94, 203–6
Smith, Pat, 278
Smith, William A., **99**
Smith College, 482
Smithson, Helga, 599, 601
Society for Pediatric Radiologists, 284
Society for Pediatric Research, 75, 388, 413
Society for Public Health Education, 563
Sockrider, Marianna, 312
South, Mary Ann, 126, 398–400
Southern Society of Pediatric Research, 578
Southwest Cancer Chemotherapy Study Group (SWCCSG), 361–62
Southwest Oncology Group (SWOG), 362
Southwest Pediatric Nephrology Study Group (SPNSG), 587, 591
Southwestern Poliomyelitis Respiratory Center, 60, 64, 262, 393, 551, 553
Special Projects of Regional and National Significance (SPRANS), 604–5, 611, 612
Speer, Michael, 489–91
Spencer, William A., 64, 393, 551, 553, 555
Spencer, Winifred, 278
Spina Bifida Association of the Gulf Coast, 638
Spock, Benjamin, 484
Squire, Charlie, 291
St. John's School, 527
St. Joseph's Hospital, 485, 624
St. Joseph's Infirmary, 3
St. Jude Research Hospital, 374
St. Louis Children's Hospital, 58, 75, 77, 127, 260–62, 442, 509, 558, 563
St. Luke's Episcopal Hospital, 8, 18, 19–20, 27, 29–36, 38–40, 42, 44, 47, 85–87, **98, 102,** 106, 112, 145, 150, 153, 160, 175, 196, 199, 209, 214, 216–18, 220, 221, 222, 225, 237, 244, 276, 281–84, 286–87, 298–99, 314, 315, 325, 339, 484–85, 488–89, 492–94, 496–97, 531–34, 569, 581, 583, 620–21, 623, 629, 635
Stal, Samuel, 632
Stalin, Joseph, 607
Standard & Poor's, 54
Stanford University, 229, 287, 578, 585
Starke, Jeff, 411, 414
Starling, Kenneth A., 363
Stavins, Cheryl, 535
Stein, Fernando, 247–48, 250, 253, 354–56
Sterling Chemicals, Inc., 519
Sterling Group Inc., 519
Steuber, C. Philip, 370–73
Stokes, John, 598
Stokes, Pamela, 596–99, 617–19
Stokes, Shirley, 596–99

Stool, Joseph, 59, **98**
Strong Memorial Hospital, 324
Sung, Bin, 163
SuperKids Mobile Pediatric Clinic, 433–34
Surgeon General's Conference (1987), 609
Surgeon General's Workshop on Children with
    HIV Infection and Their Families, 124
Surgical Treatment of Congenital Heart Disease, 219
Sustaining Club, 435
Sutow, W. W., 365
Swann, John W., 520
Sweet, L. K., 482
Sylvester, Ruth, 31–32, 532–33, 537, 538

Taber, Larry, 400, 403, 405, 410
Tanner, David, 127–28
Taos Hospital, 478
Taussig, Helen B., **111**, 167–68, 174, 178, 186,
    188, 212, 215
Taylor, Fred M., 64, 70–71, **98**, 427–28
TCH Insurance Co., Ltd., 52
TCH System, Inc., 52
TeamMates, 446–47, 450
Tellepsen, Howard T., 20, **99**
Tellepsen Construction Company, 20, 99
Temple University School of Medicine, 482
Teng, C. T., 283, 384
Teruya, Jun, 590
Texas Association of Staff Directors of Volunteer
    Services, 150
Texas Center for Fetal Surgery, 635
Texas Children's Asthma Center, 138, 311–12,
    560, 564
Texas Children's Cancer Center and Hematology
    Service, 117, 357–58, 375–79, 382, 540
Texas Children's Community Health Centers, 634
Texas Children's Foundation, 13–17, 19, 21, 22,
    65, 66, 425
Texas Children's Health Centers, 544
Texas Children's Health Plan, 52
Texas Children's Heart Center, 184, 187, 188,
    230–37
Texas Children's HIV Center, 134, 136, 137
Texas Children's Home Health Services, 52
Texas Children's Hospital, 3–640
Texas Children's Hospital Foundation, **97**
Texas Children's Hospital Pediatric Associates,
    376. *See also* Texas Children's Pediatric
    Associates
Texas Children's International, 52
Texas Children's Newborn Center, 635
Texas Children's Pediatric Associates, 52, 376,
    544
Texas Children's Sleep Center, 522
Texas Health and Human Service Commission,
    614
Texas Heart Association, 169
Texas Heart Institute, 33–35, 39, 106, 175–76,
    180, 183–84, 218–27, 236, 298, 632
Texas Hospital Association, 8, 150
Texas Institute for Rehabilitation and Research
    (TIRR), 465, 555, 557, 559–60. *See also*

Institute for Rehabilitation and Research
    (TIRR)
Texas Medical Center, 5–6, 8–9, 14–15, 19–21,
    24, 25, 34, 35, 43, 45, 46, 53, 54, 58, 60, 65,
    66, 71, 73, 85, 87, 98, 144, 145, 174, 212,
    216, 218, 276, 353, 368, 372, 373, 405, 412,
    423, 429, 437, 465, 482, 493, 510–11, 611,
    639
Texas Pediatrics Society, 579, 614
Texas Rehabilitation Commission, 470
Texas State Cancer Hospital, 4
Texas State Department of Health, 463. *See also*
    Department of Health (Texas)
Texas Tech University Health Sciences Center,
    461, 475
Textbook of Pediatric Infectious Diseases, 84, 407,
    413
Thetas, 377
Thomas, Albert, 13
Thomas, Don, 365
Tilbor, Adrienne, 316
Tinklepaugh, Jill, 163–67, 188–90
Tinklepaugh, Karly, 163–67, 188–90
Tinklepaugh, Kestly, 163–67, 188–90
Tinklepaugh, Scott, 163–67, 188–90
Tinklepaugh, Shelby, 166
Tinklepaugh, Taylor, 166
Titanic, 285
Towbin, Jeffrey A., 180, 184, 186–88
Travis, Luther, 264, 266, 572
Travolta, John, 400
Treadwell-Deering, Diane, 451
Trentin, John, 365
Tropical Storm Allison, 54
Tulane University, 10
Tumor Institute, 365
Turner Neonatal Intensive Care Unit (Hermann
    Hospital), 46
*Twenty-five Years of Progress in the Medical
    Treatment of Pediatric and Congenital Heart
    Disease,* 177

U.S. News & World Report, 92
United Fund, 10
United States Army Research Institute of
    Infectious Diseases, 75
United States Congress, 389, 520, 581, 604
United States Department of Agriculture (USDA),
    81, 87, 118, 271, 323, 327
United States Department of Health and Human
    Services, 305
United States Immigration Service, 483
United States Public Health Service, 13, 134
University of Alabama in Birmingham, 181
University of Alabama School of Medicine, 405
University of Arkansas, 181
University of California, 558, 582
University of California at Los Angeles School of
    Medicine, 84, 407
University of California, San Francisco, 584, 587
University of Cincinnati, 603, 610
University of Colorado, 58

University of Florida, 576, 606
University of Houston, 9, 10, 134, 566
University of Illinois, 508
University of Kansas, 58
University of Miami School of Medicine, 125
University of Michigan, 276, 279, 281
University of Minnesota, 175, 214, 217, 521, 574, 576
University of New Orleans, 617
University of North Carolina at Chapel Hill, 610
University of Pennsylvania, 320
University of Pittsburgh, 181, 394, 550
University of Texas, 4–5, 134, 376
University of Texas Health Science Center, 628
University of Texas in Dallas, 576
University of Texas in Houston, 182
University of Texas Medical Branch (Galveston), 226, 264, 276, 577
University of Texas Medical School, 134
University of Texas School of Public Health, 614
University of Toronto, 633
University of Utah Medical Center, 585
University of Virginia, 181
University of Washington, 580
University of Wisconsin, 196, 340
UpToDate, 413

Van Wagner, Lamaina Leigh, 25, 42, **103, 113,** 552
Vanderbilt University, 601, 602
Vargo, Thomas A., 179, 246–49
Vetter, Carol Ann, 137
Vetter, David Philip, **109,** 126–33, 136–37, 400, 471
Vetter family, 126, 130
Vietti, Theresa J., 365
Vinson, Sherry Sellers, 459–61, 473, 475–77
Vogel, Jacqueline, 196–201, 203
Voigt, Robert G., 334–35, 353

W. B. Saunders Company, 84, 407
Wagner, Milton, 284, 287, 288
Wainerdi, Richard E., 5
Walker, Barney, 278
Wallace, Bill, 264, 575
Wallace, Mark A., 43–55, 88, 89, 92, **113,** 373–73, 375, 534–35
Walt Disney Productions, 21, 28, **100–1, 107**
Walter, Carl W., 360
Ward, Margaret, 195, 199
Ward, Michael S., 428
Warren, Robert W., 610–17
Washington University School of Medicine, 57, 75, 77, 78, 79, 80, 82, 83, 127, 260, 365, 388, 402, 509, 558, 610
WATCH Fellowship, 153–54, 183
WATCH Magazine, **110,** 149–50, 195, 268, 534
Watson, James, 337
Weathers (maintenance engineer), 278
Webber, Karen, **104**
Webber, Kimberly, **104**
Weinert, Betty, 278

Weisman, Leonard E., 496–501
Weller, Thomas, 392
Wells, Amanda (pseudonym), 123–25, 136, 138–41
Welty, Steve, 506
Wesson, David E., 633–36
Western Reserve School of Medicine, 264
Western Reserve University, 575–76
Whisennand, Hartwell, 326
White, Alex, 39
White, Paul Dudley, 178
White, Ryan, 124
Wieder, Serena, 452
Wilking, Andrew P., 606, 610–11, 616
Wilkins, Lawson, 263
William Beaumont General Hospital, 508
Williams (maintenance engineer), 278
Williams, Michelle, **116**
Williams, Myrtle, 533, 536–37, 539–43
Williamson, W. Daniel, 460, 472
Wilson, Carol, 582
Wilson, Geraldine, 473
Wilson, Raphael, 126
Woman's Hospital of Texas, 401, 479
Women's Army Auxiliary Corps, 8
Women's Auxiliary, 70, 71, **104,** 108, **110,** 114, 144–57
Wood, Earl, 172
World War I, 280
World War II, 6–8, 12, 142, 143, 184, 211, 260, 280, 285, 291, 359, 389, 554, 574, 575
Wortham, Gus, 11
Wright, Jesse, 551
Wright, Randy, 535

X-Ray Diagnosis of the Alimentary Tract in Infants and Children, 283, 291

Yale University, 318, 328, 337, 610
Ybarra, Deborah, 415
Ykema, Kathy, 384–86, 415–16
Ykema, Matthew, 384–86, 414–17
Ykema, Rick (Ike), 384–86, 416
York, Byron, 576
Young, Elise C., 369
Young Chair of Pediatric Oncology, Elise C. (Baylor), 369, 373
Yow, Ellard, 391–92, 395
Yow, Martha Dukes, 64, 80, 391–92, 394–406, 410–12, 414, 428, 487

Zeller, Robert, 512
Zion, Thomas E., 465–66, 512
Zoghbi, Huda Y., 520–22, 528

APPENDIX

TEXAS CHILDREN'S HOSPITAL BOARD OF TRUSTEES 2006

BOARD OF TRUSTEES *continued*

TEXAS CHILDREN'S HOSPITAL TRUSTEES SINCE 1950

R. Bruce LaBoon
2000 – present

Ann Lents
2005 - present

J. W. Link, Jr. *†
1950 – 1984

Lawrence Marcus
1967 – 1975

Peter M. Mark
1984 – 1992

Douglas B. Marshall*†
1950 – 1967

Ben B. McAndrew III
1988 – present

A. Dossett McCullough
1967 – 2005

Edward S. McCullough
1971 – present

Ralph H. McCullough¹†
1960 – 1984

Virginia McFarland
1972 – present

William K. McGee, Jr.
1983 – present

Robert E. Meadows
1995 – present

John W. Mecom†
1960 – 1981

David L. Mendez
2002 – present

Leopold L. Meyer*†
1950 – 1982

Darrell C. Morrow
1977 – present

Robert K. Moses, Sr.†
1967 – 1978

Don R. Mullins
1977 – 1990

Philip R. Neuhaus
1971 – present

Maconda Brown O'Connor, PhD
1969 – present

Ralph S. O'Connor
1960 – 1969

George A. Peterkin, Jr.
1967 – present

Anthony G. Petrello
2002 – present

Herman P. Pressler*†
1950 – 1995

Townes G. Pressler
1979 – present

Thomas R. Reckling III
1971 – 1974

Hampton C. Robinson, M.D.†
1960 – 1988

Gary L. Rosenthal
1990 – present

L. E. Simmons
1997 – present

William A. Smith*†
1950 – 1991

Joel V. Staff
2005 - present

Lois F. Stark
1977 – present

Dick Stedman
1967 – 1971

Stuart W. Stedman
1988 – 2003

Ann B. Stern
1998 – 2002

Mike S. Stude
1971 – 1972

Y. Ping Sun
2005 - present

Brad Tucker
1996 – present

Mark A. Wallace
1989 – present

Peter S. Wareing
1982 – present

Max P. Watson
1998 – present

Frank T. Webster
1984 – 1998

Phoebe C. Welsh
1979 – present

Joe C. Wessendorff
1960 – 1973

Wesley G. West†
1950 – 1984

Gus S. Wortham†
1952 – 1976

*Charter Members
†Deceased
¹Served on the St. Luke's Episcopal Hospital Board of Directors 1952 – 1957

TEXAS CHILDREN'S HOSPITAL HISTORY COMMITTEE

1977 - 1979
Anne Baker Horton

1988
Andrea Morgan
Townes G. Pressler
Virginia McFarland
Robert L. Gerry III

1992
Robert Whittemore
Patti Rogers
Virginia McFarland
Fred M. Taylor, M.D.

1994 – 1998
Burdett S. Dunbar, M.D.
Ralph D. Feigin, M.D.
Susannah Moore Griffin
Carol Kohn
Virginia McFarland
Dace Reinholds
Patti Rogers
Fred M. Taylor, M.D.
Mark A. Wallace

1998 – 2002
Phil Caudill
Murdina M. Desmond, M.D.
Burdett S. Dunbar, M.D.
Ralph D. Feigin, M.D.
Donald J. Fernbach, M.D.
Virginia McFarland
Dace Reinholds
Patti Rogers
Fred M. Taylor, M.D.
Mark A. Wallace

2002 – 2006
Burdett S. Dunbar, M.D.
Ralph D. Feigin, M.D.
Virginia McFarland
Dace Reinholds
Patti Rogers
Lois F. Stark
Mark A. Wallace

TEXAS CHILDREN'S HOSPITAL HEADS OF DEPARTMENTS AND CHIEFS OF SERVICES, SECTIONS AND CLINICS 2006

DEPARTMENT OF MEDICINE . . . . .Sheldon L. Kaplan, M.D.
    Adolescent Medicine Service . . . . .Albert C. Hergenroeder, M.D.
    Allergy and Immunology Service .William T. Shearer, M.D., Ph.D.
    Cardiology Service . . . . .Jeffrey A. Towbin, M.D.
    Dermatology Service . . . . .Moise L. Levy, M.D.
    Developmental Pediatrics Service . . . . .Sherry Sellers Vinson, M.D., Acting
    Emergency Medicine Service . . . . .Joan E. Shook, M.D.
        Child Protection Section . . . . .Michelle Lyn, M.D.
    Endocrine-Metabolism Service . . . . .Morey W. Haymond, M.D.
    Gastroenterology, Hepatology & Nutrition Service . . . . .Mark A. Gilger, M.D.
    General Medicine Service . . . . .Brian J. Talbot, M.D.
    Genetics Service . . . . .Carlos A. Bacino, M.D.
    Hematology-Oncology Service . . . . .David G. Poplack, M.D.
    Infectious Disease Service . . . . .Sheldon L. Kaplan, M.D.
    Intensive Care Service . . . . .Larry S. Jefferson, M.D.
    Neonatology Service . . . . .Ann R. Stark, M.D.
    Neurology Service . . . . .Gary D. Clark, M.D.
    Neurophysiology Service . . . . .Gary D. Clark, M.D.
    Physical Medicine & Rehabilitation Service . . . . .Aloysia L. Schwabe, M.D.
    Psychiatry & Psychology Service . . . . .Diane E. Treadwell-Deering, M.D.
    Pulmonary Medicine Service . . . . .Dan K. Seilheimer, M.D.
    Renal Service . . . . .Eileen D. Brewer, M.D.
    Rheumatology Service . . . . .Robert W. Warren, M.D., Ph.D.

DEPARTMENT OF PATHOLOGY . . . . .Milton J. Finegold, M.D.
    General Pathology Service . . . . .Milton J. Finegold, M.D.

DEPARTMENT OF DIAGNOSTIC IMAGING . . . . .Taylor Chung, M.D.
    Nuclear Medicine Service . . . . .Warren H. Moore, M.D.
    Diagnostic Imaging Service . . . . .Taylor Chung, M.D.

DEPARTMENT OF ANESTHESIOLOGY .Dean B. Andropoulos, M.D.
    Anesthesiology Service . . . . .Dean B. Andropoulos, M.D.

HEADS OF DEPARTMENTS AND
CHIEFS OF SERVICES, SECTIONS AND CLINICS *continued*

DEPARTMENT OF SURGERY . . . . .Edmond T. Gonzales, Jr., M.D.

    Cardiovascular Service . . . . .Charles D. Fraser, Jr., M.D.

    Dental Service . . . . .Alvis Bruce Carter, D.D.S.

    General Surgery Service . . . . .David E. Wesson, M.D.

    Gynecology Service . . . . .Robert K. Zurawin, M.D.

    Hand Surgery Service . . . . .David T.J. Netscher, M.D.

    Neurosurgery Service . . . . .Robert C. Dauser, M.D.

    Ophthalmology Service . . . . .David K. Coats, M.D.

    Orthopedic Service . . . . .William A. Phillips, M.D.

        Podiatry Section . . . . .William A. Phillips, M.D.

    Otolaryngology Service . . . . .Ellen M. Friedman, M.D.

        Speech Pathology Section . . . . .Ellen M. Friedman, M.D.

    Plastic Surgery Service . . . . .Samuel Stal, M.D.

    Urology Service . . . . .Edmond T. Gonzales, Jr., M.D.

DEPARTMENT OF AMBULATORY . . . . .Rebecca T. Kirkland, M.D.

    Adolescent Medicine Clinic . . . . .Albert C. Hergenroeder, M.D.

    Allergy & Immunology Clinic . . . . .I. Celine Hanson, M.D.

    Anorectal Malformation Clinic (ARM) . . . . .Mary L. Brandt, M.D.

    Biliary Atresia Clinic . . . . .Saul J. Karpen, M.D., Ph.D.

    Birthmark Center . . . . .Moise L. Levy, M.D.

                                                 Larry Hollier, M.D., Co-Chief

    Bone Marrow Clinic . . . . .Robert A. Krance, M.D.

    Brachial-Plexus Clinic . . . . .Robert P. Cruse, D.O.

    Cancer Genetics Clinic . . . . .Sharon E. Plon, M.D.

    Cardiology Clinic . . . . .Naomi Kertesz, M.D., Acting

    Child Protective Health Clinic . . . . .Clifford O. Mishaw, M.D.

    Children's Asthma Center . . . . .Dan K. Seilheimer, M.D.

    Children's Sleep Clinic . . . . .Daniel G. Glaze, M.D.

    Clinic for Attention Problems . . . . .Judith Z. Feigin, Ed.D.

    Clinic for Diagnosis of Autistic Spectrum Disorders . . . . .Diane E. Treadwell-Deering, M.D.

                                                 Judith Z. Feigin, Ed.D.

    Cleft Palate Clinic . . . . .Samuel Stal, M.D.

    Comprehensive Epilepsy Surgery Clinic .Angus A. Wilfong, M.D.

HEADS OF DEPARTMENTS AND
CHIEFS OF SERVICES, SECTIONS AND CLINICS *continued*

DEPARTMENT OF AMBULATORY *continued*

Craniofacial Clinic . . . . .Samuel Stal, M.D.

Critical Care Clinic . . . . .Fernando Stein, M.D.

Dental Clinic . . . . .Alvis Bruce Carter, D.D.S.

Dermatology Clinic . . . . .Denise W. Metry, M.D.

Developmental Pediatrics Clinic . . . . .Sherry Sellers Vinson, M.D.

Diabetes Clinic . . . . .Morey W. Haymond, M.D.

Down Syndrome Clinic . . . . .Nirupama Madduri, M.D.

Endocrine Clinic . . . . .Morey W. Haymond, M.D.

Feeding Disorders Clinic . . . . .Carol Redel, M.D.

Fracture Clinic . . . . .William A. Phillips, M.D.

Gastroenterology Clinic . . . . .Barbara Reid, M.D.

General Medicine Clinic . . . . .Clifford O. Mishaw, M.D.

Genetics Clinic . . . . .Carlos A. Bacino, M.D.

Grow Clinic . . . . .Paula E. Sturgeon, M.D.
Angelo Giardino, M.D.

Gynecology Clinic . . . . .Robert K. Zurawin, M.D.

Hand Surgery Clinic . . . . .David T.J. Netscher, M.D.

Hearing Clinic . . . . John S. Oghalai, M.D.

Hematology Clinic . . . . .Donald H. Mahoney, M.D.

Hypertension Clinic . . . . .Daniel I. Feig, M.D.

Infectious Disease Clinic . . . . .Bonnie M. Word, M.D.

Inflammatory Bowel Disease Clinic . . . . .George D. Ferry, M.D.

International Adoption Clinic . . . . .Heidi L. Schwarzwald, M.D.

Learning Support Clinic . . . . Judith Z. Feigin, Ed.D.

Leukemia/Lymphoma Clinic . . . . .C. Philip Steuber, M.D.

Long Term Survivor Clinic . . . . .ZoAnn E. Dreyer, M.D.

Multiple Sclerosis/Muscular Dystrophy . . . . .Timothy E. Lotze, M.D.

Neonatology Graduate Clinic . . . . .Paula E. Sturgeon, M.D.

Neurofibromatosis Clinic . . . . .Sharon E. Plon, M.D.

Neurology/Blue Bird Clinic . . . . .Robert S. Zeller, M.D.

Neuro-Oncology Clinic . . . . .Murali M. Chintagumpala, M.D.

Neurosurgery Clinic . . . . .Robert C. Dauser, M.D.

Ophthalmology Clinic . . . . .David K. Coats, M.D.

Orthopaedic Surgery Clinic . . . . .William A. Phillips, M.D.

HEADS OF DEPARTMENTS AND
CHIEFS OF SERVICES, SECTIONS AND CLINICS *continued*

DEPARTMENT OF AMBULATORY *continued*

Otolaryngology Clinic . . . . .Ellen M. Friedman, M.D.

Pain Clinic . . . . .Nancy Glass, M.D.

Physical Medicine & Rehabilitation Clinic . . . . .Aloysia L. Schwabe, M.D., Acting

Plastic Surgery Clinic . . . . .Samuel Stal, M.D.

Prader-Willi Clinic . . . . .William J. Klish, M.D.

Psychopharmacology Clinic . . . . .Diane E. Treadwell-Deering, M.D.

Pediatric Surgery Clinic . . . . .Paul K. Minifee, M.D.

Pulmonary Medicine Clinic . . . . Marianna Sockrider, M.D.

Renal Clinic . . . . .Eileen D. Brewer, M.D.

Residents Primary Care Group Clinic . . . . .Jan E. Drutz, M.D.

Rheumatology Clinic . . . . .Robert W. Warren, M.D., Ph.D.

Retrovirology Clinic . . . . .Mark W. Kline, M.D.

Sickle Cell Clinic . . . . .Brigitta U. Mueller, M.D.

Scoliosis Clinic . . . . .William A. Phillips, M.D.

Skeletal Dysplasia Clinic . . . . .Brendan H. Lee, M.D.

Solid Tumor Clinic . . . . .Brigitta U. Mueller, M.D.

Spasticity Clinic . . . . .Aloysia L. Schwabe, M.D., Acting

Spina Bifida Clinic . . . . .Kathryn Ostermaier, M.D.

Sports Medicine Clinic . . . . .Albert C. Hergenroeder, M.D.

Stroke Clinic . . . . .Robert P. Cruse, D.O.

Tele-Health Clinic . . . . .Larry S. Jefferson, M.D.

Travel Medicine Clinic . . . . .Bonnie M. Word, M.D.

Urology Clinic . . . . .Edmond T. Gonzales, Jr., M.D.

Young Women's Clinic . . . . .Albert C. Hergenroeder, M.D.

ACKNOWLEDGMENTS

THIS BOOK COULD NOT EXIST WITHOUT THE PERSONAL ACCOUNTS and observations of those who actively participated in the evolving history of Texas Children's Hospital.

The compilation of more than 200 oral histories and interviews for this book has been a collaborative effort, one that began with the formation in 1977 of a history committee at Texas Children's Hospital.* Between 1977 and 1994, working under the committee's direction, a succession of interviewers—Joe Clark, Zella Maxwell, Jean E. Hardy, Charles Morrissey, and Fran Dressman—conducted 77 interviews and oral histories. Between 1994 and 1999, and again working under the committee's direction, historian and researcher Barbara J. Rozek, PhD, recorded an additional 35 oral histories. Rozek also established and maintained an extensive archival collection of documents. Writer Bryan Wirwicz briefly continued the research efforts in 1999, interviewing numerous individuals and documenting his conversations. These collective efforts represent an invaluable contribution that is essential to this book, as documented in the notes.

Additional oral histories and interviews took place in the course of the seven years, 1999–2006, that this author spent researching and writing this book. More than 70 physicians, patients, nurses, hospital executives, trustees, volunteers, and community leaders generously took the time to talk with me, many of them repeatedly. To each and every person interviewed throughout the years, I wish to express my heartfelt gratitude for both their participation and their valuable input. Quoted freely and often, their words and thoughts grace the pages of this book and represent the heart and soul of its content.

I especially wish to thank the patients and families who kindly shared

---

* See appendix.

their stories of determination, hope, and courage. Their emotional experiences help to authenticate the optimism that this book strives to bring to similarly challenged children and families all over the world. Each heartfelt message of appreciation for Texas Children's Hospital is a testament to the immeasurable impact of the loving care received, serving not only as an affirmation of the existence of the legacy, but also as an inspiration for its perpetuation.

All the patients and families I encountered left an indelible impression, as did the physicians. In particular, I will never forget the countless hours spent with the late Dr. Murdina M. Desmond, who graciously took me under her wing in 1999. She not only guided me through my initial research efforts regarding the early years at Texas Children's Hospital, but also served as my constant source of information and support throughout the process until her untimely death in 2003. With her sharp wit, keen observations, and comprehensive memory for detail, she was a constant source of information and delight. I am grateful for the opportunity to have known her.

I also received both solicited and unsolicited guidance and advice from Dr. Earl J. Brewer, Jr., who tirelessly listened to my questions, commiserated with my frustrations about spelling medical terminology, and laughed with me at my initial inability to grasp some of the simplest concepts of medicine. For his friendship, encouragement, and emotional support, I am truly thankful.

Another source of continuing guidance and inspiration was Texas Children's Hospital physician-in-chief Dr. Ralph D. Feigin, who graciously consented to numerous interviews regarding myriad subjects. I remain in constant awe of his accomplishments and abilities. For his unending patience with this writer's endless questions and for his expert assistance in producing this book, I wish to thank him formally here.

A special word of appreciation goes to Dr. Feigin's executive assistant, Carrel E. Briley, who often went out of her way to help expedite the coordination of various matters necessary for the publication of this book. Her expert guidance and assistance were invaluable.

Of immeasurable inspiration to this writer were the chiefs of service at Texas Children's Hospital who graciously took the time from their busy schedules to sit down and talk about their areas of responsibility. As they patiently explained to a novice the inner workings of their services, each demonstrated a discernable passion to care for children lovingly. Although all are teachers, theirs is an attitude that is caught, not taught, and I became incurably infected with their compassion.

Unequalled in impact on this writer was the enthusiastic encouragement and invaluable direction provided by Texas Children's Hospital president and

CEO Mark A. Wallace. Through both his words and his deeds on behalf of this book, he exemplified the legendary leadership skills for which he is so well known. For his unwavering enthusiasm, contributions, and constant support, I am most appreciative.

Without question, the successful publication of this book was the result of efforts expended by Dace Reinholds, who serves as director of governance affairs at Texas Children's Hospital. Ably assisted by senior executive secretaries Laura C. Garrett and Lauren M. Schultz, she not only helped facilitate some of the daunting logistical aspects of this book, but also did so with efficiency and professionalism. I am indebted to the three of them for their enthusiastic support, valued contributions and constant words of encouragement throughout the lengthy process.

Deserving special recognition in this space is the tenacity and dedication of the Texas Children's Hospital history committee. Since its 1977 formation, each of its members has contributed to the ongoing efforts to document and preserve the history of Texas Children's Hospital. *Legacy* is the cumulative result of that determination. A member of the history committee since 1988, Virginia McFarland steadfastly championed the idea of publishing a book about the history of Texas Children's Hospital. Her constant kind words of encouragement to this writer were greatly appreciated, as was the helpful direction and research assistance given by Patti Rogers, a member of the committee since 1992. I wish to thank them, as well as every other member of the committee, for their critical opinions, valued input, and guidance throughout the writing of this book.

Worthy of special praise for her steadfast commitment to this book is Marlene Moulder, a senior administrative secretary on the staff of Texas Children's Hospital. When she inadvertently assumed the responsibility of "keeper of the archives" in her rare spare time, she often became both my hands and my eyes during numerous research expeditions through the contents of this resource. Along with her exhaustive and repeated searches for more than a few elusive morsels of information, she enthusiastically shared an extensive knowledge of Texas Children's Hospital and never failed to offer words of encouragement throughout the seven years of this book's gestation. For all of her efforts and kindnesses, I am greatly indebted.

I also wish to recognize the countless other staff members in marketing, public relations, and the office of development at Texas Children's Hospital who assisted in the gathering of pertinent information and helped to arrange appointments and interviews. A special thank you is offered to Phil Caudill for his unwavering support and to Angela Dolder, Dawn A. Dorsey, Katy P. Gill,

Angela J. Hudson, and Anne W. Lupton for their tireless efforts on this book's behalf. There were many others, far too numerous to mention by name, who offered both assistance and encouragement and I am equally grateful to each and every one of them.

Without question, what greatly enhanced the accuracy of this book's content was the documentation of current events presented in *Developments,* a magazine produced quarterly by the Texas Children's Hospital office of development, and *WATCH Magazine*, the periodical produced since 1955 by The Auxiliary to Texas Children's Hospital. Members of The Auxiliary continue to maintain a vast collection of past issues and graciously allowed this writer to have free access. Throughout its existence at Texas Children's Hospital, members of The Auxiliary were the on-the-scene historians who documented events as they happened. They deserve recognition for their contributions and appreciation for their ongoing efforts.

For research purposes, I am particularly grateful for the longtime efforts of Tina Foster, former public relations expert at Texas Children's Hospital. She maintained and categorized another collection of *Developments* and *WATCH Magazine*, now in the archives at Texas Children's Hospital. Also utilized in research was the bound collection of every *WATCH Magazine* from 1955 to 1977 found among the papers of Dr. Russell J. Blattner, permanently housed at The John P. McGovern Historical Collections and Research Center in the Houston Academy of Medicine -Texas Medical Center Library, where archival collections focus on the development of the institutions and hospitals in the Texas Medical Center and the careers of Houston physicians. Available for scholarly research, these collections contain correspondence, speeches, reprints, financial records, photographs, and audiotapes. All were made available to this writer, for which I am greatly appreciative. A heartfelt word of thanks goes to the McGovern Center's Elizabeth Borst White and Pamela R. Cornell, who never tired of my persistent requests or of being constant sources of information and assistance.

In addition, I wish to thank the Houston Academy of Medicine - Texas Medical Center Library for allowing this writer to have remote electronic access to its vast selection of both current and archived medical journals, books, and publications. This privilege enabled the necessary research efforts to be continuous, resulting in documented medical information that is as accurate and up-to-date as possible.

Deserving my endless gratitude are Texas Children's Hospital photographers Paul Vincent Kuntz and the late Jim DeLeon, who graciously allowed me to delve through hundreds, if not thousands, of the archived images in their possession. Without their kind assistance, the job of both finding and selecting the most appropriate photographs would have been a formidable task. I thank them for their thoughtful and timesaving assistance.

I also wish to thank editor Michelle Nichols for her invaluable, expert assistance in completing this book; designer Peter Layne for his inspired layout, cover design and legendary patience; Clifford Pugh for his constructive criticism, suggestions and guidance; and Cynthia Bowman for her valued advice, constant support and much appreciated friendship.

A constant and reassuring presence on this seven-year expedition into the history of Texas Children's Hospital were Marion Alexander and Robbin Parish, who patiently listened to endless details about my research efforts and graciously read and critiqued every new chapter upon completion. The ability to share with them, as well as with other family members and friends, my newfound in-depth knowledge of Texas Children's Hospital, my wonderment about all of the medical accomplishments there and my emotional reactions to hearing firsthand accounts of the courageous patients was invigorating and immeasurably enhanced my efforts.

Most of all, I wish to express my heartfelt appreciation to and admiration of everyone at Texas Children's Hospital, both past and present, named and unnamed, whose purposeful contributions to the enduring legacy of loving care helped to create not only the history, but also the future of Texas Children's Hospital.

About the Author

Betsy Parish is a former newspaper columnist. A fifth-generation descendant of one of the pioneering families who settled Houston in 1838 and the granddaughter of a 1911 alumnus of Baylor University College of Medicine, she is an avid supporter of efforts to document and preserve the history of healthcare in Houston. This is her first book.